D1716747

Ultrasonography of the Prenatal and Neonatal Brain

Ultrasonography of the Prenatal and Neonatal Brain
Second Edition

Ilan E. Timor-Tritsch, MD
Director, Division of Ob/Gyn Ultrasound
Professor of Obstetrics and Gynecology
New York University School of Medicine
New York, New York

Ana Monteagudo, MD
Associate Professor of Obstetrics and Gynecology
New York University School of Medicine
New York, New York

Harris L. Cohen, MD
Professor and Director
Division of Ultrasound
Department of Radiology
SUNY Health Science Center at Brooklyn
Kings County and University Hospitals
Brooklyn, New York

McGraw-Hill
Medical Publishing Division

New York   Chicago   San Francisco   Lisbon   London   Madrid   Mexico City
Milan   New Delhi   San Juan   Seoul   Singapore   Sydney   Toronto

McGraw-Hill

A Division of The **McGraw·Hill** *Companies*

Ultrasonography of the Prenatal and Neonatal Brain
Second edition

1234567890 IMP/IMP 0987654321

ISBN 0-8385-8859-X

This book was set in New Century Schoolbook by The Clarinda Company
The editors were Andrea Seils and Barbara Holton.
The production supervisor was Rick Ruzycka.
The cover designer was Richard Miller.
The index was prepared by Jerry Ralya.

Imago was printer and binder.

This book is printed on acid-free paper.

Library of Congress Cataloging-in-Publication Data

Ultrasonography of the prenatal and neonatal brain / authors [i.e. editors], Ilan E. Timor-Tritsch, Ana Monteagudo, Harris L. Cohen.—2nd ed.
    p. ; cm.
  Includes bibliographical references and index.
  ISBN 0-8385-8859-X
  1. Fetal brain—Abnormalities—Ultrasonic imaging. 2. Fetal brain—Abnormalities—Diagnosis. 3. Brain—Abnormalities—Ultrasonic imaging. 4. Infants (Newborn)—Diseases—Diagnosis. I. Timor-Tritsch, Ilan E. II. Monteagudo, Ana. III. Cohen, Harris L.
  [DNLM: 1. Fetal Diseases—ultrasonography. 2. Brain—embryology. 3. Brain—growth & development. 4. Echoencephalography. 5. Infant, Newborn, Diseases—ultrasonography. WQ 209 U467 2001]
RG629.B73 U47 2001
618.3′26807543—dc21

00-063839

Contents

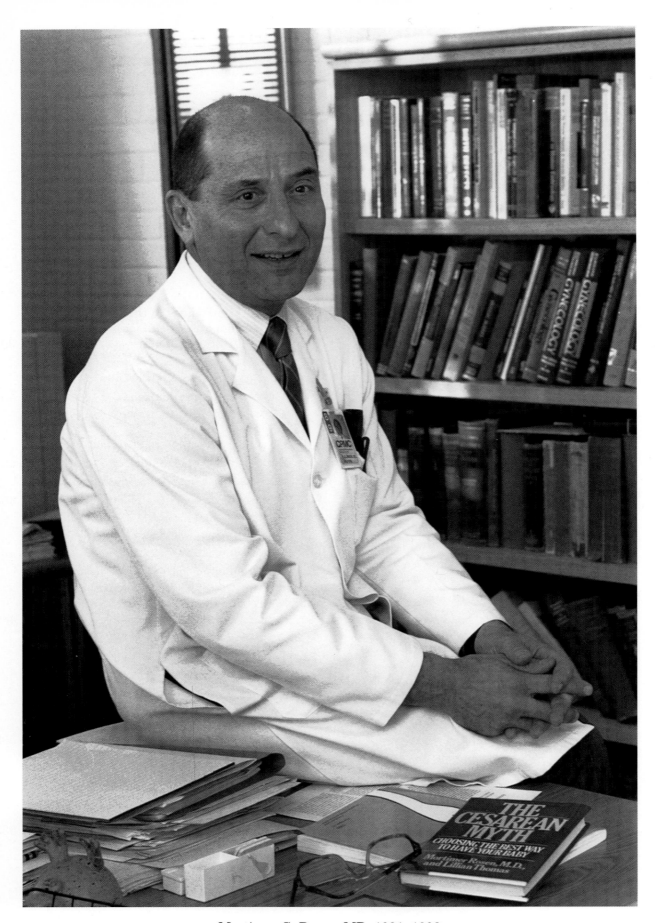

Mortimer G. Rosen, MD, 1931–1992

This book is dedicated to Mortimer G. Rosen, friend and mentor, whose early research on the fetal brain was an inspiration to me and many other young researchers struggling to understand the fetal brain. By creating the necessary clinical and scientific environment for such studies, he became very much a part of its "birth." Many years ago, probably at the beginning of his career as a perinatologist, Dr. Rosen recognized the importance of studying the human fetal brain. Surrounded by a growing group of enthusiastic scholars, including residents, maternal-fetal fellows, biomedical engineers, and biochemists, he pursued his research on one of the most difficult subjects: the physiology and the physiopathology of the fetal central nervous system.

Dr. Rosen believed that the then available systems for monitoring fetal health and well being were inadequate for predicting the intellectual functioning of the neonatal brain. He was always seeking new ways for studying the developing human brain.

When ultrasonography was introduced, Dr. Rosen was among the first to encourage its use in the study of fetal behavioral studies. When he saw the first detailed, crystal clear pictures of the prenatal central nervous system achieved by high frequency transvaginal imaging, he immediately understood the enormous potential of this laboratory technique.

His scientific integrity and skepticism stimulated us to become experts in our field, and furnish objective results to prove the clinical value of high resolution brain scanning of the fetus.

When I presented him with the outline of this book, he was not only supportive, but promised to contribute a special chapter on cerebral palsy, a subject in which he was extremely interested. This is the only time he let us down. The chapter never got further than its introduction. Mort Rosen—my mentor and friend, as well as enthusiastic supporter of our endeavors—passed away in 1992, not living long enough to see the fruits of his labors.

To you, Mort Rosen, in loving memory. I think you would be proud of this work.

Ilan E. Timor-Tritsch, MD

To my family: my son, Benjamin; my parents, Edith and Miguel; my sister, my niece, and my brother-in-law Edith A, Carolinna and Michael who inspired, supported and encouraged me.

Ana Monteagudo

To my wife, Sandra W. Cohen MD, FACP and to my children David, Lauren and Benjamin, who put up with a lot as I tilt with the windmills of academic radiology. Thanks for your help and patience.

To the memory of my parents Samuel Gozanski Cohen and Lola Esther Cohen (nee Altman) who gave me the background, desire and genes (not Levi's) that help me do what I do.

To my colleagues and mentors in pediatric imaging and diagnostic ultrasound, and to my confreres in Pediatrics, Obstetrics, Pediatric Surgery and Pathology, who have inspired, encouraged and helped me make those all-important diagnoses on those all-important and oh-so-real patients.

Harris L. Cohen, MD

Contributor List

Netta M. Blitman, MD
Assistant Professor
Director, Pediatric Radiology
State University of New York-Downstate
Brooklyn, NY

Zeev Blumenfeld, MD
Associate Professor
Reproductive Endocrinology
Department of Obstetrics Gynecology
Rambam Medical Center
The Rappaport Faculty of Medicine
Technion-Israel Institute of Technology
Haifa, Israel

Moshe Bronshtein, MD
Department of Obstetrics Gynecology
Rambam Medical Center
Haifa, Israel

Nicola Burdi, MD
Consultant
Department of Radiology
"Miulli" General Hospital
Acquaviva delle Fonti
Bari, Italy

Gilda Caruso, MD
Professor of Pathology
Institute of Pathology
University of Bari, Italy

Frank A. Chervenak, MD
Professor and Chairman
Department of Obstetrics & Gynecology
New York Presbyterian Hospital
Weill Medical College of Cornell University
New York, NY

Darleen Cioffi-Ragan, RDMS
Diagnostic Medical Sonographer
Ultrasound Division, Department of Radiology
University of Colorado, Health Sciences Center
Denver, CO

Harris L. Cohen, MD, FACR
Professor of Radiology
State University of New York-Downstate
Visiting Professor of Radiology
Johns Hopkins of Medical Institutions
Director, Division of Pediatric Imaging
Professor of Radiology
Suny-Downstate

Vincenzo D'Addario, MD
Professor and Director
4th Unit Obstetrics and Gynecology
University Medical School
Bari, Italy

Shimon Degani, MD
Senior Lecturer
Faculty of Medicine
Technion-Israel Institute of Technology
Director of Ultrasound Unit
Department of Obstetrics & Gynecology
Bani Zion Medical Center
Haifa, Israel

Pietro Falco, MD
Attending Physician
Tecnobios Institute for Prenatal Diagnosis
Bologna, Italy

Luis F. Gonçalves, MD
Clinica Materno-Fetal
Florianopolis, Brazil

Pantaleo Greco, MD
Consultant
2nd Unit of Gynecology and Obstetrics
University of Bari, Italy

Natan Haratz-Rubinstein, MD
Chief Resident
Department of Obstetrics and Gynecology
Columbia Presbyterian Medical Center
New York Presbyterian Hospital
New York, NY

Madhuri Kirpekar, MD
Associate Professor of Radiology
Department of Ultrasound
St. Luke's Roosevelt Hospital
New York, NY
Assistant Professor of Clinical Radiology
Columbia Presbyterian Medical Center
New York, NY

Michael Manco-Johnson
Professor of Radiology, OB/GYN and Medicine
Chairman, Department of Radiology
Co-Director Prenatal Diagnosis Center
University of Colorado, Health Sciences Center
Denver, CO

Patricia Mayberry, RDMS, RVT
Ultrasound Supervisor
Ob/Gyn Ultrasound Unit
New York University School of Medicine
New York, NY

Eli Maymon, MD
Visiting Scientist
Perinatology Research Branch
National Institute of Child Health and Human
    Development
Bethesda, Maryland

Laurence B. McCullough, PhD
Professor
Center for Medical Ethics and Health Policy
Baylor College of Medicine
Houston, Texas

Nicola Medicamento, MD
Consultant
Department of Neurology
Unit of Neuroradiology
University of Bari, Italy

Israel Meizner
Associate Professor of Obstetrics and Gynecology
Sackler Medical School
Tel Aviv University, Israel
Director of Obstetrics & Gynecology
    Ultrasound Unit
Rabin Medical Center
Petach-Tieva, Israel

Ana Monteagudo, MD
Associate Professor of Obstetrics & Gynecology
Director, Bellevue Ultrasound Unit
New York University School of Medicine
New York, NY

Fabiola Müller, Dr. habil.rer.nat
Formerly Research Embryologist
University of California, Davis
Davis, California

Ilse J.M. Nijhuis, MD, PhD
Registrar
Beatrix Children's Hospital
University Hospital Groningen
Groningen, The Netherlands

Jan G. Nijhuis, MD, PhD
Professor of Obstetrics
University Hospital Maastricht
Department of Obstetrics and Gynecology
AZ Maastricht, The Netherlands

Ronan O'Rahilly
Professor Emeritus of Human Anatomy and
    Neurology
University of California, Davis School of Medicine
Davis, California

Antonella Perolo, MD
Consultant
Department of Obstetrics and Gynecology
Policlinico S. Orsola-Malpighi
Bologna, Italy

Gianluigi Pilu, MD
Consultant
Department of Obstetrics and Gynecology
Policlinico S. Orsola-Malpighi
Bologna, Italy

Andrei Rebarber, MD
Assistant Professor
Division of Maternal Fetal Medicine
Department of Obstetrics and Gynecology
New York University School of Medicine
New York, NY

Maurizio Resta, MD
Consultant
Department of Neurology
Unit of Neuroradiology
University of Bari, Italy

Roberto Romero, MD
Chief, Perinatology Research Branch
National Institute of Child Health and
    Human Development
Bethesda, MD

Julian Sanchez, MD
Department of Radiology
State University of New York-Downstate
Brooklyn, NY

Gary Thieme, MD
Associate Professor of Radiology and OB/GYN
Co-Director Prenatal Diagnosis Center
University of Colorado, Health Sciences Center
Denver, CO

Ilan E. Timor-Tritsch, MD
Professor and Obstetrics & Gynecology
Director of Division of Ob & Gyn Ultrasound
New York University School of Medicine
New York, NY

Antonella Visentin, MD
Attending Physician
Tecnobios Institute for Prenatal Diagnosis
Bologna, Italy

Howard Weiner, MD
Assistant Professor
Division of Pediatric Neurosurgery
Department of Neurosurgery
New York University School of Medicine
New York, NY

Bo Hyun Yoon, MD, PhD
Associate Professor
Seoul National University
Seoul, Korea

Etan Z. Zimmer, MD
Clinical Associate Professor
Director of Obstetrics and Ultrasound
Department of Obstetrics and Gynecology
Rambam Medical Center
The Rappaport Faculty of Medicine
Technion-Israel Institute of Technology
Haifa, Israel

Foreword

Over the past few decades the continued research efforts of basic scientists and clinicians have led to extraordinary advances in the utilization of ultrasound in clinical medicine. Drs. Timor-Tritsch, Monteagudo, and Cohen have continued to explore the fetal and neonatal brain to add to our continuing knowledge to produce yet another landmark textbook. This book adds to our understanding of the role of ultrasound in the evolution of both the fetal and newborn central nervous systems. Normal development as well as central nervous system abnormalities are beautifully illustrated in this second edition. This book synthesizes basic embryology and pathophysiology into a well written and illustrated text while exploiting the latest imaging modalities. This text has further enhanced what they already contributed in the first edition. The editors are clearly the recognized authorities in this field and the contributing authors are recognized experts in the area of their contributions. This beautifully illustrated book is fascinating, concise and essential.

This text is another major contribution to medical science. I am confident it will prove to be essential to every clinician involved in prenatal diagnosis and neonatal care. This is a book that belongs in every library and clinical site where obstetrics and pediatric patients undergo ultrasound examinations. The addition of new areas and chapters in this edition, such as the role of three-dimensional imaging, both are timely and essential. The authors have already reported on the key and superior role that this modality plays in the diagnosis of many abnormalities heretofore not amenable to prenatal diagnosis by ultrasound. The introduction of topics on fetal therapy also brings new innovations and exciting new approaches that are now being undertaken in this field.

It is clear that Drs. Timor-Tritsch, Monteagudo, and Cohen have advanced their leadership in this field by yet another essential and magnificent text in this most important area of fetal and neonatal development. Along with their contributing authors, they have produced a monumental addition to our literature.

Lawrence D. Platt, M.D.
Chairman, Department of Ob/Gyn
Cedars-Sinai Medical Center
Professor and Vice Chair
UCLA School of Medicine

Preface to the Second Edition

Responding to the positive feedback to the First Edition of our book we decided to update it and expand its content. An additional reason for this decision was the amount of new and pertinent articles which have accumulated in the last 3-4 years. We wanted to review them and add most of them to the more than 1100 references we used in the First Edition.

As far as the chapters are concerned, every previously written chapter was updated and then there are several new chapters. Major changes were made in Chapters 2, 4, 5 and 8 to reflect the new clinical experience in the field of fetal neuroscan and fetal neuro-MRI. New sonographic images of commonly encountered entities were added to the previously published ones. Several rarely seen fetal neuropathologies were also illustrated and were included. All chapters were updated with the newest articles from the literature to justify the term "reference textbook," a term used by many as they mention the First Edition of the book.

Two new chapters (9 and 14) were added dealing with three-dimensional fetal and neonatal neuroscans. Pediatric neurologists and neurosurgeons rely on neonatal CT and MRI images to study the neonatal brain. So far they seemed hesitant to counsel and to plan postnatal (and prenatal) management of pathologies based upon prenatal ultrasound imaging studies. The reason was, that the prenatal images were obtained at planes unfamiliar to them. They were waiting to see the postnatal imaging studies. Since the introduction of 2D and now of 3D transfontanelle fetal neuroimaging by high frequency, high resolution ultrasound clear images can be generated in the planes which are familiar to pediatric neurologists and neurosurgeons. The expected result of these images is a better understanding of the pathologies leading to an earlier prenatal counseling and planning for postpartum management before the neonatal studies are available. We predict that the 3D fetal and neonatal brain scan will expand and will be widely employed as effective diagnostic means.

The addition of two new chapters deals with devastating diseases of the fetal brain and attempts for their correction. Chapter 16 summarizes possible causes of cerebral palsy and Chapter 18 is a description of attempts to correct neurological pathologies *in utero*. It seems that after the well known moratorium to treat diseases of the brain, while the fetus is still in the womb, there may be a place for intrauterine treatment for a well selected patient population after adequately researched surgical procedures.

The use of the icons at the side of ultrasound images, to indicate the particular plane or section at which the image was generated, was extended to several more chapters. This ensures a better understanding of the anatomy depicted.

We tried (quite successfully) to standardize the anatomic nomenclature throughout the book and based it on the latest issue of the internationally accepted *Nomina Anatomica*. Correctly or incorrectly, some terms are so deeply "embedded" in the daily use, that it may be impossible to constantly correct them. One such example is the word "hydrocephaly" (the accepted, correct way to use it) which over time was changed to "hydrocephalus" and (probably incorrectly) used in many publications. We selected to use the correct term "hydrocephalus" in all chapters.

We hope that the Second Edition of this book will contribute to the understanding and most importantly the earliest possible detection of neurological diseases of the fetus and the newborn.

Ilan E. Timor-Tritsch, MD
Ana Monteagudo, MD
Harris L. Cohen, MD

Preface to the First Edition

The concept for this book was born many years ago and was preceded by careful acquisition and selection of representative neurosonograms of normal and abnormal cases. The central nervous system is probably the most elaborate and intricate organ or system in the human body. Minute structural abnormalities can, at times, reflect major functional deficiencies. On the other hand, it would appear that at times major anatomic defects do not seem to be associated with significantly deviant function. It is extremely important to study and understand the normal and abnormal fetal and neonatal central nervous system. The central nervous system is one of the common sites of anatomical malformation in the fetus with chromosomal abnormality. The detection of anomalies within the fetal and neonatal brain is feasible using modern imaging techniques, such as ultrasound, computed tomography, and magnetic resonance imaging.

The aim of prenatal ultrasonography is to be able to reassure the pregnant patient as early as possible that fetal development is normal; or if a malformation is detected to counsel the patient about the nature of the problem. Most anomalies of the central nervous system develop early, and we have the tools to detect these as early as 10 to 16 weeks. Early detection of such central nervous system anomalies is probably the most important advance in modern perinatology. Neonatal ultrasound confirms the prenatal diagnosis. In addition, neonatal neurosonography is a powerful tool in diagnosing central nervous system pathology.

The first chapter deals with the development of the human central nervous system. Its authors are the distinguished professors Ronan O'Rahilly and Fabiola Müller, who have a lifetime of professional experience. Professor O'Rahilly not only took time to write about the embryology of the brain, but also invested valuable time in overseeing the correct anatomical terminology used throughout most of the chapters.

The vast imaging possibilities of ultrasound in general and that of transvaginal sonography in particular regarding the fetal brain, are dealt with at the beginning of our book and lead into the chapters describing the detectable pathology in the fetal and neonatal central nervous system. Because fetal and neonatal neurosonographic scanning is performed using the anterior fontanelle and other calvarial openings, the "classical" axial planes cannot be used to describe the images obtained in the fan-shaped sonographic sections. It was our goal to keep the "classic" planes in use by CT and by MRI imaging of the brain and create a separate and well defined set of planes and sections for the fetal brain imaging. A new nomenclature regarding the scanning planes of the fetal brain is introduced in Chapters 1, 2, 3, and 4.

We felt that a special and dedicated chapter dealing with biometry of the fetal brain should be included. A large number of tables and graphs as well as measurements of the fetal brain are incorporated for reference.

Because the fetal eye and the fetal face are frequently associated with brain pathology, two special chapters are devoted to these structures. Dr. Israel Meizner and Dr. Moshe Bronshtein's group from Israel have the most imaging experience in these two areas and contributed these two important chapters, which we believe are the most detailed in the literature dealing with those subjects.

Neonatal neurosonology is an established diagnostic entity which has earned its well deserved place in the armamentarium of the neuroimager since its introduction in 1979. Chapters concerning imaging of the normal and abnormal neonatal brain, and the chapter by Dr. Madhuri Kirpekar dealing with the spine, are included to form a continuum as far as the sonographic neuroimaging workup of the prenatal and neonatal CNS.

The chapter written by Gianluigi Pilu and Vincenso D'Addario and their co-workers from Italy, made a significant contribution to the book by touching on the subject of the midline brain pathologies and the recently introduced attempts to image the fetal brain using MRI.

It is hard and labor intensive to study the physiological aspects of the brain. This was successfully done by recognized authors such as Jan Nijhuis who reviewed the fetal behavioral states coordinated by the brain and by Shimon Degani and Reuven Lewinsky summarizing the clinical uses of measuring the blood flow to the central nervous system.

Finally, the ethical aspects of neurosonography are explored by Frank Chervenak, who over the years has become an authority in the field of medical ethics.

This book was written for the perinatologists, neonatologists, perinatal geneticists, as well as the imaging specialists such as radiologists, obstetricians, and sonographers who see the fetus and neonate in their clinical practice. These specialists scan the fetal and neonatal brain themselves or are directly involved with managing pregnancies with structural malformations or anomalies of the central nervous system. Special emphasis was placed on the creation of an objective and exhaustive updated review of the pertinent literature so that the reader would have a wide reference base on each subject. As far as the illustrations are concerned, the authors were encouraged to be liberal about including an unrestricted number of cases and their sonographic manifestations in their respective chapters. This may, therefore, lead to some duplication by presenting the same disease or pathology more than once. However, by allowing some deliberate repetition in depicting various cases, we, hopefully, covered the commonly occurring pathologies. We consider such occasional and repetitive presentations as one of the advantages of the text enabling the reader to be educated by the experiences of the different authors and their various points of view.

One of the particular strengths of presenting the sonograms is that we chose to include small body images so that readers could orient themselves as to how an individual sonographic view was obtained. This will, we hope, enable readers to quickly grasp and understand the actual planes used to generate the pictures.

We suggest that neuroimaging of the fetus be included in the structural evaluation of the fetus at any gestational age. We also believe that practitioners involved in fetal and/or neonatal neuroimaging will benefit from using this carefully prepared text.

Ilan E. Timor-Tritsch, MD
Ana Monteagudo, MD
Harris L. Cohen, MD

Acknowledgments

We wish to express our thanks to Christonia Joseph for the secretarial help. The professional help of Barbara Holton and her staff as well as that of Andrea Seils are greatly valued.

Ilan E. Timor-Tritsch
Ana Monteagudo

I would like to thank Benjamin Cohen for his computer consultations and to gratefully Acknowledge those who have educated me and helped me educate myself and others in the fascinating world of perinatal neurosonography. These include Drs: Bruce Markle, David Brallier, DuRee Eaton, Gwendolyn Hotson, Jack Haller, Sheldon Schechter, John Loh and E. George Kassner as well as a myriad of colleagues, sonographers, fellows and residents that I have worked with at Children's Hospital National Medical Center, Brookdale University Hospital, North Shore University Hospital-Cornell, SUNY-Downstate Medical Center, Kings County Hospital and Johns Hopkins Hospital.

Harris L. Cohen

Ultrasonography of the Prenatal and Neonatal Brain

CHAPTER ONE

Prenatal Development of the Brain

Ronan O'Rahilly
Fabiola Müller

Prenatal life can be divided conveniently into (1) the embryonic period proper, i.e., the first 8 weeks following fertilization; and (2) the fetal period, which extends to birth. The distinction between the embryonic and fetal periods is well founded and has long been established in human embryology. The embryonic period is that during which new features appear with great rapidity, whereas the fetal period is characterized more by the elaboration of existing structures. Moreover, the vast majority of congenital anomalies appear during the embryonic period. The difference is highlighted by the fact that the embryonic period has been successfully subdivided into morphological stages, whereas the fetal period has so far defied such a procedure.

The embryonic period has been divided into 23 developmental (Carnegie) stages (Table 1–1), which have been listed in detail by O'Rahilly and Müller,[1,2] in whose monograph the early development of the human embryo has been thoroughly described. Each stage, on average, lasts slightly more than 2 days. The stages are based on both external and internal morphological criteria and depend mainly on features that change rapidly, such as the number of somitic pairs, the early appearance of the eye, and the form of the developing limbs. Although it may sometimes be possible to estimate approximately a given stage on ultrasonography, the staging system is based on having an embryo "in the hand" rather than *in utero*. Moreover, very early as well as late stages can be identified precisely only by histological examination.

Although schemes have been devised to subdivide the fetal period according to either measurements or age (one of the simplest—into trimesters—is still very useful), no morphological staging system is available, largely because changes are neither sufficiently rapid nor adequately spectacular.

TERMINOLOGY

It should be pointed out that, in current usage in anatomy, practically all eponyms are now obsolete, e.g., Luschka, Magendie, Monro, Reil, Rolando, and Sylvius, which convey nothing concerning either the site or the nature of the relevant structure. The addition "of Monro" or "of Sylvius" is superfluous because there is only one interventricular foramen and only one aqueduct in the brain.

PRENATAL AGE

Just as postnatal age commences at birth, prenatal age begins at fertilization. Ovulation is sufficiently close, so that the term postovulatory has frequently been used to indicate age. Particularly since the advent of in vitro fertilization, however, age is best referred to as postfertilizational.

When a reliable menstrual history is available, or indirectly by the conventional addition of 2 weeks to the age, the duration from the first day of the last menstrual period (LMP) may be used. The duration is expressed in (post)menstrual weeks and days. This is perfectly acceptable provided that (1) the du-

1

TABLE 1–1. SUMMARY OF DEVELOPMENT OF THE CENTRAL NERVOUS SYSTEM

			Embryonic Period
Carnegie Stage	**Greatest Length (mm)**	**Approximate Age (days)**	**Key Features**
1–7	0.1–0.4	1–19	Very early embryo
8	1	23	Neural folds and groove
9	2	25	Mesencephalic flexure; rhombencephalon, mesencephalon, prosencephalon; 1–3 S
10	3	28	Fusion of neural folds begins; telencephalon and diencephalon distinguishable; Optic primordia; 4–12 S
11	3.5	29	Rostral neuropore closes; 13–20 S
12	4	30	Caudal neuropore closes; secondary neurulation begins; 21–29 S
13	5	32	Closed neural tube; primordium of cerebellum; isthmus rhombencephali; 30–? S; Fig. 1–2A
14	6	33	Pontine flexure; future cerebral hemispheres; all 16 neuromeres present
15	8	36	Five subdivisions: medulla, pons, midbrain, diencephalon, telencephalon; Figs. 1–2B; 1–3A, B; 1–4
16	10	38	Thalamus; Fig. 1–5
17	13	41	Internal and external cerebellar swellings; Fig. 1–2C
18	15	44	Future corpus striatum; interventricular foramina defined; Fig. 1–6
19	17	46	Choroid plexus of fourth ventricle
20	20	49	Choroid plexus of lateral ventricles; Figs. 1–3C, D
21	23	51	Anterior and inferior horns of lateral ventricle; circulus arteriosus complete; Fig. 1–2D
22	26	53	Internal capsule
23	29	56	Caudate nucleus and putamen; anterior commissure begins

Fetal Period		**Figs. 1–8, 1–9**
Trimester 1		Cerebellar halves unite and vermis becomes defined
		Corpus callosum is still very limited
		Aqueduct appears narrow
		Posterior horn of lateral ventricle
Trimester 2		Corpus callosum covers roof of third ventricle
		Sulci and gyri become visible on hermispheric surface
		Crura cerebri are prominent
		Hippocampal formation becomes S-shaped
		Myelinization begins in CNS
Trimester 3		Insula buried by opercula

S, pairs of somites.
Note: The greatest lengths and the postfertilizational ages given are approximate only. The latter have been revised to conform to current ultrasonic information. From data of O'Rahilly and Müller (1999).[2]

ration is designated as (post)menstrual, and (2) it is not referred to as age. At one postmenstrual week an embryo does not even exist!

In summary, two systems of designation are available: (1) age, which is postfertilizational and generally estimated; and (2) (post)menstrual duration, which, although it is not age (and should not be combined with that word), is a useful guide in clinical practice. The type of weeks being used should be specified: (1) postfertilizational weeks or weeks of age, or (2) (post)menstrual weeks. Confusion is thereby eliminated.

It has been shown that the term gestational age in the literature is either (1) not defined or (2) is used indiscriminately for postmenstrual weeks and days or for postfertilizational age.[3] The continuing confusion concerning prenatal age is unnecessary and disappears once the ambiguous and superfluous term gestational age is abandoned.

PRENATAL MEASUREMENTS

Several different measurements, such as the biparietal diameter and the ossified femoral length, are very important in later development, but the most useful datum throughout prenatal life is still the greatest length, exclusive of the (flexed) lower limbs.[4] Crown-rump (C–R) length is unsatisfactory because point C, which overlies the midbrain, is frequently difficult to locate, and point R is imprecise.

The greatest length, which is independent of fixed points, is much simpler to ascertain and is in fact what is generally measured.[5,6]

The distinction between stages and measurements should be kept clearly in mind. *The 18-mm stage* is incorrect usage, because 18 mm is merely a length, not a stage as the term is used in embryology.

The advent of ultrasonography has led to the construction of many elaborate tables of prenatal measurements related to prenatal age, or more generally to intervals since the LMP. Although not all of these tables are in agreement in detail, it can be stated with confidence that at the end of the embryonic period, when the greatest length is approximately 30 mm, the age is 8 weeks, corresponding to 10 postmenstrual weeks.

DEVELOPMENT OF THE NERVOUS SYSTEM

The development of the human nervous system is summarized here (Table 1-1). Details are available in several works, e.g., those by O'Rahilly and Müller.[7,8,9] The most detailed and precise account of the prenatal human brain, with particular emphasis on the embryonic period, is *The Embryonic Human Brain: An Atlas of Developmental Stages.*[2] That study contains a bibliography of more than 250 entries, and therefore a detailed list of references is not provided here.

PRIMARY NEURULATION

The central nervous system arises mostly from a part of the ectoderm known as the neural plate. The folding of the neural plate to form successively the neural groove and the neural tube is termed primary neurulation, and is the first visible sign of the nervous system.[2] It begins when the embryo is approximately 1 mm in length. Closure of the neural groove begins near the junction of the future brain and spinal cord. The still open ends of the developing neural tube are known as the rostral and caudal neuropores, which close successively at about 4 weeks. The closure of the rostral neuropore is bidirectional: rostrocaudal and caudorostral. Although small and variable accessory loci of fusion of the neural folds may sometimes be seen, a specific pattern of multiple sites of fusion, such as has been described in the mouse, does not occur in the human. Moreover, attempts to force the classification of neural tube defects into such a pattern are quite unconvincing. Primary neurulation is completed by the separation of neural from surface ectoderm by the interposition of mesenchyme.

SOME EARLY ANOMALIES

In diastematomyelia the spinal cord is partially split longitudinally into right and left halves that are separated by a fibrocartilaginous or bony spur in the vertebral canal. This may be a manifestation of the split notochord syndrome, which is generally attributed to persistence of the neurenteric canal, a temporary communication through the primitive node at stages 8 through 10.

Anencephaly, a partial absence of the brain and the overlying cranial vault, frequently arises from (1) failure of the rostral neuropore to close, followed by (2) protrusion of the brain (exencephaly), and finally (3) degeneration of the exposed portions.[10] The defect arises early (probably stages 8 and 9), before four postfertilizational weeks, and defective production of mesenchyme is considered to be of fundamental importance.[11]

Spina bifida may be evident *(aperta)* or concealed *(occulta)*. A cystic mass is generally present in those that are obvious and these are known as spina bifida *cystica*. Spinal and cerebral forms of neural tube defects exhibit a close parallelism, as shown in Table 1-2.

Myelomeningocele (or meningomyelocele), which may arise as a myeloschisis, is usually lumbosacral. Failure of closure of the caudal neuropore is probably a major factor, although the condition is not considered to be a simple failure of neural closure. When the caudal neuropore fails to close, fixation between neural and surface ectoderm may hinder the normal ascent of the spinal cord, which becomes tethered. When spina bifida aperta is found in the cervicothoracic region, however, the possibility of reopening of the neural tube needs to be entertained.

TABLE 1-2. NEURAL TUBE DEFECTS

Dysraphia (NTD)			
		Spinal	Cerebral
Spina Bifida	aperta	Open neural plate ↓ Myeloschisis	Open neural plate ↓ Exencephaly ↓ Anencephaly
	cystica	Myelomeningocele	Encephalocele
		Meningocele	Meningocele
	occulta	Spina bifida occulta	Cranium bifidum occultum

SECONDARY NEURULATION

Secondary neurulation is the continuing formation of the sacrococcygeal part of the spinal cord from the caudal eminence, without direct involvement of the surface ectoderm (neural plate).[2] It begins once the caudal neuropore has closed. The transition from primary to secondary neurulation is at the site of closure of the caudal neuropore. The caudal neuropore closes at the level of somitic pair 31, which corresponds to future vertebral level S2 in the embryo. Because of the ascent of the spinal cord during the fetal period, however, the site of the former caudal neuropore ascends also and corresponds to a higher vertebral level postnatally.

DEVELOPMENT OF THE BRAIN

Five to Six Postmenstrual Weeks (Three to Four Weeks of Age)

As the embryo becomes more elongated, the neural groove becomes deeper and the three major divisions are distinguishable in the folds of the completely open neural groove: the forebrain, the midbrain, and the hindbrain. The site of the midbrain is indicated by the mesencephalic flexure, which remains distinct throughout the embryonic period (Fig. 1–1). The neural tube has not yet formed and the "brain vesicles" are largely a myth. The forebrain soon becomes subdivided (earlier than previously appreciated) into the diencephalon and the telencephalon medium. The embryo is now about 3 mm in length.

Six to Seven Postmenstrual Weeks (Four to Five Weeks of Age)

When both neuropores are closed at 4 to 5 weeks after fertilization, the future ventricular system (Fig. 1–2A) no longer communicates with the amniotic cavity. At this time, in embryos of about 5 mm in length, the first (bilateral) indication of the cerebellum can be discerned.

The cerebral hemispheres (Figs. 1–2B and 1–3) then become delimited from the telencephalon medium (Figs. 1–1D, 1–2B, and 1–3). A bend, the pontine flexure (Figs. 1–1C and 1–3A), begins in the hindbrain and allows a subdivision into the metencephalon (the pons and the cerebellum) and the myelencephalon (the medulla oblongata). All five major subdivisions of the brain are then distinguishable: the telencephalon, diencephalon, mesencephalon, metencephalon, and myelencephalon (Figs. 1–1D and 1–3A). The initial development of the basal nuclei (which, by definition, are not ganglia) now takes place, and the thalami are also dis-

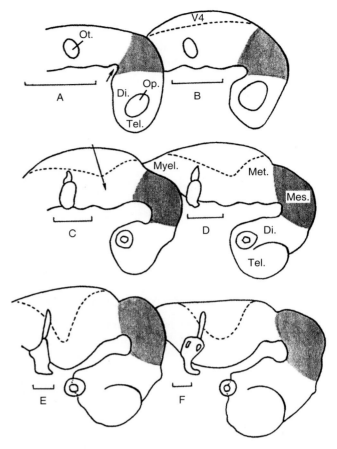

Figure 1–1. Right lateral views of the brain from about 6 to 8 postmenstrual weeks (4 to 6 weeks of age). The stages are from 12 to 18, with the omission of stage 16. The midbrain is stippled. In **A** the mesencephalic flexure *(arrow)* is already well developed and the telencephalon medium (Tel.) can be distinguished from the diencephalon (Di.). The outlines of the optic (Op.) and otic (Ot.) vesicles are shown. In **B** the fourth ventricle (V4) is indicated. In **C** the pontine flexure *(arrow)* has appeared. The optic cup has formed and the endolymphatic appendage can be seen above the closed otic vesicle. In **D** the five major subdivisions of the brain are visible: myelencephalon, metencephalon, mesencephalon, diencephalon, and telencephalon. The *(right)* cerebral hemisphere is evident. In **E** the cochlear duct is clearer. In **F** the semicircular ducts are developing. The bars represent 1 mm. Based on the authors' reconstructions.

cernible (Figs. 1–4 and 1–5). The embryo is about 6 mm in length.

Holoprosencephaly is a variable deficiency in "diverticulation" of the prosencephalon to form the cerebral hemispheres, and is usually accompanied by facial malformation. Abnormal induction by an area of future forebrain near the prechordal plate very early (stages 7 and 8) is believed to be significant.[12] The failure of lateralization may be complete

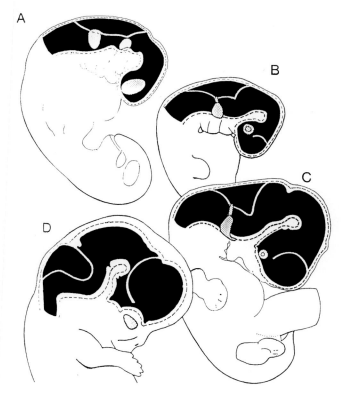

Figure 1–2. Right lateral views of the brain *(dashed lines)* in situ at **(A)** about 4½ weeks (stage 13), **(B)** 5 weeks (stage 15), **(C)** 6 weeks (stage 17), and **(D)** about 7 weeks (stage 21). The ventricular cavities are shown in black. The stippled structures are the otic vesicle, the trigeminal ganglion (shown only in **A**), and the optic vesicle, cup, and eye. In **B** all five major subdivisions of the brain can be identified: telencephalon (represented here by the right cerebral hemisphere), diencephalon (to which the optic cup is attached), mesencephalon (at the mesencephalic flexure), and metencephalon and myelencephalon. (See also Fig. 1–3A.)

(alobar holoprosencephaly), partial (semilobar), or only rostral (lobar).

Cyclopia is the occurrence within a single orbit of a median eye or (sometimes distinguished as synophthalmia) paired ocular structures.[12,13] The defective lateralization (which is not a fusion) is believed to be caused by lack of the normal inhibition of the median portion of the originally single optic field.[2] Normally the prechordal plate induces paired optic primordia very early (stages 7 and 8).

Encephalo(meningo)celes are generally in the occipital region. They are covered by skin and hence are believed to arise after closure of the neural tube, probably in the presence of mesenchymal insufficiency. Those situated anteriorly, e.g., in the fronto-ethmoidal region, constitute a separate category and are "based on a primary disturbance in

the separation of neural and surface ectoderm at the site of final closure of the rostral neuropore, "resulting" secondarily in a mesodermal defect at this site."[14]

In the Arnold-Chiari malformation, a failure of the pontine flexure to form is believed to be important in the abnormal elongation of the hindbrain. In the Dandy-Walker syndrome, maldevelopment of the rostral part of the roof of the fourth ventricle is considered to be a significant causative factor.

Seven to Eight Postmenstrual Weeks (Five to Six Weeks of Age)

The neurohypophysis (Fig. 1–3C) begins its evagination and the longitudinal fissure becomes deeper with continuing growth of the cerebral hemispheres (Fig. 1–3D). The basioccipital part of the skull is beginning to chondrify. The embryo is about 12 mm in length.

Eight to Nine Postmenstrual Weeks (Six to Seven Weeks of Age)

A feature that appears very gradually is the flattening of the insular region. The embryo is about 20 mm in length (Fig. 1–6).

Nine to Ten Postmenstrual Weeks (Seven to Eight Weeks of Age)

The falx cerebri, indicated initially by a leptomeningeal precursor, is apparent at the end of the embryonic period. Important histological differentiation takes place in the cerebral cortex and the internal capsule develops. The embryonic period proper closes at 8 weeks after fertilization, when the greatest length (exclusive of the lower limbs) is about 30 mm. Ossification is beginning in the occipital region of the skull, and the foramen magnum is definable. The anterior (frontal), posterior (occipital), and inferior (temporal) poles of the cerebral hemispheres, as well as the insula, can be detected, although they are not yet pronounced. The ventricles at this time are shown in Figure 1–7. The brain is now far more advanced morphologically than is generally appreciated, and functional considerations should be taken into account, especially in the hindbrain.

Spina bifida occulta is a normal phase of development. At the end of the embryonic period the spinal cord and the vertebral column end at the same level. Moreover, ossification has not extended dorsally, so that a total spina bifida occulta exists, and this persists into adulthood in part of the sacral region in about one-fifth of normal persons. During the fetal period, a differential shift in growth occurs

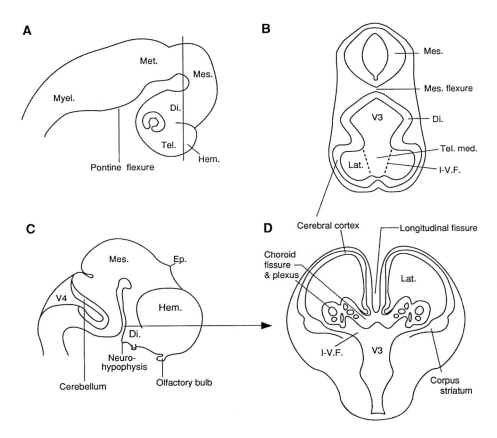

Figure 1–3. **A, B.** The brain at 5 weeks (stage 15). In **B** (the plane of which is shown in **A**) the cerebral hemispheres have begun to develop from the telencephalon medium. **C, D.** The brain at 7 weeks (stage 20). In **D** (the plane of which is shown in **C**) the wall of each hemisphere has invaginated laterally (at the choroid fissure) into the lateral ventricle to form the choroid plexus. Di., Diencephalon; Ep., epiphysis cerebri (pineal gland); Hem., cerebral hemisphere; I-V.F., interventricular foramen; Lat., lateral ventricle; Mes., mesencephalon; Met., metencephalon; Myel., myelencephalon; Tel., telencephalon; Tel.med., telencephalon medium; V3, third ventricle; V4, fourth ventricle.

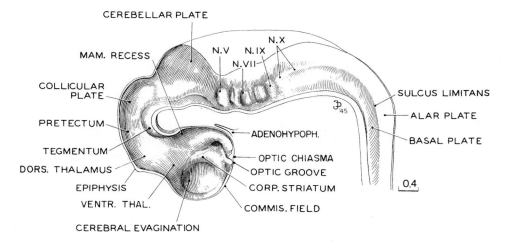

Figure 1–4. Three-dimensional reconstruction of the right half of a human brain seen from the medial side. Embryonic length, 8.3 mm. About 5 postfertilizational or 7 postmenstrual weeks (stage 15). The relatively enormous size of the ventricular system is evident. In Figures 1–4, 1–5, and 1–6, the label corpus striatum indicates its medial ventricular eminence.[2] *(From O'Rahilly and Müller, 1987,[1] with permission.)*

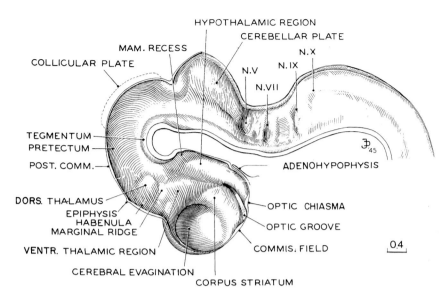

Figure 1–5. Three-dimensional reconstruction of the right half of a human brain seen from the medial side. Embryonic length, 10.1 mm. About 5 postfertilizational (7 postmenstrual) weeks (stage 16). The cerebellar plate is prominent. *(From O'Rahilly and Müller, 1987,[1] with permission.)*

whereby the conus medullaris is found at increasingly higher vertebral levels, L3 at birth and L2 or L1 in adulthood.

Spinal meningoceles may arise as herniations in the presence of a mesenchymal deficiency, probably during the time when the normal spina bifida occulta is present. Cerebral meningoceles are rare.

LATER DEVELOPMENT

The most evident external changes in the fetal period[2] are (1) the union of the cerebellar halves and the definition of the vermis; (2) the increasing concealment of the diencephalon and the mesencephalon, and (later) of a part of the cerebellum, by the cerebral hemispheres; (3) further approach of the frontal and temporal poles around the insula, which becomes increasingly buried by opercula; and (4) the appearance of sulci (lateral, central, parieto-occipital, calcarine, etc.) on the hemispheric surface at about the middle of prenatal life, at which time the cerebral peduncles become prominent. One of the most noticeable internal changes is the growth of the corpus callosum.

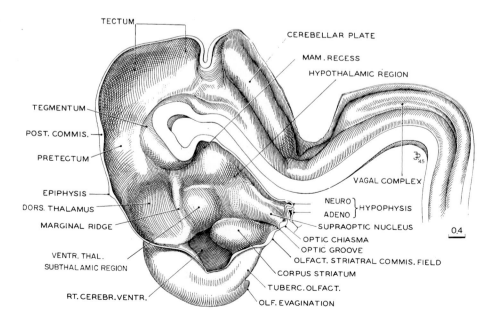

Figure 1–6. Three-dimensional reconstruction of the right half of a human brain seen from the medial side. Embryonic length, 16.8 mm. About 6 postfertilizational or 8 postmenstrual weeks (stage 18). The right cerebral *(lateral)* ventricle can be seen through the right interventricular foramen, which is still relatively wide. Between the tectum and the tegmentum of the midbrain, the large cavity is the future aqueduct. The roof of the fourth ventricle has been sectioned. *(From O'Rahilly and Müller, 1987,[1] with permission.)*

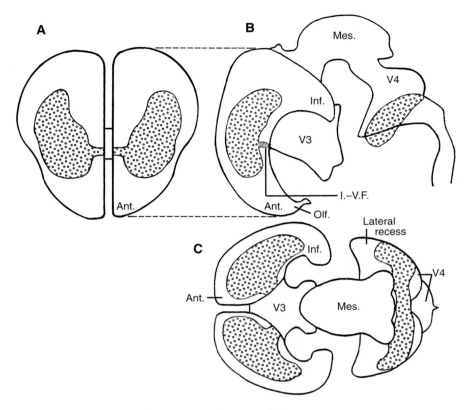

Figure 1–7. The ventricular cavities at the end of the embryonic period (stage 23, 10 postmenstrual weeks, 8 weeks of age). **A** is a dorsal view of the lateral ventricles. **B** is a left lateral view of the complete ventricular system. **C** is a dorsal view of the entire ventricular system. In each view the choroid plexuses are indicated by stippling. Ant., anterior or frontal horn; Inf., inferior or temporal horn; I-V.F., interventricular foramen; Mes., mesencephalic ventricle (the future aqueduct); Olf, "olfactory ventricle" (temporary); V3, third ventricle; V4, fourth ventricle.

THE CEREBELLUM

The cerebellum arises as a bilateral organ very early in development (at about 6½ postmenstrual weeks, i.e., 4½ weeks of age). Later in the embryonic period it projects largely into the fourth ventricle in a complicated and temporary manner (Figs. 1–4 through 1–6). Early in the fetal period, union of the two halves results in the vermis, which then develops folia and becomes largely obscured by the cerebellar hemispheres. At birth, the form of the cerebellum closely resembles that of the adult.

THE CORPUS CALLOSUM

During the fetal period three closely related structures become apparent: the corpus callosum, the underlying septum pellucidum and its cavum, and the overlying cingulate gyrus.

The commissural plate of the embryo (Fig. 1–4) gives rise early in the fetal period to the corpus callo-

sum and the anterior commissure (Fig. 1–8A). The corpus callosum, on median section, is at first merely a compact mass (Fig. 1–8B), but its length increases considerably during the second trimester (Fig. 1–8C), and the underlying portion of the commissural plate becomes thinned as the septum pellucidum.

Because the trunk of the corpus callosum is sometimes found in the absence of a genu, it has been proposed that the first part of the corpus callosum to become visible is the front portion of the trunk, which then develops bidirectionally, thereby forming the genu and the splenium.[15]

By the middle of prenatal life, the rostrum, genu, central part (not *body: corpus* already means "body"), and splenium can be distinguished clearly (Fig. 1–8D). During the second and third trimesters the corpus callosum gradually forms a solid covering over the roof of the third ventricle (except in agenesis of the corpus callosum). The corpus callosum continues to grow into the third decade of life.

A narrow cavity appears within the septum pellucidum and is known as the cavum septi pellu-

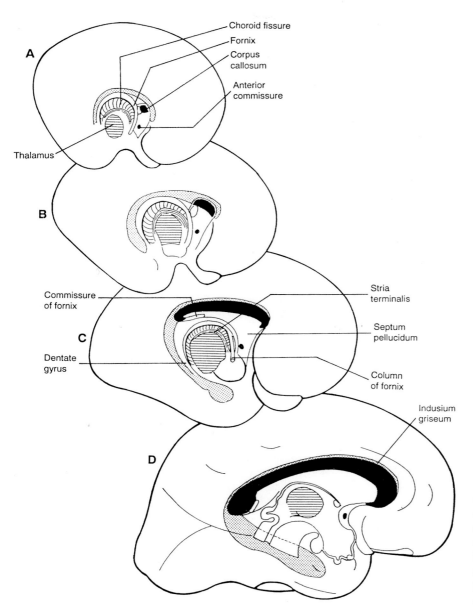

Figure 1–8. The development of the corpus callosum (shown in *black*) as seen on the medial surface of the left cerebral hemisphere at 14, 15, 19, and 30 postmenstrual weeks. The great increase in length throughout the fetal period is evident. *(From O'Rahilly and Müller, 1999,[2] with permission.)*

cidi (genitive case required!). It has been described as arising as a pocket that at first opens into the longitudinal fissure, but later becomes sealed by the rostrum of the corpus callosum. According to others, however, the cavum is formed by necrosis within the commissural mass and was never open to the subarachnoid space. The cavum can be identified during the second trimester, after which its posterior portion becomes obliterated before birth, as occurs to its anterior portion usually within a few months after birth. If the posterior portion persists, it is frequently termed the *cavum Vergae*. (See Chapter 2)

The gyrus cinguli, or cingulate gyrus, is so named because it forms a partial girdle around the corpus callosum and follows the callosal curve. It can be distinguished on the medial surface of the cerebral hemisphere during the second trimester.

Agenesis of the corpus callosum is assumed to arise already in the commissural plate or field (Fig. 1–4), which is a thickening of the embryonic lamina terminalis that appears very early (stage 12).

MYELINIZATION

Reflexes can occur while nerve fibers are still unmyelinated, and embryonic and fetal movements during the first trimester take place before the onset of myelinization. Myelinization in the central nervous system begins during the second trimester, although the cerebral hemispheres contain little myelin at birth. Myelin is deposited more rapidly during the first two postnatal years, but the process continues into adulthood.

Fibers associated with related functions tend to become myelinated at the same time, and cortical association fibers are the last to be involved. It is believed that the state of myelinization indicates the functional maturity of the brain and is correlated with psychomotor development. Magnetic resonance imaging is particularly suitable for assessing the progress of myelinization.

THE VENTRICULAR SYSTEM

The ventricles are a significant feature on ultrasonography, and their development is described briefly here. The ventricular system, including the central canal of the medulla and the spinal cord, is derived from the cavity of the neural tube.[16] During the embryonic period and the early portion of the fetal period, the walls of the brain are very thin in most regions, and hence the ventricular system is relatively very large (Figs. 1–2 and 1–9B). Later, as the walls increase in thickness, the ventricles occupy relatively less of the volume of the brain (Fig. 1–9C and D).

In the region of the rhombencephalon, the roof of the brain is already noticeably thin at about 4 to 5 weeks after fertilization, thereby indicating the fourth ventricle (Fig. 1–3C), the floor of which has become rhomboid. Extensions of the ventricle that are already detectable early become the lateral recesses (Fig. 1–7C) of the fourth ventricle. The median aperture of the fourth ventricle appears, at the earliest, at the end of the embryonic period and is almost constant from early in the fetal period. The lateral apertures appear later, probably during the second trimester.

The cavity of the midbrain (the mesencephalic ventricle) remains relatively wide throughout the embryonic period (Fig. 1–2C), at the end of which its ends become slightly constricted (Fig. 1–7B). It becomes gradually more tubular during the fetal period and would seem to justify the name *aqueduct* at the end of the first trimester.

As the cerebral hemispheres begin to develop, their cavities become the lateral ventricles (Fig. 1–3B), and the cavity of the telencephalon medium and the diencephalon becomes delimited as the third ventricle (Figs. 1–3B and D). The temporary cavities of the optic cups (the optic ventricles) and their stalks are originally evaginations of the diencephalon. The openings between the third and lateral ventricles become very gradually narrowed

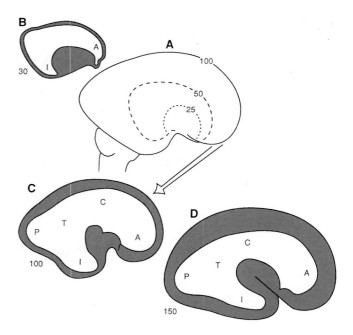

Figure 1–9. **A.** Right lateral outlines of the brain at 25 mm, 50 mm, and 100 mm GL (9½, 12, and 13 postmenstrual weeks). **B, C,** and **D** show the right lateral ventricle at 30 mm, 100 mm, and 150 mm GL (10, 13, and 19 postmenstrual weeks). A comparison of views **B, C,** and **D** shows that the wall of the hemisphere *(shaded)* is becoming thicker, and hence that the ventricle appears relatively smaller as age advances. The small evagination from the anterior horn is the temporary "olfactory ventricle." A, Anterior horn; C, central part; I, inferior horn; P, posterior horn; T, trigonum. (**A** is based on Hochstetter,[17] **B** on O'Rahilly and Müller,[2] and **C** and **D** on Westergaard.[18])

(Fig. 1–3B and D) to form the interventricular foramina (Fig. 1–6).

Growth of the corpus striatum during the last week of the embryonic period further narrows the interventricular foramen (Fig. 1–3D) and transforms the formerly spherical lateral ventricle into a characteristic C-shaped cavity (Fig. 1–9B), which extends from anterior (its frontal horn) to inferior (its temporal horn).[2, 17, 18] A number of structures in the brain (e.g., the caudate nucleus, the fornix, and the choroid plexus) follow this C-shaped growth. The posterior (occipital) horn (Fig. 1–9C) develops at about 12 postmenstrual weeks and is very obvious early in the second trimester. The following subdivisions can now be distinguished: the anterior or frontal horn, the central part (which is not really a "body"), and the trigone (frequently referred to as the atrium), from which proceed the posterior or occipital horn and the inferior or temporal horn (Figs. 1–9C and D). (Strictly speaking, the collateral trigone is the ventricular floor between the posterior and inferior horns, but the term *trigone* is commonly used for a portion of the cavity.)

Three different liquids are successively in contact with the developing brain: (1) the amniotic fluid until closure of the neuropores, (2) the ependymal fluid after closure, and (3) the cerebrospinal fluid after the formation of the choroid plexuses.

The choroid plexuses (the incorrect *plexi* is not the plural), first that of the fourth ventricle and then those of the lateral ventricles (Fig. 1–3D), develop between 8 and 9 postmenstrual weeks. The plexuses are noticeably voluminous in the lateral ventricles (Fig. 1–7) during the embryonic period and on into fetal life, as is readily seen on ultrasonography. The choroid plexus of the third ventricle develops early in the fetal period, and the interthalamic adhesion (formerly termed the massa intermedia) may develop, in some instances, before the middle of prenatal life.

Although indications of the subarachnoid space appear much earlier, the space and most of the cisternae are distinct at the end of the embryonic period, at which time the cerebellomedullary cistern (the cisterna magna) is also discernible.[19]

PLANES

The three main sets of planes used in anatomy are the horizontal and the two vertical series: coronal and sagittal. One of the sagittal planes is median.[20] There is no limit to the number of sagittal and coronal planes, so that sections are in *a*, not *the,* sagittal or coronal plane. Although frontal is frequently used

as a synonym for coronal, in strict usage the term frontal should be reserved for the antonym of occipital. A particularly important plane in the head is the orbitomeatal (Fig. 1–10D), because it is used to ensure that the head is in the standard position. For this purpose, the plane is kept horizontal. In other words, the orbitomeatal and the numerous possible horizontal planes in the adult are all parallel with each other. Strictly coronal planes can be defined as those vertical planes that are at a right angle to the orbitomeatal plane and also at a right angle to the median plane. Strictly coronal planes are necessarily parallel with one another.

It needs to be emphasized that, in anatomy and embryology in general, the unofficial word *midsagittal* should not be used for *median. Coronal* and *sagittal* refer to planes parallel to, but not necessarily through, the coronal and sagittal sutures, respectively. All planes parallel to the median plane are sagittal, so that the unofficial term *parasagittal* is redundant and should be eliminated. If necessary, a plane particularly close to the median could justifiably be termed *paramedian.*

A scheme has been prepared for the embryonic (Fig. 1–10A), fetal (Fig. 1–10B), and neonatal (Fig. 1–10C) heads, positioned in relation to the orbitomeatal plane. The situation is complicated prenatally, however, by the curvature of the body and particularly by the flexion of the head. As a result, a transverse section of the trunk (Fig. 1–10B), which would correspond to a horizontal section in the adult, is no longer parallel to the orbitomeatal plane. Similarly, "coronal" planes (of the adult type)

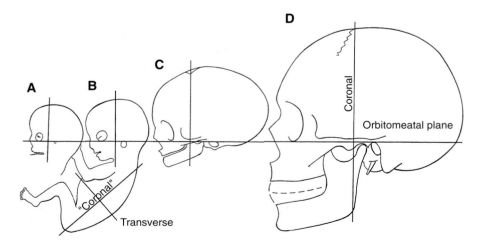

Figure 1–10. Left lateral views of the developing head, showing the orbitomeatal plane and examples of the many possible coronal planes. **A,** At the end of the embryonic period (stage 23) showing the orbitomeatal plane as determined from graphic reconstructions by the authors. **B,** A fetus of 10 postfertilizational weeks illustrating that transverse and "coronal" planes through the trunk differ considerably from horizontal and coronal planes through the head. **C,** A neonatal skull showing a coronal plane through the anterior fontanelle. **D,** An adult skull showing a coronal plane through the bregma.

in the prenatal trunk differ considerably from those in the head, i.e., from vertical planes at a right angle to the orbitomeatal (Fig. 1–10B).

The above-mentioned differences are important in discussions of the imaging of the prenatal brain. A further complication arises because many of the planes used in prenatal ultrasonography are oblique, as will be explained in Chapter 2.

SUMMARY

The various features of the brain, including numerous nuclei and tracts not mentioned here, first appear very early, during the embryonic period, which has been stressed in this chapter. Indeed, 167 features of the brain that appear during the first 7 weeks after fertilization have been listed by O'Rahilly and Müller[2] (See their appendix.) Hence, when a structure is first seen in vivo and in utero by current imaging techniques, it should not only be understood but also clearly indicated that this is usually much later than the actual situation elucidated by human embryology.

REFERENCES

1. O'Rahilly R, Müller F. *Developmental Stages in Human Embryos, Including a Revision of Streeter's "Horizons" and a Survey of the Carnegie Collection.* Washington, DC: Carnegie Institution of Washington, 1987. Publication 637.
2. O'Rahilly R, Müller F. *The Embryonic Brain: An Atlas of Developmental Stages.* 2nd ed. New York: Wiley-Liss; 1999.
3. O'Rahilly R, Müller F. Prenatal ages and stages: Measures and errors. *Teratology.* 2000, 61:382–384.
4. O'Rahilly R, Müller F. Embryonic length and cerebral landmarks in staged human embryos. *Anat Rec.* 1984;209:265–271.
5. Böhmer S, Bruhns T, Degenhardt F, et al. Vergleich von vagino- und abdominosonographischen Messergebnissen mit embryologischen Wachstumskurven der Frühschwangerschaft. *Geburtsh Frauenheilk,* 1993;53:792–799.
6. Wisser J, Dirschedl P, Krone S. Estimation of gestational age by transvaginal sonographic measurement of greatest embryonic length in dated human embryos. *Ultrasound Obstet Gynecol.* 1994;4:457–462.
7. O'Rahilly R, Müller F. *Human Embryology and Teratology.* 3rd ed. New York: Wiley-Liss, 2000, in press.
8. Müller F, O'Rahilly R. The timing and sequence of appearance of neuromeres and their derivatives in staged human embryos. *Acta Anat.* 1997;158:83–99.
9. O'Rahilly R, Müller F. A summary of the initial development of the human nervous system. *Teratology.* 1999;60:39–41.
10. Müller F, O'Rahilly R. Cerebral dysraphia (future anencephaly) in a human twin embryo at stage 13. *Teratology.* 1984;30:167–177.
11. Müller F, O'Rahilly R. The development of anencephaly and its variants. *Am J Anat.* 1991;190:193–218.
12. Müller F, O'Rahilly R. Mediobasal prosencephalic defects, including holoprosencephaly and cyclopia, in relation to the development of the human forebrain. *Am J Anat.* 1989;185:391–414.
13. O'Rahilly R, Müller F. Interpretation of some median anomalies as illustrated by cyclopia and symmelia. *Teratology.* 1989;40:409–421.
14. Hoving E W. *Frontoethmoidal Encephaloceles.* Groningen: Rijksuniversiteit; 1993.
15. Kier EL, Truwit CL. The normal and abnormal genu of the corpus callosum. *Am J Neuroradiol.* 1996;17:1631–1641.
16. O'Rahilly R, Müller F. Ventricular system and choroid plexuses of the human brain during the embryonic period proper. *Am J Anat.* 1990;189:285–302.
17. Hochstetter F. *Beiträge zur Entwicklungsgeschichte des menschlichen Gehirns.* I. Teil. Vienna: Deuticke; 1919.
18. Westergaard E. The lateral cerebral ventricles of human fetuses with a crown rump length of 26–178 mm. *Acta Anat.* 1971;79:409–421.
19. O'Rahilly R, Müller F. The meninges in human development. *J Neuropathol Exp Neurol.* 1986;45:588–608.
20. O'Rahilly R. Making planes plain. *Clin Anat.* 1996;10:128–129.

CHAPTER
TWO

Normal Two-Dimensional Neurosonography of the Prenatal Brain

Ilan E. Timor-Tritsch
Ana Monteagudo

Problems of the central nervous system (CNS) can range from very simple, i.e., merely a variance of the normal, to the most devastating diseases incompatible with life. It is important to recognize these anomalies as the fetus is scanned throughout gestation, starting very early in the first trimester to late in the third.

The prerequisite for differentiating normal from abnormal structures is a thorough knowledge of the CNS anatomy. It is beyond the scope of this and the following chapters to teach the reader advanced neuroanatomy; however, special emphasis is placed on describing basic but sufficiently detailed sonographic neuroanatomy to recognize structures seen by transabdominal (TAS) or transvaginal sonography (TVS). Those interested in scanning the fetal brain to detect deviations from the norm should first refresh their knowledge of neuroanatomy.

However, it is not sufficient to know only the anatomy of the full-term fetal or neonatal brain. Dealing with the sonographic anatomy and pathology of the fetal brain requires an additional dimension that is of the utmost importance for correctly evaluating the CNS at various prenatal ages of the fetus, i.e., knowledge of the evolution of structures from about 6 to 7 postmenstrual weeks to the time of birth. Almost all organs and organ systems are in place by the end of the embryonic period. However, only at approximately 14 to 16 postmenstrual weeks

would some of them—the heart and the kidneys, for example—perform almost at the level of perfection found in the final month.

All that most organs do during the fetal period is increase in size. The brain, on the other hand, undergoes major developmental changes almost until the last several postmenstrual weeks of intrauterine life. Good examples of this are the changes in the size of the ventricles; the appearance and completion of the development of the corpus callosum; and the deepening, branching, multiplying, and growth of the sulci and the gyri. It is therefore essential to understand the development of various parts of the prenatal brain in order to evaluate it and differentiate abnormal from normal development.

We deal with the prenatal brain throughout several chapters of this book. This chapter deals with normal anatomy as viewed by sonography, emphasizing the development of the fetal brain from 6 to 7 postmenstrual weeks to term. Of course, the CNS starts to develop at much earlier prenatal ages. However, at these very early prenatal ages, probably up to 7 postmenstrual weeks, the tiny structures still cannot be recognized by presently used ultrasonographic technologies. These methods were dealt with in Chapter 1, on the embryology and development of the early prenatal brain. This chapter, therefore, will begin with the description of the sonographic appearance of the CNS starting at 6 to 7 postmenstrual weeks.

The reader's expectation for this chapter should be limited to enhancing one's understanding of the normal prenatal brain anatomy before engaging in the diagnostic process and describing its pathology.

ULTRASOUND EQUIPMENT

The customary ultrasound equipment is used in imaging the prenatal brain. The two types of ultrasound probes employed are the transabdominal and transvaginal ultrasound transducer probes. Imaging the fetal brain depends on penetration of the sound waves as well as acoustic impedance of the tissues along the sound path. The acoustic impedances of most biologic tissues are similar. Therefore, only a small fraction of the sound is bounced back at each of these interfaces. The sound is thus successfully transmitted to deeper tissues, which can then be imaged. The soft tissue–bone interface is an exception to this rule. Bone has a much higher impedance; thus, at the interface, due to the reflected sound, a very strong echo is produced. The sound energy reflected back is significant, and only a fraction of the attenuated sound waves are transmitted penetrating to deeper structures. To illustrate the magnitude of this effect, the acoustic impedance of bone is about 7 times that of water or soft tissues in the fetal body. Imaging of structures behind bone therefore becomes problematic because an acoustic shadow is created. As the fetal skull bones thicken and calcify during the course of gestation, fewer and fewer sound waves penetrate to enable imaging of the brain.

Imaging is also frequency dependent. The higher the frequency is, the better the resolution of the picture. However, the "price we pay" for increased picture resolution is reduced penetration or the reduced "half-intensity depth." The latter describes the ability of sound to penetrate and is expressed as the thickness of the tissues at which the sound intensity is reduced by half. This half-intensity depth decreases with increased frequency, correlates well with the attainable imaging depth, and is greatly dependent on the medium in which it travels. Excellent through-transmission of sound in fluids such as blood or even in body tissue results from their weak sound-absorbing properties. However, bone and air strongly attenuate the intensity of sound. It is clear that the high acoustic impedance of the skull bone, as well as its property to attenuate the intensity of sound, greatly influences the way the brain can be imaged inside its bony case.

It was necessary to find imaginative ways to scan the fetal as well as the neonatal brain. By nature, transabdominal probes use lower frequencies to obtain deeper penetration and greater half-intensity depth. This is one way to penetrate beyond the bony skull. Another way is to scan through "windows" of the skull. These windows are, of course, the fontanelles. The younger the fetus is, the larger the fontanelles. Since these fontanelles measure about 1 to 2 cm in width, it is natural that sector or curvilinear scanners having a small footprint yield a better picture of the fetal and neonatal brain. These special transducers yield images that are of diagnostic value, even if they are acquired via the transabdominal route.

Another inventive way to scan the fetal brain is to use extremely high-frequency probes, such as 6.5 to 7.5 or even 9 MHz. Such probes are used in transvaginal gynecologic scanning. If the fetus is in the vertex presentation, it is relatively easy to maneuver the fetal head and the vaginal transducer into a position from which the device can "see" through a fontanelle. If this is successfully achieved, extremely clear pictures of the fetal brain from 13 postmenstrual weeks to term can be obtained.

Lately, we became aware of another possibility to obtain a limited access to the brain using the

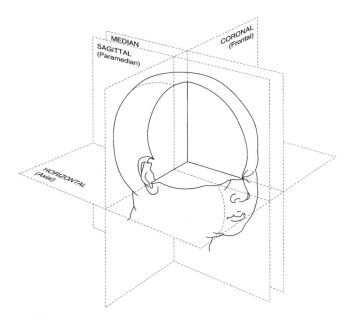

Figure 2–1. The "classical" planes used in the imaging of the fetal brain. The vertical planes are either coronal or sagittal. One of the latter is the median plane. There are infinite numbers of coronal and sagittal (paramedian) planes. As far as fetal neurosonography is concerned, the coronal and sagittal planes are reached through the anterior fontanelle in a fetus presenting with the vertex. Several sections through each plane can be generated. The horizontal (axial) planes are classically achieved by transabdominal or 3D scanning.

transvaginal probe: This rather narrow but still open "window" is the space between the two parietal bones; namely, the sagittal suture. By placing the footprint of the vaginal probe over the sagittal suture, a satisfactory picture of the mid-brain structures in the median plane can be obtained. Because of the narrow nature of this space, it is almost impossible to obtain an image of lateral structures.

Transabdominal scanning of the fetal brain can, in certain cases, yield clear and clinically diagnostic images. However, the younger the fetus is, or the smaller the structure in question is that must be scrutinized, the more the transabdominal probes will be at increasing handicap as opposed to the higher-resolution transvaginal probes. Under matched conditions the transvaginal probes, which operate at higher frequency, produce better and clinically more useful pictures.[1]

Lately electronically steered transducers can improve image quality obtained by the abdominal route. This modality employs compound scanning techniques.

SCANNING CONCEPT

Fetal brain scanning has emerged from the vast experience gained with neurosonographic imaging of the neonate. The fetal as well as the neonatal head is scanned using the three main body coordinates: the sagittal, coronal (frontal), and horizontal axial planes (Fig. 2–1). Initially, scanning of the neonatal brain was done through the temporal region, obtaining axial sections.[2–9] To achieve this imaging, lower-frequency transducers were used. Two factors contributed significantly to the improved resolution of one neonatal scan: the higher-frequency ultrasound

transducers (mainly the sector and the small-footprint curvilinear probes) and use of the anterior fontanelle as an acoustic window. The pictures obtained are in the median, paramedian, and different coronal, as well as oblique, sections.[10–19] It should be stated at the outset that TAS of the fetal brain usually provides axial and coronal sections. However, it is extremely difficult or almost impossible to obtain sagittal sections (Fig. 2–2). At times, though, sagittal sections are needed for the imaging of different pathognomonic features and diseases of the brain. Transvaginal scanning through the anterior fontanelle provides us with such median and paramedian as well as different coronal and oblique sections, much like neonatal scanning (Fig. 2–3).[20] An additional advantage of scanning the fetal brain using TVS is that the scanning planes obtained are *identical,* and therefore *comparable to those performed in the neonate.* Continuity of follow-up and comparison between fetal and neonatal scans are then possible by the pediatric neurologists and neurosurgeons. The input of these consultants is therefore relevant even in the prenatal period.

An issue of some importance is that fetal neuroimaging requires the use of an end-firing, symmetrical, in-axis (or in-line) vaginal probe. Using an end-firing, off-axis vaginal probe makes symmetrical imaging of the brain and maneuvering of the probe extremely cumbersome (Fig. 2–4). The orientation process is also affected, with regard to its speed, simplicity, and teaching. Most off-axis probes require constant use of the left–right orientation key on the control panel to correctly display orientation on the picture.

Recently, Blaas et al.[20a] have described the use of the 3D sonographic probe. The development of the

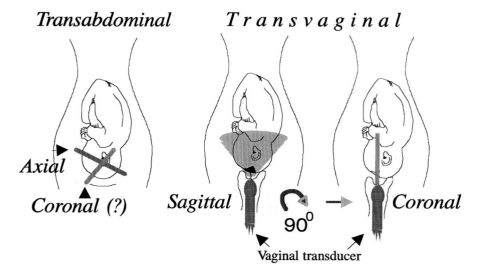

Figure 2–2. Schematic illustration of fetal neuroscanning routes. The transabdominal and the 3D routes classically provide axial or coronal, but rarely sagittal, views. The transvaginal approach rarely yields axial views. However, sagittal and coronal planes are typically obtained.

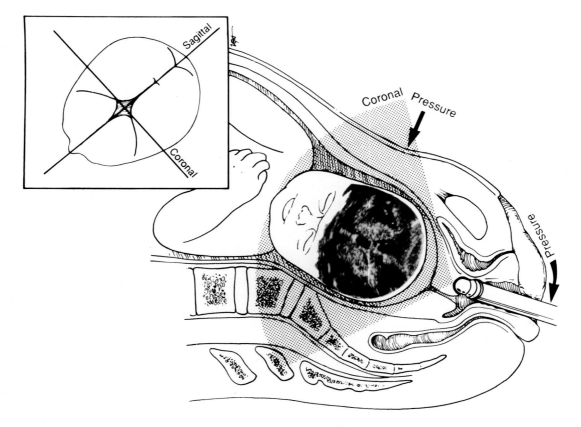

Figure 2–3. Schematic drawing depicting the technique of transvaginal sonography during the second and third trimesters. *Inset:* The relationship of the anterior fontanelle to the transvaginal transducer is demonstrated. *(From Monteagudo and colleagues, 1991,[20] with permission.)*

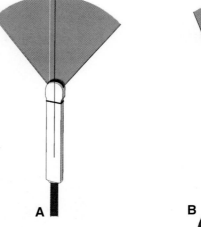

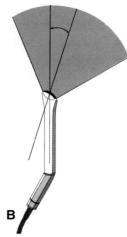

Figure 2–4. The different scanning planes of the transvaginal probes most often used. **A.** Transvaginal fetal neuroscans are imaged best with an end-firing, symmetrical, in-axis probe. **B.** The tilted, off-axis scanning plane generated by a curvilinear transvaginal probe. In order to scan both hemispheres at the same time, the shaft of the probe must be moved from side to side. This may be uncomfortable for the patient, or may simply be impossible. At times, the probe must be rotated 180° to direct the scanning plane to the other hemisphere.

three different structures in the brain were defined using this technique (Fig. 2–5). The information obtained by this "spatial scan" is stored in the computer and enables the user to obtain the different pictures, creating not only the classical coronal, sagittal, and axial planes but also selected planes to highlight anatomy and pathology. Until the 3D technology becomes universally available and widely used, we must mentally re-create the necessary planes and sections. Thus, knowledge of neuroanatomy remains an important issue. Chapter 9 discusses three-dimensional neurosonography.

Another technique that can be used to better describe the anatomy of the fetal brain are the color flow studies. If color flow studies are to be used, a textbook on neuroanatomy, namely, that on the arterial and venous network of the fetal brain, should initially be studied. Color flow studies may become important when anatomic structures such as space-occupying lesions, degenerative changes, or hemorrhages of the brain are examined. An additional area still under investigation is the physiology of the blood supply to the brain. This is covered in Chapter 14.

SCANNING TECHNIQUE

Because TAS is easy to perform and is used routinely by those who engage in ultrasonography of the fetus, it seems redundant to describe its technique. Transvaginal scanning of the fetal brain, however, requires more experience and is skill dependent; therefore, we describe it here in detail.

Obviously, due to its small size, the embryonic and early fetal CNS requires the use of a high-resolution transvaginal ultrasound probe.[21–29] The CNS structures seen in the first trimester are described later.

Scanning the fetal brain in the second and third trimesters via the vaginal route requires the same safety guidelines used for the customary speculum or palpatory examination during pregnancy. If these can be performed safely in the second trimester, there is no contraindication to insertion of the vaginal probe for scanning the fetal brain. Of course, as stated before, the fetus must be in the cephalic presentation. At times, when it is of the utmost importance to obtain accurate and more detailed information regarding a disease state, or if an additional sagittal view would significantly contribute to the diagnostic process, it may be important to consider external cephalic version of the fetus. When a second-trimester fetus is scanned, such a change in the fetal presenting part can be brought about without effort or can occur spontaneously.

Transvaginal neuroscanning can be used as early as 10 to 14 postmenstrual weeks. Its technique

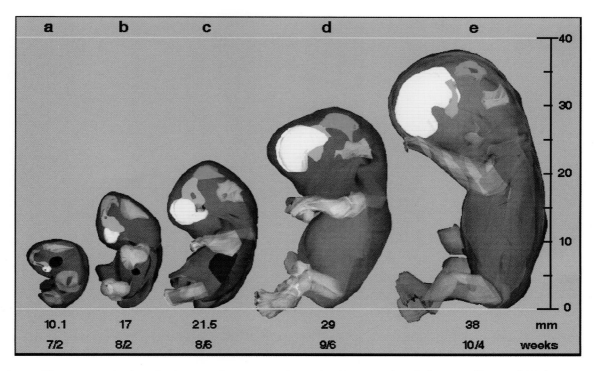

Figure 2–5. In vivo 3D ultrasound reconstructions of embryos and early fetuses. (From ref. 20a).

is relatively simple.[20, 23, 30, 31] The transvaginal probe is prepared in the customary fashion, covering it with a clean condom or one of the digits of a surgical rubber glove after contact gel has been applied to the tip of the probe and finally, applying some lubricating (K-Y) gel onto the covered tip, making it ready for vaginal insertion. Lately, due to increasing reports of latex allergies in the population, special prelubricated polyvinyl vaginal probe covers became available. The patient should be in the lithotomy position, preferably lying on a gynecologic examination table. Constantly following the image created by the advancing probe on the monitor, the first structure to be viewed (and evaluated as well as measured) is the cervix. The tip of the probe is typically placed on top of the anterior cervical lip. If the patient's bladder is full and displaces the fetal head upward, the patient should be asked to void before the examination proceeds.

To obtain a clear image of the fetal brain, it may be necessary to maneuver the probe and/or the fetal head into the most convenient position. This will be achieved if the axis of the probe and the median plane of the fetal brain (i.e., the falx cerebri) are in line (Fig. 2–3). Usually, the operator must use both hands to point the probe to the anterior fontanelle and hold the fetal head in the desired position. Unless skilled help is available to freeze the image and

trigger the recording device, a foot pedal is necessary to perform all of the necessary tasks at the same time. An active fetus may be extremely hard to stabilize by the abdominally placed second hand of the operator. To wait for the fetus to enter a quiet sleep state (state IF) (see Chapter 11) may be a time-consuming option. However, the scanning of an almost motionless fetus in deep sleep does have its dividends.

ORIENTATION AND SCANNING PLANES

In addition to the previously mentioned advantages and disadvantages of TAS and TVS of the fetal CNS, another caveat should be introduced. At times, it is hard or too time-consuming to obtain perfect planes and classical sections of the brain using TVS. This is, of course, a result of the somewhat limited mobility of the vaginal probe and/or the almost constantly moving fetus. Sometimes the fetal head position is such that it prevents the imaging of clear planes. Complementing the scan with an attempt at TAS, rescheduling the scan, or simply allowing the patient to walk for some time may improve the results.

Figure 2–1 depicts the three well-known classical planes of the body, in terms of its planes and sections. These are described below. Additional terms used in the orientation process are *rostral* or

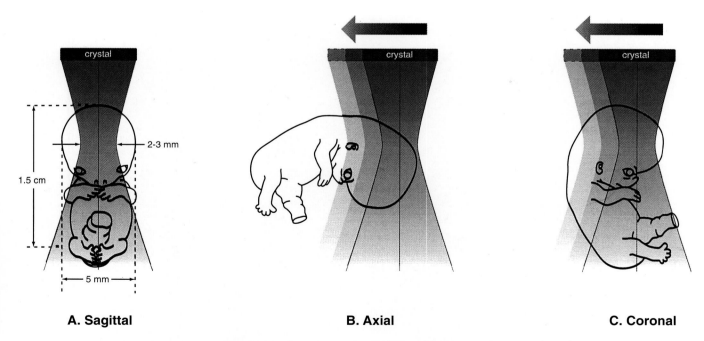

A. Sagittal **B. Axial** **C. Coronal**

Figure 2–6. The effect of slice thickness, or the third dimension of ultrasound imaging, is demonstrated. **A.** Due to the slice thickness, even at the focal point, a scan in the median plane may include the entire width of the embryonic head. **B, C.** In axial or coronal planes two or three sections may be possible. Starting with the fetal period, an increasing number of sections become feasible.

anterior (toward the face); *occipital, posterior,*or *nuchal* (toward the back); *left lateral* or *right temporal* (toward the respective ear); *caudal, basal,* or *inferior* (toward the base of the skull); and *medial* (toward the middle). It should be noted that the sagittal plane traversing the middle of the body is termed MEDIAN Plane (and not "mid sagittal"). (See Chapter 1)

Scanning Before Twelve Postmenstrual Weeks

Ultrasonographic images of the embryonic (up to 9 postmenstrual weeks) or fetal period is heavily dependent on several factors. The *resolution,* which, in turn, is a function of the *frequency* at which the crystals operate. The frequency and, in some ways, the *diameter* of the piezoelectric crystal determine the *"slice thickness."* The thicker the slice that is insonated and imaged, the more information is "collapsed" into the two-dimensional picture seen on the screen. This slice thickness may, in many cases, be several millimeters. In the case of a 7- or 8-postmenstrual week embryonic brain, the median imaging plane may include the entire "width" of the head due to the relatively thick imaging slice (Fig. 2–6A). This is true even for a 6.5-MHz transvaginal transducer. In the axial or coronal planes it may be possible to obtain several sections due to the somewhat larger size of the growing embryo (Figs. 2–6B and C).

Around 9 postmenstrual weeks the size of the embryonic head becomes large enough to yield several sections in each of the three cardinal planes. Due to the small head size, the sections can be obtained in almost a perfect parallel fashion. This becomes increasingly difficult later in pregnancy, as discussed in subsequent sections.

It should also be clear that the terms *axial (horizontal)* and *coronal (frontal) planes* refer to the trunk and become somewhat unclear if applied to the anteflexed embryonic head. Therefore, a coronal plane of the trunk would be axial of the flexed head. It is our understanding, therefore, that the term *axial* in an embryo of 8 to 10 postmenstrual weeks is a plane parallel with the base of the skull or the orbitomeatal plane (see Chapter 1). A coronal plane of the same fetus is one at 90° to the axial plane (Fig. 2–7).

If for any reason (e.g., research or clinical observation) it is necessary to image the brain in the first trimester, the observer should place the region of interest rigorously into the exact focal point of the transducer. Thus, it is essential to be knowledgeable about the respective transducer specifications in order to generate high-quality images.

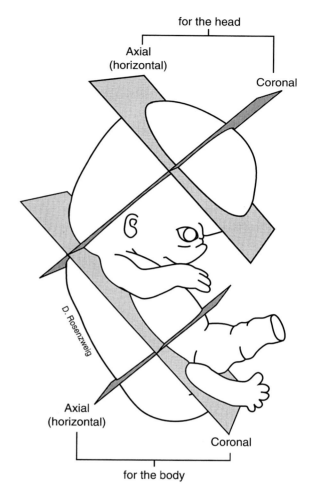

Figure 2–7. Due to the flexed posture of the embryonic or early fetal head, the plane that is coronal as far as the trunk is concerned becomes an axial plane when applied to the brain. In the same way, if an axial or transverse section of the trunk is applied to the head, it generates a coronal section of the brain.

Scanning After Twelve Postmenstrual Weeks

With its increasing size, the developing fetal brain becomes progressively "available" for high-frequency (6.5- to 9.0-MHz) TVS. The pictures obtained in the different scanning planes are of diagnostic quality. In other words, *major* diseases of the CNS can be diagnosed, starting at 12 to 13 postmenstrual weeks.

With regard to scanning the fetal brain after 12 weeks—but definitely after 14 to 15 postmenstrual weeks—it is at this point that the thickening skull bones attenuate the high-frequency sound waves of the vaginal probe to a very low level, making imaging from any randomly selected direction increasingly impossible. This is the time at which the window to the fetal brain, i.e., the fontanelle, becomes important. This relatively narrow gateway for the

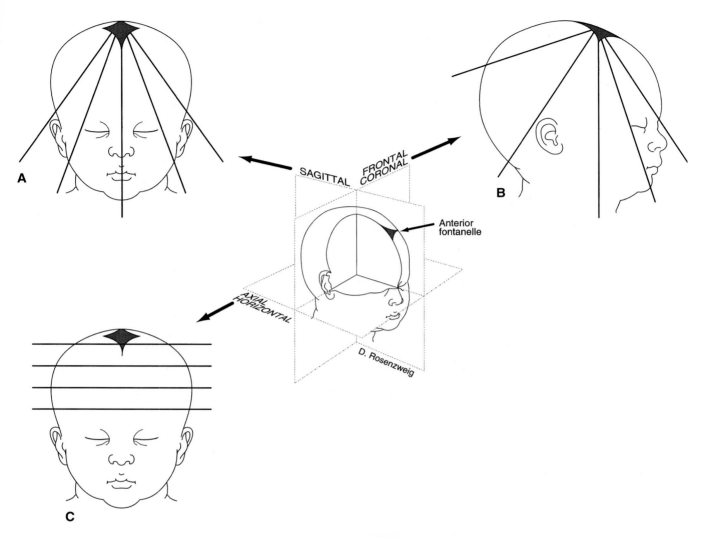

Figure 2–8. Scan through the anterior fontanelle. **A.** The limited motion of the probe within the vagina allows the median plane to be visualized, whereas on each side of it the planes are oblique and *not* parallel, and therefore cannot be regarded as strictly sagittal. **B.** Similarly, a coronal plane can be obtained, whereas those in front of and behind it are oblique planes, *not* subsequent coronal planes. **C.** The horizontal planes can be achieved using the transabdominal approach.

sound waves forces certain restrictions on the sonologist or sonographer. First, the tip of the transducer must be kept over the fontanelle or the sagittal suture, to achieve the full scanning potential of the sound output. Second, the different scanning sections in the sagittal, coronal, and oblique planes should be generated by tilting the transducer back and forth (Fig. 2–8). These successive sections, due to the reasons mentioned, are not parallel to each other in any given plane, as, for example, the shifting but always parallel planes of computed tomography or magnetic resonance imaging.

This transfontanelle scanning by TVS, common to prenatal and neonatal brain scanning, is really performed in a "radial" fashion. Some of the sagittal

as well as coronal sections are therefore oblique-sagittal and oblique-coronal sections. In the "sagittal" plane, then, left and right oblique sections, and in the "coronal" plane occipital and frontal oblique sections, are generated (Fig. 2–8).

It is important to understand that in order to scan the fetus presenting with the vertex, the free motion of the vaginal probe is restricted by the anatomic limits of the vagina. Only very few "classical" and "pure" planes can therefore be achieved: the *median* and one *coronal* plane. In the sagittal planes (to use the best approximation), because of the fan-shaped, radial scanning sections, several *left* and *right oblique* planes can be generated on each side of the median plane (Fig. 2–8). In the coronal plane (once again, to use the best approximation) in front of or behind the coronal plane several *frontal* and *occipital oblique* sections can be generated (Fig. 2–8).

If several sections are created, the three-dimensional anatomy should be re-created mentally by the observer, using these consecutive sections. As mentioned before, this "mental processing" will be less and less necessary by the introduction of three-dimensional multiplanar imaging. 3D imaging of the fetal brain will also eliminate the "radiating" planes since all planes will be parallel with each other. (See Chapter 9)

If the second- or third-trimester fetus assumes a rather asynclitic head position, it is sometimes possible to obtain axial planes. The same is true if the head assumes a flexed occipito-anterior position. A detailed study of the posterior fossa should be performed as soon as this presentation is detected. After some time, due to fetal movement, this presenting anatomy may shift away, not to return for the duration of the examination.

As the examination proceeds, we have observed certain conventions in orientation. This serves to introduce a systematic way of displaying the images.

In the sagittal planes the fetal face or the frontal direction should be almost uniformly oriented to the left of the picture. This will orient the posterior fossa and the occipital structures toward the right side of the screen. Likewise, if the lateral ventricles are imaged using these planes, the anterior horn should point toward the left and the posterior horn toward the right side of the monitor.

In the coronal planes the pictures should be taken in such a manner that the fetus should "face, or look right at, the examiner." This means that by convention—as is customary in imaging laboratories—the right side of the brain will appear on the left side of the screen, whereas the left side of the prenatal brain will point toward the right of the picture. If no annotation is to be seen on a hard copy, it is assumed that the above-described orientations of the prenatal brain sections in the coronal planes were observed. It seems best, however, to indicate the orientation of the left or right side on at least one of the images. *This annotation of the left or right side becomes crucial if an asymmetrical or unilateral lesion is detected.*

BRAIN DEVELOPMENT AND SONOANATOMY FROM SIX POSTMENSTRUAL WEEKS TO TERM

This section deals with the sonoembryology and sonoanatomy of the prenatal brain as it appears and as a continuous function of structural development.

It should be clear that parts of the prenatal brain exist and are in different developmental stages even *before* they can be imaged by ultrasonography. This is particularly true for brain structures revealed by a scan performed during the first 12 to 14 postmenstrual weeks of pregnancy. The structure may well be in place, but due to its size and location, the angle of insonation may not be obvious to the observer. Other structures develop later as a normal process, and because of this they are not seen on early scans.

We present here the normal embryonic and fetal neurosonology in two sections. The first subsection deals with the period up to 9 postmenstrual weeks. The second section comprises the weeks following the ninth postmenstrual week. This is an entirely arbitrary partition. Starting from the 13th postmenstrual week, some of the structures imaged by high-frequency transvaginal transducers are of clinically usable quality. This is also the time after which multiple and clearly discernible brain sections can be obtained using the standard planes.[22]

Scanning the Embryonic Central Nervous System (Six to Nine Postmenstrual Weeks)

To better understand the development of the embryonic brain, the reader is referred to Chapter 1. After reading that chapter a clearer perception of the sonographically visualized structures will be possible.

As concerns the age of the embryos and fetuses, the arguments and debates are well known and well documented. Chapter 1 provides the tools to understand the different views. Table 2–1 contains the embryonic and fetal age conversions, which will allow quick reference for those who would like to rely on the date of the last menstrual period (LMP) to calculate age as well as for those who are used to expressing age in weeks or days from fertilization (if such a date is known).[32] O'Rahilly and Müller[33] indicated that points C and R of the crown–rump length (CRL) (Fig. 2–9) are imprecise and frequently are difficult to determine. They emphasized that the best single measurement is the greatest length (GL), exclusive of the lower limbs, and its determination is practicable in both the embryonic and fetal periods. [Subsequently, Goldstein[34] expressed concern about measuring the longest diameter of the developing embryo sonographically, calling it the crown–rump length.] This measurement, according to the study, does not follow the curvature of the curled-up embryonic body. Therefore, it actually measures the longest diameter (i.e., the GL of O'Rahilly and Müller[33])—or the size of the embryo. Goldstein[34] proposed the term *early embryonic size* (EES) for the sonographic measurement. Table 2–1

TABLE 2–1. CONVERSION TABLE FOR EMBRYONIC AND FETAL AGE AND SIZE

Postmenstrual Week	Time From LMP (Weeks and Days)	Time From Fertilization (Weeks and Days)	Days From Fertilization	Crown–Rump Length (cm)[a]	EES (mm)
7th	6 + 0 to 6 + 6	4 + 0 to 4 + 6	~28–34	0.42–0.81	1–6
8th	7 + 0 to 7 + 6	5 + 0 to 5 + 6	~35–41	0.89–1.38	7–13
9th	8 + 0 to 8 + 6	6 + 0 to 6 + 6	~42–48	1.47–2.08	14–20
10th	9 + 0 to 9 + 6	7 + 0 to 7 + 6	~49–55	2.19–2.92	[b]
11th	10 + 0 to 10 + 6	8 + 0 to 8 + 6	~56–62	3.05–3.89	[b]
12th	11 + 0 to 11 + 6	9 + 0 to 9 + 6	~63–69	4.04–5.00	[b]
13th	12 + 0 to 12 + 6	10 + 0 to 10 + 6	~70–76	5.17–6.25	[b]
14th	13 + 0 to 13 + 6	11 + 0 to 11 + 6	~77–83	6.43–7.63	[b]

LMP, Last menstrual period; EES, early embryonic size.[34]
[a]After Robinson, 1973.[32]
[b]EES measurements of embryonic length are used up to 25 mm or 68 ± 3 base from LMP.

also contains the EES measurements and their conversions to embryonic age.

Returning to the work of O'Rahilly and Müller,[33] it is clear that the C point (the crown), which, in stages 13 to 20 (6 to 9½ weeks from the LMP), is at the point where an imaginary line drawn along the mesencephalic flexure would touch the surface of the embryo, just above the middle of the midbrain (see Fig. 2–9), is hard to find sonographically. Even if it can be determined, the CRL would yield a smaller length than the GL or the EES of Goldstein.[34] Figure 2–9 depicts how the "C point" changes location throughout development from stage 13 to stage 20. Only at stage 23 (9 to 9½ postmenstrual weeks) do the CRL and GL (or EES) become identical as clinically used measurements.

Using the presently available ultrasound machines, the earliest scan to depict any brain structure can be performed at 7 postmenstrual weeks (5 weeks, or 35 days, from fertilization). At this age one or several sonolucent areas can be detected in the rostral end (cephalic pole) of the embryo. The detail of the image depends on the resolution of the equipment used.

If attempts are made to image details of the CNS before this embryonic age, a clear fetal pole, at times adjacent to the yolk sac, can be seen (Figs. 2–10 through 2–12A).[35] However, sagittal as well as coronal sections do not yield distinct structures. At times, a tiny sonolucency is seen in the rostral part of the embryo. The nature of this structure is unknown. The parallel lines of the somites (from which the vertebrae are derived) are discernible at or slightly before 7 postmenstrual weeks (Figs. 2–11 and 2–12B).

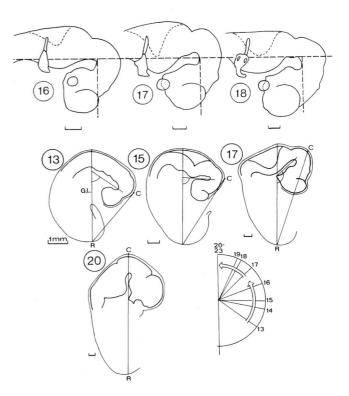

Figure 2–9. The outlines of four embryos (right lateral views) with the brain superimposed. The embryos are shown at stages 13, 15, 17, and 20, respectively, and are 4½, 5, 6, and 7 weeks in age, or at 6½, 7, 8, and 9 postmenstrual weeks. In the first three examples the greatest length (GL) is larger than the crown–rump (C–R) length, whereas the two measurements coincide in the fourth. The last drawing (stages 13 to 23) is a scheme to summarize the "ascent" of point C until the C–R length comes to equal the GL. *(From O'Rahilly and Müller, 1984,[33] with permission.)*

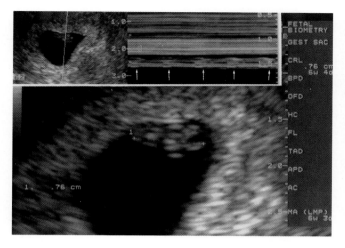

Figure 2–10. Transvaginal ultrasonographic image at 6 weeks 3 days from the last menstrual period LMP (crown–rump length, 7.6 mm). No brain structure could be detected. The heart beats are marked on the M-mode trace.

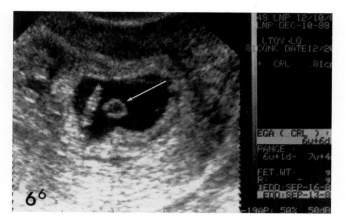

Figure 2–11. Coronal section of the embryo 6 weeks 6 days after the last menstrual period, measuring 8.1 mm. Note the arrangement of the somites in pairs, representing the future vertebral column. The yolk sac is marked with an *arrow. (From Timor-Tritsch and colleagues, 1991,[35] with permission.)*

Blaas and colleagues[28, 29] studied the brain structures, starting with an embryo with a CRL of 12 mm (7 weeks 3 days from the LMP). They described the possibility of imaging the cerebral hemispheres (telencephalic vesicles), rhombencephalon, and diencephalon (Fig. 2–13). In embryos with a CRL of 16 mm (8 weeks from the LMP), these structures become better defined. Thus, the interventricular foramina (Monro) can be seen (Fig. 2–14).

Our group has scanned well-dated embryos from *7 to 10 weeks* from the LMP and evaluated the structures imaged. A 6.5-MHz mechanical transvaginal transducer was used. At 7 weeks 3 days (from the LMP) in the sagittal and axial/coronal planes, we could see the mesencephalon and the rhombencephalon (Figs. 2–15A and B). Figure 1–4 in Chapter 1 represents a sagittal section of the embryonic brain at a comparable age.

At *8 weeks 1 day* and *8 weeks 3 days* from the LMP (Figs. 2–16 and 2–17), the structures appear clearer and flexures of the brain, such as the mesencephalic and pontine flexures, were located. The coronal sections revealed the rhombencephalon with regard to the major divisions. Figure 1–4 in Chapter 1 depicts a median section of the brain at 8 weeks 3 days after the LMP. The subdivisions of the brain (Fig. 2–18) could not yet be sufficiently discerned by TVS.[36] Because of the small size of the embryonic head (about $1 \times 1 \times 1.5$ cm), only one or, at most, two sections could be obtained in each plane.

At *8 weeks 5 days* from the LMP (Fig. 2–19), the embryo starts to "unfold."[22] The mesencephalic flexure is almost in axis with the longitudinal body axis.

The cavities of the ventricular system are clearly identifiable. Subdivisions such as the telencephalon, diencephalon, metencephalon, and myelencephalon are seen sonographically not only on sagittal but also on coronal sections.

Observations by Blaas and associates[28, 29] are consistent with those described above. Figures 2–20 and 2–21 show an almost paramedian sagittal section and a coronal section of embryos with a 17- and 18-mm CRL (about 8½ weeks from the LMP). In addition to the already described structures, the choroid fold and—slightly later, at 8 weeks 5 days from the LMP—the first sighting of the choroid plexus were reported (Fig. 2–22). On the same picture, these investigators suggested that cerebellar thickening was also seen. Only days later, at 9 weeks 3 days from the LMP (with a CRL of 25 mm), a better image of the choroid plexus and the cerebellum was seen (Fig. 2–23).

From about 9 weeks from the LMP, there is a significant change in the TVS evaluation of the fetus as a whole, and particularly of the CNS. Due to their gradual development and increase in size, more structures are better seen. The development of the tortuous, fluid-filled ventricular system is readily imaged in the median plane (Fig. 2–24). The subdivisions as well as the serially connected cavities appear on both the sagittal and coronal planes. Suddenly, it seems that many more sections can be generated in almost each of the three cardinal planes (Fig. 2–24A).[22]

The different parts of the ventricular system are visible at this time. A study of the median sec-

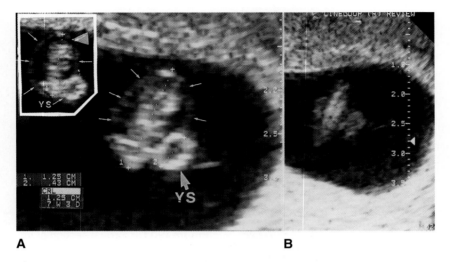

Figure 2–12. Embryo at 7 weeks 3 days from the last menstrual period (crown–rump length, 12.5 mm). **A.** Coronal section. The cephalic pole points upward on the picture and shows a sonolucent structure. The yolk sac (YS) is situated outside the amnion *(small arrows)*. *Inset:* Sagittal section showing the cephalic sonolucent structure *(arrowhead)*. **B.** The two distinct lines of the vertebral column on a posterior coronal section are evident.

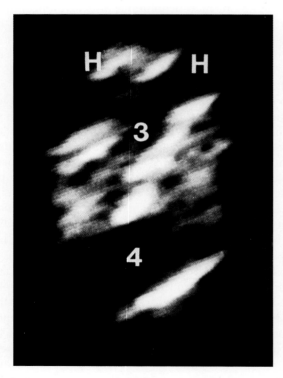

Figure 2–13. Transverse/oblique section through the rhombencephalon (4), diencephalon (3), and cerebral hemispheres (H) of an embryo (crown–rump length of 12 mm at 7 postmenstrual weeks 3 days). The bilateral evaginations of the hemispheres are clearly seen. There is still a wide opening to the third ventricle. *(From Blaas and colleagues, 1994,[28] with permission.)*

tion of the embryo at 9 weeks and 5 days from the LMP is depicted in Figure 2–24B. The sonolucent chain of the ventricular system winds itself around the two most prominent solid structures: the echogenic pontine flexure and the mesencephalic flexure. This age marks the stage (Carnegie stage 23) at which the latter points at the "crown" of the head and the true CRL can be measured reliably.[33,34] The first rostral sonolucent structure on this image is the diencephalon. Following the diencephalon, in the caudal direction, are the mesencephalon, the metencephalon, the myelencephalon, and finally, the part of the medulla that contains the central canal. On a paramedian section the relatively large choroid plexus in the lateral ventricle is depicted (Fig. 2–25B). At this age the choroid plexus fills the entire lateral (telencephalic) ventricle. On coronal as well as axial sections, the falx is seen as an echogenic structure. If the choroid plexus and the falx are imaged by TVS, the age of the embryo must be at least 9 postmenstrual weeks. A reasonably high-quality and high-frequency vaginal probe is necessary to detect the falx, the different ventricles, and the choroid plexus at or around 9 to 9½ postmenstrual weeks.

The Developing and Maturing Fetal Brain

The development of the embryonic brain was previously described. As detailed in Chapter 1, the embryonic period lasts up to 8 weeks from fertilization,

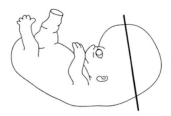

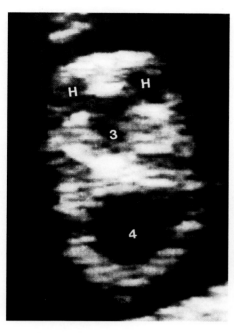

Figure 2–14. Transverse/oblique section through the rhombencephalon (4), diencephalon (3), and cerebral hemispheres (H) of an embryo (crown–rump length of 16 mm at 8 postmenstrual weeks 0 days). The borders between the cerebral hemisphere and the third ventricle (3) remain relatively small and start to develop into the interventricular foramina. *(From Blaas and colleagues, 1994,[28] with permission.)*

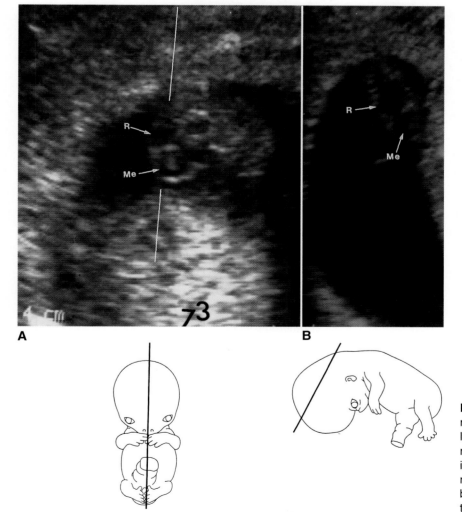

A   **B**

Figure 2–15. A. Median section at 7 postmenstrual weeks 3 days (crown–rump length, 13 mm). R, Rhombencephalon; Me, mesencephalon. **B.** Coronal section showing the tapered, sonolucent shape of the mesencephalon. This image was generated by scanning along the plane, marked with the *white line* in **A.**

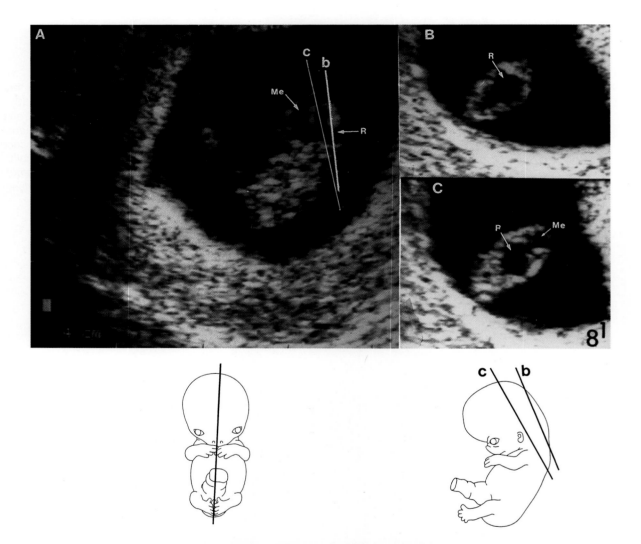

Figure 2–16. At 8 weeks 1 day from the last menstrual period (crown–rump length, 16 mm), the ventricular system becomes evident with the use of a 6.5-MHz probe. **A.** Median section showing the following structures: mesencephalon (Me) and rhombencephalon. The *white lines* marked *b* and *c* show the coronal sections used to obtain images **B** and **C** at the level of the rhombencephalon (R) and a small portion of the mesencephalon (Me), respectively.

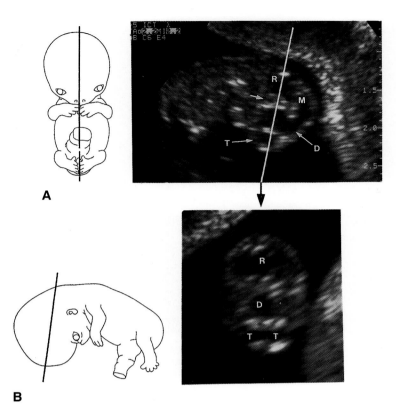

A

B

Figure 2–17. At 8 weeks 2 days from the last menstrual period (CRL, 17 mm), an image similar to that in Figure 2–15 can be obtained. However, this time the plane represented by the *white line,* placed in an almost axial fashion, shows a slightly different picture than that in Figure 2–8B. R, rhombencephalon; Me, mesencephalon; D, diencephalon; T, telencephalon. The *arrow* points to the cephalic flexure.

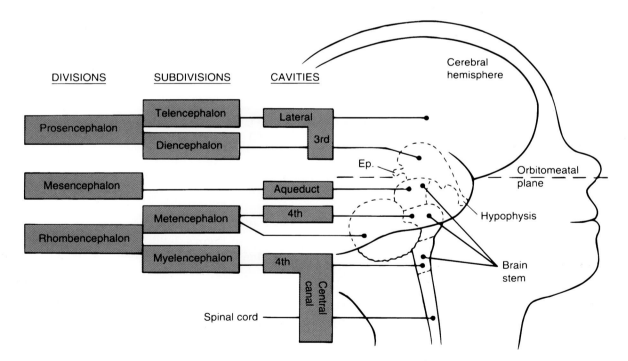

Figure 2–18. The divisions, subdivisions, and cavities seen in an infant's brain. The metencephalon consists of the cerebellum and the pons. The myelencephalon is the medulla oblongata. The brain stem comprises the midbrain, pons, and medulla. The third ventricle is mainly diencephalic, but is partly telencephalic. The central canal is mainly in the spinal cord, but is partly in the medulla. All of these parts are present by 5 postfertilizational (7 postmenstrual) weeks. The subdivisions and the cavities can be detected by high-frequency transvaginal sonography, but only from about 8 to 8½ postmenstrual weeks. *(From O'Rahilly and Müller, 1992,[36] with permission.)*

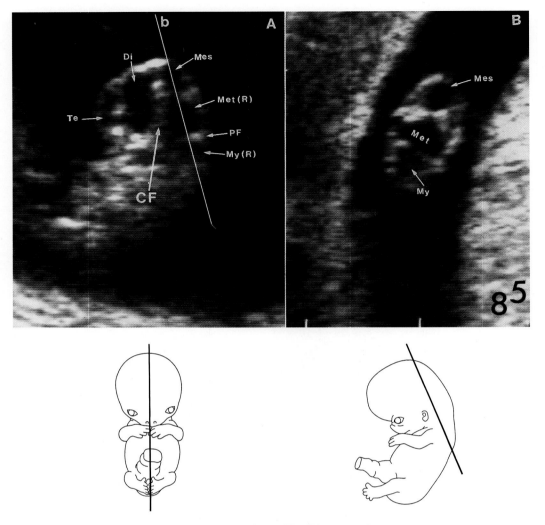

Figure 2–19. Median and coronal (posterior oblique) sections of an embryo at 8 postmenstrual weeks and 5 days (crown–rump length, 20 mm). **A.** Median section showing the following structures: telencephalon (Te), diencephalon (Di), and mesencephalon (Mes). The metencephalon (Met) and myelencephalon (My) are parts of the rhombencephalon (R). The two main flexures, pontine (PF) and mesencephalic (CF), are also seen. **B.** Coronal oblique section through line *b*. *(Modified from Timor-Tritsch and colleagues, 1991,[22] with permission.)*

or roughly 10 postmenstrual weeks. Following this, the fetal period starts, which lasts until delivery takes place. From a sonographic standpoint there is definitely no visible quantitative reason for this qualitative change. There is a constantly increasing number of detectable structures from 8 postmenstrual weeks on, without any significant increase at or around the cutoff age at which the name changes from *embryo* to *fetus*.

From 10 postmenstrual weeks on, three axial, three sagittal, and three or four coronal sections in each of these cardinal planes of the fetal head can be obtained.[30]

A three-dimensional model created by computer and based on serial two-dimensional slice scans of fetuses at 8 to 10 postmenstrual weeks is depicted in Figure 2–26. The Norwegian group from Trondheim produced such computer-generated "casts" of the well-delineated ventricular system, which enabled a close study of this system as it changed shape between 8 and 12 postmenstrual weeks.[37] Until an ultrasound system becomes widely available to re-create the different brain structures in a three-dimensional fashion, we will have to rely on our own mental re-creation of fetal structures in general, and the brain in particular. To perform such a complex task in our own brain, serial sections of the structure in question must be generated and examined during every scanning session. A similar series of horizontal (axial) slices

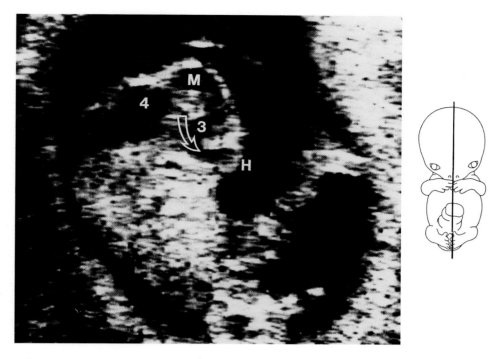

Figure 2–20. Paramedian sagittal section at 8½ postmenstrual weeks (crown–rump length, 17 mm). This section includes the hemisphere (H), rhombencephalon (4), mesencephalon (M), and diencephalon (3). The circlelike hemisphere (H) should not be misinterpreted as the orbit. The *open arrow* indicates the connection between the lateral and third ventricles. *(From Blaas and colleagues, 1994,[28] with permission.)*

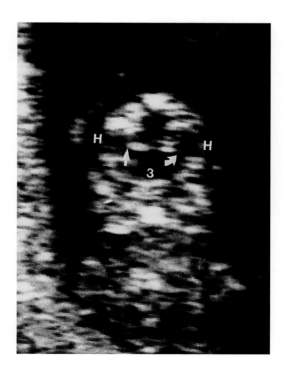

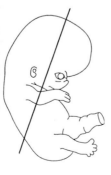

Figure 2–21. Coronal section showing the cerebral hemisphere (H) and the third ventricle (3) (crown–rump length of 18 mm at approximately 8½ postmenstrual weeks). The *curved arrow* points to the interventricular foramina; the *straight arrow* indicates the choroid folds, which are the first sign of the developing choroid plexus. *(From Blaas and colleagues, 1994,[28] with permission.)*

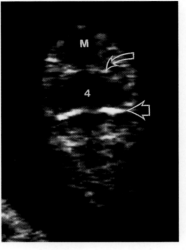
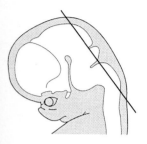

Figure 2–22. Coronal section at 8 postmenstrual weeks and 5 days (crown–rump length, 20 mm), showing the rhombencephalon. The structures seen are the mesencephalon (M), the cerebellar thickening *(open curved arrow),* the fourth ventricle (4), and the choroid plexus *(open straight arrow). (Courtesy of Blaas, Department of Obstetrics and Gynecology, National Center for Fetal Medicine, Trondheim University Hospital, Trondheim, Norway.)*

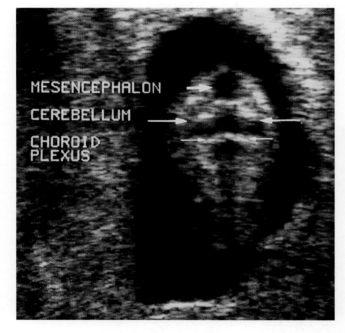
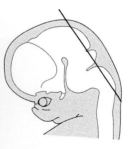

Figure 2–23. Coronal section at 9 postmenstrual weeks and 3 days, showing the rhombencephalon (crown–rump length, 25 mm). The mesencephalon, cerebellum, and choroid plexus are marked. *(Courtesy of Blaas, Department of Obstetrics and Gynecology, National Center for Fetal Medicine, Trondheim University Hospital, Trondheim, Norway.)*

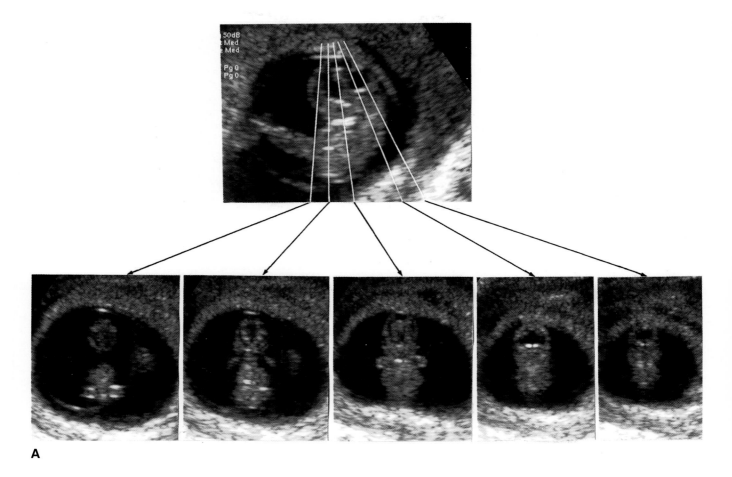

A

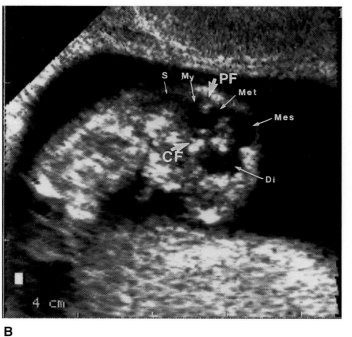

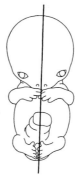

B

Figure 2–24 A. At 9 postmenstrual weeks and 1 day it is possible to acquire multiple sections in the clanical planes. This picture illustrates 5 coronal sections obtained using a high frequency transvaginal probe at this age. **B.** Median section 9 postmenstrual weeks and 5 days (crown–rump length, 28 mm). The sonolucent and progressively tortuous ventricular system is imaged. Di, diencephalon; Mes, mesencephalon; Met, metencephalon; My, myelencephalon; S, the entrance to the central canal; CF, mesencephalic flexure; PF, pontine flexure. *(Modified from Timor-Tritsch and colleagues, 1991,[22] with permission.)*

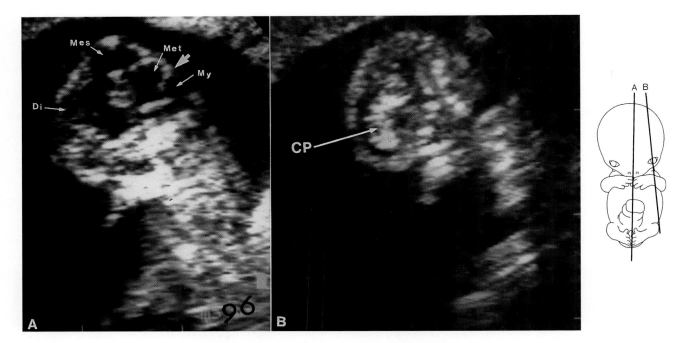

Figure 2–25. Median and paramedian sections at 9 postmenstrual weeks 6 days (crown–rump length, 32 mm). **A.** Median section. The structures seen are the diencephalon (Di), mesencephalon (Mes), metencephalon (Met), pontine flexure *(large white arrow),* and myelencephalon (My). **B.** Paramedian section. For the first time, a well-developed cerebral hemisphere containing the choroid plexus (CP) is depicted. *(From Timor-Tritsch and colleagues, 1991,[22] with permission.)*

is depicted in Figure 2–27. From these images it is obvious that the choroid plexus of the 11- to 11½-postmenstrual week fetus almost fills the available space within the lateral ventricle. If the gain control is increased, the high brightness of the choroid enables the detection of cysts as small as 2 to 3 mm, should they exist. The falx is sufficiently echoreflective, and therefore easily seen. In addition, the third ventricle, the tentorium, the posterior fossa, and the cerebellum and its peduncles leading to the midbrain can be imaged (Figs. 2–27 and 2–28). On a very low axial section the foramen magnum can also be seen (Fig. 2–27).

It seems that the presence of the third ventricle can clearly be seen on axial scans at 11, 12, and even 13 postmenstrual weeks (Figs. 2–27 through 2–29). However, on serial scans at 14 and 16 postmenstrual weeks (Figs. 2–30 through 2–34), the space is progressively taken up by the expanding thalamus.

A significant change first noted at 11 to 12 postmenstrual weeks is the relative increase of the anterior tip of the anterior horns of the lateral ventricles. Note the sonolucent area marked *AH* in Figure 2–28 in a fetus at almost 12 postmenstrual weeks. This is

the anterior horn of the lateral ventricle and it is difficult to overlook. For the next 2 to 3 weeks it will remain relatively large (Figs. 2–29, 2–30, 2–35, and 2–36). Two simultaneous processes occur from 11 to 16 to 18 postmenstrual weeks: the choroid plexuses of the lateral ventricles "moves back" on top of the thalamus into its final place—the body and the atrium of the lateral ventricle—and progressive growth of the cerebral cortex slowly decreases the size of the horn. Indeed, toward term the anterior horns become slitlike.

At around 14 to 16 postmenstrual weeks the slowly but constantly growing and thickening skull bones present an increasing obstacle for the high-frequency sound waves that, until this age, have created images of the fetal CNS in a rather unrestricted fashion. The solution to this problem is to use the anterior fontanelle (Fig. 2–37) as an acoustic window to continue scanning of the fetal brain. As mentioned previously, scans obtained via the anterior fontanelle do not provide *parallel* sections in the coronal or sagittal plane. These sections are generated radiating in an oblique fashion with their apex at the fontanelle, as shown in Figure 2–8 as well as in other figures in this chapter.

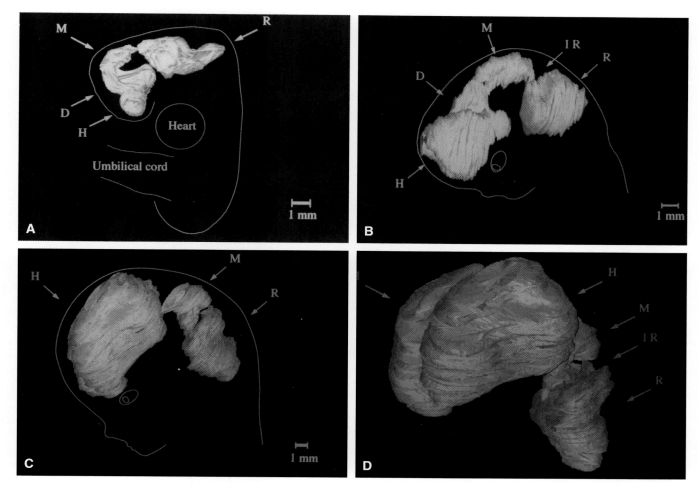

Figure 2–26. Three-dimensional representation of the embryonic and fetal ventricular system. **A.** Lateral view of the brain cavities in an embryo of 13-mm crown–rump length (CRL). The outline shows the embryonic shape, with the head and the umbilical cord. **B.** Lateral view of the brain cavities in an embryo of 24-mm CRL. The outline shows the embryonic head and eye. **C.** Lateral view of the brain cavities in a fetus of 40-mm CRL. The outline shows the fetal head and eye. **D.** Oblique view of the brain cavities in a fetus of 40-mm CRL. H, Cerebral hemisphere; D, diencephalon; M, mesencephalon; R, rhombencephalon; IR, isthmus rhombencephali. *(From Blaas and colleagues, 1995,[38] with permission.)*

Coronal Planes

Using the anterior fontanelle as a sonic window, a few perfect midcoronal and a series of oblique coronal sections, from anterior to posterior, can be obtained.

For easier understanding, but even more so for clearer clinical use, three main groups of sections through the above-mentioned planes are described. The three main groups are the frontal, midcoronal, and occipital sections (Table 2–2).[38, 39] Each of these may have two or three possible subsections. Their importance is discussed later.

Sonographic Anatomic Landmarks

Because of extensive changes in the size and location of several anatomic landmarks that are well seen sonographically, it is practical to clearly separate two age groups. One is the age group from 12 to 18 postmenstrual weeks; the second is above at least 18 but clearly above 20 weeks. The groups require partitioning because before 18 postmenstrual weeks the frontal horn extends frontally and is evident on any of the anterior (frontal) coronal sections.

The sonographically identifiable anatomic landmarks in the coronal sections group are listed in

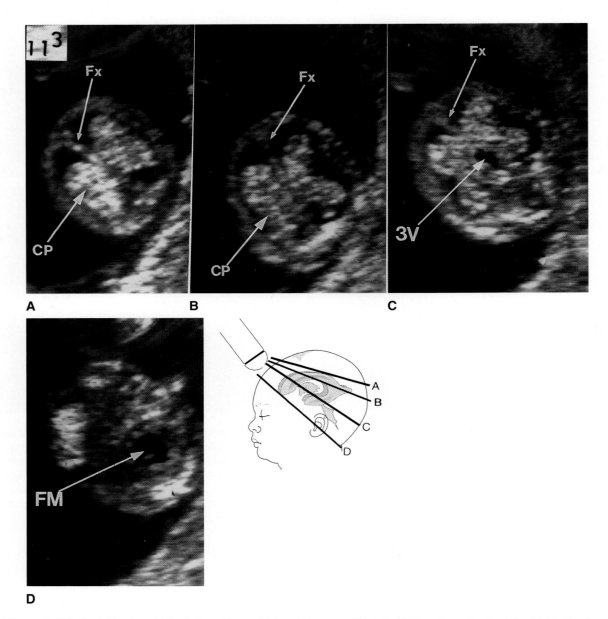

Figure 2–27. Serial horizontal (axial) sections at 11 postmenstrual weeks 3 days, from the top *(far left)* to the base of the skull *(far right).* The third ventricle (3V) and the foramen magnum (FM) are seen. CP, Choroid plexus; Fx, falx. *(Modified from Timor-Tritsch and colleagues, 1991,[37] with permission.)*

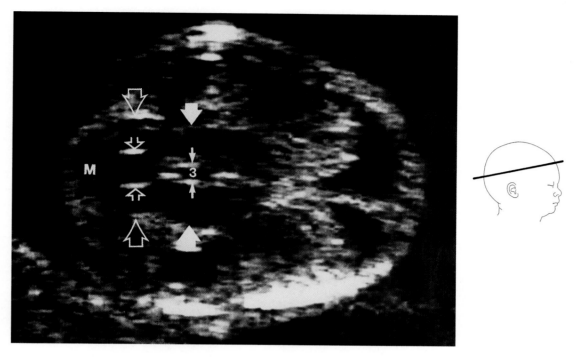

Figure 2–28. Horizontal (axial) section through the head of a fetus at 11 postmenstrual weeks and 6 days (crown–rump length, 49 mm). The view is of the diencephalon *(bold arrows)* and its narrow third ventricle (3), and through the mesencephalon *(large open arrows; M),* with its wide cavity *(small open arrows).* AH, anterior horns. *(From Blaas and colleagues, 1994,[28] with permission.)*

Table 2–2. These landmarks are listed as subdivisions of the following structures: skull, brain ventricles, cavities, choroid plexus, midbrain, cerebellum, and meninges. Their presence on all of these sections is indicated.[38]

There are several cardinal landmarks, i.e., those that, if present on a specific plane, are clear markers of the plane in question. Such anatomic markers are the *orbits,* the *passage of the choroid plexus into the third ventricle through the interventricular foramina (Monro),* and the *posterior horns.* The presence of these structures indicates unequivocally that the section was taken at the Frontal–2, Midcoronal–2, and Occipital–1 sections, respectively. These cardinal landmarks are highlighted in Table 2–2 for easier understanding.

There is also a typical and unique clustering of several structures throughout each of the sections. Such a clustering indicates that the section was obtained at a specific and well-defined section. For example, if on a coronal section the orbits and the anterior horns are seen (without the choroid plexus), this can exclusively apply to the Frontal–2 section. On the other hand, if one seeks out the Midcoronal–2 section, one would search for an image con-

taining the cross section of the corpus collusum, the choroid plexus containing lateral ventricles, the cavum septi pellucidi, the thalami, as well as the falx, all seen at the same time. Only this one specific section is consistent with the Midcoronal–2 section. This concept holds true for all the specific and unique sections obtained in the two general planes.[38]

Based on these easily recognized sonographic landmarks and the typical picture generated, we refer to the Frontal–2 section as "the steer's head configuration" (Figs. 2–29; 2–30B; 2–37A, B, and C; and 2–38B). The Occipital–1 section resembles the "owl's eye configuration" (Figs. 2–31E, 2–33B, 2–38A, 2–39B, 2–40B, and 2–40D).

Structures Seen on Coronal Sections
1. FRONTAL SECTIONS: At 12 to 18 postmenstrual weeks both Frontal–1 and –2 images contain the widely open anterior horns of the lateral ventricles. The Frontal–2 section contains the orbits (steer's head configuration). Later during gestation, the Frontal–1 (more anterior frontal) section "cuts" through the white matter only. The longitudinal fissure and the subarachnoid space containing the superior sagittal sinus are present (Fig. 2–38A–C).

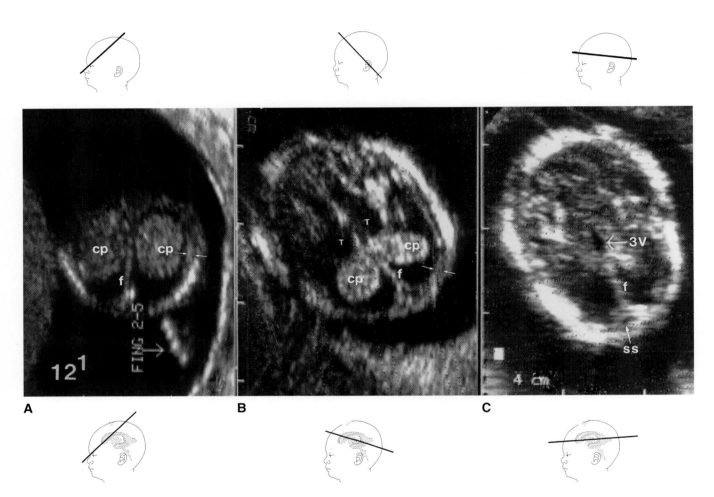

A   **B**   **C**

Figure 2–29. At 12 postmenstrual weeks 1 day, a frontal oblique section **(A)** shows the falx and the choroid plexus. Axial sections **(B, C)** reveal the hyperechoic choroid plexus (cp) on top of the thalamus (T) in the lateral ventricles. Only a thin cerebral cortex mantle is still seen between the *small arrows*. The third ventricle (3v), the falx (f), and the frontal part of the sagittal sinus (SS) are also seen. *(Modified from Timor-Tritsch and colleagues, 1991,[22] with permission.)*

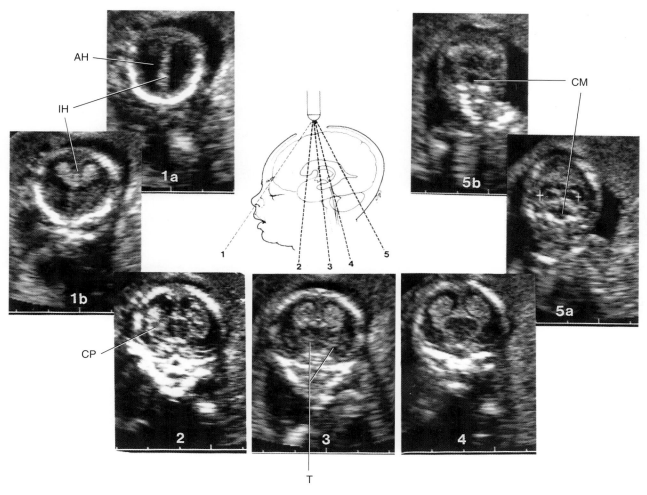

Figure 2–30. Serial brain sections at 14 postmenstrual weeks. **1A, 1B.** Frontal oblique sections, showing the longitudinal fissure (IH) and the anterior horns (AH). Somewhat more posteriorly **(1B),** the choroid plexus appears (C). In sections **2** through **4** (midcoronal sections) the changing relationship of the choroid plexus (C) to the thalamus (T) can be seen. **5A** and **5B** are more posterior occipital oblique sections showing the cisterna magna (CM) and a bicerebellar diameter measurement of the cerebellum. *(From Timor-Tritsch and Monteagudo, 1991,[23] with permission.)*

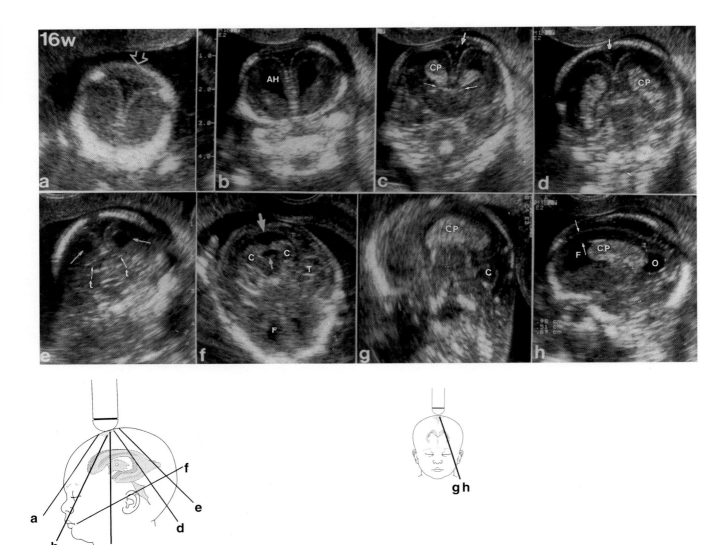

Figure 2–31. Serial scans of the fetal brain at 16 postmenstrual weeks. **A.** An extreme anterior frontal–1 section (see Table 2–2) almost tangential to the fetal skull, showing the wide opening of the anterior fontanelle *(open arrow).* **B.** Frontal–2 section. The cortex and the white matter around the anterior horns are becoming progressively thicker. The sonolucency of the anterior horn (AH) is outstanding. The subarachnoid space is marked by the *white arrow.* **C.** Mid-coronal section. The choroid plexus (CP) and its connection through the interventricular foramina *(small white arrows)* are shown. The *midline arrow* indicates the falx. **D.** Midcoronal–3 section through the antrum of the lateral ventricles, which are filled entirely by the choroid plexus (CP). The *arrow* indicates the falx. **E.** Occipital–1 section. The posterior horns are marked by the *small white arrows.* The tentorium (t) is also indicated. **F.** Horizontal section. The sonolucent cisterna magna is highlighted by the *large white arrow.* The cerebellum (C) and the fourth ventricle *(small white arrow)* are shown. The anterior horns (F) and the inferior horns (T) are visible using this section. **G.** An oblique section highlighting the choroid plexus (C) and one of the cerebellar hemispheres (C). **H.** Right oblique–1 section with the anterior horn (F), posterior horn (O), and choroid plexus (C) situated above the thalamus (T). The thick mass of the brain tissue is indicated by the two *small arrows.*

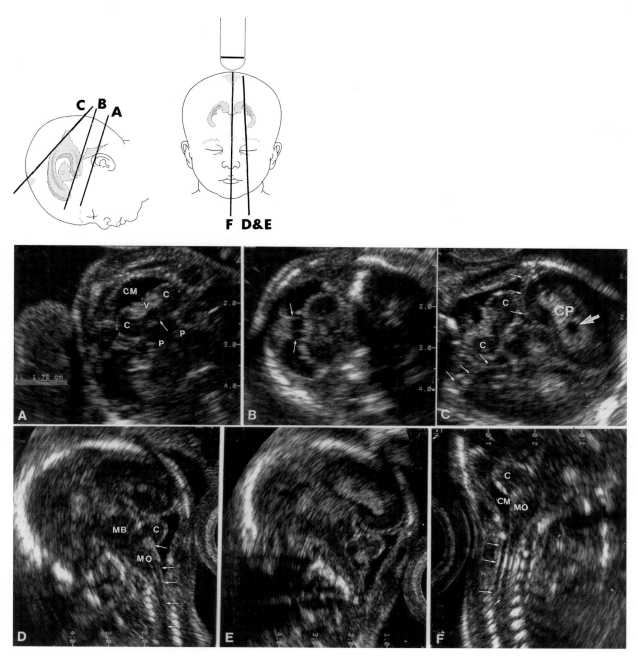

Figure 2–32. These series of horizontal and sagittal sections are part of the workup of the posterior fossa in a normal fetus at 16 postmenstrual weeks. **A.** "Low" horizontal section. The cerebellum (C) measures 1.78 cm, and the cisterna magna measures 0.66 cm. Note the inferior pedunculi (P), the hyperechoic lower portion of the vermis (V), and the fourth ventricle *(small arrow).* **B.** The somewhat higher horizontal section of the posterior fossa, highlighting the small, threadlike structures of the arachnoid membrane *(small arrows).* **C.** This is a higher, composite horizontal/coronal section that shows the tentorium *(small arrows).* The cerebellum (C) and the choroid plexus (C) with a tiny choroid plexus cyst *(small white arrow).* **D.** Almost median section showing the midbrain (MB), medulla oblongata (MO), hyperechoic vermis *(small single arrow),* and cerebellum (C). The *tiny arrow* points toward the medulla. This section clearly shows the upper portion of the medulla *(multiple small arrows).* **E.** Paramedian section. The structures are similar to those indicated in **D. F.** Median section of the suboccipital region, highlighting the cerebellum (C), cisterna magna (CM), medulla oblongata (MO), and spinal cord *(small arrows).*

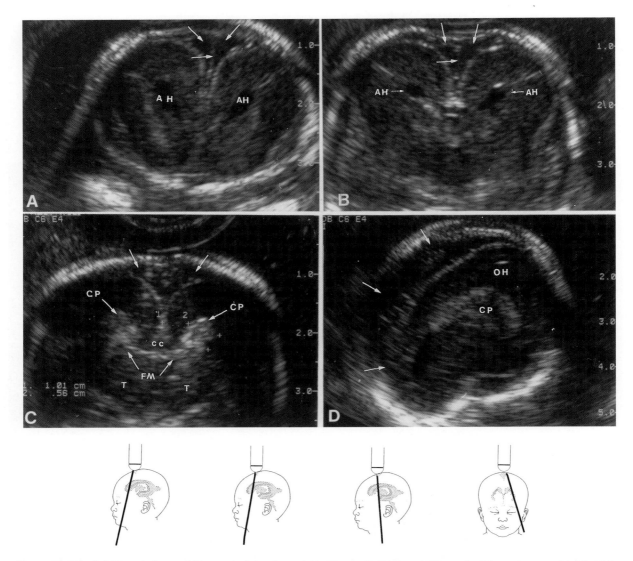

Figure 2–33. Additional views of the same fetus imaged in Figure 2–31. In addition, all of these images highlight the subarachnoid space. **A.** Frontal–2 section. **B.** Midcoronal–1 section. **C.** Midcoronal–2 section. **D.** Left oblique–1 section. The subarachnoid space is highlighted by *small white arrows* in all of these sections. AH, Anterior horn; F, falx; CC, corpus callosum; FM, interventricular foramina; CP, choroid plexus; T, thalamus; OH, posterior horn. The two measurements in **C** are the distance from the midline to the tip of the anterior horn *(1)* and the depth of the anterior horn *(2).* These are normal for this age.

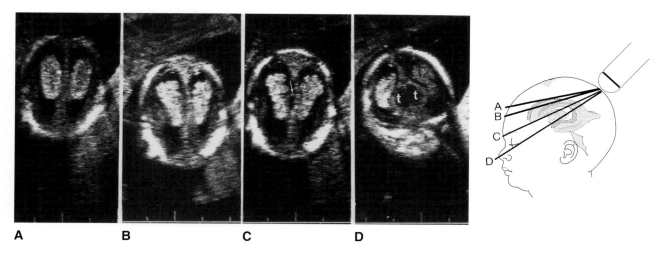

Figure 2–34. Structural evaluation of the fetal brain at 15 postmenstrual weeks. Systematic scanning of the lateral ventricles and the choroid plexus can be performed using several horizontal or oblique planes. The cavity of the septum pellucidum (*arrow* in **C**) and the thalami (t in **D**) are shown. *(From Timor-Tritsch and colleagues, 1995,[39] with permission.)*

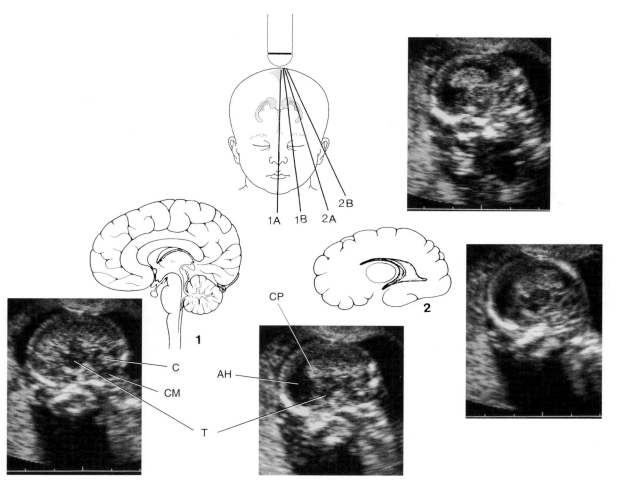

Figure 2–35. Median, paramedian and left oblique sections at 14 postmenstrual weeks. **1A.** Median section showing the thalamus (T), the hypoechoic cerebellum (C), and the posterior cisterna magna (CM). **1B.** Slightly more lateral paramedian sagittal section showing the relationship between the anterior horn (AH) and the choroid plexus (C) and the thalamus (T). **2A, 2B.** Left oblique views also depicting the posterior horn (OH). *(From Timor-Tritsch and Monteagudo, 1991,[23] with permission.)*

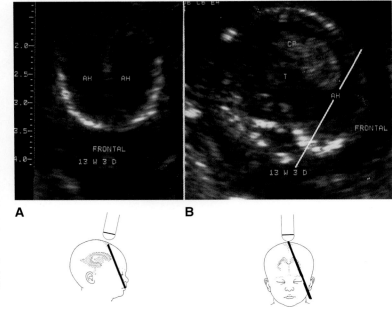

Figure 2–36. This image depicts the anterior part of the fetal brain at 13 weeks and 3 days from the last menstrual period. The importance of this image is to show the relatively large and sonolucent anterior horns (AH). **A.** Frontal slightly slanted section taken at the plane shown by the *white line* in **B.** Note the ample free space, which is normal at this age. **C.** Left oblique section showing the thalamus (T), on top of which the hyperechoic choroid plexus (CP) is seen.

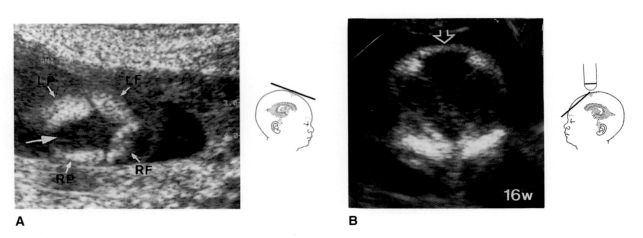

Figure 2–37. Images of the fetal skull bones and the fontanelles and sutures at approximately 16 and at 20 post-menstrual weeks. **A.** Tangential view of the main fontanelle *(arrow)* through which transvaginal scanning of the fetal brain is performed, i.e., the anterior fontanelle. The left and right frontal and parietal bones are also seen (LF, RF, LP, and RP, respectively). **B.** An anterior coronal (almost tangential) section of the fetal skull showing the anterior fontanelle *(arrow)*.

Frontal–2 is the typical "steer's head configuration" and should contain only continuous white matter with the anterior horns. The longitudinal fissure is seen (Figs. 2–39A and 2–41A).

2. MIDCORONAL SECTIONS: The distinct midcoronal sections can be separated. The common denominator of all three is that the anterior horn, with or without the choroid plexus, as well as the corpus callosum is seen on all three midcoronal sections. These are almost true coronal sections because they are close to each other and are generated by a very slight tilt of the probe from the classical coronal plane.

Structures seen in the *Midcoronal–1* plane are the laterally and upward slanted frontal horn of the lateral ventricle, the corpus callosum, the interventricular septum, and the cavum septi pellucidi between the heads of the caudate nuclei (Figs. 2–30-2, 2–33B, 2–39D and 2–41B).

TABLE 2–2. THE CORONAL PLANES.

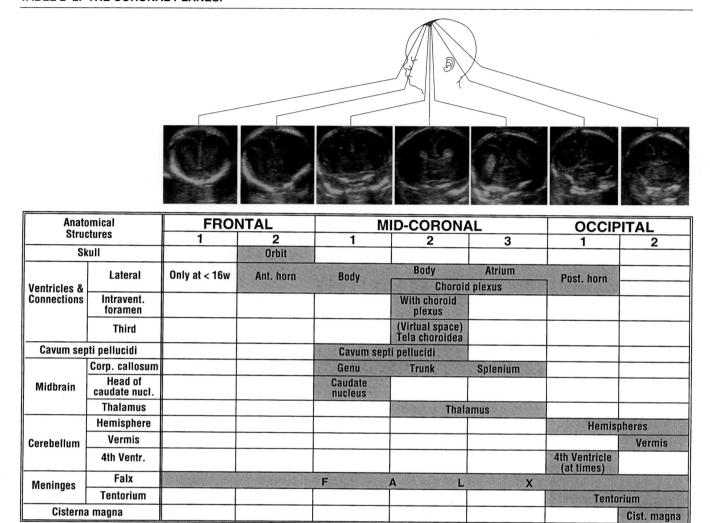

Anatomical Structures		FRONTAL		MID-CORONAL			OCCIPITAL	
		1	2	1	2	3	1	2
Skull			Orbit					
Ventricles & Connections	Lateral	Only at < 16w	Ant. horn	Body	Body	Atrium	Post. horn	
					Choroid plexus			
	Intravent. foramen				With choroid plexus			
	Third				(Virtual space) Tela choroidea			
Cavum septi pellucidi				Cavum septi pellucidi				
Midbrain	Corp. callosum			Genu	Trunk	Splenium		
	Head of caudate nucl.			Caudate nucleus				
	Thalamus				Thalamus			
Cerebellum	Hemisphere						Hemispheres	
	Vermis							Vermis
	4th Ventr.						4th Ventricle (at times)	
Meninges	Falx			F A L X				
	Tentorium						Tentorium	
Cisterna magna								Cist. magna

This table summarizes the brain structures imaged on each of the consecutive frontal, midcoronal, and occipital sections.
From Timor-Tritsch et al.[38] with permission.

Structures seen in the *Midcoronal–2* plane are the lateral ventricles (body) containing the echogenic choroid plexuses, their extension through the interventricular foramina (of Monro) into the space between the thalami (virtual space of the third ventricle), the cavum septi pellucidi below the corpus callosum, the longitudinal fissure, the budding (at 28 postmenstrual weeks) or the developed (after 31 to 32 postmenstrual weeks) cingulate gyrus and sulcus, and the triangular subarachnoid space containing the superior sinus (Figs. 2–30-3, 2–31C, 2–33C, 2–38A, B & C 3, 2–29C and 2–41C).

Structures seen in the *Midcoronal–3* plane are the lateral ventricles (body) containing the choroid plexuses; at times, the slightly echogenic choroid plexus of the third ventricle between the thalami; the corpus callosum; the longitudinal fissure; and the cingulate gyrus and sulcus. Also, toward term, the secondary and tertiary branches of the cingulate sulcus can be imaged (Figs. 2–30-4, 2–38C-4, and 2–39D).

3. OCCIPITAL SECTIONS: The occipital oblique sections may be the hardest to obtain.[20, 22, 31, 38] If circumstances permit, two distinct sections can be obtained. The *Occipital–1* section displays the typical owl's eye configuration because the cortical and white matter is seen in a symmetrical fashion surrounding the sonolucent and almost perfectly round posterior horns, above the V-shaped subarachnoid space and below the tentorium and the hemispheres of the cerebellum. At times, the fourth ventricle and

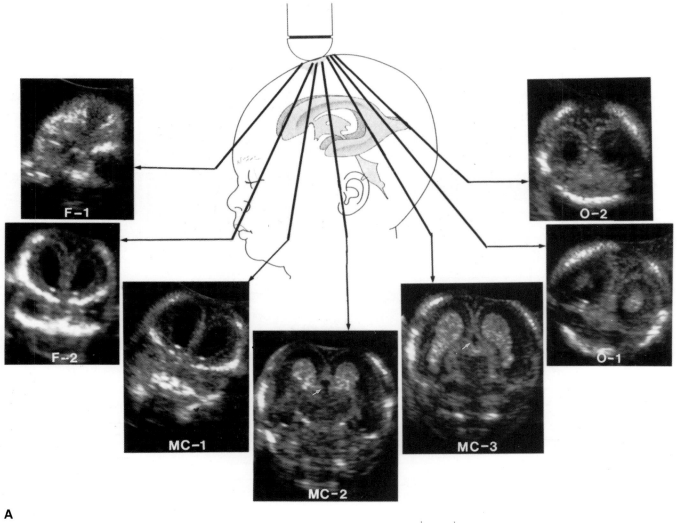

Figure 2–38. A. Serial "coronal" sections at 16 postmenstrual weeks from frontal to occipital. Note the anterior fontanelle on F–1, the wide open anterior horns on F–2 and on MC–1. The incipient cavum septi pellucidi *(arrows)* are seen on MC–2 and on MC–3. F, Frontal; MC, midcoronal; O, occipital. **B.** The Median (M) and Oblique–1 (OB–1) sagittal sections of the same fetus at 16 postmenstrual weeks. Note that the corpus callosum is not yet developed and that the lateral ventricles are relatively large on the OB–1 section.

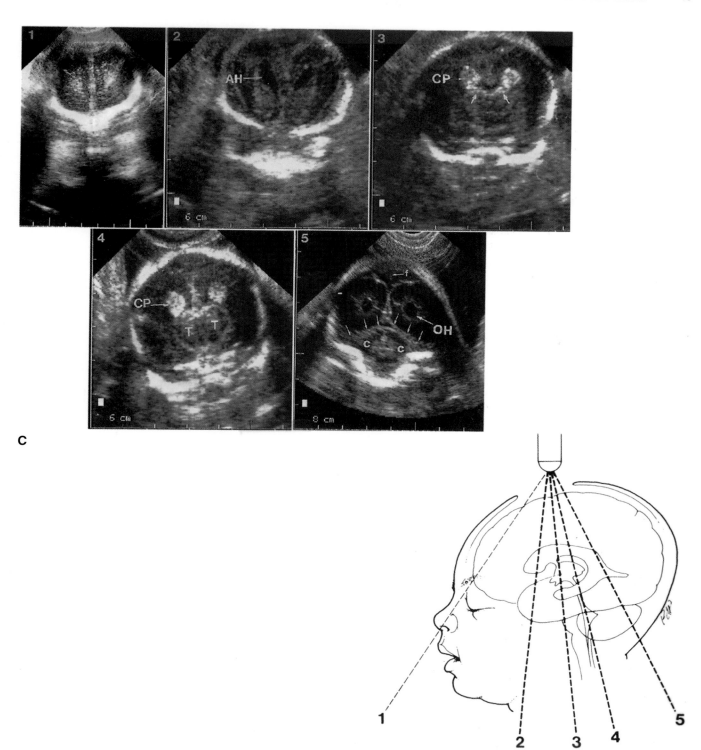

Figure 2–38. C. Serial "coronal" brain sections at 18 postmenstrual weeks. **(1)** Frontal–1 section through the white matter. **(2)** Frontal–2 section through the anterior horns (AH). **(3)** Midcoronal–2 section through the choroid plexus (CP) and the interventricular foramina (two *small arrows*) and the thalamus (T). **(4)** Midcoronal–3 section through the choroid plexus (C) and the thalamus (T). **(5)** Occipital–1 section through the posterior (occipital) horn (OH). The *arrows* indicate the tentorium. C, Cerebellum; f, falx. *(Modified from Timor-Tritsch, Monteagudo, 1991,[23] with permission.)*

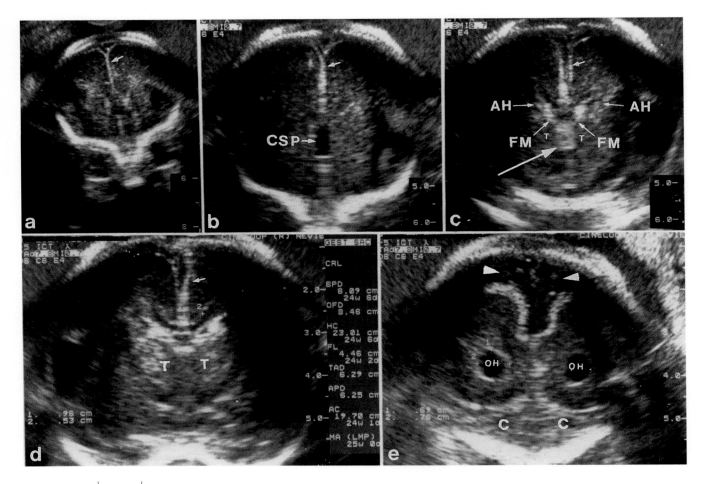

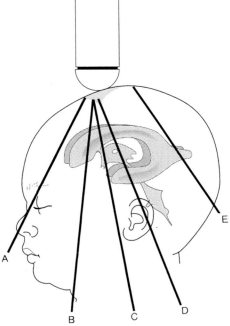

Figure 2–39. Serial transvaginal coronal sections at 25 postmenstrual weeks: **(A)** Frontal–1, **(B)** Frontal–2, **(C)** Mid-coronal–2, **(D)** Midcoronal–3, and **(E)** Occipital–1. The longitudinal fissure is indicated by *small arrows.* CSP, cavum septi pellucidi; AH, anterior horn; T, thalamus; FM, interventricular foramina; OH, posterior horn; C, cerebellum. The *long arrow* in **C** indicates the choroid plexus within the third ventricle between the thalami; the *arrowheads* point to the subarachnoid space.

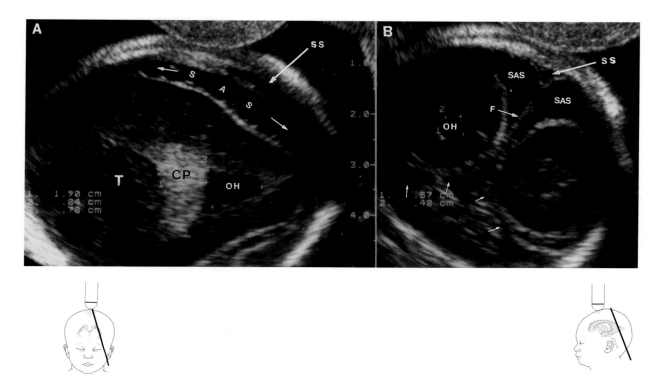

Figure 2–40. At 18 postmenstrual weeks this brain was scanned in **(A)** the left Oblique–1 and **(B)** the Occipital–1 planes. The conventional measurements that can be taken of the lateral ventricle and the posterior horn are shown. These measurements are within the normal range. T, Thalamus; CP, choroid plexus; OH, posterior (occipital) horn; SAS, subarachnoid space; F, falx; SS, sagittal sinus. The *small arrows* indicate the tentorium.

the hyperechoic vermis are seen (Figs. 2–30-5A, 2–31E, 2–38-C5, 2–39E, and 2–40D).

The *Occipital–2* section is the most posterior one. Rarely seen, however, it contains the tip (smallest sonolucent circle) of the posterior horn and the tentorium, below which the cerebellar hemispheres, vermis, and cerebellomedullary cistern (the cisterna magna) are seen (Fig. 2–30-5B).

A faster way to scan the fetal brain in the coronal plane is to use one each of the frontal, midcoronal, and occipital sections. On the *Frontal–1* section, besides its symmetrical picture, one should *not* see the anterior horns (these are seen on this section in the case of ventriculomegaly). The *Midcoronal–2* section should contain the corpus callosum and the left and right thalami, and the choroid plexus should fill the body of the lateral ventricle, proceeding through the interventricular foramina. The *Occipital–1* section should show the normal-sized posterior horn (see its normal measurements in Chapter 3), and the tentorium and the cerebellum should fill the posterior fossa. This abbreviated scanning algorithm should not take more than several minutes.

Sagittal Planes

As opposed to the coronal section, in which the right and left hemispheres are scrutinized simultaneously, sagittal sections are different. After the image in the median plane is obtained, the right and left hemispheres should be scanned using right and left paramedian or oblique sections.

Table 2–3 contains the pertinent images and the structures seen on each of the following structures.

1. MEDIAN SECTION: The hallmark of the median section is the corpus callosum and, below it, the sonolucent cavum septi pellucidi. In addition, the thalamus, the head of the caudate nucleus, their thin covering tela choroidea, parts of the midbrain, and posteriorly, the hyperechoic vermis are depicted (Figs. 2–42-1, 2–43A, 2–44, and 2–45).

Recognition of these structures on this section at 14 postmenstrual weeks is dependent on the quality and resolution of the transducer (Fig. 2–34-1A).

The appearance of the corpus callosum is age dependent and is discussed below. As an example, at 16 postmenstrual weeks (Fig. 2–38B) the corpus callosum is not yet evident.

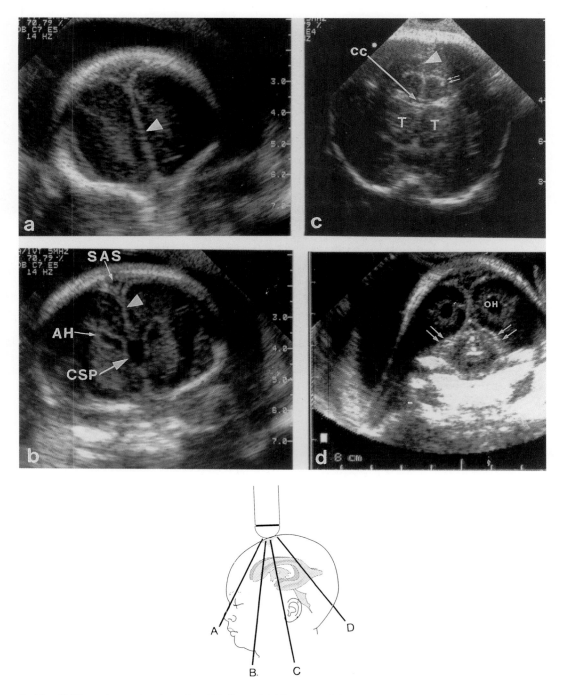

Figure 2–41. At 32 postmenstrual weeks: **(A)** Frontal Oblique–1, **(B)** Midcoronal–1, **(C)** Midcoronal–2, and **(D)** Occipital Oblique–1 sections are shown. Note that the longitudinal fissure *(arrowheads)* in **C** displays the branching of the cingulate gyrus (two *arrows*). In **D** the tentorium is highlighted with *small double arrows*. SAS, Subarachnoid space containing the superior sagittal sinus; CSP, cavum septi pellucidi; AH, anterior horn; T, thalamus; CC, corpus callosum; OH, posterior (occipital) horn.

TABLE 2–3. SUMMARY OF THE BRAIN STRUCTURES IMAGED ON EACH OF THE CONSECUTIVE MEDIAN, OBLIQUE–1, AND OBLIQUE–2 SECTIONS

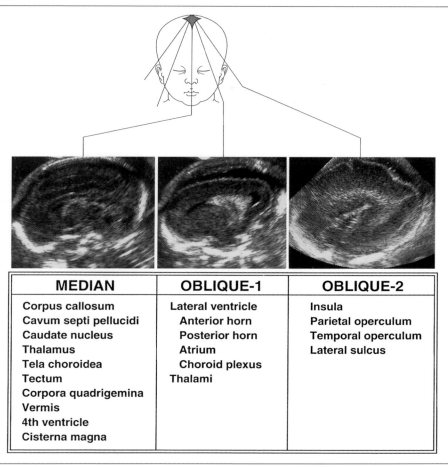

MEDIAN	OBLIQUE-1	OBLIQUE-2
Corpus callosum	Lateral ventricle	Insula
Cavum septi pellucidi	Anterior horn	Parietal operculum
Caudate nucleus	Posterior horn	Temporal operculum
Thalamus	Atrium	Lateral sulcus
Tela choroidea	Choroid plexus	
Tectum	Thalami	
Corpora quadrigemina		
Vermis		
4th ventricle		
Cisterna magna		

From Timor-Tritsch, et al.,[38] with permission.

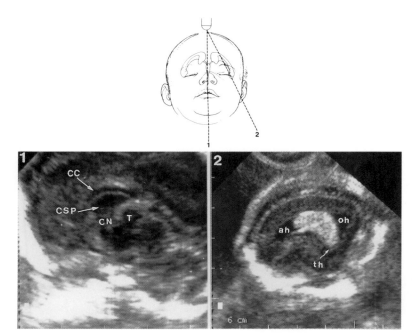

Figure 2–42. (1) Median and. (2) left Oblique–1 sections at 18 postmentstrual weeks. CC, Corpus callosum; CSP, cavum septi pellucidi; CN, caudate nucleus; T, thalmus; ah, anterior horn; CP, choroid plexus; oh, posterior (occipital) horn; lh,lateral horn. *(Modified from Timor-Tritsch and Monteagudo, 1991,[23] with permission.)*

At times, as a function of the transducer (age dependent) or the depth at which it is situated, the fourth ventricle and the cerebellomedullary cistern become visible (Figs. 2–43A and 2–45).

2. OBLIQUE–1 (RIGHT AND LEFT) SECTIONS: The Oblique–1 sections should be obtained on the right as well as the left side. Although the sizes of the ventricles in both hemispheres should be the same, slight discrepancies in size are common. These sagittal sections are of importance and should never be overlooked. Lately, using 3D fetal neuroscanning techniques, we have named such oblique planes as: *the 3-horn views,* because it enables the viewer to evaluate the anterior, posterior, and the inferior horns on the same section. (See Chapter 9)

At 14 postmenstrual weeks the anterior horn is relatively large and the posterior horn is barely de-veloped and difficult to image (Figs. 2–31H, 2–34-2A, and 2–35A and B). At times, the inferior horn is visible in normal fetuses at this age (Fig. 2–42-2). Later, these sections should *not* contain the inferior horn of the lateral ventricle (Fig. 2–31D), because this horn is barely open in a normal brain.

At or after 18 postmenstrual weeks on this section, the anterior horn progressively decreases in size. Toward term it may not be visible at all. The choroid plexus fills the entire antrum above the thalamus. The posterior horn increases its relative size and is quite easily imaged (Figs. 2–40A and 2–43B).

3. OBLIQUE–2 (RIGHT AND LEFT) SECTIONS: If, after scanning through the sagittal planes, the scanning plane of the transducer is further tilted toward the fetal ears, almost tangential scans of the cere-

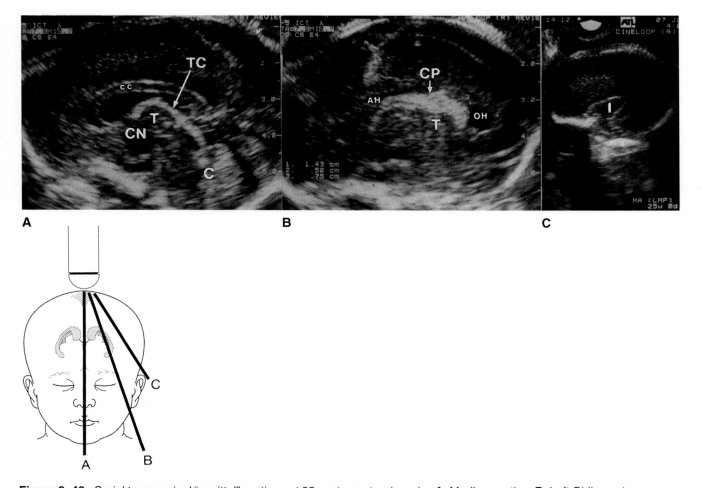

Figure 2–43. Serial transvaginal "sagittal" sections at 25 postmenstrual weeks. **A.** Median section. **B.** Left Oblique–1 section. **C.** Left Oblique–2 and extremely lateral section through the still-gaping lateral sulcus, showing the insula. CC, corpus callosum; CN, caudate nucleus; TC, tela choroidea; T, thalamus; C, vermis of the cerebellum; C, choroid plexus; AH, anterior horn; OH, posterior horn; I, insula.

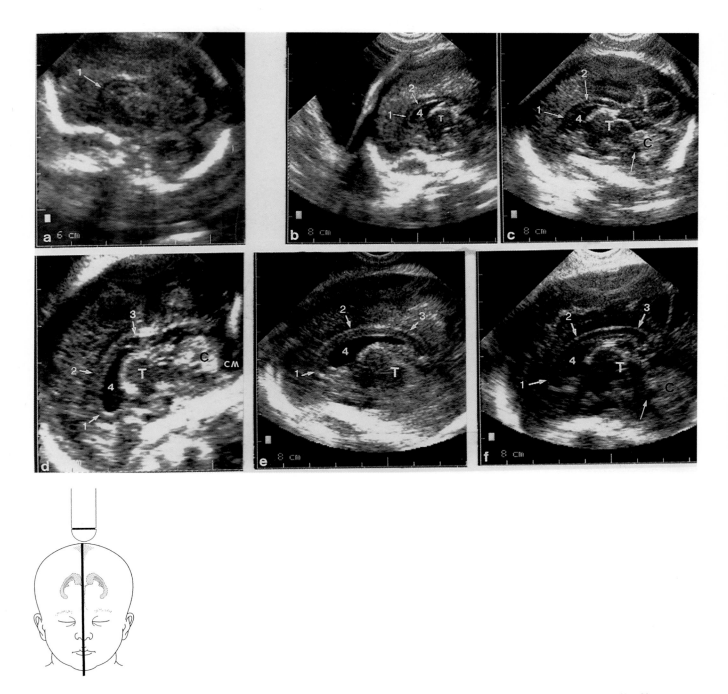

Figure 2–44. Transvaginal median images depicting the development of the corpus callosum at **(A)** 18, **(B, C)** 22, **(D)** 23, and **(E, F)** 28 postmenstrual weeks. C, Cerebellum; 1, genu of the corpus callosum; 2, central part (trunk) of the corpus callosum; 3, splenium of the corpus callosum; 4, cavum septi pellucidi; 5, cavum vergae; T, thalamus; CM, cisterna magna. The *white arrows* in **C** and **F** indicate the fourth ventricle. *(Modified from Timor-Tritsch and Monteagudo, 1991,[23] with permission.)*

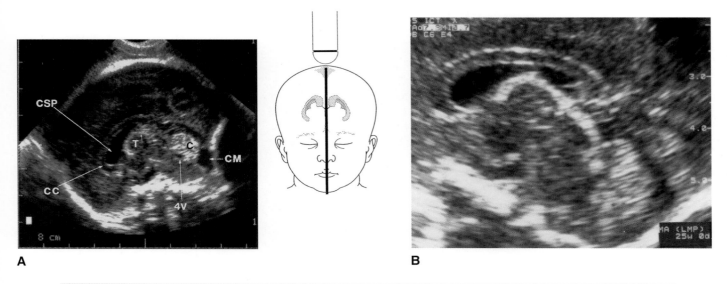

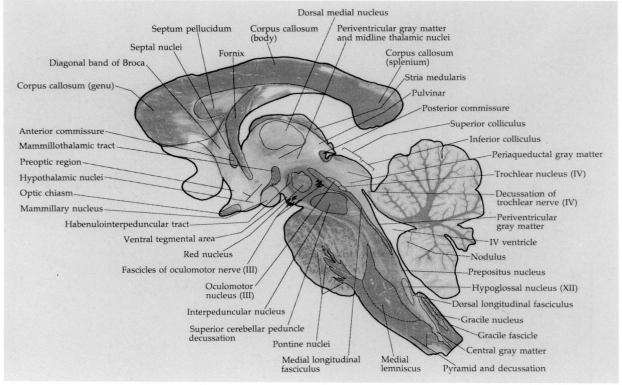

C

Figure 2–45. Sonographically identifiable central structures of the fetal brain at 25 and 28 postmenstrual weeks. **A.** This transvaginal median section shows the fully developed corpus callosum (CC), the cavum septi pellucidi (CSP), the thalamus (T), the tela choroidea of the third ventricle *(small arrow),* the vermis of the cerebellum (c), the fourth ventricle (4V), and the cisterna magna (CM) at 28 postmenstrual weeks' gestation. **B.** Focused median section of the fetal brain at 25 postmenstrual weeks. No annotations were made to identify structures. The image is presented for comparison with the drawing and properly annotated picture in **C. C.** The anatomic structures of the midbrain. *(From Martin, 1989,[40] with permission.)*

bral hemispheric surfaces are obtained. Typical on this section is the still widely gaping lateral sulcus (of Sylvius), which appears as if the capital letter V were lying on its side. The apex of the V points toward the occiput (Fig. 2–43C). The more advanced the age, the more closed the lateral fissure becomes. Between the two "legs" of the letter V, the tangentially "touched" insula is imaged. The upper lip of the V-shaped edges of the fissure is called the parietal operculum; the lower lip is the temporal operculum.

Horizontal (Axial) Planes

At times—in the early second trimester—the fetus turns conveniently into a position in which an axial view is most revealing. The thin bone of the skull is still thin enough to enable meaningful TVS scrutiny of the brain.

The horizontal planes allow the gathering of information on two important aspects of brain anatomy. The first is the examination of the entire choroid plexus of the lateral ventricles (Fig. 2–37) using different ascending sections. The second is a careful look at the posterior fossa using a posteriorly tilted axial plane (Figs. 2–53, 2–57, and 2–58). The images of the posterior fossa are discussed subsequently.

Having pioneered the fetal transfontanelle neuroscan using the high-frequency transvaginal ultrasound probe, we are aware of the following.

1. The sections and/or planes obtained through the anterior fontanelle, using conventional two-dimensional transvaginal neurosonography, were adopted emulating the neonatal transfontanelle approach. All sections are obtained by placing the footprint of the vaginal probe on the anterior fontanelle and the sections therefore "radiate" from one point: the fontanelle. Almost each plane, except the median and one coronal plane, is angled or is oblique, therefore are not parallel to each other. Fanning the probe from anterior-to-posterior to obtain the coronal sections and from side-to-side for the sagittal sections results in the desired planes.

2. In contrast to the two-dimensional technique, when a volume of the fetal brain is obtained by using the three-dimensional transvaginal ultrasound probes through the anterior fontanelle, the volume of the fetal brain can now be se-

quentially sectioned at demand in all three classical orthogonal planes these planes are parallel to each other. These planes are therefore comparable to those sections obtained using serial tomograms by CT or MRI.

3. Using the three-dimensional volume scans, it is easy to render scanning planes that are almost impossible to obtain as a routine procedure. An example is the rendering of axial sections.

Although, we use extensively the two-dimensional fetal transfontanel neuroscan initiated by us, we are increasingly aware of the new and more advanced technique to examine the fetal brain by the three-dimensional technique. Due to this awareness, we included a separate chapter on this new and emerging technique. (See Chapter 9)

Ventricular System

The fetal cerebral ventricular system, as far as ultrasonography is concerned, consists of the following interconnecting structures and their parts (Fig. 2–46): the *lateral ventricles*—anterior (frontal) horn, body, atrium, posterior (occipital) horn, and inferior (temporal) horn—and the *interventricular foramina* (of Monro)—third ventricle, cerebral aqueduct (of Sylvius), fourth ventricle, median aperture (of Magendie), and lateral apertures (of Luschka).

The lateral ventricles are situated in parallel fashion within both cerebral hemispheres. They have three horns—anterior, posterior, and inferior—a body, and a triangular atrium. Even though this is the correct nomenclature of the three horns of the lateral ventricles, on some of the pictures the old nomenclature (frontal, occipital, and temporal horns) may still appear.

The embryology of the cerebral ventricles was touched on in Chapter 1 as well as in this chapter.

The different parts of the lateral ventricle undergo extensive change in their shape and size. The lateral ventricles are at first relatively very large (Fig. 1–7 in Chapter 1) and gradually become more slender during the fetal period. The posterior horn is the last to appear (Fig. 1–7 in Chapter 1) and is the most variable. Three examples of casts by Day[41] are shown in Figure 2–47. They are from fetuses at 12, 18, and 32 weeks, respectively. Because we are currently dealing with a more precise evaluation of the lateral ventricles using TVS, it is important to look at these three representative pictures of the casts at 12, 18, and 32 postmenstrual weeks (Fig. 2–47). It seems that they match, in general, the sonographic

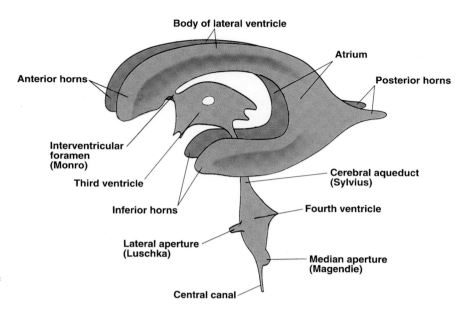

Figure 2–46. The ventricular system of the brain, seen from the left side.

evaluation of the lateral ventricles performed with high-frequency transvaginal transducers. The conclusions of Day's study were (1) the posterior horn develops late in relation to the anterior and inferior horns, (2) the lateral ventricles become progressively more slender in proportion, and (3) the difference in size between homologous ventricles is not as great in the fetus as in the adult, especially in the posterior horn.

The lateral ventricles are the most obvious when ultrasonography of the fetal brain is undertaken. As the largest of all ventricles, they were quite readily seen by the relatively low-frequency transabdominal probes. The diagnosis of ventriculomegaly and hydrocephaly was established by measuring the size of the body of the lateral ventricle on the axial transabdominal picture. The term *lateral ventricle–hemisphere width* ratio was coined to objectively measure ventricular size. The change in this ratio throughout normal gestation was followed up and reported.[42–50] By looking at the published graphs, it is obvious that the relative size of the lateral ventricular width decreases rapidly from about 70% at 18 postmenstrual weeks to 30% at around 28 weeks and stays constant at this level thereafter.

One of the problems of ventricular measurements by TAS is the lack of standardization. "Obviously normal" and "clearly abnormal" lateral ventricles do not seem to require measurements. However, borderline cases would probably benefit from a quantitative determination of size. Continuous follow-up of a case with suspected ventriculomegaly would also require the values to be put on a conventional graph.

There is, however, another pitfall—namely, that different authors measure distances from and to different echogenic "lines" within the head.

The last and probably the most important drawback of conventional transabdominal imaging of the fetal brain is, at times, the problem of ineffective imaging of the hemisphere close to the transducer (Fig. 2–48). This incomplete picture is the reason for a large number of referrals to imaging centers.

If more sophisticated and better ultrasound machines are used (e.g. compound scanning transducers) and operated by knowledgeable examiners, the transabdominal images have the capability to produce pictures of the fetal brain with a high degree of resolution (Fig. 2–49).

Hertzberg and colleagues[52] questioned the validity of these echogenic "lines" mentioned above, postulating that they do not correspond to the walls of the lateral ventricles. In a more recent article, the same author suggests that for a correct measurement of the lateral ventricle on an axial view, the examiner should make "a direct attempt to find the medial wall of the ventricle."[52]

Cardoza and coworkers[48] tried to measure selectively the width of the lateral ventricular atrium according to increasing fetal age. These measurements remained relatively constant throughout gestation (Table 2–4), at a value of 7.6 ± 0.6 mm. This group suggested that atrial diameters above 10 mm (above +4 standard deviations) should raise suspicion of ventriculomegaly. Other graphs, tables, and nomograms to measure distances from the lateral and medial walls of the lateral ventricles are now

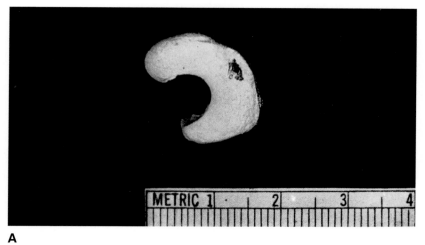

A

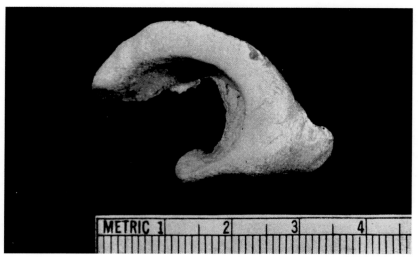

B

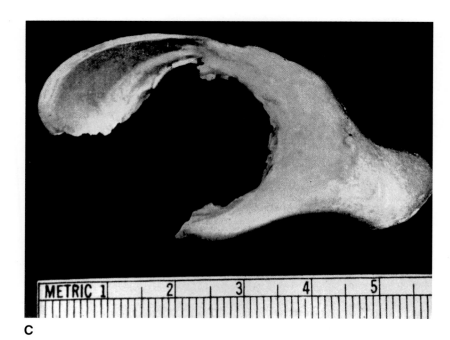

C

Figure 2–47. The development of the human fetal lateral ventricles at **(A)** 12, **(B)** 18, and **(C)** 32 postmenstrual weeks. *(From Day, 1959,[41] with permission.)*

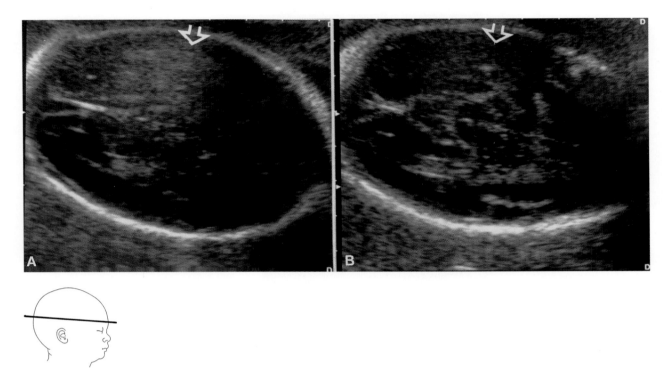

Figure 2–48. (A, B) Two axial sections of the brain at 26 postmenstrual weeks, showing the obscured near field due to ineffective transabdominal imaging of the hemisphere close to the transducer *(open arrows).*

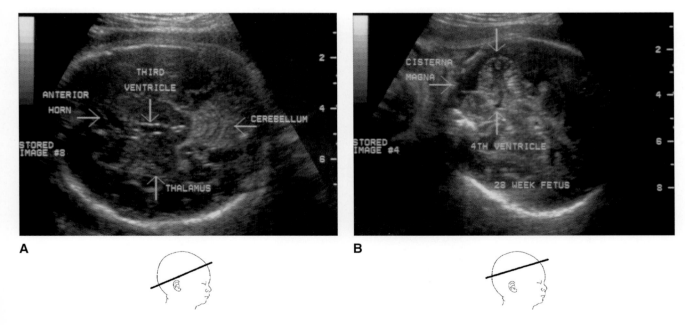

Figure 2–49. The more advanced technology of the transabdominal transducer allows visualization of very fine detail of the cerebellum as well as the fourth and third ventricles at 28 postmenstrual weeks.

TABLE 2–4. DIAMETER OF THE NORMAL LATERAL VENTRICULAR ATRIUM AS A FUNCTION OF POSTMENSTRUAL AGE

Postmenstrual Weeks	Mean ± SD (mm)	Range (mm)
14–20	7.6 ± 0.7	6.0–9.0
21–25	7.7 ± 0.5	7.0–9.0
26–30	7.5 ± 0.7	6.5–9.0
31–38	7.6 ± 0.5	7.0–8.5

Adapted from Cardoza and colleagues, 1988,[48] with permission.

available[53–56] (see also Chapter 5). All of these, however, still use the axial views of the head obtained by TAS. Indeed, newer equipment has helped in identifying the above-mentioned components of the lateral ventricles to serve as reproducible landmarks for the measurements. Reece and Goldstein[57] tried to standardize the axial planes obtained by TAS by introducing three successive scanning planes (Levels I, II, and III) at the intersection of different intracranial brain structures. Unfortunately (as in the case of all transabdominal scanning approaches) abdominal thickness of the patient, mounting bone thickness and low transducer frequencies will almost always yield less resolution, hence, a relatively poor fetal neuroscan as opposed to TVS of the brain. However, once the technique of transvaginal neurosonography is observed and mastered, there is no doubt that it will be increasingly used until it will almost entirely replace the transabdominal route, provided that the fetus is in vertex presentation.[20, 22, 23, 30, 31] At times, as mentioned before, it may become important to perform cephalic version to the vertex presentation, of a fetus presenting with the breech, for more accurate studies.

Measurements of the *anterior horn–hemispheric width* ratio were reported on by Campbell in 1979.[58] This ratio decreases from 60% at week 14 to 40% at 21 postmenstrual weeks. Another ratio—that of the frontal horn to the hemispheric width—was measured by Goldstein and collaborators.[54] This ratio diminishes from 50% to 28% from 15 postmenstrual weeks to term. In addition, the size of the frontal lobe can be measured on the TAS picture. Because this measurement correlates with fetal size, it was used to detect microcephaly.[59]

The *atrium* of the lateral ventricles has also been the subject of numerous studies and serial measurements by various authors. Sonographically, it is easy to recognize the atrium because it contains a large part of the choroid plexus present in the lateral ventricular system. The distance, measured typically on an axial plane, is that from the falx to the lateral wall of the atrium.[55] As usual, the ratio

between this distance and the hemispheric width was proposed as a sensitive indicator of abnormality. This ratio decreases from 60% to 30% from 15 postmenstrual weeks to 24 weeks.[60] From 27 postmenstrual weeks to term, the same ratio remains fairly constant, at values of 0.56 to 0.51.[45] Pilu and associates[55] suggested that the size of the atrium remains relatively constant across gestation, at about 7 ± 1.3 mm, and this is due to the thickening of the parenchyma. This increase in the brain mass is expressed—according to this group—by the slow but constantly increasing distance between the falx and the lateral atrial wall.

The *posterior horn* is an extremely important structure. It is considered to be the most sensitive indicator of incipient ventriculomegaly. This horn of the lateral ventricle was somewhat neglected in the literature. The reason may be that it is rather hard to obtain a consistently good-quality image of the posterior horn for purposes of measurement. It is interesting that in a study concentrating on several measurements of the lateral cerebral ventricles to detect impending poor fetal outcome, the most significant increase in size was that of the posterior horn. However, this was not given great importance.[61] Chapter 3 discusses the importance of measuring the size of the posterior horn as well as two ratios in which the size of the posterior horn is compared to the thickness of the choroid plexus within the atria.

The *inferior horn* extends from the atrium into the temporal lobe. After emerging from the atrium, the horn turns slightly toward the inferior and lateral direction, ending in the center of the temporal lobe (Fig. 2–46). The lateral position of this horn is less obvious before 14 to 16 postmenstrual weeks, when the Oblique–1 section may include all three horns, i.e., anterior, posterior, and inferior. As mentioned before, we refer to this section as to *the 3-horn view*. After 16 postmenstrual weeks the Oblique–1 section "cuts" through the anterior and occipital horns but definitely does not include the inferior horn, which, as stated, is slightly lateral to this plane. Based on our experience, if after 16 postmenstrual weeks all three horns are clearly imaged on the paramedian sagittal section, ventriculomegaly should be seriously considered.

The *third ventricle* is relatively well imaged in the first and early second trimesters (Figs. 2–27 through 2–29). However, as gestation progresses, it becomes filled with the choroid plexus (tela choroidea) of the third ventricle and is considered a virtual space. The two contralateral thalami touch each other at the point of the interthalamic adhesion (massa intermedia). Denkhaus and Winsberg[42] claimed to be able to measure the width of the third ventricle on axial TAS images. They suggested a table that lists the width of this ventricle at 2.5 mm at a biparietal diameter of 2.3 cm, increasing to 8.2 mm at term. It is unclear from this report whether or not they saw the choroid plexus within the third ventricle. They also attributed no importance to the clinical value of a change in the size of this ventricle with respect to the diagnosis of antenatal hydrocephaly. Our observation is to the contrary; and this is touched on in the chapter on the pathology of the fetal brain (Chapter 4).

The *fourth ventricle* can quite easily be seen using a median plane or an axial section using the occipital approach (Figs. 2–31F, 2–32A, 2–44, and 2–45).

Foramina and the Aqueduct

As mentioned already, a pair of narrow *interventricular foramina* connect the body of the lateral ventricles with the third ventricle. These tiny connections would certainly elude the scanning sound waves if an extremely echogenic structure, namely, the choroid plexus, did not highlight them. These connections were reportedly detected as early as 8½ postmenstrual weeks (Figs. 2–20 and 2–21) by the Trondheim group.[28] The interventricular foramina (of Monro) are clearly visible from 14 to 16 postmenstrual weeks on and mark the most typical coronal (Midcoronal–2) section of the fetal brain (Figs. 2–31C, 2–33C, 2–38-3, and 2–39C).

The *cerebral aqueduct* (of Sylvius), the connection between the third and fourth ventricles, was not reported to be detected by ultrasonography of the normal fetal brain. This may soon change using three-dimensional imaging when a special plane to detect and study this extremely thin structure can be created by the multiplanar capability of this technique.

Using a posterior (occipital) axial or median approach, the *median aperture* (of Magendie) can be seen (Fig. 2–44). This aperture is wide open before 16 postmenstrual weeks and is more easily detected before 20 postmenstrual weeks than after. This aperture becomes wide open in cases of abnormal dilatations of the cerebellomedullary cistern (the cisterna magna) and the fourth ventricle (see Chapter 4).

Choroid Plexus

An integral part of the ventricular system is a complex tissue dedicated to the production of cerebrospinal fluid (CSF): the choroid plexuses. This structure is found in all lateral ventricles.

The choroid plexuses consists of villi in large numbers, the outer (ventricular) surface of which is covered by a single-layered, modified cuboidal epithelium (ependyma). The inner layer is a stromal core derived from the pia. The capillaries found in each of these villi are the major source of CSF production.

Embryologically, the choroid plexus develops from the anteriorly located ventricles, more precisely, from their medial and upper wall. The stroma as well as the covering pia is derived from the mesenchyme. Even though the choroid plexus is present from 6 to 7 postmenstrual weeks on, it takes several weeks until it becomes large and echogenic enough to be detected by a high-frequency transvaginal probe. At 8 to 8½ postmenstrual weeks, it is small in size and already significantly echogenic (Figs. 2–21 through 2–23). Starting from the ninth postmenstrual week, it is consistently seen on the two sides of the falx within the lateral ventricles. It can be said that it is the most striking sonographic intracranial structure well beyond the end of the first trimester. At 9 to 11 postmenstrual weeks, the choroid plexus fills both entire lateral ventricles (Figs. 2–45, 2–27, and 2–29). As pregnancy progresses, their relative size compared to the lateral ventricular size decreases. They "move" posteriorly and assume their permanent anatomic site within the atrium, "hugging" the thalami from posterior and above (Figs. 2–30 through 2–32, 2–34, and 2–35). Their posterior contour is smooth. If they lose their regular contours, one should suspect an adjacent intraventricular hemorrhage. An obviously thin or dangling choroid plexus should arouse suspicion of ventriculomegaly or hydrocephaly. The *tela choroidea* is the thin choroid plexus layer covering the thalami, extending into the third ventricle (Figs. 2–39C and 2–43). The choroid plexus of the fourth ventricle is probably extremely difficult to image. Therefore, to our knowledge, it is not mentioned in the pertinent literature.

It should be emphasized that the choroid plexus may give rise to tumors such as choroid plexus papilloma and carcinoma.

The *cavum septi pellucidi* and its posterior part, the *cavum vergae,* are not strictly part of the ventricular system. If found at autopsies of infants and adults, they are generally considered insignificant. The cavum septi pellucidi and the cavum vergae are, in fact, the same structure, the former located anteriorly and the latter positioned posteriorly to a vertical plane formed by the columns of the fornix. The two usually communicate with each other (Fig. 2–50A and B). The presence or absence of the cavum septi pellucidi as a function of age was studied by Shaw and Alvord.[62] Dissecting the brains of 374 normal subjects, they found that 100% of the premature infants had a cavum septi pellucidi wider than 1 mm. The cavum vergae closes first, well before term, and the cavum septi pellucidi starts to close just before term. Table 2–5 also shows that at 6 months of age only 12% of the brains had a recognizable cavum. This group did not report on the age of the premature infants.

Jones et al[63] measure the width of the cavum septi pellucidi from 19 to 42 weeks in 608 fetuses. They found that this measurement increased gradually to 27 weeks when it plateaued until term.

Larroche and Bandey[64] noted that the cavum vergae is typically absent at birth. This was observed following pneumoencephalographic studies in neonates.

The cava form simultaneously with the corpus callosum. The appearance of the cava on ultrasonographic images is also limited to the first detection of the corpus callosum, i.e., at about 17 to 18 postmenstrual weeks. At term, as mentioned before, these spaces become almost obliterated.

Even though it will be mentioned in detail later in this chapter when we describe the arteries of the brain, we have to mention here the pericallosal artery. This artery closely follows the corpus callosum. As a matter of fact, three structures and their development are closely interrelated: the corpus callosum; above it, the pericallosal artery; and below it, the cavum septi pellucidi. This parallel development of these three structures becomes important when deviant development of the corpus callosum is discussed.

The cavum septi pellucidi is best imaged on the Median (Figs. 2–42 through 2–45) and the Midcoronal–1 and –2 (Figs. 2–39 and 2–41B) sections. Two lateral walls separate this structure from the anterior horns of the lateral ventricles (Fig. 2–41B). Failing to detect these lateral walls should arouse suspicion of disease such as agenesis of the corpus callosum, septo-optic dysplasia, schizencephaly, hydrocephaly, and porencephaly, among others.[65]

Corpus Callosum

The corpus callosum is one of the important structures of the brain, connecting the right and left hemispheres. In fact, it is the largest interconnecting structure and consists of myelin-coated nerve fibers that cross the median plane. It forms the roof of the cavum septi pellucidi and the cavum vergae. The development of these structures (i.e., the corpus callosum and the cava) is closely linked. Because the roof of the cavum septi pellucidi is the corpus callosum itself, it is clear that if there is no roof, there is no cavum.

If the corpus callosum is scanned through the anterior fontanelle, the sound waves meet this structure at almost a right angle. The sonographic picture in the Median plane of the developed corpus callosum is that of two parallel echogenic lines with a sonolucent strip of about 3 to 5 mm between them. The upper line is generated by the deepest points of the longitudinal fissure. The lower echogenic line is the roof of the cavum septi pellucidi and the cavum vergae. The pericallosal artery closely follows the upper boundary of the corpus callosum. The Midcoronal–1 and –2 sections depict this commissural structure as a semilunar structure.

After understanding the anatomy and the sonographic presentation of the corpus callosum in the various scanning planes, its development should be discussed. The corpus callosum is a relatively late-developing structure reported to develop between the 12th and 18th postmenstrual weeks.[66, 67] It is also known that it develops in an anterior-to-posterior direction,[64] but this development can be followed sonographically.[20, 23, 67–69] (See Chapter 1)

In Figures 2–30 and 2–34, which represent coronal and sagittal sections of fetuses at 14 postmenstrual weeks, it is not yet possible to discern the corpus callosum. At 16 postmenstrual weeks the first hint of its sonographic appearance is present (Figs. 2–31B and 2–33B and C). At 18 postmenstrual weeks (Figs. 2–38 and 2–42) the anterior portion of the genu and almost all of the central part is seen. Figure 2–44 depicts images of the corpus callosum from 18 to 28 postmenstrual weeks.

At 22 to 23 postmenstrual weeks, the Median section shows the totally formed corpus callosum (see Fig. 2–45). This structure has four parts, from anterior to posterior: the rostrum, the genu (knee), the trunk, and the splenium.

The importance of knowing this developmental pattern is because, at times, and for various reasons, the development of the corpus callosum is incomplete.[67, 68, 70] Such a partial agenesis of the corpus callosum appears on the sonographic image as if it had been "caught" at an early stage of the development. The lack of development of this structure is discussed in Chapter 5.

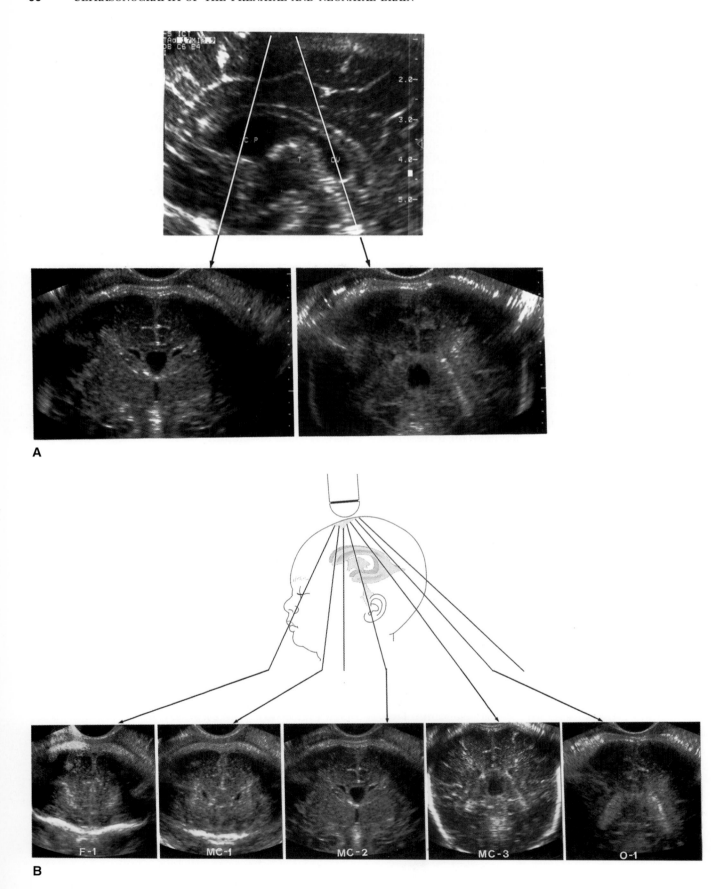

A

B

TABLE 2–5. INCIDENCE OF OPEN CAVUM SEPTI PELLUCIDI AS A FUNCTION OF AGE

Age	Percentage Present
Premature	100
Full term to 7 days	97
8 days to 1 month	85
6 month to 16 years	12

After Shaw and Alvord, 1969,[62] with permission.

Subarachnoid Spaces and Cisterns

Scanning the normal fetal brain, spaces of different shapes and sizes are seen between the cortex and the bony skull or between structures of the brain itself. Fine cords of the arachnoid, delicate blood vessels, and probably arachnoid granulations produce a variety of echoes within this space (Figs. 2–32B, 2–39B through E, 2–51, and 2–52). Figures 2–51 and 2–52 show an ultrasonographic image and a drawing of the subarachnoid space.

Early in pregnancy, it is rare to detect subarachnoid spaces. However, around 14 to 16 postmenstrual weeks, they can be revealed using high-frequency TVS (Figs. 2–31 through 2–33, 2–40, 2–51, and 2–53). The relative sizes of these spaces decrease as pregnancy advances. In a study by Laing and colleagues,[71] 122 fetuses from 21 to 40 postmenstrual weeks were scanned (transabdominally). A "subdural space" was sought on a "transaxial" scan. Eighty-three percent of the fetuses with this subdural space were less than 30 postmenstrual weeks, whereas 77% lacking this sign were older than 30 weeks. All of the fetuses were normal at birth. These investigators concluded that if a wide subarachnoid space is seen in late pregnancy, it should be investigated following birth, since a prominent space may predispose a neonate to subdural hematoma.[72]

It is possible that Laing's group[71] studied the space immediately adjacent to the lateral sulcus (of Sylvius). This fluid-filled space was also studied by Jeanty and collaborators.[73] The latter came to the conclusion that the structure (i.e., the cortex) below the internal table of the bone overlapping this area in which the pulsations of the middle cerebral artery is seen should be termed the *insula* and not the *Sylvian fissure*. Such an area is shown in Figure 2–54.

The subarachnoid space overlying the insula is also shown in the subsection dealing with the sulci, fissures, and gyri in this chapter.

It is worth discussing the echoes appearing within the subarachnoid space seen in Figure 2–51. These may be cross-sections of vessels; however, on color Doppler and power Doppler scans, these do not demonstrate flow. An additional hypothesis is that they may represent cross-sections of arachnoid granulations (see Fig. 2–52).

Several *cisterns* in the subarachnoid space can be seen by neurosonography of the fetal brain. The cisterns are scattered around as well as within the folds of the brain. We could not detect cisterns such as that of the *lamina terminalis* or the *chiasmatic, interpeduncular,* and *pontine cisterns*. So far, the largest one, the *cerebellomedullary cistern* (cisterna magna), and, at times, the superior (interpeduncular) cistern below the cerebellum and the *quadrigeminal cistern* and the bilateral *cisterna ambiens* above the cerebellum have been imaged by ultrasonography.[74]

The cisterna magna has been seen as early as 12 to 14 postmenstrual weeks (Figs. 2–30, 2–34, 2–36, and 2–55). From 14 postmenstrual weeks on, it is easy to visualize this relatively large sonolucent structure in the posterior fossa (Figs. 2–31, 2–32, 2–45, 2–48, and 2–53).

As mentioned before, using a posterior (occipital) approach and a transvaginal probe, some of the fine details of the posterior fossa and the cisterna magna as well as the quadrigeminal cistern can be revealed (Fig. 2–56). The connection between the fourth ventricle and the cisterna magna through the median aperture can also be seen if the correct section and plane can be applied (Figs. 2–57 through 2–60).

The exact anatomy of the posterior fossa, but more so the connections between the fourth ventricle and the cisterns around the cerebellum (e.g., the cisterna magna), should be well known to those engaging in neurosonography of the fetal posterior fossa. Variations in the size of these CSF-filled spaces are not uncommon. The size of the cisterna magna in normal neonates was measured and ranges between 3 and 8 mm, with a mean value of 4.5 mm.[71] As opposed to an increase in the size of this space due to disease, there is also restriction of

Figure 2–50. The cavum vergae in the brain of this normal 28 week fetus is the posterior part of the cavum septi pellucidi. **A.** The two lower images were generated along the white lines seen on the median plane. The anterior section "cuts" through the cavum septi pellucidi (CP). The posterior coronal section highlights the cavum vergae (CV). **B.** The systematic scanning using the transfontanelle approach reveals the normal cavum septi pellucidi on the MC–2 plane and the still open cavum vergae on the MC–3 plane. This study uses the sequential "coronal" planes.

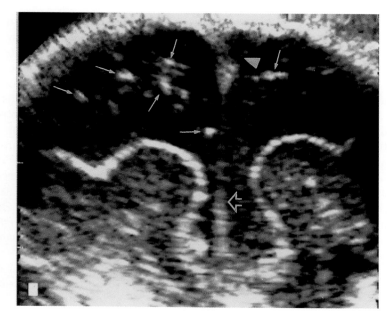

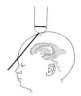

Figure 2–51. The subarachnoid space is shown on this Frontal–1 section. The *small arrows* indicate the hyperechoic structures thought to represent cross-sections of blood vessels or arachnoid granulations in the subarachnoid space. The *open arrow* indicates the falx; the *arrowhead* marks the sagittal sinus.

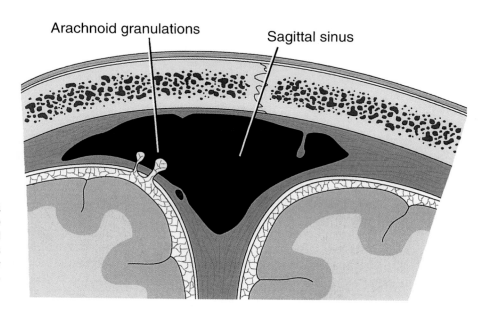

Arachnoid granulations

Sagittal sinus

Figure 2–52. Schematic drawing of a similar section depicted in Figure 2–49, showing the subarachnoid space and the arachnoid granulations bulging into the areas supplied by blood and which drain the cerebrospinal fluid.

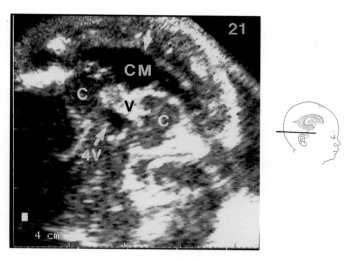

Figure 2–53. Axial section of the posterior fossa in a normal fetus at 21 postmenstrual weeks. CM, Cisterna magna; C, cerebellum; V, vermis; 4V, fourth ventricle.

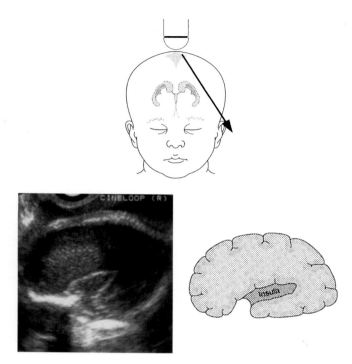

Figure 2–54. Left Oblique–2 section through the insula. Pulsations of the middle cerebral artery may be detected by scanning through this view.

this cistern due to pathology (Arnold–Chiari type II malformation). It is therefore of the utmost importance that this space be examined in the context of the entire CNS.

The use of high-frequency (possibly through the transvaginal route) transducers is probably warranted, along with sound knowledge of the anatomy and neuropathology of this region.

At times, only TAS of the ventricular system is feasible (e.g., with breech or transverse positions of the fetus). In such a case one should be familiar with nomograms developed for atrial measurements. One of these nomograms was suggested by Pilu and coworkers.[55] After conducting a prospective study of 171 normal pregnancies from 15 postmenstrual weeks to term, the following were found: (1) The atrial width remained fairly constant during pregnancy (0.69 ± 0.13 cm = 2 standard deviations). (2) Significant relationships were found between the cerebroatrial distance (Fig. 2–61) and age (R^2 = 0.936; P = 0.0001) and between the cerebroatrial distance and the biparietal diameter as well as between the atrial width–cerebroatrial distance ratio and age.

It is hard to compare ventricular measurements taken on axial sections using TAS with those obtained on paramedian sagittal sections using TVS. In spite of this, it seems that the general trend, e.g., the very slow increase of fetal atrial size seen using the two methods, is comparable.[49]

Posterior Fossa and Upper Spinal Cord

Transvaginal sonographic examination of the posterior fossa is feasible using a variety of approaches

and scanning planes. All of them are useful and informative.

After 10 to 12 postmenstrual weeks several larger structures of this anatomic area, such as the cerebellar hemispheres and the cisterna magna, are discernible (Figs. 2–30-5A and 2–55). At 16 to 18 postmenstrual weeks the posterior fossa lends itself to excellent imaging (Figs. 2–31F and 2–32). Studying the infratentorial region reveals the following structures: the cisterna magna, with fine, linear echoes of the arachnoid; the hemispheres, with their hyperechoic cortex; the extremely hyperechoic vermis; the pons; the fourth ventricle; and, on a median section, the connection between the fourth ventricle and the cisterna magna, i.e., the median aperture (Magendie).

The late closure of the cerebellar vermis, toward the 18th postmenstrual week, was documented by Bromley et al[75] using transabdominal scanning. Using the transfontanelle approach, we have noted several fetuses with even later "closure" of the vermis, with normal neonatal outcome.

For easier orientation the posterior fossa is depicted in the following figures: *horizontal (axial) sections*—Figures 2–31F; 2–32A, B, and D; 2–48C and D; 2–53; 2–59; and 2–60A and B; *coronal sections*—Figures 2–30-5A, 2–38-5, and 2–55; and *median* and

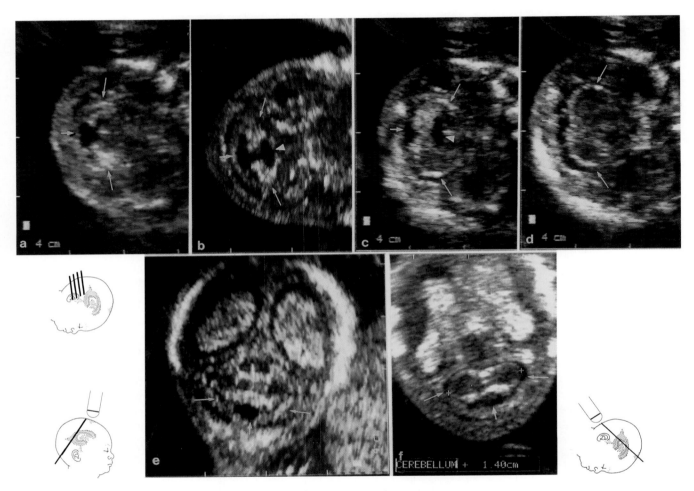

Figure 2–55. Structural evaluation of the brain at 15 postmenstrual weeks. The posterior fossa and the cerebellum are studied on these serial sections. The two *slanted arrows* on both sides of the cerebellum throughout the six images point to the two cerebral hemispheres. **a.** Low axial section depicting the cisterna magna *(small arrow).* **b.** The higher axial plane reveals the widening cisterna magna *(small arrow)* and the lower pole of the fourth ventricle *(arrowhead).* **c.** A somewhat "higher" axial section shows the hemispheres and the fourth ventricle *(arrowhead).* **d.** This is the highest of the axial sections depicting the cerebellum at the level where the bicerebellar diameter measurement is usually taken. Note the hyperechoic cortex surrounded by sonolucent cerebrospinal fluid and the low echogenicity of the medulla. **e.** Coronal section showing the cisterna magna *(small white arrow* in the median plane), the inverted-funnel-shaped tentorium (two *black arrows*), and the choroid plexus (cp). **f.** A combined oblique axial–coronal section showing the bicerebellar diameter, which measures 1.4 cm. The *small arrow* in the midline indicates the cisterna magna. *(From Timor-Tritsch and colleagues, 1995,[39] with permission.)*

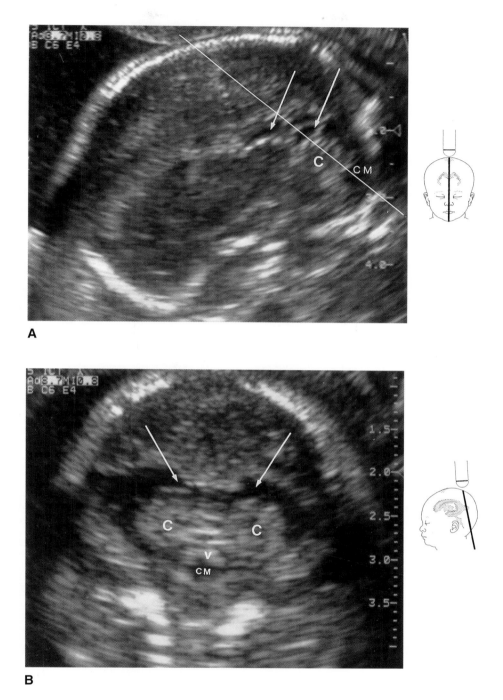

Figure 2–56. The cisterns around the cerebellum in a normal fetus at 17 postmenstrual weeks. **A.** Median section. The two *arrows* indicate the quadrigeminal cisterns. C, Cerebellum; CM, cisterna magna. **B.** Coronal view obtained along the *white line* in **A.** The two *arrows* point to the cisterna ambiens above the cerebellar hemispheres. Note the generous amount of cerebrospinal fluid around the cerebellar hemispheres (C). A small segment of the cisterna magna (CM) is also shown below the vermis (V).

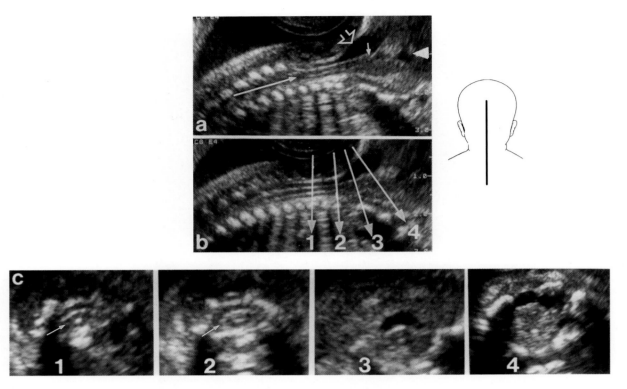

Figure 2–57. A, B. Median sections through the posterior fossa and the upper portion of the spinal cord. The *open arrow* indicates the cisterna magna; the *small arrow,* the medulla oblongata; and the *arrowhead,* the fourth ventricle (at 17 postmenstrual weeks). **B** is similar to **A,** the *arrows* and the *numbers* showing the levels at which the cross-sections shown in **C** were taken. **(1, 2)** These sections were taken at the cervical level. The *arrow* indicates the spinal cord. **(3, 4)** These sections were obtained at the level of the medulla oblongata.

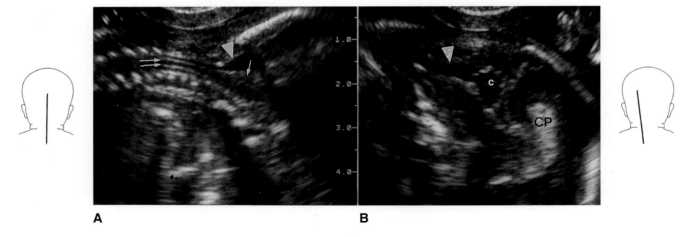

Figure 2–58. Imaging the upper spinal cord and the posterior fossa at 18 postmenstrual weeks. **A.** Median section. The *small arrow* indicates the medulla oblongata; the *arrowhead,* the cisterna magna; the *double arrow,* the spinal cord. **B.** Paramedian section through the cerebellar hemisphere (C) and the posterior horn of the lateral ventricle with the choroid plexus (CP).

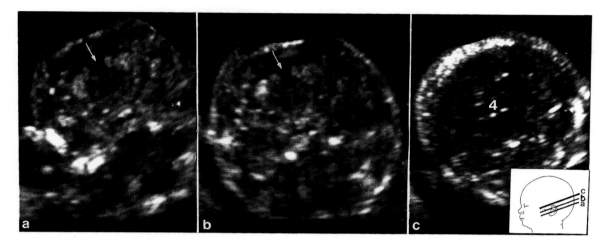

Figure 2–59. Anatomy of the cerebellum and the vermis in the posterior fossa at 15 to 16 postmenstrual weeks. **A.** A low almost-axial section reveals the open communication (Magendie) between the cerebello medullary cistern (cisterna magna) and the fourth ventricle *(arrow)*. **B.** A somewhat higher section still shows the communication. **C.** The highest of the three sections demonstrates that the vermis at this level is already present.

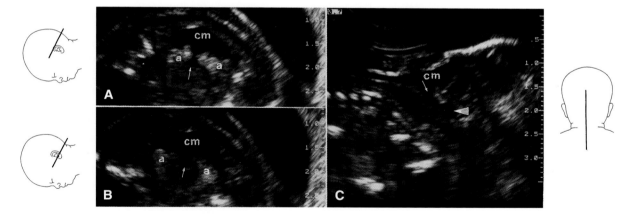

Figure 2–60. Anatomy of the posterior fossa at 19 postmenstrual weeks and 4 days. **A, B.** Two parallel axial sections demonstrating the still partially open connection between the cisterna magna (cm) and the median aperture of the fourth ventricle *(small arrows)*. The slightly more echogenic lowermost portions of the two cerebellar hemispheres are evident. The *arrowhead* indicates the fourth ventricle. a, Amygdala. **C.** Median section. The *white line* is the plane along which the two axial sections in **A** and **B** were taken. p, Pons; c, cerebellum. The *arrowhead* marks the fourth ventricle.

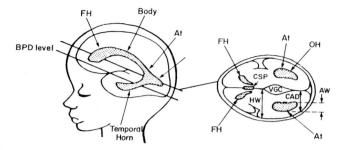

Figure 2–61. Schematic representation of a sagittal view of the fetal ventricular system at a level slightly above that normally used for obtaining the biparietal diameter. FH, Frontal horn; At, atrium; OH, occipital horn; CSP, cavum septi pellucidi; HW, hemispheric width; CAD, cerebroatrial distance; VGC, cerebral vein of Galen; AW, atrial width. *(From Pilu and colleagues, 1989,[55] with permission.)*

sagittal sections—Figures 2–31G, 2–32D through F, 2–43A, 2–45, 2–57A and B, 2–58A and B, and 2–60.

Figures 2–32F, 2–57, 2–58, and 2–60B depict the upper spinal cord. To achieve a good view of the posterior fossa and the upper spinal cord, the transducer should ideally be over the nuchal area of the fetus. It is obvious that such views are not always possible. Gentle manipulation of the fetal position using the abdominally placed second hand of the scanning person, in combination with equally gentle touching with the tip of the vaginal probe, may ease the fetus into the desired position.

By knowing the normal anatomy of the posterior fossa, early detection of pathology (e.g., Dandy–Walker cysts, atrophy of the vermis, and posterior cephalocele) is feasible as early as 10 to 11 postmenstrual weeks.

Because the size of the cerebellum is easy to image on axial as well as coronal sections, this structure has been discussed in detail by various authors. The bicerebellar (lateral edge–to–lateral edge) measurement has been plotted and published by several centers.[76,77]

Sulci, Fissures, and Gyri

Examination of the sulci, fissures, and gyri is one of the many instances when fetal neuroimaging is fashioned after that of the neonatal brain scanning by ultrasonography.

Neuropathologists and pediatric neurologists use sequential sulcal and gyral developments as a clinical estimate of fetal age, particularly between 22 and 34 postmenstrual weeks.[78–83] Deformities or delayed development of the cingulate gyrus may predict disease in the immediate neighborhood of this structure.[84]

In spite of the fact that rather crude timing of the fetal age is possible, based on the developmental stages of the gyri and the sulci, it seems that perinatologists may never have to rely on these markers to determine age. However, it may, at times, be important to assess cortical maturation and development as well as diseases that affect formation of the cerebral cortex.

Performing antenatal neurosonography enables us to evaluate some of the sulci, fissures, and gyri of the developing fetal brain. Before these structures are shown as they progressively appear on the ultrasound screen, a list of the major sulci, fissures, and gyri of the mature human brain is shown in Figures 2–62 through 2–67. These images depict the mature brain in normal neonates. The next step is to examine the sequential appearance of the sulci, fissures, and gyri as a function of increasing fetal age, expressed in weeks from the LMP. Tables 2–6 and 2–7 were compiled using data from Chi and associates.[85] This group examined photographs of 507 brains and serial sections of 209 brains from pathological specimens of fetuses 10 to 44 weeks from the LMP. They concluded that many gyri become well defined within a short period (between 26 and 28 postmenstrual weeks). Thereafter, only a few gyri develop. During the last trimester the gyri and the sulci become more prominent and deep, giving rise to secondary and tertiary gyri.

In 1977, a study examining 80 brains ranging in age from 22 postmenstrual weeks to 1 month of postnatal life was published by Dorovini-Zis and Dolman.[86] They concluded that at 22 postmenstrual weeks the cerebral hemispheres are smooth and the lateral sulci on both sides are wide open. The parietooccipital and calcarine fissures are present on the medial surface. By 24 postmenstrual weeks the central sulcus begins to form and the cingulate sulcus is seen. By 26 postmenstrual weeks deepening of these fissures and sulci occurs. A great growth spurt takes place between 28 and 30 postmenstrual weeks. The sulci and the gyri deepen and become more branched. Figure 2–66 depicts the development of the sulci and the gyri as described in the work of Dorovini-Zis and Dolman.[86]

Slagle's group[80] studied the development of the cingulate sulcus in preterm infants by performing cranial ultrasonographic scans. Two hundred eleven infants from 24 to 40 postmenstrual weeks were studied on their third postnatal day of life. These investigators identified five patterns: (1) a discontinuous line of the sulcus appears, (2) a continuous line appears, (3) first branches of the primary sulcus appear (marginal ramus), (4) multiple branches of the primary sulcus appear, and (5) multiple branches

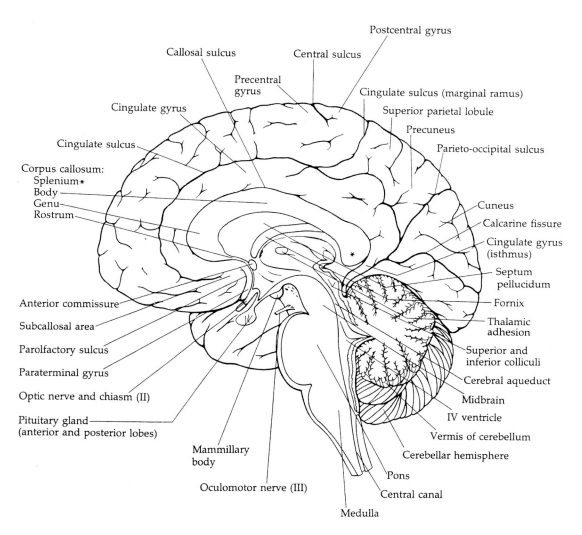

Figure 2–62. Medial surface of the cerebral hemisphere and median section through the diencephalon, brain stem, cerebellum, and rostral spinal cord of a mature brain. The sulci and the gyri and other major structures of the medial cerebral surface are shown. *(From Martin, 1989,[40] with permission.)*

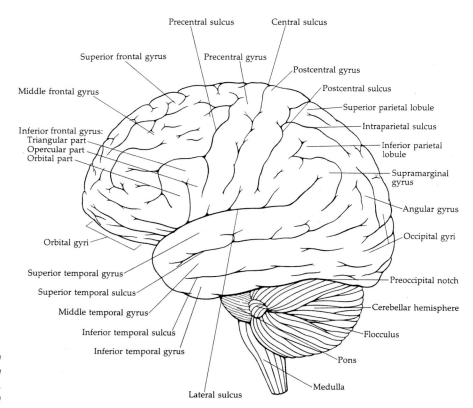

Figure 2–63. Lateral surface of the cerebral hemisphere, emphasizing the gyri and the sulci of a mature brain. *(From Martin, 1989,[40] with permission.)*

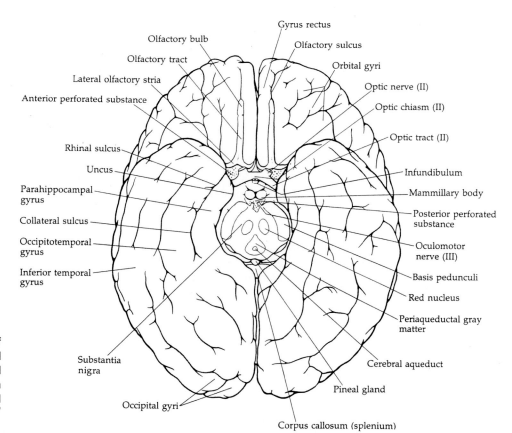

Figure 2–64. Inferior surface of the cerebral hemispheres and the diencephalon. The gyri and the sulci are marked. The brain stem is transected at the rostral midbrain. *(From Martin, 1989,[40] with permission.)*

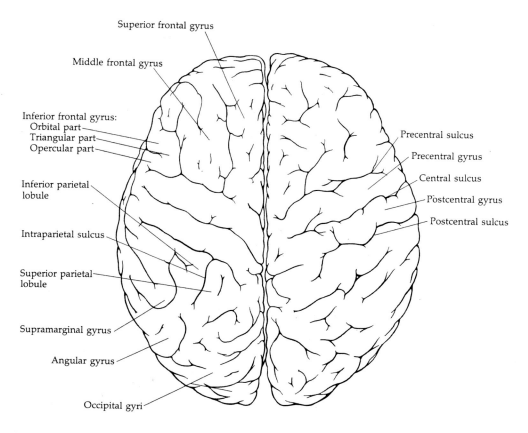

Figure 2–65. Gyri and sulci of the superior surface of the cerebral hemisphere. *(From Martin, 1989,[40] with permission.)*

appear and merge with other sulci, giving the surface a "cobblestone" appearance.

Figure 2–67 depicts the sequential appearance of these five patterns. The first pattern appeared at 24 postmenstrual weeks, the first straight line was seen at 26 ± 2 postmenstrual weeks, first branching appeared at 32 ± 3 postmenstrual weeks, multiple branches occurred at 34 ± 3 postmenstrual weeks, and the cobblestone pattern appeared after 38 postmenstrual weeks. This study suggested that cingulate sulcus maturation occurs in a predictable pattern (Fig. 2–68). Slagle and colleagues[84] also studied 30 infants with evidence of brain damage. These infants showed significant delay in the postnatal development of the cingulate sulcus.

Our observations of the developing cortex using transvaginal ultrasonography focused on three readily available planes. The first was the median plane, which touches the medial aspect of the cerebral hemisphere and scans along the longitudinal fissure. The second available plane is a midcoronal plane at the level of the anterior horns. The third is an extreme lateral right or left oblique plane "touching" almost tangentially the upper surface of the cerebral hemispheres, emphasizing the lateral sulcus and the insula.

We focused on the following sulci and fissures: on the median plane the cingulate sulcus with its marginal ramus, the posterior occipital sulcus, and the calcarine sulcus; and on the coronal plane the longitudinal fissure, with its progressive branching of the cingulate sulcus. Finally, on the lateral sagittal section we examined the shape of the lateral sulcus and the underlying insula. Figures 2–69 through 2–71 clearly show progressive deepening and branching as well as curving of the different fissures and sulci and the appearance of the insula, respectively. Relative flatness of the cortex is present until 24 to 25 postmenstrual weeks, with widely gaping longitudinal fissures, calcarine, posterior occipital fissures, and lateral sulcus (insula). At 28 to 30 postmenstrual weeks significant depth and branching of the sulci and fissures occur. Between 30 and 36 postmenstrual weeks more secondary branching develops, and at 38 postmenstrual weeks the tertiary branching is seen.

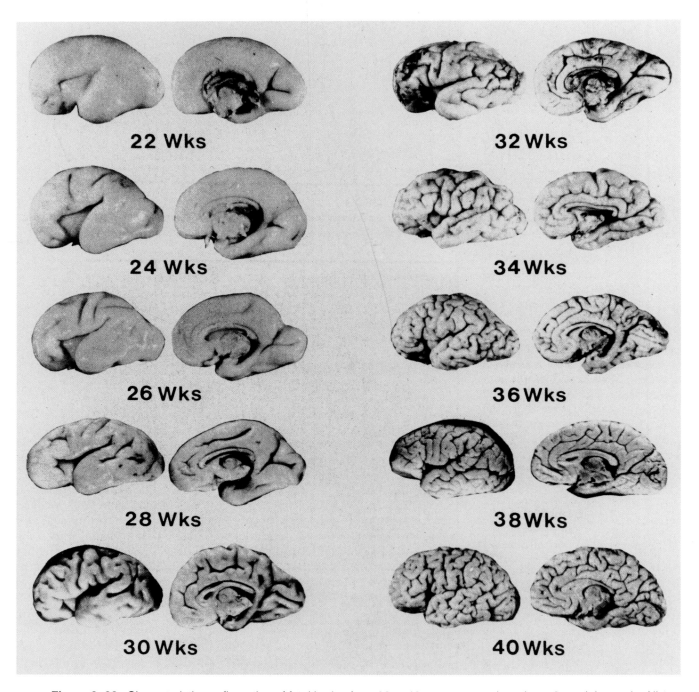

22 Wks

24 Wks

26 Wks

28 Wks

30 Wks

32 Wks

34 Wks

36 Wks

38 Wks

40 Wks

Figure 2–66. Characteristic configuration of fetal brains from 22 to 40 postmenstrual weeks at 2-week intervals. All brains have been brought to the same size. *(From Dorovini-Zis and Dolman, 1977,[86] with permission.)*

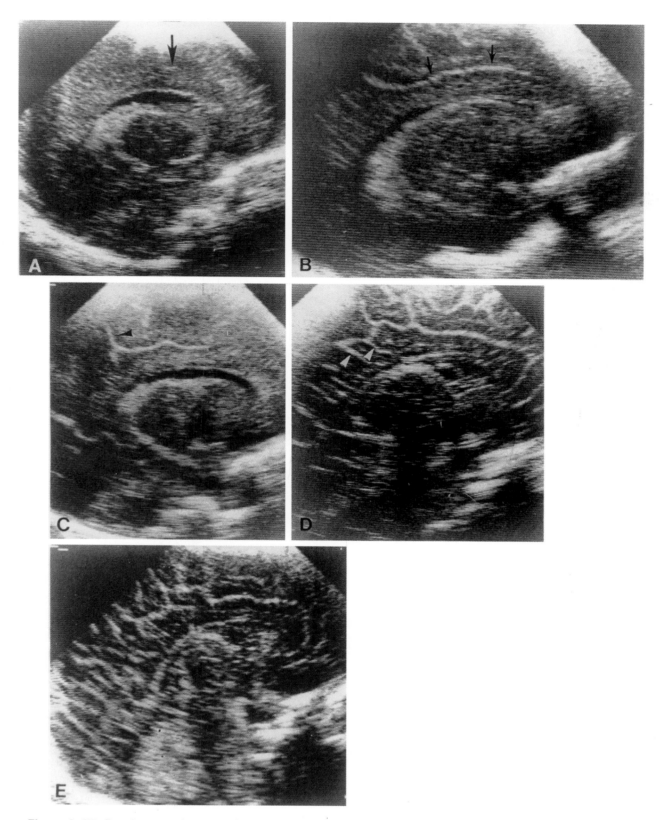

Figure 2–67. Developmental stages of the cingulate sulcus. Paramedian sonograms demonstrating five developmental stages: **(A)** the presence of one or more discontinuous linear echoes *(arrow);* **(B)** continuity—a single continuous linear echo *(arrows);* **(C)** first branch—perpendicular echo of the primary sulcus *(arrowhead);* **(D)** multiple branches—additional branches off the primary sulcus *(arrowheads);* and **(E)** "cobblestone" pattern branches from the cingulate sulcus, merging with other cortical sulci. *(From Slagle and colleagues, 1989,[84] with permission.)*

TABLE 2–6. TEMPORAL DEVELOPMENT OF THE CEREBRAL HEMISPHERES

Gestational Age* (No. Examined)	Sulci and Fissures	Gyri
10–15 weeks (n = 6)	Interhemispheric fissure, sylvian fissure, transverse cerebral fissure, callosal sulcus	—
16–19 weeks (n = 13)	Parieto-occipital fissure, olfactory sulcus, circular sulcus, cingulate sulcus, calcarine fissure	Gyrus rectus, insula, cingulate gyrus
20–23 weeks (n = 41)	Rolandic sulcus, collateral sulcus, superior temporal sulcus	Parahippocampal gyrus, superior temporal gyrus
24–27 weeks (n = 46)	Prerolandic sulcus, middle temporal sulcus, postrolandic sulcus, interparietal sulcus, superior frontal sulcus, lateral occipital sulcus	Prerolandic gyrus, middle temporal gyrus, postrolandic gyrus, superior and inferior parietal lobules, superior and middle frontal gyri, superior and inferior occipital gyrus, cuneus and lingual gyrus, fusiform gyrus
28–31 weeks (n = 36)	Inferior temporal sulcus, inferior frontal sulcus	Inferior temporal gyrus, triangular gyrus, medial and lateral orbital gyrus, callosomarginal gyrus, transverse temporal gyrus, angular and supramarginal gyrus, external occipitotemporal gyrus
32–35 weeks (n = 29)	Marginal sulcus Secondary superior, middle, and inferior frontal; superior and middle temporal; superior and inferior parietal; prerolandic and postrolandic, superior and inferior occipital sulci and gyri; insular gyri	Paracentral gyrus
36–39 weeks (n = 31)	Secondary transverse and inferior temporal and cingulate sulci and gyri; tertiary superior, middle, and inferior frontal and superior and inferior parietal sulci and gyri	Anterior and posterior orbital gyri
40–44 weeks (n = 29)	Secondary orbital, callosomarginal, and insular sulci and gyri; tertiary inferior temporal and superior and inferior occipital gyri and sulci	

After Chi and colleagues, 1977,[85] with permission.
*Postmenstrual weeks.

The clinical significance of these observations is still not clear. It may be possible to establish whether the cortex progresses along a well-defined and age-dependent pattern. It may also be feasible to detect diseases of the fetal brain that are expressed by a delayed or nonexistent maturational process.

The sonographic appearance of the sulci and the fissures is dependent on the higher-echogenicity pia mater (pachymeninx) and the pia–arachnoid complex, also called the "soft brain covering" or the leptomeninx. Note that the high echogenicity of the choroid plexus is due to the highly vascular and abundant presence of the pia mater. The highly echogenic leptomeninx or the choroid plexus in close proximity to the CSF generates a highly visible interface, which appears as bright echoes. The *dura* is prominent in those places where it protrudes into the brain to separate structures. These two dura-containing places are the falx (Figs. 2–27, 2–30, 2–31, 2–33, 2–38, 2–39, 2–41, 2–50, and 2–55) and the tentorium (Figs. 2–31, 2–38, 2–40, and 2–41). The *pia* closely follows the surface of the cortex. Wherever a fissure or a sulcus is present, the pia (and, at times, the arachnoid) closely follows, making this a sonographically easily recognized structure. In the case of the cerebellar cortex, and even more so the vermis of the cerebellum, which have extremely abundant and tightly folded gyri and sulci, the sonographic image shows extremely bright echoes. The sonographic hallmark of the vermis is its easily recognizable high echogenicity, due to the repeatedly infolded double layers of leptomeninges (Figs. 2–32, 2–44, 2–45, 2–48, 2–53, 2–59, and 2–60).

It is hard to image sonographically the convexity of the cerebral hemisphere. Thus, it is rare to see a small area of the tangential picture of the gyri and the sulci. However, the medial surface of the cere-

TABLE 2–7. REGIONAL DEVELOPMENT OF THE CEREBRAL HEMISPHERES

Lobe	Fissures and Sulci	Weeks*	Gyri	Weeks
Frontal	Interhemispheric fissure	10	Gyrus rectus	16
	Transverse cerebral fissure	10	Insula	18
	Callosal sulcus	14	Cingulate gyrus	18
	Sylvian fissure	14	Prerolandic gyrus	24
	Olfactory sulcus	16	Superior frontal gyrus	25
	Circular sulcus	18	Middle frontal gyrus	27
	Cingulate sulcus	18	Triangular gyrus	28
	Rolandic sulcus	20	Medial and lateral orbital gyrus	28
	Prerolandic sulcus	24	Callosomarginal gyrus	28
	Superior frontal sulcus	25	Anterior and posterior orbital gyrus	36
	Inferior frontal sulcus	28		
Parietal	Interhemispheric fissure	10	Cingulate gyrus	18
	Transverse cerebral fissure	10	Postrolandic gyrus	25
	Sylvian fissure	14	Superior parietal lobule	26
	Parieto-occipital fissure	16	Inferior parietal lobule	26
	Rolandic sulcus	20	Angular gyrus	28
	Postrolandic sulcus	25	Supramarginal gyrus	28
	Interparietal sulcus	26	Paracentral gyri	35
Temporal	Sylvian fissure	14	Superior temporal gyrus	23
	Superior temporal sulcus	23	Parahippocampal gyrus	23
	Collateral sulcus	23	Middle temporal gyrus	26
	Middle temporal sulcus	26	Fusiform gyrus	27
	Inferior temporal sulcus	30	Inferior temporal gyrus	30
			External occipitotemporal gyrus	30
			Transverse temporal gyrus	31
Occipital	Interhemispheric fissure	10	Superior occipital gyri	27
	Calcarine fissure	16	Inferior occipital gyri	27
	Parieto-occipital sulcus	16	Cuneus	27
	Collateral sulcus	23	Lingual gyrus	27
	Lateral occipital sulcus	27	External occipitotemporal gyrus	30

After Chi and colleagues, 1977,[85] with permission.
*Postmenstrual weeks.

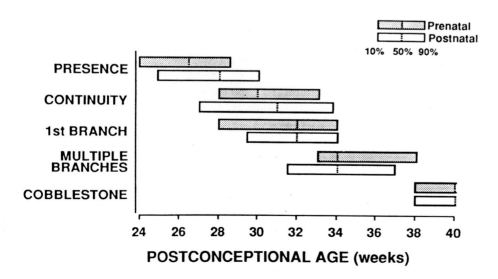

Figure 2–68. Developmental sequence of the cingulate sulcus. Shown is a comparison of the 10%, 50%, and 90% levels of prenatal *(stippled bars)* and postnatal *(open bars)* development of the cingulate sulcus. There was no difference in cingulate sulcus landmark timing between prenatal (determined on initial sonograms of 211 infants of 24 to 40 postmenstrual weeks' gestational age) and postnatal development (determined on serial ultrasound examinations from week 1 of age to 40 weeks' postconceptual age in the 144 infants born at less than 32 weeks' postmenstrual age). *(From Slagle and colleagues, 1989,[84] with permission.)*

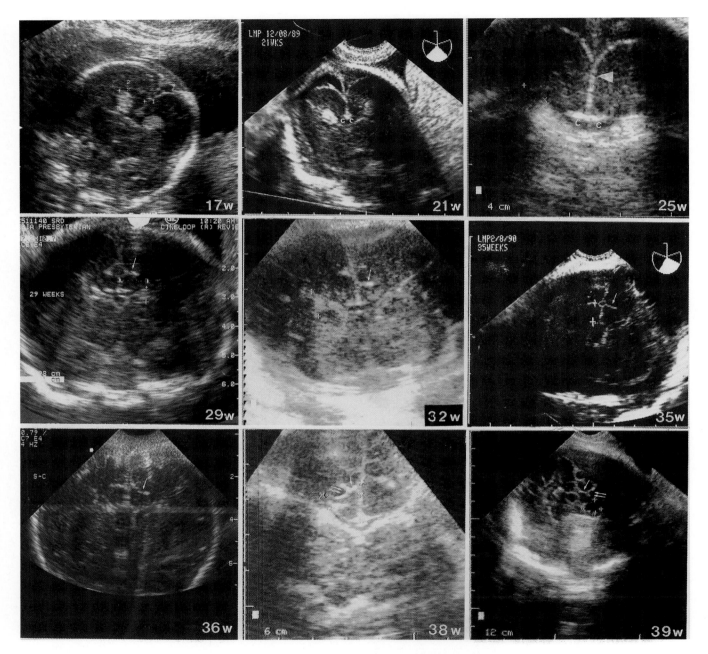

Figure 2–69. Development of the sulci and the gyri. Coronal sections (usually midcoronal–2) from 17 to 39 postmenstrual weeks are depicted. Note that at first the straight line of the longitudinal fissure (*arrowhead* shown at 25 postmenstrual weeks). At 25 to 28 postmenstrual weeks (not shown) the first indentation of the cingulate sulcus (*small single arrow*) appears and remains evident up to 36 weeks. At 37 to 38 postmenstrual weeks secondary and, finally, tertiary branches appear (*small double arrows*). CC, Corpus callosum; CG, cingulate gyrus.

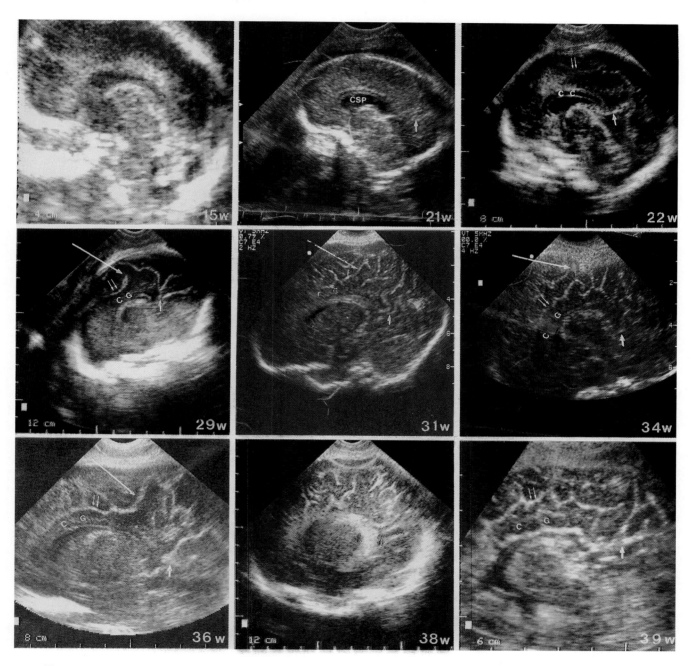

Figure 2–70. Development of the fissures, sulci, and gyri. The median sections from 15 to 39 postmenstrual weeks show the first appearance of the cingulate gyrus (CG) and the cingulate sulcus *(small double arrows)* at 22 post-menstrual weeks and the calcarine fissure and the parieto-occipital sulcus *(arrow)* at 21 postmenstrual weeks. Note the progressive appearance of the "cobblestone" gyral pattern, fully recognizable at 38 to 39 postmenstrual weeks. The *long arrow* points to the callosomarginal sulcus. CC, Corpus callosum; CG, cingulate gyrus.

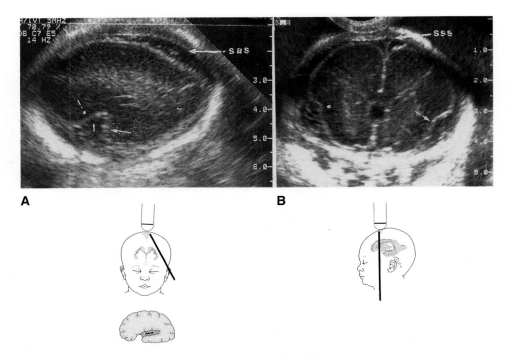

A   B

Figure 2–71. The insula, lateral sulcus, and subarachnoid space at 25 postmenstrual weeks. **A.** On the left Oblique–2 extremely lateral sagittal section the subarachnoid space (sas), the operculum *(arrows),* and the insula are shown. **B.** On the Midcoronal–1 plane the subarachnoid space surrounding the superior sagittal sinus (sss) and the insula *(arrows)* are depicted.

bral hemisphere along the longitudinal fissure is quite easily imaged by ultrasonographic techniques. It is this flat surface where good images of the cortex are obtained.

Fetal and neonatal sulcal examination by ultrasonography is a noninvasive and convenient method to assess cerebral maturation. This cerebral maturation has, so far, been proven only in neonates. However, if the proper methodology is developed for use in fetal neurosonology, it may prove to be useful.

Imaging the Blood Vessels of the Fetal Brain

At times, lesions of the fetal brain can be better understood if the blood supply to that area is known or if the presence or absence of a known blood vessel would indicate the specific lesion in question. For example, the pericallosal artery is present if the corpus callosum is developed. Its absence supports the diagnosis of agenesis of the corpus callosum. The CNS is dependent on continuous uninterrupted blood flow. Even relatively short cessation of this flow causes severe anatomic lesions of the region to which the supply of oxygen and various nutrients was cut off.

The arterial blood supply to the brain comes from the anterior and posterior circulations.[40, 87]

The anterior circulation is derived from the internal carotid arteries. The posterior circulation is fed by the vertebral arteries, which join at the level of the pontomedullar junction to give rise to a single basilar artery in the median plane. These two circulations interconnect on the inferior as well as the cortical surface of the brain. The hemispheres are supplied predominantly by the anterior circulation. The midbrain and the medulla derive their blood supply from the posterior circulation (Fig. 2–72A).

Internal Carotid Artery

The course of the internal carotid artery may be considered in four main parts: cervical, petrous, cavernous, and cerebral. The cervical part enters the carotid canal in the petrous part of the temporal bone. The petrous part is closely related to the internal and middle ear. At the foramen lacerum the petrous part ascends and then enters the cavernous sinus. The cavernous part passes forward along the side of the sella turcica and pierces the dural roof of the sinus. The cerebral part turns backward and, at the medial end of the lateral sulcus, divides into the anterior and middle cerebral arteries: (1) the ophthalmic artery, (2) the posterior communicating artery, (3) the anterior choroid artery, (4) the anterior cerebral artery, (5) and the middle cerebral artery. (Fig. 2–72b)

The course of the vertebral artery may be considered in four parts: cervical, vertebral, suboccipital, and intracranial. The suboccipital part passes through the foramen magnum. At the lower border of the pons, the two right and left vessels unite to form the basilar artery. The main paired branches of the basilar artery are (1) the anterior inferior cerebellar artery, (2) the superior cerebellar artery, and (3) the posterior cerebral artery.

Two major communicating arteries connect the anterior and posterior circulations into a polygonal system of vessels. The reason for these large anastomoses is probably to regulate blood supply at times of an occlusion of either system.

The ringlike communicating system of the blood vessels on the basis of the brain surrounding the pineal body and the mamillary bodies is called the circulus arteriosus, described by Willis (Fig. 2–73). It is built from the following sources and arteries: (1) the anteriorly turning *right* and *left anterior cerebral arteries;* (2) the *internal carotid arteries;* (3) the *anterior communicating artery,* connecting the previously mentioned arteries (an unpaired arterial link; on the two sides both *posterior communicating arteries* link); (4) the two *middle cerebral arteries* (as mentioned, arising from the anterior circulation); and (5) the *posterior cerebral arteries.*

The medial surface of the hemisphere, as far as the blood supply is concerned, is important to mention because it can be scrutinized using ultrasound waves. Figure 2–72 is a graphic representation of the main branches of the arteries supplying blood to these areas. The anterior cerebral arteries give rise to the *frontal polar* and *medial orbitofrontal* arteries. After the left and right anterior cerebral arteries are linked by the anterior communicating artery, the *pericallosal artery* emerges; proceeding on top (on the dorsal surface) of the corpus callosum, it turns upward and ends in the precuneal artery, turning on to the outer surface of the hemispheres.

The *callosomarginal artery* arises from the pericallosal artery at the level of the genu of the corpus callosum and runs in the depth of the cingulate sulcus, above the cingulate gyrus. This artery also turns upward and ends in its marginal branch: the paracentral artery. The callosomarginal artery gives off several branches, which, when turning upward, supply the gyri above this area.

The *posterior cerebral artery* branches into the *parieto-occipital* and *calcarine arteries* (which are found in the sulci bearing the same name) as well as the *posterior pericallosal artery.*

The *middle cerebral artery* takes its course to the laterally situated lateral sulcus (of Sylvus), to reach the lateral surface of the hemispheres (Fig. 2–74). This artery has a rather indirect course because it must pass over the insular surface and the temporal, parietal, and frontal lobes before it reaches the lateral surface of the hemispheres. The middle cerebral artery also feeds the nuclei of the midbrain through the lenticulostriate arteries, among others.

Venous drainage of the CNS is achieved in two ways. (1) One way is the direct route or the direct drainage into the systemic circulation. The lower part of the medulla and the vertebral column return their share of the blood by this direct way. (2) Most other areas of the brain collect the blood into major *dural sinuses,* such as the *superior sagittal sinus,* the straight sinus (which also drains the great cerebral vein (of Galen), the inferior sagittal sinus, two transverse sinuses, the superior petrosal sinus, and the cavernous sinus, to name the major ones. The dural sinuses are also responsible for resorbing the CSF.

The ventricles and the subarachnoid spaces contain CSF. About two thirds of this fluid is secreted by the choroid plexus located along the different ventricles. About one third of the fluid is contributed by the brain capillaries adjacent to the open spaces on the surface of the brain. In adults about 500 mL of fluid is formed and then reabsorbed by the dural sinuses through arachnoid granulations.

The CSF flows from the ventricles toward the interventricular foramina and joins the fluid arising from the third ventricle (Fig. 2–75). Then the fluid flows along the cerebral aqueduct and, reaching the fourth ventricle, continues to the two lateral apertures and a single median aperture, which drain the fluid into the *cisterns.* The CSF then spreads through the cisterns and surrounds the hemispheres along the subarachnoid spaces. After reaching the arachnoid granulations, it is reabsorbed in the dural sinuses, as mentioned.

Sonographic Appearance of the Cerebral Blood Vessels

The cerebral circulation can be documented at 8 postmenstrual weeks (Fig 2–76) in the form of discrete pulsations of the interacerebral part of the largest vessel: the internal carotid artery.[88] The visualization rate of obtaining intracranial blood flow using TVS at the eighth postmenstrual week was 50 percent[88] (Fig. 2–77). This detection rate for the middle cerebral artery became 71 percent at 9 postmenstrual weeks (Fig. 2–78), 83 percent at 10 weeks (Fig. 2–79), and finally, 100 percent at 11 to

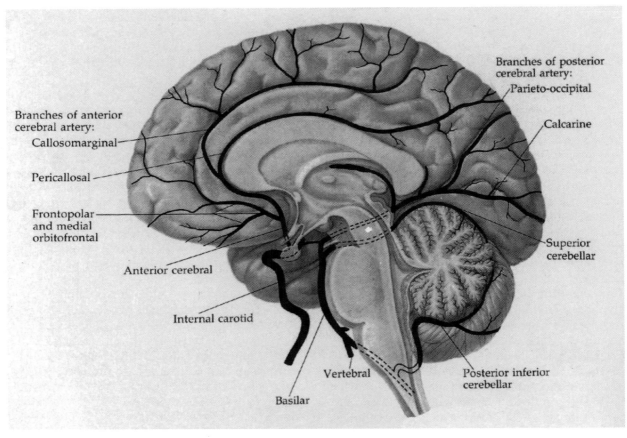

A

Figure 2–72.   A. The courses of the three cerebral arteries are illustrated as viewed from the medial surface. *(From Martin, 1989,[40] with permission.)*

18 weeks of the pregnancy (Fig. 2–78). Van den Wijngard and associates[89] reported a 91 percent detection rate for the middle cerebral artery in the second and third trimesters. The literature reflects on the better identification of the intercerebral arteries in the first trimester of pregnancy by the TVS method.

As pregnancy progresses, an increasing number of new vessels can be detected using color Doppler or power Doppler studies. Figure 2–80 demonstrates the change in the number of the detectable vessels from 15 to 19 and to 25 postmenstrual weeks.

Sonographic detection of the brain arteries, but most importantly that of the middle cerebral artery, has practical implications. The middle cere-bral artery caries the largest volume of blood to the hemispheres.[83] This artery can be imaged almost throughout its entire course, using different scanning planes. On the axial plane its origin is clear by looking at the circulus arteriosus (of Willis) (Fig. 2–81). The next segment can be followed using a Midcoronal–1 section (Figs. 2–82 and 84). The anterior branches of this artery are seen on the Median or very slightly parasagittal sections (Fig. 2–83).

With regard to predicting blood flow to the brain of normal as well as growth-regarted fetuses, studies of the middle cerebral arteries were performed mostly using transabdominal ultrasound Doppler techniques. Lately, the transvaginal route

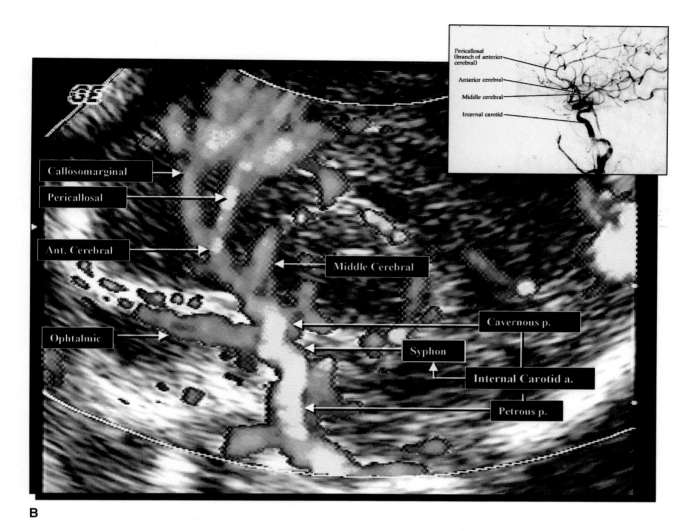

Figure 2–72. **B.** Transvaginal color (power) Doppler image showing the arterial circulation of some of the anterior branches of the internal carotid artery. The picture was obtained through the anterior fontanelle at 17 postmenstrual weeks using a slightly paramedian plane.

has become an alternate route to approaching the cerebral vessels, provided that the fetus is in the vertex presentation. The implications as well as the technique of these Doppler studies are discussed in Chapter 17.

A new imaging technology developed in the last few years is the color power angiography, or power Doppler imaging of flow. This technique is extremely sensitive, even to low or high velocities, and is not influenced by the direction of flow. The images appear as if on a real angiogram of the vascular tree. A few of these images are included here.

As far as the sonographic appearance and location of the internal carotid artery are concerned, these can be seen using color flow Doppler tech-

niques and turning mostly to the axial sections (Fig. 2–81) as well as the coronal sections (Fig. 2–82).

On the median section in the sagittal plane the following arteries can also be recognized: (1) the pericallosal and callosmarginal arteries, turning upward and ending in their marginal branches (Figs. 2–72B, 2–80, 2–83, and 2–84A); (2) at times, the parieto-occipital branch of the posterior cerebral artery; and (3) on the extreme lateral Oblique–2 section, a segment of the middle cerebral artery.

On the coronal sections the following arteries are seen: (1) on the Frontal–2 section, the branches of the right and left anterior cerebral arteries and the first segments of the callosomarginal and pericallosal arteries; (2) on a Midcoronal–1 section, the

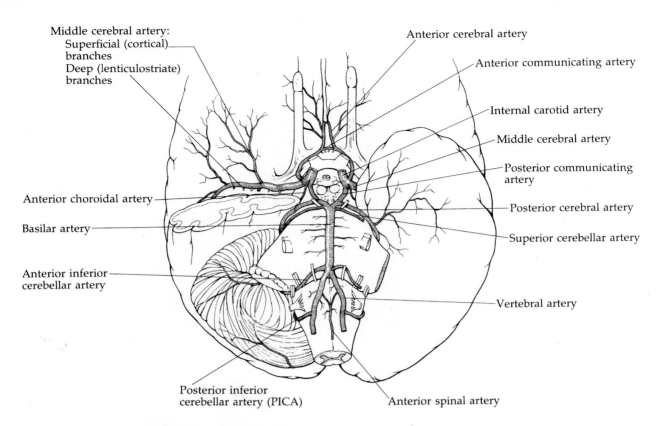

Middle cerebral artery:
  Superficial (cortical) branches
  Deep (lenticulostriate) branches

Anterior cerebral artery

Anterior communicating artery

Internal carotid artery

Middle cerebral artery

Posterior communicating artery

Posterior cerebral artery

Superior cerebellar artery

Anterior choroidal artery

Basilar artery

Anterior inferior cerebellar artery

Vertebral artery

Posterior inferior cerebellar artery (PICA)

Anterior spinal artery

Figure 2–73. Diagram of the ventral surface of the brain stem and the cerebral hemispheres, illustrating the key components of the anterior (carotid) circulation and the posterior (vertebral–basilar) circulation. The anterior portion of the temporal lobe is removed to illustrate the course of the middle cerebral artery through the lateral sulcus and the penetrating branches (lenticulostriate arteries). The circulus arteriosus (of Willis) is formed by the anterior communicating artery, the two posterior communicating arteries, and the three cerebral arteries. *(From Martin, 1989,[40] with permission.)*

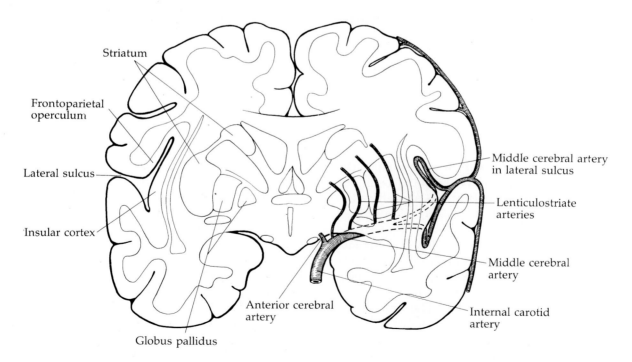

Striatum

Frontoparietal operculum

Lateral sulcus

Insular cortex

Middle cerebral artery in lateral sulcus

Lenticulostriate arteries

Middle cerebral artery

Internal carotid artery

Anterior cerebral artery

Globus pallidus

Figure 2–74. Course of the middle cerebral artery through the lateral sulcus and along the insular and opercular surfaces of the cerebral cortex is shown on a schematic coronal section.

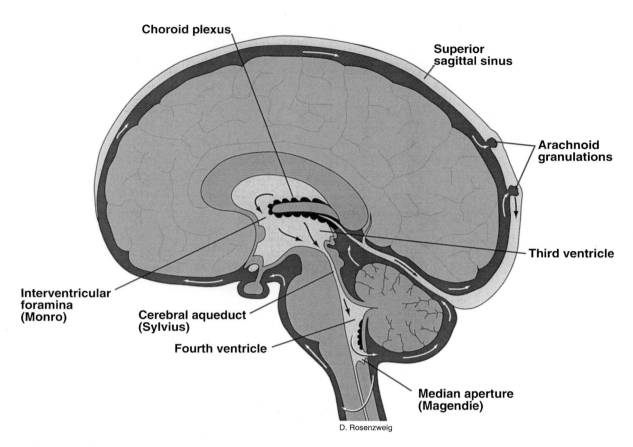

Figure 2–75. Schematic representation of the cerebrospinal fluid circulation, using a median sagittal plane.

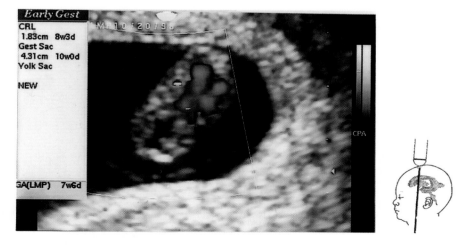

Figure 2–76. Only the middle cerebral arteries could be seen at 7 postmenstrual weeks and 6 days (from the LMP) using power Doppler.

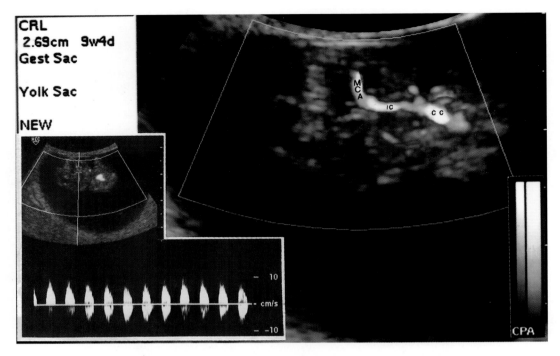

Figure 2–77. At 9 postmenstrual weeks and 4 days (from the LMP), the common carotid artery (CC), the internal carotid artery (IC), and the prominent middle cerebral artery (MCA) can be detected by power Doppler. Note that there is still no diastolic flow detectable in the middle cerebral artery *(inset)*.

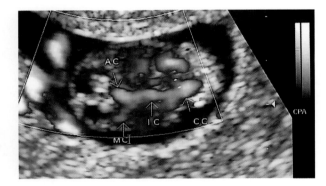

Figure 2–78. At 10 postmenstrual weeks and 2 days (from the LMP), the anterior cerebral artery (AC) can be seen in addition to the previously seen common carotid artery (CC), internal carotid artery (IC), and the middle cerebral artery (MC).

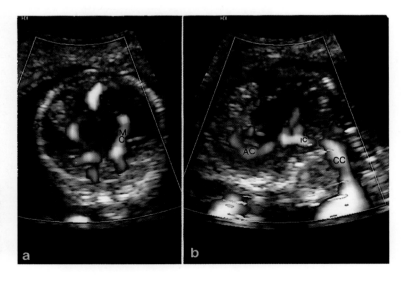

Figure 2–79. At 13 postmenstrual weeks, almost all main brain vessels can be found and imaged by power Doppler interrogation **(a)** coronal section and **(b)** sagittal section. MC, middle cerebral artery; CC, common carotid artery; IC, internal carotid artery; AC, anterior cerebral artery.

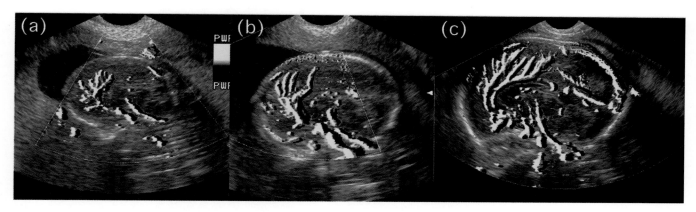

Figure 2–80. Gestational change of the brain circulation **(a)** 15 postmenstrual weeks, **(b)** 19 postmenstrual weeks, and **(c)** 25 postmenstrual weeks.

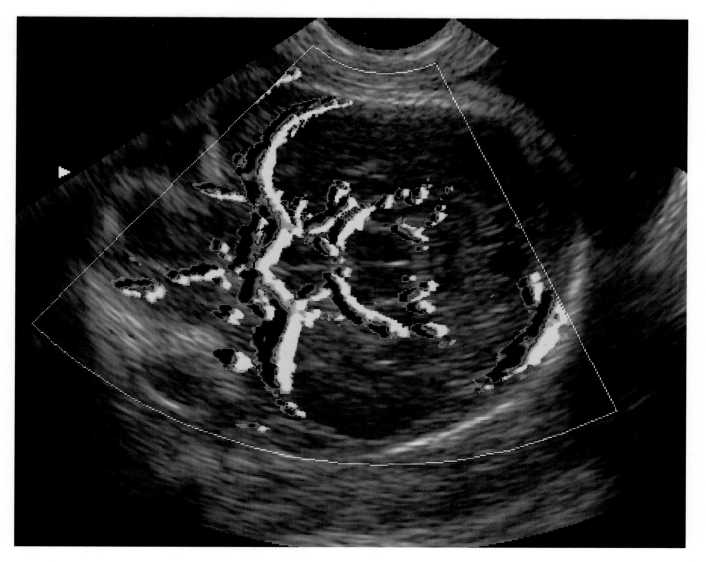

Figure 2–81. Power Doppler scan of the circle of Willis. *(Courtesy of RK Pooh MD. Clinical Research Institute, National Zentsui Hospital, Japan).*

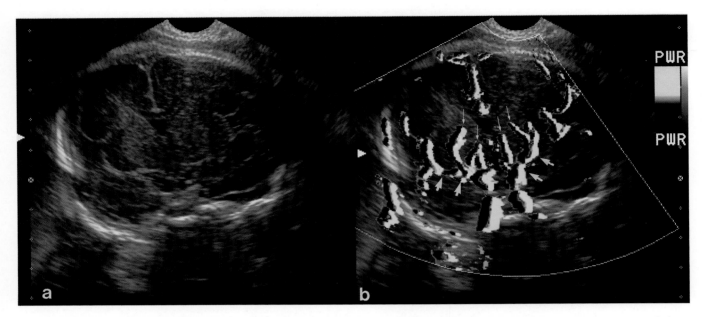

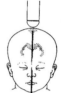

Figure 2–82. On the Midcoronal–1 section the gray scale image **(a)** is depicting the brain anatomy. Turning on the power Doppler **(b)** the lentricular branches *(small arrow)* of the middle cerebral artery (arrows) are shown *(Courtesy of RK Pooh MD. Clinical Research Institute, National Zentsui Hospital, Japan).*

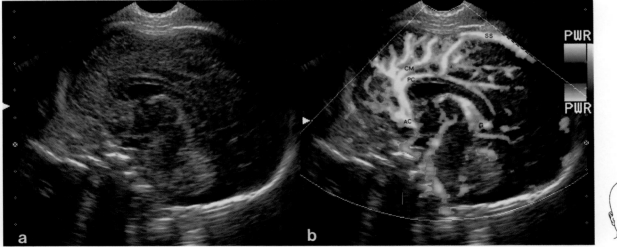

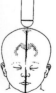

Figure 2–83. On the Median section, the gray scale image **(a)** is showing the brain anatomy. Turning on the power Doppler shown. AC, anterior cerebral artery; PC, pericallosal artery; CM, callosomarginal artery; SS, superior sagittal sinus; G, vein of Galen. *(Courtesy of RK Pooh MD. Clinical Research Institute, National Zentsui Hospital, Japan).*

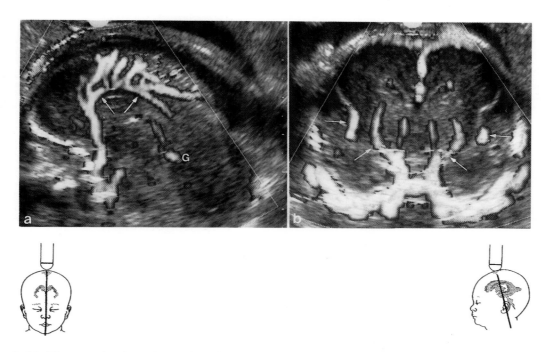

Figure 2–84. The most basic work-up of the fetal vascular supply is compressed in these two images, **(a)** on the median section the pericallosal artery *(two arrows)* and the great cerebral vein (of Galen) (G) have to be documented, and **(b)** on the Midcoronal–1 or –2 section the symmetrical blood supply to the midbrain and the insula (by the middle cerebral arteries) have to be documented *(arrows)*.

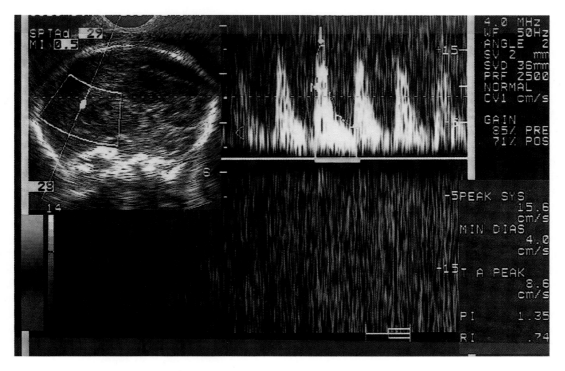

Figure 2–85. Any of the arteries can be interrogated, with regard to their blood flow properties, by placing the gate (sample volume) over a segment of it. In this example the waveform, velocities, and resistance indices of the callosomarginal artery are displayed.

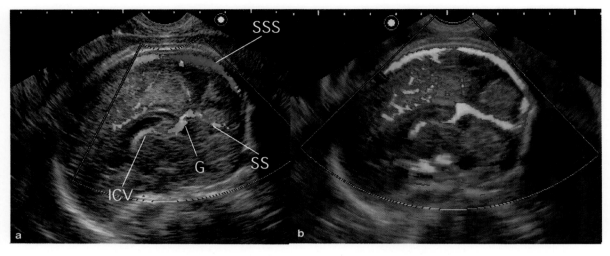
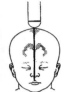

Figure 2–86. Intracerebral venous circulation in the median section **(a)** color and **(b)** power Doppler images. Superior sagittal sinus (SSS), internal cerebral vein (ICV), great cerebral vein (of Galen) (G), and straight sinus (SS) are demonstrated. *(Courtesy of RK Pooh MD. Clinical Research Institute, National Zentsui Hospital, Japan.*

main, upward-turning midcerebral artery (Fig. 2–82B); (3) on a Midcoronal–2 section, the middle cerebral and upward-pointing branches of the anterior cerebral arteries in the interhemispheric area; and (4) on a Midcoronal–1, –2, and –3 section, branches of the middle cerebral and posterior cerebral arteries (Figs. 2–82 and 2–84B).

In the last several years, three-dimensional imaging of the fetal brain became possible. Using the transfontanelle approach in selected cases, we were able to obtain a volume scan of the brain using the power Doppler modality. This is useful in cases in which is important to trace the pericallosal artery to establish diagnosis related to the presence or the absence of the corpus callosum. It is also possible to follow the course of a displaced artery by the multiplanar three-dimensional volume scan, scrolling through the volume. This aspect will be discussed in Chapter 9.

Any time an artery is detected by color Doppler studies, a flow study with regard to velocities and resistance to flow can be undertaken. Here, an example of a flow pattern of the callosomarginal artery is shown (Fig. 2–85). An entire chapter is devoted to the subject of flow studies of the cerebral vasculature (Chapter 17).

Venous Drainage of the Central Nervous System

Two routes are present for collecting the blood from the brain. One drains the blood into the systemic circulation. The spinal cord and part of the medulla follow this path. The other structure drains into the dural sinuses. These low-pressure drainage channels run between layers of the dura and finally meet in an area called the confluence of sinuses within the skull in the area of the occipital pole. After the blood reaches confluence, it flows into the internal jugular vein via the transverse sinus and the sigmoid sinus.

Sonographically, it would probably be possible to detect the various sinuses. However, at this time, disease of very few of these sinuses pertinent to the fetal period has been reported. The superior sagittal sinus is easy to image by fetal neurosonography (Fig. 2–83). We were also able to detect the venous system in the median plane, built up from the inferior sagittal sinus flowing into the great cerebral vein (of Galen), continuing through the straight sinus (Fig. 2–86). This area may develop an aneurysm; therefore, its location on the median sagittal section should be familiar to the imaging specialist.

SUMMARY

Neurosonography of the fetus and the neonate is an informative and noninvasive as well as inexpensive modality which is of great benefit in clinical diagnosis. As technology improves and our understanding of sonoanatomy of the fetal and neonatal brain widens, the distinction between normal and abnormal, as far as anatomy is concerned, becomes increasingly possible. Anomalies and disease of the developing brain area are quite common. In order to diagnose a deviation from what is normal, it is important to understand and recognize the normal brain as it forms, develops, grows, and matures, reaching its almost final anatomy at birth.

This chapter has not only presented the developmental landmarks of the embryonic and fetal CNS but also suggested new ways to study it systematically.

The introduction of TVS in fetal neurosonography adds an additional and powerful tool to the diagnostic algorithm, increasing diagnostic precision considerably in patients suspected of having an anatomically abnormal fetal CNS. In the future, this technique will probably be used routinely in all pregnant patients to examine the developing brain, the same way we now examine other fetal organs and organ systems.

REFERENCES

1. Kossoff G, Griffith KA, Dixon CE. Is the quality of transvaginal images superior to transabdominal ones under matched conditions? *Ultrasound Obstet Gynecol.* 1991;1:29–35.
2. Kossoff G, Garret WJ, Radavaniovich G. Ultrasonic atlas normal brain of infant. *Ultrasound Med Biol.* 1974;1:259–266.
3. Garret WJ, Kossoff G, Jones RF. Ultrasonic cross-sectional visualization of hydrocephalus in infants. *Neuroradiology.* 1975;8:279–288.
4. Lees RF, Harrison RB, Sims TL. Gray scale ultrasonography in the evaluation of hydrocephalus and associated abnormalities in infants. *Am J Dis Child.* 1978;132:376–378.
5. Babcock DS, Han BK, LeQuesne GW. B-mode gray scale ultrasound of the head in the newborn and young infant. *AJR.* 1980;134:457–468.
6. Skolnick ML, Rosenbaum AE, Matzuk T, et al. Detection of dilated cerebral ventricle in infants: A correlative study between ultrasound and computed tomography. *Radiology.* 1979;131:447–451.
7. Haber K, Wachter RD, Christenson PC, et al. Ultrasonic evaluation of intracranial pathology in infants: A new technique. *Radiology.* 1980;134:173–178.
8. Vlieger M. Evaluation of echoencephalography. *J Clin Ultrasound.* 1980;8:38.
9. Johnson ML, Rumack CM. Ultrasonic evaluation of the neonatal brain. *Radiol Clin North Am.* 1980; 18:117–131.
10. Ben-Ora A, Eddy L, Hatch G, et al. The anterior fontanelle as an acoustic window to the neonatal ventricular system. *J Clin Ultrasound.* 1980;8:65–67.
11. Dewbury KC, Aluwihare APR. The anterior fontanelle as an ultrasound window for study of the brain: A preliminary report. *Br J Radiol.* 1980;53:81–84.
12. Grant EG, Schelligner D, Borts FT, et al. Real-time sonography of the neonatal and infant head. *AJR.* 1981;136:265–270.
13. Slovis TL, Kuhns LR. Real-time sonography of the brain through the anterior fontanelle. *AJR.* 1981;136: 277–286.
14. Edwards MK, Brown DL, Muller J, et al. Cribside neurosonography: Real-time sonography for intracranial investigation of the neonate. *AJR.* 1981;136:271–276.
15. Pigadas A, Thompson JR, Grube GL. Normal infant brain anatomy: Correlated real-time sonograms and brain specimens. *AJNR.* 1981;2:339–344.
16. Harwood-Nash DC, Flodmark O. Diagnostic imaging of the neonatal brain: Review and protocol. *AJNR.* 1982;3:103–115.
17. Cremin BJ, Chilton SJ, Peacock WJ. Anatomical landmarks in anterior fontanelle ultrasonography. *Br J Radiol.* 1983;56:517.
18. Richardson DJ, Grant EG. Scanning techniques and normal anatomy. In: Grant GE, ed. *Neurosonography of the Preterm Neonate.* New York: Springer-Verlag; 1986:1–24.
19. Naidich TP, Yousefzadeh DK, Gusnard DA. II: The neonatal head. Sonography of the normal neonatal head. Supratentorial structures: State-of-the-art imaging. *Neuroradiology.* 1986;28:408–427.
20. Monteagudo A, Reuss ML, Timor-Tritsch IE. Imaging the fetal brain in the second and third trimesters using transvaginal sonography. *Obstet Gynecol.* 1991;77:27–32.
20a. Blaas HG, Eik-Nes SH, Berg S, Torp H. In vitro three dimensional ultrasound reconstructions of embryos and early fetuses. Lancet 1993;352:1182–1186.
21. Timor-Tritsch IE, Farine D, Rosen MG. A close look at early embryonic development with the high-frequency transvaginal transducer. *Am J Obstet Gynecol.* 1988; 159:676–681.
22. Timor-Tritsch IE, Monteagudo A, Warren WB. Transvaginal ultrasonographic definition of the central nervous system in the first and early second trimesters. *Am J Obstet Gynecol.* 1991;164:747–753.
23. Timor-Tritsch IE, Monteagudo A. Transvaginal sonographic evaluation of the fetal central nervous system. *Obstet Gynecol Clin North Am.* 1991; 18:713–748.
24. Warren WB, Timor-Tritsch IE, Peisner DB, et al. Dating the early pregnancy by sequential appearance of embryonic structures. *Am J Obstet Gynecol.* 1989; 161:747–753.
25. Timor-Tritsch IE, Peisner DB, Raju S. Sonoembryology: An organ-oriented approach using a high-frequency vaginal probe. *J Clin Ultrasound.* 1990; 18:286–298.
26. Achiron R, Achiron A. Transvaginal ultrasonic assessment of the early fetal brain. *Ultrasound Obstet Gynecol.* 1991;1:336–344.
27. Kushnir U, Shalev J, Bronstein M, et al. Fetal intracranial anatomy in the first trimester of pregnancy: Transvaginal ultrasonographic evaluation. *Neuroradiology.* 1989;31:222–225.
28. Blaas HG, Eik-Nes SH, Kiserud T, et al. Early development of the forebrain and midbrain: A longitudinal ultrasound study from 7 to 12 postmenstrual weeks of gestation. *Ultrasound Obstet Gynecol.* 1994;4:183–192.
29. Blaas HG, Eik-Nes SH, Kiserud T, et al. Early development of the hindbrain: A longitudinal ultrasound

study from 7 to 12 weeks of gestation. *Ultrasound Obstet Gynecol*. 1995;5:151–160.

30. Monteagudo A, Timor-Tritsch IE, Reuss, ML, et al. Transvaginal sonography of the second- and third-trimester fetal brain. In: Timor-Tritsch IE, Rottem S, eds. *Transvaginal Sonography*. 2nd ed. New York: Chapman & Hall, 1991. pp 393–426.

31. Monteagudo A, Timor-Tritsch IE, Moomjy M. Nomograms of the fetal lateral ventricles using transvaginal sonography. *J Ultrasound Med*. 1993;5:265–269.

32. Robinson HP. Sonar measurements of fetal crown–rump length as means of assessing maturity in the first trimester of pregnancy. *Br Med J*. 1973; 4:28–31.

33. O'Rahilly R, Müller F. Embryonic length and cerebral landmarks in staged human embryos. *Anat Rec*. 1984;209:265–271.

34. Goldstein SR. Embryonic ultrasonographic measurements: Crown–rump length revisited. *Am J Obstet Gynecol*. 1991;165:497–501.

35. Timor-Tritsch IE, Blumenfeld Z, Rottem S. Sonoembryology. In: Timor-Tritsch IE, Rottem S, eds. *Transvaginal Sonography*. 2nd ed. New York: Chapman & Hall; 1991:241.

36. O'Rahilly R, Müller F. *Human Embryology and Teratology*. New York: Wiley–Liss; 1992.

37. Blaas HG, Eik-Nes SH, Kiserud T, et al. Three-dimensional imaging of the brain cavities in human embryos. *Ultrasound Obstet Gynecol*. 1995;5:228–232.

38. Timor-Tritsch IE, Monteagudo A. Transvaginal fetal neurosonography: Standardization of the planes and sections by anatomic landmarks. *Ultrasound Obstet Gynecol*. 1996; 8:42–47.

39. Timor-Tritsch IE, et al. Sonoembryology in the structural evaluation of the fetus from 6 to 16 weeks. In: Reed GB, Claireaux AE, Cockburn F, Eds. *Diseases of the Fetus and Newborn*. 2nd ed. London: Chapman & Hall; 1995:897–917.

40. Martin JH, ed. *Neuroanatomy: Text and Atlas*. New York: Elsevier; 1989.

41. Day WR. Casts of foetal lateral ventricles. *Brain*. 1959;82:109–115.

42. Denkhaus H, Winsberg F. Ultrasonic measurement of the fetal ventricular system. *Radiology*. 1979;131: 781–787.

43. Johnson ML, Dunne MG, Mack LA, et al. Evaluation of fetal intracranial anatomy by static and realtime ultrasound. *J Clin Ultrasound*. 1980;8:311.

44. Horbar J, Leahy K, Lucey J. Ultrasound identification of lateral ventricular asymmetry in the human neonate. *J Clin Ultrasound*. 1983;11:67.

45. Hadlock FP, Deter RL, Park SK. Real-time sonography: Ventricular and vascular anatomy of the fetal brain in utero. *AJR*. 1981;136:133–137.

46. Jeanty P, Dramaix-Wilmet M, Delbeke D, et al. Ultrasonic evaluation of fetal ventricular growth. *Neuroradiology*. 1981;21:127–133.

47. Pretorius DH, Rose JA, Manco-Johnson ML. Exclusion of fetal ventriculomegaly with a single measurement of the width of the lateral ventricular atrium. *Radiology*. 1988;169:711.

48. Cardoza JD, Goldstein RB, Filly RA. Exclusion of fetal ventriculomegaly with a single measurement of the width of the lateral ventricular atrium. *Radiology*. 1988;169:711.

49. Chinn DH, Callen PW, Filly RA. The lateral ventricle in early second trimester. *Radiology*. 1983;148: 529–531.

50. Lustig-Gillman I, Snyder JR, Silverman F, et al. Sonographic anatomy of the fetal cerebral ventricles, with reference to the early diagnosis of hydrocephaly. *J Perinat Med*. 1984;12:185–191.

51. Hertzberg BS, Sowie JD, Burder PC, et al. The three lines: Origin of a sonographic landmark in the fetal head. *AJR*. 1987;149:1009–1012.

52. Hertzberg BS, Kliewer MA, Bovie JD: Fetal cerebral ventriculomegaly: Misidentification of the true medial boundary of the ventricle at US. *Radiology*. 1997;205:813–816.

53. Siedler DE, Filly RA. Relative growth of the higher brain structures. *J Ultrasound Med*. 1987;6: 573–576.

54. Goldstein I, Reece EA, Pilu G, et al. Sonographic evaluation of the normal developmental anatomy of fetal cerebral ventricles. I: The frontal horn. *Obstet Gynecol*. 1988;72:588–592.

55. Pilu G, Reece EA, Goldstein I, et al. Sonographic evaluation of normal developmental anatomy of the fetal cerebral ventricles. II: The atria. *Obstet Gynecol*. 1989;73:250–256.

56. Goldstein I, Reece EA, Pilu G, et al. Sonographic evaluation of the normal developmental anatomy of the fetal cerebral ventricles. IV: The posterior horn. *Am J Perinatol*. 1990;7:79–83.

57. Reece EB, Goldstein I. Three-level view of fetal brain imaging in the prenatal diagnosis of congenital anomalies. *Matern Fetal Med*. 1999:8:249–52.

58. Campbell S. Diagnosis of fetal abnormalities by ultrasound. In: Milunsky A, ed. *Genetic Disorders and the Fetus*. New York: Plenum; 1979:431–467.

59. Goldstein I, Reece EA, Pilu G, et al. Sonographic assessment of the fetal frontal lobe: A potential tool for the prenatal diagnosis of microcephaly. *Am J Obstet Gynecol*. 1988;158:1057–1062.

60. Campbell S, Pearce JM. Ultrasound visualization of congenital malformations. *Br Med Bull*. 1983;39: 322–331.

61. Mahony BS, Nyberg DA, Hirsch JH, et al. Mild idiopathic lateral cerebral ventricular dilatation in utero: Sonographic evaluation. *Radiology*. 1988;169: 715–721.

62. Shaw CM, Alvord EC. Cava septi pellucidi and vergae: Their normal and pathological states. *Brain*. 1969;92:213–224.

63. Jou HJ, Shyu MK, Wu SC, et al. Ultrasound measurement of the fetal cavum septi pellucidi. *Ultrasound Obstet Gynecol*. 1998;12:419–421.

64. Larroche JC, Bandey J. Cavum septi lucidi, cavum vergae, cavum veli interpositi: Cavités de la ligne médiane. Etude anatomique et pneumoencéphalographique dans la période néo-natale. *Biol Neonat*. 1961;3:193–236.

65. Kostovic I, Lukinovic N, Judas M, et al. Structural basis of the developmental plasticity in the human cerebral cortex: The role of the transient subplate zone. *Metab Brain Dis.* 1989;4:17–23.

66. Lemire RJ, Loeser JD, Leech RW, et al. *Normal and Abnormal Development of the Human Nervous System.* New York: Harper & Row; 1975:260–277.

67. Pilu G, Sandri F, Perolo A, et al. Sonography of fetal agenesis of the corpus callosum: A survey of 35 cases. *Ultrasound Obstet Gynecol.* 1993;3:318–329.

68. Comstock CH, Culp D, Gonzales J. Agenesis of the corpus callosum in the fetus: Its evolution and significance. *J Ultrasound Med.* 1985;4:613–616.

69. Malinger G, Zakut H. The corpus callosum: Normal fetal development as shown by transvaginal sonography. *AJR.* 1993;161:1041–1043.

70. Guibert-Tranier F, Piton J, Billerey L, et al. Agenesis of the corpus callosum. *J Neuroradiol.* 1982;9:135.

71. Laing FC, Stamler CE, Jeffrey BR. Ultrasonography of the fetal subarachnoid space. *J Ultrasound Med.* 1983;2:29–32.

72. Kapila A, Trice J, Spies WG, et al. Enlarged cerebrospinal fluid in infants with subdural hematoma. *Radiology.* 1982;142:669–672.

73. Jeanty P, Chervenak FA, Romero R, et al. The sylvian fissure: A commonly mislabeled cranial landmark. *J Ultrasound Med.* 1984;3:15–18.

74. Mahony BS, Callen PW, Tilly RA. The fetal cisterna magna. *Radiology.* 1984;153:73–76.

75. Bromley B, Nadel AS, Parker S, Estroff JA, Benacerraf BR. Closure of the cerebellar vermis: Evaluation with second trimester US. *Radiology.* 1994;193: 761–763.

76. Goldstein I, Reece EA, Pilu G, et al. Cerebellar measurements with ultrasonography in the evaluation of fetal growth and development. *Am J Obstet Gynecol.* 1987;156:1065–1069.

77. Hill LM, Quzick D, Fried J, et al. The transverse cerebellar diameter in estimating gestational age in the large-for-gestational-age fetus. *Obstet Gynecol.* 1990; 75: 983–992.

78. Turner OA. Growth and development of the cerebral cortical pattern in man. *Arch Neurol Psychol.* 1948; 59:1.

79. Dooling EC, Chi JG, Gilles FH. Telencephalic development, changing gyral patterns. In: Gilles FH, ed. *The Developing Human Brain.* Boston: Wright–PSG; 1983:94.

80. Worthen NJ, Gilbertson V, Lau C. Cortical sulcal development seen on sonography: Relationship to gestational parameters. *J Ultrasound Med.* 1986: 5:153.

81. Salamon G, Raynaud C, Regis J, et al. *Magnetic Resonance Imaging of the Pediatric Brain: An Anatomical Atlas.* New York: Raven; 1990.

82. Hansen PE, Ballesteros MC, Soila K, et al. MR imaging of the developing human brain, part 1. Prenatal development. *Radiographics.* 1993:13:21.

83. Naidich TP, Graut JL, Altman N, et al. The developing cerebral surface: Preliminary report on the patterns of sulcal and gyral maturation—Anatomy, ultrasound, and magnetic resonance imaging. *Neuroimaging Clin North Am.* 1994;4:201–240.

84. Slagle TA, Oliphant M, Gross SJ. Cingulate sulcus development in preterm infants. *Pediatr Res.* 1989; 26:598–602.

85. Chi JG, Dooling EC, Gilles FH. Gyral development of the human brain. *Ann Neurol.* 1977;1:86–93.

86. Dorovini-Zis K, Dolman CL. Gestational development of the brain. *Arch Pathol Lab Med.* 1977;101: 192–195.

87. O'Rahilly R. *Anatomy, a Regional Study of Human Structure.* 5th ed. Philadelphia: WB Saunders; 1986.

88. Predanic M, Zudenigo D, Funduk-Kurjak B, et al. Assessment of early normal pregnancy. In: Kurjak A, ed. *An Atlas of Transvaginal Color Doppler: The Current State of the Art.* London: Parthenon Publishing; 1994:51–69.

89. Van den Wijngard JAG, Groanengerg IAL, Wladimiroff JW, et al. Cerebral Doppler ultrasound of the human fetus. *Br J Obstet Gynaecol.* 1989;96: 845–849.

CHAPTER
THREE

Biometry of the Fetal Brain

Ana Monteagudo
Nathan Haratz-Rubinstein
Ilan E. Timor-Tritsch

Prenatal diagnosis should be instituted accurately and early enough to achieve an excellent level of care of the obstetric patient. Ultrasonography, with its increasing resolution and image quality, is making it easier for health care providers to make appropriate management decisions. Assessing whether a structure is normal or abnormal may not always be feasible, but if doubt exists regarding its normalcy, it must be carefully and diligently pursued. In addition, several measurements, such as the biparietal diameter (BPD) and the head circumference (HC), can also be used to determine the gestational age of a fetus, especially during the first half of pregnancy. Correct estimation of gestational age is of paramount importance because adequate management of both low- and high-risk obstetric populations relies heavily on knowing the precise gestational age.

The tables in this chapter have been compiled from the literature for the sole purpose of serving as an easy reference against which measurements can be compared. An attempt has been made to include as many tables of different parameters as possible. These tables, assembled in a single chapter, will allow the sonographer or sonologist to more easily make the differentiation between normal and abnormal measurements, without having to search different textbooks and articles for a particular measurement.

This chapter is divided into four main sections. The first, crown–rump length (CRL), although not a brain or head measurement, is included to provide a means of predicting embryonic or fetal age. This parameter is of obvious importance, and prevents the need to turn to another source.

The second section, dealing with head measurements, can be used not only to date the pregnancy but also to aid in the diagnosis of microcephaly and alterations in fetal head shape. In addition, this section also includes measurements of orbital diameters, which can be of help in the diagnosis of eye pathology.

The third section provides a variety of tables concerning the different portions of the fetal ventricular system, mainly for the purpose of making early diagnosis of ventriculomegaly possible. Congenital hydrocephaly is one of the most frequently described anomalies, with an incidence of 0.3 to 1.5 per 1000 births. The importance of in utero detection of this anomaly cannot be overemphasized. This section also includes tables that we have generated using the transvaginal–transfontanelle approach to the fetal brain using 5- to 7.5-MHz transvaginal probes. These tables enhance and complement the widely accepted transabdominally generated tables, therefore advancing the field of fetal neurosonography and giving new meaning to the term *"early" diagnosis.*

The fourth and final section includes measurements of other intracranial structures, such as the thalami, basal nuclei, cerebellum, and cerebellomedullary cistern. These can assist the sonographer or sonologist in the diagnosis of pathologies such as Dandy–Walker and Arnold–Chiari malformations.

In conclusion, this chapter attempts to provide the reader with a unique reference guide to fetal brain measurements.

Crown–Rump Length

DEFINITION

The CRL represents the longest measurable length of the embryo or fetus, excluding the inferior limbs or the yolk sac.[1,2]

HOW TO MEASURE IT (FIG. 3–1)

In a longitudinal scan the CRL is measured from a point immediately over the middle of the midbrain (crown) to the embryonic or fetal rump. O'Rahilly and Müller[1] have suggested that from 28 to 44 postovulatory days (6 to 8.5 menstrual weeks,* or Carnegie stages 13 to 18) the maximal longitudinal length of the embryo is not truly represented by the CRL, but by what they called the greatest length. This is explained by the fact that during these stages the normal flexion of the embryonic head locates the middle of the midbrain below the highest point of the head. As pregnancy advances, the head extends, making the middle of the midbrain match the highest point of the head and thus becoming a true "crown" reference point (see Chapters 1 and 2).

COMMENTS

Although the CRL is obviously not a measurement of the brain, it will be included in this chapter as a reference for the assessment of estimated age, a parameter of utmost importance when evaluating the embryo and the fetus, and one against which most biometry tables are plotted. The validity of this parameter for determination of age in the first trimester has been widely reported in the literature.[2–4] The average of three measurements should be used to diminish random errors in the technique. The variability in predicting postmenstrual age with the CRL changes over time, with a reported range of error of ±8% of the estimate.[2] Possible factors contributing to this range are (1) normal biologic variation in fetal size, (2) variation in the times

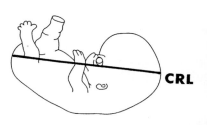 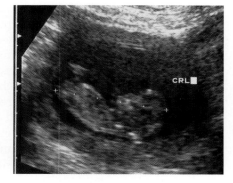

Figure 3–1.

---

*Fetal and embryonic age is described here in reference to postmenstrual weeks. Postovulatory age is approximately 2 weeks less than postmenstrual age.

of ovulation and fertilization, and (3) errors attributed to the measurement technique.[3] Nevertheless, the CRL remains the "gold standard" measurement for dating pregnancy in the first trimester, with the exception of in vitro fertilization cases (Tables 3–1 and 3–2).

Recently, Blaas and colleagues[5] have described the use of three-dimensional transvaginal sonography to outline in detail the outer contours of embryos at 7 to 10 weeks of gestation. Using this technique, they have been able to describe the contours of the brain cavities as well as calculate volumes that corresponded well to the descriptions from classic human embryology.

TABLE 3–1. NOMOGRAM OF THE SONOGRAPHICALLY DETERMINED CROWN–RUMP LENGTH AS A FUNCTION OF GESTATIONAL AGE

Postmenstrual Gestational Age (weeks + days)	Crown–Rump Length (mm)		Postmenstrual Gestational Age (weeks + days)	Crown–Rump Length (mm)	
	Mean	2 SD		Mean	2 SD
6 + 2	6.7	2.9	10 + 2	35.5	6.9
6 + 3	7.4	3.1	10 + 3	36.9	7.0
6 + 4	8.0	3.2	10 + 4	38.4	7.2
6 + 5	8.7	3.4	10 + 5	39.9	7.3
6 + 6	9.5	3.5	10 + 6	41.4	7.4
7 + 0	10.2	3.7	11 + 0	43.0	7.6
7 + 1	11.0	3.8	11 + 1	44.6	7.7
7 + 2	11.8	3.9	11 + 2	46.2	7.9
7 + 3	12.6	4.1	11 + 3	47.8	8.0
7 + 4	13.5	4.2	11 + 4	49.5	8.1
7 + 5	14.4	4.4	11 + 5	51.2	8.3
7 + 6	15.3	4.5	11 + 6	52.9	8.4
8 + 0	16.3	4.6	12 + 0	54.7	8.6
8 + 1	17.3	4.8	12 + 1	56.5	8.7
8 + 2	18.3	4.9	12 + 2	58.3	8.8
8 + 3	19.3	5.1	12 + 3	60.1	9.0
8 + 4	20.4	5.2	12 + 4	62.0	9.1
8 + 5	21.5	5.3	12 + 5	63.9	9.3
8 + 6	22.6	5.5	12 + 6	65.9	9.4
9 + 0	23.8	5.6	13 + 0	67.8	9.5
9 + 1	25.0	5.8	13 + 1	69.8	9.7
9 + 2	26.2	5.9	13 + 2	71.8	9.8
9 + 3	27.4	6.0	13 + 3	73.9	10.0
9 + 4	28.7	6.2	13 + 4	76.0	10.1
9 + 5	30.0	6.3	13 + 5	78.1	10.2
9 + 6	31.3	6.5	13 + 6	80.2	10.4
10 + 0	32.7	6.6	14 + 0	82.4	10.5
10 + 1	34.0	6.7			

From Robinson HP, Fleming Fee A Critical Evaluation of Sonar "Crown Rump Length" Measurements. Br J Obstet Gynecol, 1975;82:702. With permission.

TABLE 3–2. PREDICTED MENSTRUAL AGE FROM CROWN–RUMP LENGTH MEASUREMENTS

CRL (cm)	MA (weeks)	CRL (cm)	MA (weeks)	CRL (cm)	MA (weeks)
0.2	5.7	4.2	11.1	8.2	14.2
0.3	5.9	4.3	11.2	8.3	14.2
0.4	6.1	4.4	11.2	8.4	14.3
0.5	6.2	4.5	11.3	8.5	14.4
0.6	6.4	4.6	11.4	8.6	14.5
0.7	6.6	4.7	11.5	8.7	14.6
0.8	6.7	4.8	11.6	8.8	14.7
0.9	6.9	4.9	11.7	8.9	14.8
1.0	7.2	5.0	11.7	9.0	14.9
1.1	7.2	5.1	11.8	9.1	15.0
1.2	7.4	5.2	11.9	9.2	15.1
1.3	7.5	5.3	12.0	9.3	15.2
1.4	7.7	5.4	12.0	9.4	15.3
1.5	7.9	5.5	12.1	9.5	15.3
1.6	8.0	5.6	12.2	9.6	15.4
1.7	8.1	5.7	12.3	9.7	15.5
1.8	8.3	5.8	12.3	9.8	15.6
1.9	8.4	5.9	12.4	9.9	15.7
2.0	8.6	6.0	12.5	10.0	15.9
2.1	8.7	6.1	12.6	10.1	16.0
2.2	8.9	6.2	12.6	10.2	16.1
2.3	9.0	6.3	12.7	10.3	16.2
2.4	9.1	6.4	12.8	10.4	16.3
2.5	9.2	6.5	12.8	10.5	16.4
2.6	9.4	6.6	12.9	10.6	16.5
2.7	9.5	6.7	13.0	10.7	16.6
2.8	9.6	6.8	13.1	10.8	16.7
2.9	9.7	6.9	13.1	10.9	16.8
3.0	9.9	7.0	13.2	11.0	16.9
3.1	10.0	7.1	13.3	11.1	17.0
3.2	10.1	7.2	13.4	11.2	17.1
3.3	10.2	7.3	13.4	11.3	17.2
3.4	10.3	7.4	13.5	11.4	17.3
3.5	10.4	7.5	13.6	11.5	17.4
3.6	10.5	7.6	13.7	11.6	17.5
3.7	10.6	7.7	13.8	11.7	17.6
3.8	10.7	7.8	13.8	11.8	17.7
3.9	10.8	7.9	13.9	11.9	17.8
4.0	10.9	8.0	14.0	12.0	17.9
4.1	11.0	8.1	14.1	12.1	18.0

CRL, Crown–rump length; MA, menstrual age.

From Hadlock FP, Shah YP, Kanon DJ, Lindsey JV. Fetal crown–rump length: Reevaluation of relation to menstrual age (5–18 weeks) with high-resolution real time US. Radiology 1992;182:501–505. With permission.

Head Measurements
Biparietal Diameter

DEFINITION

The BPD represents the widest transverse dimension of the fetal head.

HOW TO MEASURE IT (FIG. 3–2)

The fetal head should be imaged in a horizontal (axial) plane. The transducer should be tilted to match the angle of inclination of the head in the vertical axis of the fetus so that a horizontal section can be obtained. This is recognized by the appearance of the midline echo and the widest fetal head diameter at right angles with it. The transducer should then be rotated (following the position of the fetal spine) until the head appears as an ovoid and a small anechoic area is detected in the midline, one third of the distance from the sinciput.[6] According to Hadlock and colleagues,[7] this plane represents a section along the suboccipital–bregmatic axis, angled about 40°, to the canthomeatal line. Intracranial landmarks that should be recognized in an anterior-to-posterior fashion are (see Fig. 3–2 for abbreviations) the falx cerebri (F); the cavum septi pellucidi (CSP), which corresponds to the midline anechoic area described by Campbell and Thoms[5]; the cerebral peduncles (P); and again, the falx cerebri in the midline. Laterally, one should be able to recognize, depending on the age of the fetus, the anterior horns (AH) of the lateral ventricles, the hypoechoic thalami (T), and the choroid plexus (CP) in the atrium (A) of each lateral ventricle. Halfway between the thalami and the calvarium, a linear echo corresponding to the insula (I) can be seen, with the pulsating middle cerebral artery within. Once the correct plane has been identified, the calipers should be placed at the outer surface of the skull table nearest the transducer and at the inner margin of the opposite skull table, with gain settings adjusted so that the width of the skull table nearer the transducer is 3 to 5 mm.

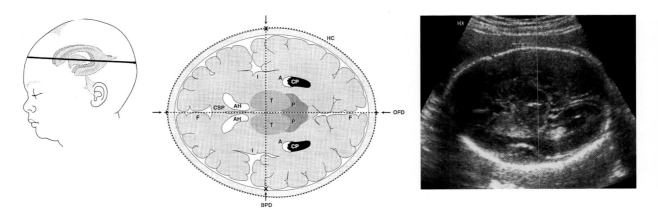

Figure 3–2.

COMMENTS

The BPD was one of the first sonographic parameters used to estimate fetal age.[8] The BPD has been demonstrated to be a reliable predictor of menstrual age in the first half of pregnancy, being the most accurate between 12 and 18 (±1.2) weeks. As pregnancy progresses, the BPD loses its power to correctly predict gestational age, with a margin of error of ±3.2 weeks at 36 to 42 weeks (Tables 3–3 and 3–4).[9]

The observed variation in the third trimester has been related to (1) technical errors in imaging, (2) genetic variations in head size in fetuses of equal age, and (3) differences in the times of ovulation and fertilization during the menstrual period.

TABLE 3–3. PREDICTED FETAL BIPARIETAL DIAMETER AT SPECIFIC MENSTRUAL AGES

Menstrual Age (weeks)	Biparietal Diameter (cm)	Menstrual Age (weeks)	Biparietal Diameter (cm)
12.0	1.7	26.0	6.5
12.5	1.9	26.5	6.7
13.0	2.1	27.0	6.8
13.5	2.3	27.5	6.9
14.0	2.5	28.0	7.1
14.5	2.7	28.5	7.2
15.0	2.9	29.0	7.3
		29.5	7.5
15.5	3.1	30.0	7.6
16.0	3.2	30.5	7.7
16.5	3.4	31.0	7.8
17.0	3.6	31.5	7.9
17.5	3.8	32.0	8.1
18.0	3.9	32.5	8.2
18.5	4.1	33.0	8.3
19.0	4.3	33.5	8.4
19.5	4.5	34.0	8.5
20.0	4.6	34.5	8.6
20.5	4.8	35.0	8.7
21.0	5.0	35.5	8.8
21.5	5.1	36.0	8.9
22.0	5.3	36.5	8.9
22.5	5.5	37.0	9.0
23.0	5.6	37.5	9.1
23.5	5.8	38.0	9.2
24.0	5.9	38.5	9.2
24.5	6.1	39.0	9.3
25.0	6.2	39.5	9.4
25.5	6.4	40.0	9.4

After Hadlock and colleagues, 1984,[8] with permission.

TABLE 3–4. ASSESSMENT OF GESTATIONAL AGE FROM THE BIPARIETAL DIAMETER

Biparietal Diameter (mm)	Gestational Age (weeks + days)		
	5th Percentile	50th Percentile	95th Percentile
10	7 + 0	10 + 1	13 + 1
11	7 + 2	10 + 2	13 + 3
12	7 + 3	10 + 4	13 + 4
13	7 + 5	10 + 5	13 + 5
14	7 + 6	10 + 6	14 + 0
15	8 + 1	11 + 1	14 + 1
16	8 + 2	11 + 2	14 + 3
17	8 + 4	11 + 4	14 + 4
18	8 + 5	11 + 5	14 + 6
19	9 + 0	12 + 0	15 + 0
20	9 + 1	12 + 2	15 + 2
21	9 + 3	12 + 3	15 + 3
22	9 + 4	12 + 5	15 + 5
23	9 + 6	12 + 6	16 + 0
24	10 + 1	13 + 1	16 + 1
25	10 + 2	13 + 3	16 + 3
26	10 + 4	13 + 4	16 + 5
27	10 + 6	13 + 6	17 + 0
28	11 + 0	14 + 1	17 + 1
29	11 + 2	14 + 3	17 + 3
30	11 + 4	14 + 4	17 + 5
31	11 + 6	14 + 6	18 + 0
32	12 + 1	15 + 1	18 + 1
33	12 + 3	15 + 3	18 + 3
34	12 + 4	15 + 5	18 + 5
35	12 + 6	16 + 0	19 + 0
36	13 + 1	16 + 2	19 + 2
37	13 + 3	16 + 4	19 + 4
38	13 + 5	16 + 6	19 + 6
39	14 + 0	17 + 1	20 + 1
40	14 + 2	17 + 3	20 + 3
41	14 + 4	17 + 5	20 + 5
42	14 + 6	18 + 0	21 + 0
43	15 + 1	18 + 2	21 + 2
44	15 + 3	18 + 4	21 + 4
45	15 + 6	18 + 6	21 + 6
46	16 + 1	19 + 1	22 + 1
47	16 + 3	19 + 3	22 + 4
48	16 + 5	19 + 5	22 + 6
49	17 + 0	20 + 1	23 + 1
50	17 + 3	20 + 3	23 + 3
51	17 + 5	20 + 5	23 + 6
52	18 + 0	21 + 0	24 + 1
53	18 + 2	21 + 3	24 + 3
54	18 + 5	21 + 5	24 + 5
55	19 + 0	22 + 0	25 + 1

Continued.

TABLE 3–4. ASSESSMENT OF GESTATIONAL AGE FROM THE BIPARIETAL DIAMETER—Cont'd

Biparietal Diameter (mm)	Gestational Age (weeks + days)		
	5th Percentile	50th Percentile	95th Percentile
56	19 + 2	22 + 3	25 + 3
57	19 + 5	22 + 5	25 + 6
58	20 + 0	23 + 1	26 + 1
59	20 + 3	23 + 3	26 + 3
60	20 + 5	23 + 6	26 + 6
61	21 + 1	24 + 1	27 + 1
62	21 + 3	24 + 4	27 + 4
63	21 + 6	24 + 6	27 + 6
64	22 + 1	25 + 2	28 + 2
65	22 + 4	25 + 4	28 + 5
66	22 + 6	26 + 0	29 + 0
67	23 + 2	26 + 2	29 + 3
68	23 + 5	26 + 5	29 + 5
69	24 + 0	27 + 1	30 + 1
70	24 + 3	27 + 3	30 + 4
71	24 + 6	27 + 6	30 + 6
72	25 + 1	28 + 2	31 + 2
73	25 + 4	28 + 5	31 + 5
74	26 + 0	29 + 0	32 + 1
75	26 + 3	29 + 3	32 + 4
76	26 + 6	29 + 6	32 + 6
77	27 + 1	30 + 2	33 + 2
78	27 + 4	30 + 5	33 + 5
79	28 + 0	31 + 1	34 + 1
80	28 + 3	31 + 3	34 + 4
81	28 + 6	31 + 6	35 + 0
82	29 + 2	32 + 2	35 + 3
83	29 + 5	32 + 5	35 + 6
84	30 + 1	33 + 1	36 + 2
85	30 + 4	33 + 4	36 + 5
86	31 + 0	34 + 0	37 + 1
87	31 + 3	34 + 3	37 + 4
88	31 + 6	35 + 0	38 + 0
89	32 + 2	35 + 3	38 + 3
90	32 + 5	35 + 6	38 + 6
91	33 + 2	36 + 2	39 + 2
92	33 + 5	36 + 5	39 + 6
93	34 + 1	37 + 1	40 + 2
94	34 + 4	37 + 5	40 + 5
95	35 + 0	38 + 1	41 + 1
96	35 + 4	38 + 4	41 + 4
97	36 + 0	39 + 0	42 + 1
98	36 + 3	39 + 4	42 + 4
99	37 + 0	40 + 0	43 + 0

From Jeanty P. Fetal biometry. In Fleischer AC, Romero R, et al. The Principles and Practice of Ultrasonography in Obstetrics and Gynecology. 4th ed. 1991. East Norwalk, CT: Appleton & Lange, p. 100, with permission.

Sonographic measurement of the BPD may be misleading if the fetal head shape is abnormal. It has been postulated that extrinsic factors such as breech presentation and oligohydramnios can alter fetal head shape.[10,11] In an attempt to identify variations in the shape of the fetal skull which might adversely affect the potential of the BPD in estimating age, Hadlock and associates[12] developed the so-called cephalic index (CI). When this parameter is abnormal, other measurements, such as the HC, abdominal circumference, or femur length, should be used to predict fetal age.

Cephalic Index

DEFINITION

The CI is the relationship between the short and long axes of the fetal skull, measured at the level of the BPD.

HOW TO MEASURE IT

The widest transverse and longitudinal (occipitofrontal diameter [OFD]) dimensions of the fetal skull at the level of the BPD are measured from outer margin to outer margin. The CI can then be calculated using the following simple equation:

$$CI = \text{short axis (transverse)/long axis (OFD)} \times 100$$

COMMENTS

The clinical application of the CI lies in its property to discriminate between the normal fetal head shape and the head that is abnormal enough to alter fetal age estimation based on the BPD. Thus, in situations that may modify the fetal head shape, e.g., oligohydramnios and breech presentation,[13,14] other parameters, such as the HC, should be used.

Hadlock and coworkers[12] suggested that the CI is constant throughout gestation, with a mean value of 78.3 and a standard deviation (SD) of 4.4. A CI greater than 1 SD from the mean (under 74 or over 83) was found to be associated with a significant change in the BPD measurement expected for any given age. Using the CI, certain variations in the shape of the fetal skull, such as dolichocephaly (CI below 74) and brachycephaly (CI above 84), have been described.[12]

More recently, Gray and collaborators[15] have proposed that the CI varies with advancing age (Table 3–5). These authors also suggested that the normal CI range is within 1 SD of the mean, with a sensitivity of 84% and a false-positive rate of 35% for detection of a misleading BPD value.

TABLE 3–5. CEPHALIC INDEX: MEAN AND NORMAL RANGE

Week	Mean Cephalic Index	−1 SD	+1 SD
14	81.5	77.8	85.3
15	81.0	77.3	84.8
16	80.5	76.8	84.3
17	80.1	76.4	83.9
18	79.7	76.0	83.5
19	79.4	75.7	83.2
20	79.1	75.4	82.9
21	78.8	75.1	82.6
22	78.6	74.9	82.4
23	78.4	74.7	82.2
24	78.3	74.6	82.0
25	78.1	74.4	81.9
26	78.0	74.3	81.8
27	78.0	74.3	81.8
28	78.0	74.3	81.8
29	78.0	74.3	81.8
30	78.1	74.4	81.9
31	78.2	74.5	82.0
32	78.3	74.6	82.1
33	78.5	74.8	82.3
34	78.7	75.0	82.5
35	78.9	75.2	82.7
36	79.2	75.5	83.0
37	79.5	75.8	83.3
38	79.9	76.2	83.7
39	80.3	76.6	84.1
40	80.7	77.0	84.5

From Gray and colleagues, 1989,[15] with permission.

Head Circumference

DEFINITION

The HC represents the outer perimeter of the fetal calvarium measured at the level of the BPD.

HOW TO MEASURE IT

The correct anatomic plane that should be used to measure the HC corresponds to the axial plane described by Campbell and Thoms,[5] previously delineated in the section on BPD. Ideally, the formula for the circumference of an ellipse should be used.[16]

$$HC = \sqrt{(\text{transverse diameter})^2 + (\text{longitudinal diameter})^2/2} \times \Pi$$

Both transverse and longitudinal diameters should be outer-to-outer distances (as for the CI). Adequate calculation of the HC can also be made using the formula[17] [D1 + D2] × 1.57.

The HC can also be measured along the outer perimeter of the calvarium, using a map measurer or electronic digitizer, as originally described by Hadlock's group.[18] The calculation of a circumference from two diameters is equivalent to the electronically digitized perimeter measurement, although the probability of technical errors between these techniques exists.[16]

COMMENTS

The HC was originally described as a useful index to estimate fetal age in cases in which variations in head shape (e.g., dolichocephaly or brachycephaly) adversely affected the accuracy of the BPD.[19] Several authors have demonstrated that the HC is a better predictor of fetal age than the BPD.[20–22] This is because the HC is more shape independent, and thus is less prone to be affected by molding of the fetal head (Tables 3–6 and 3–7).

TABLE 3–6. PREDICTED HEAD CIRCUMFERENCE AT SPECIFIC MENSTRUAL AGES

Menstrual Age (weeks)	Head Circumference (cm)	Menstrual Age (weeks)	Head Circumference (cm)
12.0	6.8	26.5	25.1
12.5	7.5	27.0	25.6
13.0	8.2	27.5	26.1
13.5	8.9	28.0	26.6
14.0	9.7	28.5	27.1
14.5	10.4	29.0	27.5
15.0	11.0	29.5	28.0
15.5	11.7	30.0	28.4
16.0	12.4	30.5	28.8
16.5	13.1	31.0	29.3
17.0	13.8	31.5	29.7
17.5	14.4	32.0	30.1
18.0	15.1	32.5	30.4
18.5	15.8	33.0	30.8
19.0	16.4	33.5	31.2
19.5	17.0	34.0	31.5
20.0	17.7	34.5	31.8
20.5	18.3	35.0	32.2
21.0	18.9	35.5	32.5
21.5	19.5	36.0	32.8
22.0	20.1	36.5	33.0
22.5	20.7	37.0	33.3
23.0	21.3	37.5	33.5
23.5	21.9	38.0	33.8
24.0	22.4	38.5	34.0
24.5	23.0	39.0	34.2
25.0	23.5	39.5	34.4
25.5	24.1	40.0	34.6
26.0	24.6		

After Hadlock and colleagues, 1984,[9] with permission.

TABLE 3–7. ASSESSMENT OF GESTATIONAL AGE FROM THE HEAD CIRCUMFERENCE

Head Perimeter (mm)	Gestational Age (weeks + days)		
	5th Percentile	50th Percentile	95th Percentile
80	10 + 5	12 + 4	14 + 2
84	11 + 0	12 + 5	14 + 4
88	11 + 2	13 + 0	14 + 6
92	11 + 4	13 + 2	15 + 0
96	11 + 6	13 + 4	15 + 2
100	12 + 1	13 + 6	15 + 4
104	12 + 3	14 + 1	15 + 6
108	12 + 5	14 + 3	16 + 1
112	13 + 0	14 + 5	16 + 3
116	13 + 2	15 + 0	16 + 5
120	13 + 4	15 + 2	17 + 0
124	13 + 6	15 + 4	17 + 2
128	14 + 1	15 + 6	17 + 5
132	14 + 3	16 + 1	18 + 0
136	14 + 5	16 + 4	18 + 2
140	15 + 0	16 + 6	18 + 4
144	15 + 3	17 + 1	18 + 6
148	15 + 5	17 + 3	19 + 2
152	16 + 0	17 + 6	19 + 4
156	16 + 3	18 + 1	19 + 6
160	16 + 5	18 + 3	20 + 1
164	17 + 0	18 + 6	20 + 4
168	17 + 3	19 + 1	20 + 6
172	17 + 5	19 + 3	21 + 2
176	18 + 0	19 + 6	21 + 4
180	18 + 3	20 + 1	21 + 6
184	18 + 5	20 + 4	22 + 2
188	19 + 1	20 + 6	22 + 4
192	19 + 3	21 + 2	23 + 0
196	19 + 6	21 + 4	23 + 3
200	20 + 2	22 + 0	23 + 5
204	20 + 4	22 + 2	24 + 1
208	21 + 0	22 + 5	24 + 3
212	21 + 2	23 + 1	24 + 6
216	21 + 5	23 + 3	25 + 2
220	22 + 1	23 + 6	25 + 4
224	22 + 4	24 + 2	26 + 0
228	22 + 6	24 + 5	26 + 3
232	23 + 2	25 + 0	26 + 6
236	23 + 5	25 + 3	27 + 2
240	24 + 1	25 + 6	27 + 4
244	24 + 4	26 + 2	28 + 0
248	25 + 0	26 + 5	28 + 3
252	25 + 3	27 + 1	28 + 6
256	25 + 6	27 + 4	29 + 2
260	26 + 1	28 + 0	29 + 5
264	26 + 4	28 + 3	30 + 1
268	27 + 1	28 + 6	30 + 4

Continued.

TABLE 3–7. ASSESSMENT OF GESTATIONAL AGE FROM THE HEAD
CIRCUMFERENCE—Cont'd

Head Perimeter (mm)	Gestational Age (weeks + days)		
	5th Percentile	50th Percentile	95th Percentile
272	27 + 4	29 + 2	31 + 0
276	28 + 0	29 + 5	31 + 3
280	28 + 3	30 + 1	31 + 6
284	28 + 6	30 + 4	32 + 2
288	29 + 2	31 + 0	32 + 6
292	29 + 5	31 + 4	33 + 2
296	30 + 1	32 + 0	33 + 5
300	30 + 5	32 + 3	34 + 1
304	31 + 1	32 + 6	34 + 5
308	31 + 4	33 + 3	35 + 1
312	32 + 1	33 + 6	35 + 4
316	32 + 4	34 + 2	36 + 0
320	33 + 0	34 + 6	36 + 4
324	33 + 4	35 + 2	37 + 0
328	34 + 0	35 + 5	37 + 4
332	34 + 4	36 + 2	38 + 0
336	35 + 0	36 + 5	38 + 4
340	35 + 3	37 + 2	39 + 0
344	36 + 0	37 + 5	39 + 4
348	36 + 4	38 + 2	40 + 0
352	37 + 0	38 + 5	40 + 4
356	37 + 4	39 + 2	41 + 0
360	38 + 0	39 + 6	41 + 4
364	38 + 4	40 + 2	42 + 1

From: Jeanty P. Fetal biometry. In Fleischer AC, Romero R, Manning FA, Jeanty P, James AE. The Principles and Practice of Ultrasonography in Obstetrics and Gynecology. 4th ed. 1991. East Norwalk, CT: Appleton & Lange, p. 102, with permission.

TABLE 3–8. VARIABILITY IN PREDICTING MENSTRUAL AGE USING THE BIPARIETAL DIAMETER
AND THE HEAD CIRCUMFERENCE

Fetal Parameters	Subgroup Variability (±2 SD) in Weeks				
	12–18 Weeks	18–24 Weeks	24–30 Weeks	30–36 Weeks	36–42 Weeks
Biparietal diameter	±1.19	±1.73	±2.18	±3.08	±3.20
Head circumference	±1.19	±1.48	±2.06	±2.98	±2.70

After Hadlock and colleagues, 1984,[9] with permission.

As with other parameters, such as the BPD, the variability for estimation of age via the HC progressively increases with advancing menstrual age, ranging from ±1.19 at the 12- to 18-week interval to ±2.70 at the 36- to 42-week interval (Table 3–8).[9]

The HC has also been used in equations developed to estimate fetal weight,[23] to monitor normal fetal growth as well as intrauterine growth restriction,[24,25] and for the diagnosis of microcephaly (Table 3–9). Microcephaly

TABLE 3–9. MEANS AND STANDARD DEVIATIONS OF THE HEAD CIRCUMFERENCE AS A FUNCTION OF GESTATIONAL AGE

Week	Mean	Head Circumference (mm): SD Below Mean				
		−1	−2	−3	−4	−5
20	175	160	145	131	116	101
21	187	172	157	143	128	113
22	198	184	169	154	140	125
23	210	195	180	166	151	136
24	221	206	191	177	162	147
25	232	217	202	188	173	158
26	242	227	213	198	183	169
27	252	238	223	208	194	179
28	262	247	233	218	203	189
29	271	257	242	227	213	198
30	281	266	251	236	222	207
31	289	274	260	245	230	216
32	297	283	268	253	239	224
33	305	290	276	261	246	232
34	312	297	283	268	253	239
35	319	304	289	275	260	245
36	325	310	295	281	266	251
37	330	316	301	286	272	257
38	335	320	306	291	276	262
39	339	325	310	295	281	266
40	343	328	314	299	284	270
41	346	331	316	302	287	272
42	348	333	319	304	289	275

After Chervenak and colleagues, 1984,[28] with permission.

is a clinical syndrome characterized by an abnormally small head. Most authors agree that the diagnosis of microcephaly should be suspected when the HC is 3 SD below the mean for a given gestational age.[26–28] Nevertheless, the antenatal accuracy for the diagnosis of microcephaly using this parameter has been reported to be as low as 56.2%.[28] To overcome this low performance, other measurements, such as the frontal lobe distance and the thalamic frontal lobe distance, have been proposed.[29] Other typical features of microcephalic fetuses, such as a cone-shaped head, a large face, large ears, and a sloping forehead ("birdhead"),[29] as well as associated anomalies such as ventricular enlargement, porencephaly, and cephaloceles,[28] should be carefully searched. Some investigators have postulated that a reduction in blood supply to the underdeveloped cerebral hemispheres in fetuses with microcephaly could be detected with color Doppler and power Doppler imaging.[30]

As the nomograms for HC require knowledge of the accurate fetal age and this information is not always available, the use of ratio such as the HC–to–femur length ratio has the advantage of reducing dependence on reliable age evaluation (Table 3–10).[28] This ratio assumes that limb growth is not affected in fetuses with microcephaly, which might not always be the case.

TABLE 3–10. MEANS AND STANDARD DEVIATIONS OF THE FEMUR LENGTH: HEAD CIRCUMFERENCE RATIOS AS A FUNCTION OF GESTATIONAL AGE

Week	Mean	SD Below Mean				
		−5	−4	−3	−2	−1
20	0.180	0.107	0.122	0.137	0.152	0.167
21	0.190	0.111	0.126	0.141	0.156	0.171
22	0.190	0.115	0.130	0.145	0.160	0.175
23	0.190	0.118	0.133	0.148	0.163	0.178
24	0.200	0.121	0.136	0.151	0.166	0.181
25	0.200	0.123	0.138	0.153	0.168	0.183
26	0.200	0.125	0.140	0.155	0.170	0.185
27	0.200	0.127	0.142	0.157	0.172	0.187
28	0.200	0.129	0.144	0.159	0.174	0.189
29	0.200	0.130	0.145	0.160	0.175	0.190
30	0.210	0.131	0.146	0.161	0.176	0.191
31	0.210	0.132	0.147	0.162	0.177	0.192
32	0.210	0.134	0.149	0.164	0.179	0.194
33	0.210	0.135	0.150	0.165	0.180	0.195
34	0.210	0.136	0.151	0.166	0.181	0.196
35	0.210	0.138	0.153	0.168	0.183	0.198
36	0.210	0.140	0.155	0.170	0.185	0.200
37	0.220	0.142	0.157	0.172	0.187	0.202
38	0.220	0.144	0.159	0.174	0.189	0.204
39	0.220	0.147	0.162	0.177	0.192	0.207
40	0.230	0.151	0.166	0.181	0.196	0.211
41	0.230	0.155	0.170	0.185	0.200	0.215
42	0.230	0.160	0.175	0.190	0.205	0.220

After Chervenak and colleagues, 1984,[28] with permission.

Orbital Diameters: Inner Orbital Diameter, Outer Orbital Diameter, and Ocular Diameter

DEFINITION

The inner orbital, or interorbital, diameter (IOD) is defined as the distance between the medial border of one orbit and the medial border of the opposite orbit. The outer orbital diameter (OOD), or biorbital diameter, is defined as the distance between the lateral border of one orbit and the lateral border of the opposite orbit.[31] The ocular diameter corresponds to the distance between the medial border and the lateral border of a single orbit.

HOW TO MEASURE IT (FIG. 3–3)

To measure the orbital diameters, an axial plane slightly caudad to the BPD is commonly used. The criteria used for this section are (1) a symmetrical sec-

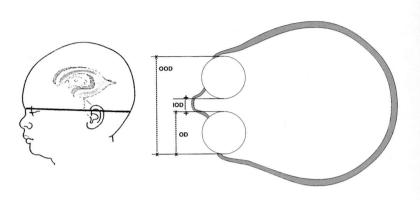 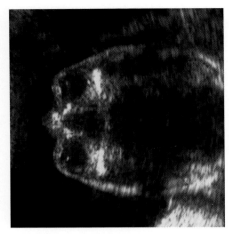

Figure 3–3.

tion, (2) both eyes imaged and of equal diameter, and (3) the largest possible diameter of the eyes.[32] Measurements of orbital diameters can also be accomplished using a coronal plane, approximately 2 cm posterior to the glabella–alveolar line.[31]

COMMENTS

The study of the orbital diameters should help in the diagnosis of hypotelorism, hypertelorism, and microphthalmos. Trout and colleagues[33] have found that in cases of hypotelorism, both the IOD and the OOD clearly fall below 2 SD of the mean. In cases of hypertelorism, the IOD fell above the 95th percentile, whereas the OOD measurement fell within normal limits but near the 95th percentile. Hypotelorism has been associated with chromosomal anomalies (trisomy 13, trisomy 21, 18p−, 5p−, and 14q+), holoprosencephaly, Meckel–Gruber syndrome, microcephaly, maternal phenylketonuria, and others.[32–34] Hypertelorism can occur as an isolated defect but has also been associated with a long list of malformations and syndromes, such as frontal, ethmoidal, or sphenoidal meningoencephalocele; median cleft syndrome; and craniosynostosis.[34]

Mayden and associates[31] developed nomograms of orbital measurements as a function of the BPD, which are taken as a classical reference to which newer data are compared (Table 3–11). More recently[33] nomograms for orbital diameters as a function of age have been published because the authors felt that some patients could have pathological intracranial conditions that might alter the BPD, making this measurement less reliable (Table 3–12).

Microphthalmos can be suspected when the orbital diameter falls below the 5th percentile for age (Table 3–13). Because this is a statistical definition, careful examination of the intraorbital anatomy as well as detection of associated anomalies is warranted. Conditions associated with microphthalmos include chromosomal (trisomies 13 and 18 and trisomy 9 mosaic), environmental (fetal toxoplasmosis, rubella, varicella, and alcohol syndrome and maternal phenylketonuria), and multiple syndromes (e.g., frontonasal dysplasia, Fraser syndrome, Lenz's syndrome, and Fanconi's syndrome).[35]

TABLE 3–11. NOMOGRAM FOR EVALUATION OF THE INNER AND OUTER ORBITAL DIAMETERS IN THE FETUS VERSUS BIPARIETAL DIAMETER

Biparietal Diameter (cm)	Inner Orbital Diameter (cm)	Outer Orbital Diameter (cm)
1.9	0.5	1.3
2.0	0.5	1.4
2.1	0.6	1.5
2.2	0.6	1.6
2.3	0.6	1.7
2.4	0.7	1.7
2.5	0.7	1.8
2.6	0.7	1.9
2.7	0.8	2.0
2.8	0.8	2.1
2.9	0.8	2.1
3.0	0.9	2.2
3.1	0.9	2.3
3.2	0.9	2.4
3.3	1.0	2.5
3.4	1.0	2.5
3.5	1.0	2.6
3.6	1.0	2.7
3.7	1.1	2.7
3.8	1.1	2.8
4.0	1.2	3.0
4.2	1.2	3.1
4.3	1.2	3.2
4.4	1.3	3.2
4.5	1.3	3.3
4.6	1.3	3.4
4.7	1.3	3.4
4.8	1.4	3.5
4.9	1.4	3.6
5.0	1.4	3.6
5.1	1.4	3.7
5.2	1.4	3.8
5.3	1.5	3.8
5.4	1.5	3.9
5.5	1.5	4.0
5.6	1.5	4.0
5.7	1.5	4.1
5.8	1.6	4.1
5.9	1.6	4.2
6.0	1.6	4.3
6.1	1.6	4.3
6.2	1.6	4.4
6.3	1.7	4.4
6.4	1.7	4.5
6.5	1.7	4.5
6.6	1.7	4.6
6.7	1.7	4.6
6.8	1.7	4.7

Continued.

TABLE 3–11. NOMOGRAM FOR EVALUATION OF THE INNER AND OUTER ORBITAL DIAMETERS IN THE FETUS VERSUS BIPARIETAL DIAMETER—Cont'd

Biparietal Diameter (cm)	Inner Orbital Diameter (cm)	Outer Orbital Diameter (cm)
6.9	1.7	4.7
7.0	1.8	4.8
7.1	1.8	4.8
7.3	1.8	4.9
7.4	1.8	5.0
7.5	1.8	5.0
7.6	1.8	5.1
7.7	1.8	5.1
7.8	1.8	5.2
7.9	1.9	5.2
8.0	1.9	5.3
8.2	1.9	5.4
8.3	1.9	5.4
8.4	1.9	5.4
8.5	1.9	5.5
8.6	1.9	5.5
8.8	1.9	5.6
8.9	1.9	5.6
9.0	1.9	5.7
9.1	1.9	5.7
9.2	1.9	5.8
9.3	1.9	5.8
9.4	1.9	5.8
9.6	1.9	5.9
9.7	1.9	5.9

From Mayden and colleagues, 1982,[31] with permission.

TABLE 3–12. NOMOGRAM FOR EVALUATION OF THE INNER AND OUTER ORBITAL DIAMETERS IN THE FETUS VERSUS GESTATIONAL AGE

Gestational Age (weeks)	Inner Orbital Diameter (mm)			Outer Orbital Diameter (mm)		
	5th Percentile	50th Percentile	95th Percentile	5th Percentile	50th Percentile	95th Percentile
13	4	7	10	12	16	20
14	5	8	11	14	18	22
15	5	8	11	17	21	25
16	6	9	12	19	23	27
17	7	10	13	21	25	29
18	8	11	14	24	27	31
19	8	11	14	26	30	34
20	9	12	15	28	32	36
21	10	13	16	30	34	38
22	10	13	16	32	36	40
23	11	14	17	33	37	41
24	12	14	17	35	39	43
25	12	15	18	37	41	45
26	13	16	19	39	43	47
27	13	16	19	40	44	48

Continued.

TABLE 3–12. NOMOGRAM FOR EVALUATION OF THE INNER AND OUTER ORBITAL DIAMETERS IN THE FETUS VERSUS GESTATIONAL AGE—Cont'd

Gestational Age (weeks)	Inner Orbital Diameter (mm)			Outer Orbital Diameter (mm)		
	5th Percentile	50th Percentile	95th Percentile	5th Percentile	50th Percentile	95th Percentile
28	14	17	20	42	46	50
29	14	17	20	43	47	51
30	15	18	21	45	49	52
31	15	18	21	46	50	54
32	16	19	22	47	51	55
33	17	20	23	48	52	56
34	17	20	23	49	53	57
35	18	21	24	50	54	58

From Trout and colleagues, 1994,[33] with permission.

TABLE 3–13. NOMOGRAM FOR EVALUATION OF THE OCULAR DIAMETER VERSUS GESTATIONAL AGE

Gestational Age (weeks)	Ocular Diameter (mm)		
	5th Percentile	50th Percentile	95th Percentile
11	—	—	—
12	1	3	6
13	2	4	7
14	3	5	8
15	4	6	9
16	5	7	9
17	5	8	10
18	6	9	11
19	7	9	12
20	8	10	13
21	8	11	13
22	9	12	14
23	10	12	15
24	10	13	15
25	11	13	16
26	12	14	16
27	12	14	17
28	13	15	17
29	13	15	18
30	14	16	18
31	14	16	19
32	14	17	19
33	15	17	19
34	15	17	20
35	15	18	20
36	16	18	20
37	16	18	21
38	16	18	21
39	16	19	21
40	16	19	21

From Romero and colleagues, 1988,[34] with permission.

The Ventricular System

For practical purposes, we have divided the analysis of the ventricular system depending on the sonographic modality used, e.g., transabdominal or transvaginal.

Transabdominal Sonography
LATERAL VENTRICULAR WIDTH–HEMISPHERIC WIDTH RATIO

DEFINITION

The lateral ventricular width–hemispheric width ratio (LVW/HW) represents the percentage of the whole cerebral hemisphere that corresponds to the lateral ventricle, measured in an axial plane.

HOW TO MEASURE IT (FIG. 3–4)

The widths of the lateral ventricles and the hemispheres are measured in a plane parallel to the BPD, but slightly closer to the top of the head. In this section the lateral ventricles (LV) appear as two linear echoes, roughly parallel to the midline. The LVW is then measured as the distance from the midline to the first echoes of the lateral ventricles. This measurement is thus slightly greater than that of the actual lateral ventricle, because it does not use its medial wall as the internal landmark. The HW is the largest distance between the midline and the inner edge of the skull, measured perpendicular to the midline. To avoid tilting errors, one should be able to recognize both lateral ventricles as being equal in size.[36]

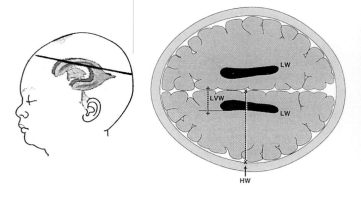

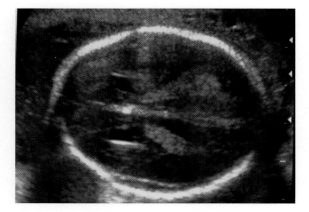

Figure 3–4.

COMMENTS

The normal LVW/HW ratio at 15 weeks can be as high as 71%, with a mean of 56% and a range of 40% to 71%. By 37 postmenstrual weeks, the mean is 29%, with a range of 24% to 34% (Table 3–14). These data reflect the rapid growth of the cerebral hemispheres as pregnancy progresses, making the LVW/HW decrease with advancing age.[37]

The LVW/HW ratio was developed to monitor ventricular growth in an attempt to provide an early diagnosis of hydrocephaly in a time when the classical diagnosis of intrauterine hydrocephaly relied on the finding of a BPD greater than 11 cm or a head-to-abdomen ratio greater than 2.[38] Although this ratio provided a way to diagnose hydrocephaly up to 2 months before the BPD was pathologically enlarged,[36] other parameters, such as the width of the lateral ventricular atrium.[37] More recently, transvaginal neurosonography, can evaluate the fetal ventricular system in a much more accurate way and somewhat earlier.

One of the major drawbacks of the LVW/HW ratio is that echogenic "lines" previously used to delineate the ventricular walls are, instead, reflections from small venous structures deep in the fetal white matter.[39] Also, the wide SD of this ratio renders it ineffective for detecting early ventricular dilatation.[40]

TABLE 3–14. NOMOGRAM FOR EVALUATION OF THE LATERAL VENTRICULAR WIDTH–HEMISPHERIC WIDTH RATIO

Menstrual Age (weeks)	Lateral Ventricular Width (LVW) (cm)	Hemispheric Width (HW) (cm)	Ratio LVW/HW (% ±2 SD)
15	0.75	1.4	56 (40–71)
16	0.86	1.5	57 (45–69)
17	0.85	1.5	52 (42–62)
18	0.83	1.8	46 (40–52)
19	—	—	—
20	0.82	1.9	43 (29–57)
21	0.76	2.2	35 (27–43)
22	0.82	2.6	32 (26–38)
23	0.83	2.5	33 (24–42)
24	0.83	2.7	31 (23–39)
25	1.1	3.0	34 (26–42)
26	0.9	3.0	30 (24–36)
27	0.9	3.0	28 (23–34)
28	1.1	3.3	31 (18–45)
29	1.0	3.4	29 (22–37)
30	1.0	3.4	30 (26–34)
31	1.0	3.4	29 (23–36)
32	1.1	3.6	31 (26–36)
33	1.1	3.4	31 (25–37)
34	1.1	3.8	28 (23–33)
35	1.1	3.8	29 (26–31)
36	1.1	3.9	28 (23–34)
37	1.2	4.1	29 (24–34)
Term	1.2	4.3	28 (22–33)

From Johnson and colleagues, 1980,[37] with permission.

ANTERIOR (FRONTAL) HORN OF THE LATERAL VENTRICLES AND CAVUM SEPTI PELLUCIDI

DEFINITION

The anterior horn corresponds to the portion of the lateral ventricles anterior to the interventricular foramen.

The cavum septi pellucidi (CSP) is a closed cavity in the brain, located on the midline of the transverse plane between the two leaves of septum pellucidum, which separate the lateral ventricles.

HOW TO MEASURE IT (FIG. 3–5)

To allow proper visualization of the anterior horn with transabdominal sonography, a horizontal (axial) scanning plane parallel and slightly anterior to that for the BPD should be used. In this section one should be able to recognize, in an anterior-to-posterior fashion, the anterior horns (AH), the cavum septi pellucidi (CSP), and the atria of the lateral ventricles (A). The cerebrofrontal horn distance (CFHD) can then be measured from the midline echo to the lateral wall of the anterior horn distal to the transducer. It should be kept in mind that from about 30 postmenstrual weeks on, the lumen of the anterior horns is very hard to visualize, and only its lateral aspect is defined. The frontal HW is measured from the leading edge of the midline echo to the inner aspect of the fetal calvarium at the point of maximal HW.[41]

COMMENTS

The relative size of the anterior horns decreases with advancing gestational age. This was demonstrated by Goldstein and coworkers,[41] who found that, in spite of an increasing CFHD throughout pregnancy, the CFHD/HW ratio decreases throughout gestation, from 50% at 15 menstrual weeks to 28% at term (Tables 3–15 and 3–16). These findings correlate with previous reports[42] and are related to the fact that the internal lumina of the ventricles are progressively reduced and molded by the growth of the basal nuclei, the corpus striatum, and the knee of the corpus callosum.

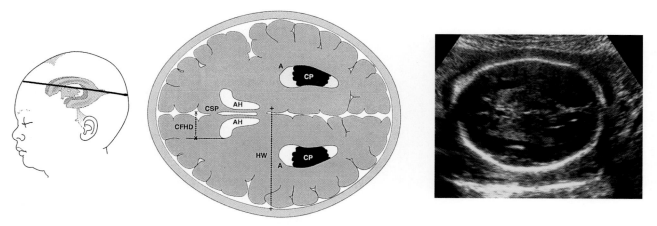

Figure 3–5.

TABLE 3–15. NOMOGRAM OF THE CEREBROFRONTAL HORN DISTANCE THROUGHOUT PREGNANCY (CM)

Gestational Age (weeks)	Mean ± 2 SD	Percentile 10th	50th	90th
15	0.7 ± 0.10	0.6	0.7	0.9
16	0.8 ± 0.12	0.5	0.8	1.0
17	0.9 ± 0.16	0.7	0.9	1.2
18	0.8 ± 0.05	0.8	0.9	0.9
19	0.8 ± 0.10	0.7	0.8	0.9
20	0.8 ± 0.10	0.7	0.8	1.0
21	0.8 ± 0.08	0.7	0.8	0.9
22	0.8 ± 0.07	0.7	0.8	0.9
23	0.9 ± 0.10	0.7	0.8	1.0
24	0.8 ± 0.07	0.7	0.9	0.9
25	0.8 ± 0.05	0.7	0.8	0.8
26	0.9 ± 0.11	0.8	1.0	1.1
27	1.0 ± 0.17	0.8	1.0	1.2
28	0.9 ± 0.13	0.8	0.9	1.1
29	1.0 ± 0.09	0.9	1.0	1.1
30	1.0 ± 0.12	0.8	1.0	1.2
31	1.0 ± 0.16	0.8	1.0	1.3
32	1.1 ± 0.08	1.0	1.1	1.2
33	1.1 ± 0.12	0.9	1.1	1.2
34	1.1 ± 0.13	0.9	1.0	1.2
35	1.2 ± 0.15	1.0	1.1	1.4
36	1.2 ± 0.10	1.1	1.2	1.3
37	1.1 ± 0.00	1.1	1.1	1.1
38	1.2 ± 0.06	1.2	1.2	1.3
39	1.3 ± 0.19	1.0	1.3	1.4
40	1.2 ± 0.00	1.2	1.2	1.2

From Goldstein and colleagues, 1988,[41] with permission.

The septae pellucidae are two thin, translucent leaves that extend from the anterior part of the body, the genu, and the rostrum of the corpus callosum to the superior surface of the fornix. They begin to develop at 10 to 12 weeks of gestation and reach an adult form by the 17th week of gestation (Table 3–17).[43] They are also part of the limbic system and are important relay stations, which are linked with the main hippocampus and hypothalamus. For a more extensive review of the sonographic diagnosis of CSP abnormalities, see Chapter 5.

ATRIUM OF THE LATERAL VENTRICLES

DEFINITION

The atrium, or the trigone, is the triangular portion of the lateral ventricle that is connected anteriorly to the body, posteriorly to the posterior horn, and inferiorly to the inferior horn. The width of the lateral ventricular atrium

TABLE 3–16. NOMOGRAM OF THE FRONTAL HEMISPHERIC WIDTH THROUGHOUT PREGNANCY

Gestational Age (weeks)	Mean ± 2 SD (cm)	Percentile		
		10th	50th	90th
15	1.5 ± 0.11	1.3	1.5	1.6
16	1.6 ± 0.12	1.5	1.7	1.8
17	1.7 ± 0.10	1.6	1.8	1.9
18	2.0 ± 0.07	1.9	2.0	2.1
19	2.1 ± 0.09	2.0	2.1	2.2
20	2.2 ± 0.10	2.1	2.3	2.3
21	2.3 ± 0.09	2.2	2.3	2.5
22	2.5 ± 0.07	2.4	2.5	2.6
23	2.7 ± 0.13	2.5	2.7	2.9
24	2.8 ± 0.10	2.6	2.9	2.9
25	3.0 ± 0.04	3.0	3.0	3.1
26	3.1 ± 0.11	3.0	3.3	3.4
27	3.3 ± 0.12	3.1	3.3	3.4
28	3.4 ± 0.09	3.3	3.5	3.5
29	3.6 ± 0.15	3.4	3.6	3.8
30	3.7 ± 0.20	3.4	3.8	3.9
31	3.9 ± 0.19	3.6	3.9	4.2
32	3.9 ± 0.17	3.5	3.9	4.1
33	4.0 ± 0.10	3.8	4.0	4.1
34	4.1 ± 0.18	3.8	4.2	4.2
35	4.4 ± 0.34	3.9	4.4	4.8
36	4.4 ± 0.13	4.2	4.4	4.5
37	4.4 ± 0.00	4.4	4.4	4.4
38	4.3 ± 0.22	4.1	4.3	4.6
39	4.6 ± 0.14	4.5	4.5	4.8
40	4.4 ± 0.00	4.4	4.4	4.4

From Goldstein and colleagues, 1988,[41] with permission.

TABLE 3–17 MEAN WIDTH AND STANDARD DEVIATION (SD) OF THE CAVUM SEPTI PELLUCIDI (CSP) AT VARIOUS GESTATIONAL AGES IN 608 FETUSES.

Gestational Age (weeks)	−2 SD	−1 SD	Mean Width (mm)	+1SD	+2 SD	n
19–20	2.08	2.74	3.40	4.06	4.7	43
21–22	2.60	3.33	4.06	4.81	5.52	104
23–24	3.02	3.88	4.74	5.60	6.46	92
25–26	3.96	4.76	5.56	6.36	7.16	36
27–28	4.12	5.27	6.42	7.57	8.72	18
29–30	4.37	5.29	6.11	7.13	8.05	24
31–32	4.43	5.47	6.51	7.55	8.59	77
33–34	4.04	5.26	6.48	7.70	8.92	116
35–36	4.37	5.41	6.45	7.49	8.53	55
37–38	3.81	5.09	6.37	7.65	8.93	27
39–40	4.64	5.47	6.30	7.13	7.96	10
41–42	3.62	4.55	5.48	6.41	7.34	6

Reproduced with permission from Jou HJ, Shyu MK, Wu SC, Chen SM, Su CH, Hsieh FJ. Ultrasound measurement of the fetal cavum septi pellucidi. Ultrasound Obstet Gynecol 1998;12:419–421.[43]

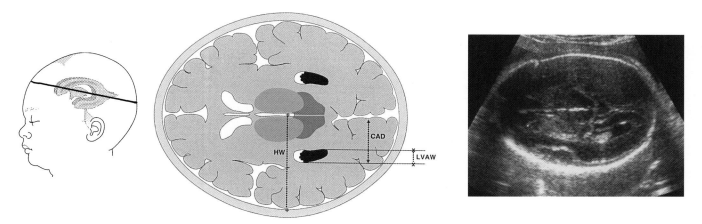

Figure 3–6.

(LVAW) is the widest dimension of the atrium of the lateral ventricles that can be measured in an axial plane.

HOW TO MEASURE IT (FIG. 3–6)

The atrium (A) of the lateral ventricles can be measured near the axial plane previously described for the BPD.[39] It can be easily recognized by the presence of the highly echogenic choroid plexus (CP) within it, marking the lateral wall of the ventricle farther from the transducer. The electronic calipers are then placed using an outer-to-inner (leading edge–to–leading edge) technique. Other parameters that can be used to evaluate the ventricular atrium are the cerebroatrial distance (CAD), atrial width/HW ratio, atrial width/CAD ratio, and CAD/HW ratio. The CAD is measured in the same plane as the distance between the midline and the outer border of the atrial lumen. The HW corresponds to the distance between the midline and the inner border of the calvarium.

COMMENTS

The ventricular atrium is a structure easily recognized due to the presence within of the choroid plexus, which is among the most noticeable intracranial landmarks. During the second and third trimesters, the choroid plexus normally fills the atrium of the lateral ventricles, touching the lateral ventricular walls. Ventricular enlargement can thus be suspected when a separation of 3 mm or more can be measured between the ventricular surface of the choroid plexus and the adjacent ventricular wall.[44]

The LVAW is an excellent measurement for verifying the state of the ventricular system. It is age independent, with a mean of 7.6 mm, which remains stable with little change (SD of 0.6 mm) throughout gestation, certainly a very useful feature for any parameter used to evaluate a normal fetal structure (Table 3–18). For practical purposes, a normal upper limit of 10 mm for atrial width has been established.[45,46] Another advantage of this measurement is its low reported intra- and interobserver variability.[39] Other authors[47] prefer morphological criteria, such as the shrunken appearance of the choroid plexus in hydrocephaly, rather than absolute measurements for estimation of the cerebral ventricles.

TABLE 3–18. DIAMETER OF THE LATERAL VENTRICULAR ATRIUM ACCORDING TO GESTATIONAL AGE

Gestational Age (weeks)	Lateral Ventricular Atrium Diameter (mm)	
	Mean ± SD	Range
14–20	7.6 ± 0.7	6.0–9.0
21–25	7.7 ± 0.5	7.0–9.0
26–30	7.5 ± 0.7	6.5–9.0
31–38	7.6 ± 0.5	7.0–8.5
All	7.6 ± 0.6	6.0–9.0

After Cardoza and colleagues, 1988,[39] with permission.

TABLE 3–19. NOMOGRAM OF THE CEREBROATRIAL DISTANCE THROUGHOUT PREGNANCY

Gestational Age (weeks)	Mean ± SD (cm)
15–17	1.16 ± 0.08
18–20	1.35 ± 0.09
21–23	1.45 ± 0.10
24–26	1.59 ± 0.13
27–29	1.81 ± 0.14
30–32	1.96 ± 0.17
33–35	2.04 ± 0.15
36–38	2.15 ± 0.21
39–40	2.36 ± 0.15

From Pilu and colleagues, 1989,[49] with permission.

Typically, a reverberation artifact from the fetal calvarium obscures the ventricle closest to the transducer, but variations in the angle of the beam and maternal position can make visualization of this ventricle possible.[44] Both atria should be visualized if the uncommon but reported[48] possibility of unilateral ventriculomegaly is to be ruled out in the atria closest to the transducer.

The CAD increases as pregnancy progresses, reflecting the steady growth of the cerebral hemispheres (Table 3–19). The decreasing atrial width/HW, atrial width/CAD, and CAD/HW ratios (Tables 3–20 through 3–22) indicate that the relative size of the atria decreases with brain growth, probably due not to an actual decrease in its size, which is relatively constant, but to growth of brain tissue throughout fetal life.[49]

POSTERIOR (OCCIPITAL) HORN OF THE LATERAL VENTRICLES

DEFINITION

The posterior or occipital horn of the lateral ventricles represents the posterior continuation of the atria of the lateral ventricles.

TABLE 3–20. NOMOGRAM OF THE ATRIAL WIDTH–HEMISPHERIC WIDTH RATIO VERSUS GESTATIONAL AGE

Gestational Age (weeks)	Mean ± 2 SD (%)
15	49 ± 10
16	47 ± 9
17	46 ± 6
18	42 ± 8
19	35 ± 8
20	20 ± 8
21	33 ± 6
22	27 ± 6
23	23 ± 8
24	22 ± 8
25	20 ± 4
26	21 ± 4
27	19 ± 6
28	18 ± 6
29	16 ± 2
30	14 ± 2
31	17 ± 4
32	15 ± 6
33	17 ± 4
34	15 ± 4
35	17 ± 6
36	13 ± 4
37	13 ± 4
38	13 ± 4
39	14 ± 2
40	14 ± 2

From Pilu and colleagues, 1989,[49] with permission.

TABLE 3–21. NOMOGRAM OF THE ATRIAL WIDTH–CEREBROATRIAL DISTANCE RATIO THROUGHOUT PREGNANCY

Gestational Age (weeks)	Mean ± 2 SD (cm)	Percentile 10th	Percentile 50th	Percentile 90th
15	0.59 ± 0.086	0.50	0.60	0.70
16	0.70 ± 0.060	0.58	0.72	0.75
17	0.67 ± 0.101	0.53	0.66	0.81
18	0.63 ± 0.058	0.57	0.61	0.71
19	0.56 ± 0.071	0.50	0.53	0.69
20	0.54 ± 0.766	0.42	0.53	0.64
21	0.54 ± 0.043	0.50	0.53	0.62
22	0.48 ± 0.048	0.40	0.50	0.54
23	0.44 ± 0.079	0.31	0.43	0.56
24	0.43 ± 0.094	0.27	0.46	0.57
25	0.37 ± 0.388	0.31	0.39	0.41
26	0.39 ± 0.380	0.35	0.41	0.44
27	0.36 ± 0.067	0.28	0.35	0.44
28	0.37 ± 0.095	0.26	0.35	0.50

Continued.

TABLE 3–21. NOMOGRAM OF THE ATRIAL WIDTH–CEREBROATRIAL DISTANCE RATIO THROUGHOUT PREGNANCY—Cont'd

Gestational Age (weeks)	Mean ± 2 SD (cm)	Percentile 10th	50th	90th
29	0.31 ± 0.063	0.20	0.32	0.41
30	0.29 ± 0.046	0.21	0.28	0.35
31	0.34 ± 0.059	0.24	0.37	0.40
32	0.30 ± 0.064	0.17	0.32	0.40
33	0.36 ± 0.070	0.27	0.35	0.44
34	0.30 ± 0.600	0.24	0.27	0.39
35	0.36 ± 0.072	0.29	0.33	0.47
36	0.28 ± 0.043	0.23	0.29	0.33
37	0.25 ± 0.043	0.25	0.25	0.25
38	0.29 ± 0.038	0.27	0.28	0.35
39	0.28 ± 0.034	0.25	0.27	0.32
40	0.33 ± 0.330	0.33	0.33	0.33

From Pilu and colleagues, 1989,[49] with permission.

TABLE 3–22. NOMOGRAM OF THE CEREBROATRIAL DISTANCE–HEMISPHERIC WIDTH RATIO THROUGHOUT PREGNANCY

Gestational Age (weeks)	Mean ± 2 SD (cm)	Percentile 10th	50th	90th
15	0.82 ± 0.090	0.71	0.80	1.00
16	0.73 ± 0.069	0.64	0.71	0.86
17	0.70 ± 0.062	0.61	0.70	0.76
18	0.70 ± 0.055	0.60	0.72	0.75
19	0.65 ± 0.014	0.63	0.65	0.67
20	0.63 ± 0.610	0.55	0.62	0.75
21	0.66 ± 0.046	0.60	0.67	0.73
22	0.60 ± 0.044	0.52	0.61	0.65
23	0.58 ± 0.050	0.54	0.56	0.67
24	0.54 ± 0.040	0.46	0.54	0.59
25	0.58 ± 0.033	0.55	0.57	0.62
26	0.57 ± 0.033	0.53	0.57	0.63
27	0.57 ± 0.025	0.53	0.57	0.60
28	0.51 ± 0.054	0.44	0.49	0.57
29	0.55 ± 0.040	0.51	0.54	0.62
30	0.51 ± 0.050	0.46	0.50	0.61
31	0.53 ± 0.050	0.46	0.53	0.60
32	0.54 ± 0.056	0.46	0.52	0.60
33	0.52 ± 0.042	0.45	0.53	0.58
34	0.30 ± 0.060	0.24	0.27	0.39
35	0.52 ± 0.034	0.48	0.53	0.57
36	0.49 ± 0.024	0.46	0.49	0.52
37	0.57 ± 0.024	0.57	0.57	0.57
38	0.53 ± 0.038	0.48	0.53	0.59
39	0.54 ± 0.026	0.52	0.53	0.57
40	0.50 ± 0.026	0.50	0.50	0.50

From Pilu and colleagues, 1989,[49] with permission.

TABLE 3–25. EQUATIONS OF THE REGRESSIONS, INCLUDING THE 95% PREDICTION INTERVALS

Independent Variable	Dependent Variable	Equations
Hemispheres		
Gestational age	Length	$y = (-3.34 + 0.62x \pm 1.96 \times 0.26)^2$
Gestational age	Width	$y = (-1.45 + 0.33x \pm 1.96 \times 0.21)^2$
Gestational age	Depth	$y = (-1.25 + 0.34x \pm 1.96 \times 0.22)^2$
Choroid plexus of the lateral ventricles		
Gestational age	Length	$y = (-3.99 + 0.63x \pm 1.96 \times 0.29)^2$
Gestational age	Width	$y = (-1.71 + 0.32x \pm 1.96 \times 0.21)^2$
Gestational age	Height	$y = (-1.55 + 0.32x \pm 1.96 \times 0.19)^2$
Diencephalon		
Gestational age	Length	$y = -2.15 + 0.575x \pm 1.96 \times 0.63$
Gestational age	Width	$y = 1.63 - 0.07x \pm 1.96 \times 0.24$
Gestational age	Height	$y = -0.87 + 0.28x \pm 1.96 \times 0.34$
Mesencephalon		
Gestational age	Length	$y = -0.32 + 0.42x \pm 1.96 \times 0.54$
Gestational age	Width	$y = 0.54 + 0.1x \pm 1.96 \times 0.28$
Gestational age	Height	$y = 0.01 + 0.16x \pm 1.96 \times 0.28$

The gestational age is based on the date of the last menstrual period.

TABLE 3–26. MEAN SIZE AND 95% PREDICTION INTERVALS OF THE RHOMBENCEPHALIC STRUCTURES

Gestational Age (weeks + days)	Rhombencephalon (mm)			Cerebellum (mm)		Choroid Plexus (mm)	
	Length	Width	Depth	Width	Height	Width	Height
7 + 0	3.8 (2.2–5.3)	2.1 (0.6–3.7)	1.5 (0.4–2.6)				
8 + 0	3.9 (2.3–5.4)	3.1 (1.5–4.7)	2.1 (1.0–3.2)				
9 + 0	4.0 (2.5–5.6)	3.8 (2.2–5.4)	2.5 (1.5–3.6)	4.8 (3.0–7.1)	1.4 (0.7–2.1)	3.2 (1.8–4.6)	1.1 (0.6–1.6)
10 + 0	4.1 (2.6–5.7)	4.3 (2.7–5.8)	2.9 (1.8–3.9)	5.8 (3.8–8.3)	1.7 (1.0–2.4)	3.5 (2.1–4.9)	1.1 (0.6–1.6)
11 + 0	4.3 (2.7–5.8)	4.5 (2.9–6.1)	3.1 (2.0–4.2)	6.9 (4.7–9.6)	2.1 (1.4–2.8)	3.8 (2.4–5.2)	1.2 (0.7–1.7)
12 + 0	4.4 (2.8–5.9)	4.5 (2.9–6.1)	3.2 (2.2–4.3)	8.1 (5.7–11.0)	2.5 (1.8–3.2)	4.1 (2.7–5.6)	1.3 (0.8–1.8)

From Blaas and colleagues, 1995,[54] with permission.

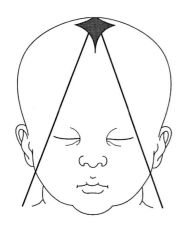
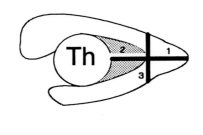
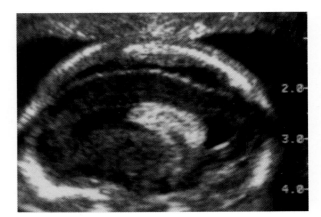

Figure 3–17.

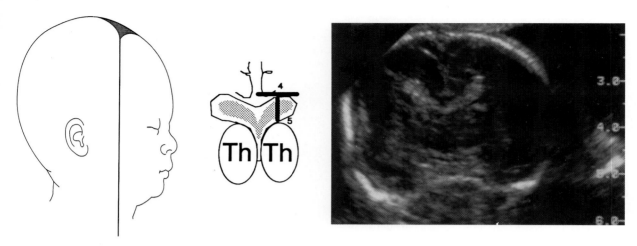

Figure 3–18.

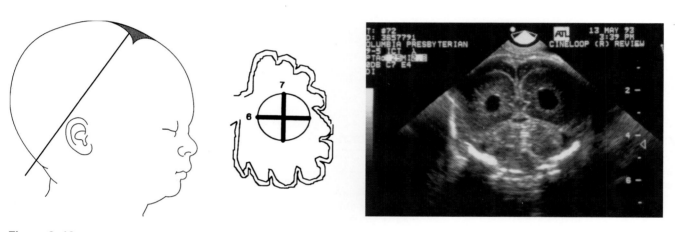

Figure 3–19.

is in a nonvertex presentation and the transabdominal scan is suboptimal, an external cephalic version may be considered in selected cases. Usually, end-firing probes with frequencies of 5 or 7.5 MHz are used.[57,58] Oblique and coronal planes can be used to measure the cerebral ventricles in the following fashion.[2]

DESCRIPTION OF MEASUREMENTS

Number	Plane	Measurement
1	Oblique–1 (Fig. 3–17)	Thalamus–choroid plexus interface to the tip of the posterior (occipital) horn (TCP–TOH)
2		Choroid plexus thickness (CPT)
3		Posterior (occipital) horn height (OHH)
4	Midcoronal–2 (Fig. 3–18)	Midline to the upper edge of the lateral ventricle (MUELV)
5		Depth of the lateral ventricle (DLV)
6	Occipital–1 (posterior coronal) (Fig. 3–19)	Width of the posterior (occipital) horn (WOH)
7		Height of the posterior (occipital) horn (HOH)
Ratio		Thalamus to tip of posterior horn (TCP–TOH)/choroid plexus thickness (CPT)
Ratio		Posterior horn height (oblique plane) (OHH)/choroid plexus thickness (CPT)

COMMENTS

In 1989, Kushnir and colleagues[59] proposed the use of transvaginal sonography to examine certain biometric parameters (CRL, BPD, HC, LVW, and HW) in a group of 50 patients whose pregnancies were between 12 and 14 gestational weeks. In 1991, our group[54] described for the first time the feasibility of the routine transvaginal sonographic evaluation of the fetal brain during the second half of pregnancy. With this approach, using the anterior fontanelle, images of diagnostic quality of the intracranial anatomy can be obtained. The differentiation between normal and pathological brain structures is easier and avoids the disadvantages of the transabdominal route. Such disadvantages may be (1) the inadequate visualization of the cerebral hemispheres due to reverberation artifacts, a deeply engaged fetal head, or maternal obesity and abdominal scarring; and (2) the presence of pseudohydrocephalus, unilateral hydrocephalus, and pseudoepidural artifact, which are detected using conventional axial planes.[60]

Using this technique, nine nomograms of the fetal lateral ventricles were developed and evaluated using the sagittal and coronal planes (Tables 3–26 through 3–36). The occipital plane is usually the hardest to image due to maternal discomfort while maneuvering the probe. Measurements such as the TCP–TOH, OHH, and MUELV increased in a linear fashion as pregnancy advanced. Measurements such as the CPT, DLV, WOH, HOH, and the ratios TCP–TOH/CPT and OHH/CPT demonstrated little, if any, association with gestational age.[60]

One of the major applications of these nomograms is the early diagnosis of hydrocephaly. Two early changes have been described. The first is the dilatation of the posterior horn in an up-and-down fashion, where the resistance to the cerebrospinal fluid (CSF) pressure is least,[61,62] and second is the squeezed appearance of the choroid plexus, probably as a result of the increasing CSF pressure.[63] In our experience[58] measurement of the choroid plexus alone was not discriminatory, but when its thickness was used as a denominator in the two ratios, it became a very sensitive measurement. We propose that although all seven measurements may add important clinical information, evaluation of the OHH (number 3) in the Oblique–1 plane and measurements of the lateral ventricle and the HOH (numbers 5 and 7) in the Midcoronal–2 and Occipital–1 planes are the best markers of early ventricular dilatation. If a single plane had to be chosen as the first-line indicator of ventriculomegaly with the transvaginal route, the Oblique–1 plane should be selected because in this plane the OHH can be obtained and the two ratios can be calculated.[58]

Transvaginal neurosonography not only has a place in the diagnosis of ventricular dilatation, but also can be of invaluable help in diagnosing almost any type of congenital central nervous system anomaly.[64] The sonographic planes described can also be used for evaluating the appearance and development of the corpus callosum. By 18 weeks of gestation, all the components of the corpus callosum are present and can be visualized on transvaginal sonography in approximately 95% of cases (Table 3–27).[65] Transvaginal sonography provides an excellent method for direct examination of this structure, allowing for the diagnosis of anomalies such as agenesis and hypogenesis as well as more subtle findings associated with "callosal thinning," particularly in cases of infection, periventricular leukomalacia, inborn errors of the metabolism, and anomalies of neuronal migration.

TABLE 3–27.

Gestational Age (weeks)	Length (mm)	Thickness (mm)		
		Genu	*Body*	*Splenium*
18–19	16.9 ± 2.4	2.2 ± 0.5	1.3 ± 0.1	2.1 ± 0.1
20–21	20.6 ± 4.4	2.3 ± 0.6	1.6 ± 0.1	2.1 ± 0.1
22–23	23.3 ± 3.0	2.7 ± 0.6	1.7 ± 0.2	3.1 ± 0.2
24–25	29.8 ± 2.3	3.0 ± 0.6	1.9 ± 0.3	3.0 ± 0.3
26–27	33.7 ± 2.4	3.5 ± 0.6	2.0 ± 0.2	3.3 ± 0.6
28–29	25.8 ± 2.8	4.0 ± 0.7	2.0 ± 0.4	4.0 ± 0.8
30–31	36.8 ± 1.4	4.2 ± 0.5	2.1 ± 0.4	4.1 ± 0.7
32–33	39.1 ± 4.3	4.5 ± 1.2	2.5 ± 0.6	4.2 ± 0.8
34–35	40.6 ± 6.4	4.6 ± 0.5	2.5 ± 0.5	4.4 ± 0.8
36–37	41.9 ± 3.5	5.0 ± 0.4	2.5 ± 0.4	4.4 ± 1.3
38–39	43.0 ± 4.2	4.8 ± 0.7	2.6 ± 0.5	4.4 ± 0.6
40–42	44.0 ± 3.8	4.8 ± 0.4	2.6 ± 0.5	4.4 ± 0.7

Modified after: Malinger G, Zakut H. The corpus callosum: Normal fetal development as shown by transvaginal sonography. AJR 1993;161:1041–1043.[65]

TABLE 3–28. THALAMUS TO THE TIP OF THE POSTERIOR HORN

Estimated Gestational Age (weeks)	5th Percentile (mm)	50th Percentile (mm)	Percentile 95th (mm)
14	6.06	13.34	20.62
15	6.47	13.75	21.03
16	6.87	14.15	21.43
17	7.27	14.55	21.83
18	7.68	14.96	22.24
19	8.08	15.36	22.64
20	8.49	15.77	23.05
21	8.89	16.17	23.45
22	9.29	16.57	23.85
23	9.70	16.98	24.26
24	10.10	17.38	24.66
25	10.51	17.79	25.07
26	10.91	18.19	25.47
27	11.31	18.60	25.88
28	11.72	19.00	26.28
29	12.12	19.40	26.68
30	12.53	19.81	27.09
31	12.93	20.21	27.49
32	13.34	20.62	27.90
33	13.74	21.01	28.30
34	14.14	21.42	28.70
35	14.55	21.83	29.11
36	14.95	22.23	29.51
37	15.36	22.64	29.92
38	15.76	23.04	30.32
39	16.16	23.44	30.72
40	16.57	23.85	31.13

TABLE 3–29. CHOROID PLEXUS THICKNESS

Estimated Gestational Age (weeks)	5th Percentile (mm)	50th Percentile (mm)	95th Percentile (mm)
14	4.41	8.89	13.37
15	4.48	8.96	13.44
16	4.55	9.03	13.51
17	4.62	9.10	13.58
18	4.69	9.17	13.65
19	4.76	9.24	13.72
20	4.83	9.31	13.79
21	4.90	9.38	13.86
22	4.97	9.45	13.93
23	5.04	9.52	14.00
24	5.11	9.59	14.07
25	5.18	9.66	14.14
26	5.25	9.73	14.21
27	5.32	9.80	14.28
28	5.39	9.87	14.34
29	5.45	9.93	14.41
30	5.52	10.00	14.48
31	5.59	10.07	14.55
32	5.66	10.14	14.62
33	5.73	10.21	14.69
34	5.80	10.28	14.76
35	5.87	10.35	14.83
36	5.94	10.42	14.90
37	6.00	10.49	14.97
38	6.08	10.56	15.04
39	6.15	10.63	15.11
40	6.22	10.70	15.18

TABLE 3–30. POSTERIOR HORN HEIGHT

Estimated Gestational Age (weeks)	5th Percentile (mm)	50th Percentile (mm)	95th Percentile (mm)
14	1.97	6.91	11.85
15	2.20	7.14	12.08
16	2.42	7.36	12.30
17	2.64	7.58	12.53
18	2.87	7.81	12.75
19	3.09	8.03	12.97
20	3.32	8.26	13.20
21	3.54	8.48	13.42
22	3.76	8.70	13.64
23	3.99	8.93	13.87
24	4.21	9.15	14.09
25	4.43	9.37	14.31
26	4.66	9.60	14.54
27	4.88	9.82	14.76
28	5.11	10.05	14.98
29	5.33	10.27	15.21
30	5.55	10.49	15.43
31	5.78	10.72	15.66
32	6.00	10.94	15.88
33	6.22	11.16	16.10
34	6.45	11.39	16.33
35	6.67	11.61	16.55
36	6.90	11.84	16.78
37	7.12	12.06	17.00
38	7.34	12.28	17.22
39	7.57	12.51	17.45
40	7.79	12.73	17.67

TABLE 3–31. MIDLINE TO THE UPPER EDGE OF THE LATERAL VENTRICLE

Estimated Gestational Age (weeks)	5th Percentile (mm)	50th Percentile (mm)	95th Percentile (mm)
14	3.95	8.39	12.83
15	4.19	8.63	13.07
16	4.44	8.88	13.32
17	4.68	9.12	13.56
18	4.93	9.37	13.81
19	5.17	9.61	14.05
20	5.42	9.86	14.30
21	5.67	10.11	14.55
22	5.91	10.35	14.79
23	6.16	10.60	15.04
24	6.40	10.84	15.28
25	6.65	11.09	15.53
26	6.89	11.33	15.77
27	7.14	11.58	16.02
28	7.39	11.83	16.27
29	7.63	12.07	16.51
30	7.98	12.32	16.76
31	8.12	12.56	17.00
32	8.37	12.81	17.25
33	8.62	13.06	17.50
34	8.86	13.30	17.74
35	9.11	13.55	17.99
36	9.35	13.79	18.23
37	9.60	14.04	18.48
38	9.84	14.28	18.72
39	10.09	14.53	18.97
40	10.34	14.78	19.22

TABLE 3–32. DEPTH OF THE LATERAL VENTRICLE

Estimated Gestational Age (weeks)	5th Percentile (mm)	50th Percentile (mm)	95th Percentile (mm)
14	2.25	5.49	8.73
15	2.18	5.42	8.66
16	2.11	5.35	8.59
17	2.04	5.28	8.52
18	1.97	5.21	8.45
19	1.91	5.15	8.39
20	1.84	5.08	8.32
21	1.77	5.00	8.25
22	1.70	4.94	8.18
23	1.63	4.87	8.11
24	1.56	4.80	8.04
25	1.49	4.73	7.97
26	1.42	4.66	7.90
27	1.35	4.59	7.83
28	1.28	4.52	7.76
29	1.23	4.45	7.69
30	1.14	4.38	7.62
31	1.07	4.31	7.55
32	1.00	4.24	7.48
33	0.93	4.17	7.41
34	0.87	4.11	7.35
35	0.80	4.04	7.28
36	0.73	3.97	7.21
37	0.66	3.90	7.14
38	0.59	3.83	7.07
39	0.52	3.76	7.00
40	0.45	3.69	6.93

TABLE 3–33. WIDTH OF THE POSTERIOR HORN

Estimated Gestational Age (weeks)	5th Percentile (mm)	50th Percentile (mm)	95th Percentile (mm)
14	1.23	5.53	9.83
16	1.31	5.61	9.91
17	1.36	5.66	9.96
18	1.40	5.70	10.00
19	1.44	5.74	10.04
20	1.48	5.78	10.08
21	1.52	5.82	10.12
22	1.56	5.86	10.16
23	1.60	5.90	10.20
24	1.65	5.95	10.25
25	1.69	6.00	10.29
26	1.73	6.03	10.33
27	1.77	6.07	10.37
28	1.82	6.12	10.42
29	1.86	6.16	10.46
30	1.90	6.20	10.50
31	1.94	6.24	10.54
32	1.98	6.28	10.58
33	2.02	6.32	10.62
34	2.07	6.37	10.67
35	2.10	6.40	10.71
36	2.15	6.45	10.75
37	2.19	6.49	10.79
38	2.23	6.53	10.83
39	2.28	6.58	10.88

TABLE 3–34. HEIGHT OF THE POSTERIOR HORN

Estimated Gestational Age (weeks)	5th Percentile (mm)	50th Percentile (mm)	95th Percentile (mm)
14	0.70	5.80	10.90
16	0.94	6.04	11.14
17	1.06	6.16	11.26
18	1.18	6.28	11.38
19	1.30	6.40	11.50
20	1.42	6.52	11.62
21	1.54	6.64	11.74
22	1.66	6.76	11.86
23	1.78	6.88	11.98
24	1.90	7.00	12.10
25	2.02	7.12	12.22
26	2.15	7.25	12.35
27	2.27	7.37	12.47
28	2.39	7.49	12.59
29	2.51	7.61	12.71
30	2.63	7.73	12.83
31	2.75	7.85	12.95
32	2.87	7.97	13.07
33	2.99	8.09	13.19
34	3.11	8.21	13.31
35	3.23	8.33	13.43
36	3.34	8.45	13.55
37	3.47	8.57	13.67
38	3.59	8.69	13.79
39	3.71	8.80	13.91

TABLE 3–35. RATIO OF THE THALAMUS TO THE TIP OF THE OCCIPITAL (POSTERIOR) HORN TO CHOROID PLEXUS THICKNESS

Estimated Gestational Age (weeks)	5th Percentile (mm)	50th Percentile (mm)	95th Percentile (mm)	Estimated Gestational Age (weeks)	5th Percentile (mm)	50th Percentile (mm)	95th Percentile (mm)
14	0.50	1.55	2.60	28	0.95	1.99	3.05
15	0.54	1.59	2.64	29	0.98	2.03	3.08
16	0.57	1.62	2.68	30	1.00	2.06	3.11
17	0.59	1.65	2.70	31	1.04	2.09	3.14
18	0.63	1.68	2.73	32	1.07	2.12	3.17
19	0.66	1.71	2.76	33	1.10	2.15	3.20
20	0.69	1.74	2.79	34	1.14	2.19	3.24
21	0.73	1.78	2.83	35	1.17	2.22	3.27
22	0.76	1.81	2.86	36	1.20	2.25	3.30
23	0.79	1.84	2.89	37	1.23	2.28	3.33
24	0.82	1.87	2.92	38	1.26	2.31	3.36
25	0.85	1.90	2.95	39	1.29	2.34	3.39
26	0.88	1.93	2.98	40	1.32	2.37	3.42
27	0.91	1.96	3.01				

TCP–TOH, Thalamus to the tip of the occipital horn; CPT, choroid plexus thickness.

TABLE 3–36. RATIO OF THE OCCIPITAL (POSTERIOR) HORN HEIGHT TO THE CHOROID PLEXUS THICKNESS

Estimated Gestational Age (weeks)	5th Percentile (mm)	50th Percentile (mm)	95th Percentile (mm)
14	0.02	0.85	1.68
15	0.04	0.86	1.69
16	0.05	0.88	1.71
17	0.07	0.90	1.72
18	0.84	0.91	1.74
19	0.10	0.93	1.75
20	0.12	0.94	1.77
21	0.13	0.96	1.79
22	0.15	0.97	1.80
23	0.16	0.99	1.82
24	0.18	1.00	1.83
25	0.19	1.02	1.85
26	0.21	1.04	1.87
27	0.23	1.05	1.88
28	0.24	1.07	1.90
29	0.26	1.09	1.91
30	0.27	1.10	1.93
31	0.29	1.12	1.94
32	0.31	1.13	1.96
33	0.32	1.15	1.98
34	0.24	1.16	1.99
35	0.35	1.18	2.00
36	0.37	1.20	2.02
37	0.38	1.21	2.04
38	0.40	1.23	2.06
39	0.42	1.24	2.07
40	0.43	1.26	2.09

OHH, Occipital horn height; CPT, choroid plexus thickness.

Other Intracranial Structures
Thalamus, Basal Nuclei–Insula,
and Temporal Operculum

DEFINITIONS

The thalamus is a diencephalic structure separated from the epithalamus by the epithalamic sulcus and from the hypothalamus by the hypothalamic sulcus. It develops rapidly on each side and bulges into the cavity of the third ventricle, molding and reducing its size. In most brains (70%) the thalami fuse in the midline, forming a bridge of gray matter called the massa intermedia.[66]

The basal nuclei are an arbitrary group that includes the corpus striatum, the amygdaloid body, and the claustrum. The corpus striatum and the claustrum are telencephalic structures, whereas the amygdaloid body is of diencephalic origin. From a clinical point of view, the subthalamic nucleus and the substantia nigra are added, to complete the basal structures affected pathologically in the so-called extrapyramidal motor diseases.[67]

The temporal operculum corresponds to the caudal end of the temporal lobe, growing forward and downward to form the posterocaudal edge of the lateral sulcus. The insula is a portion of the cerebral cortex buried by the folds of frontal, parietal, and temporal cortices that form the walls of the lateral sulcus.[68]

HOW TO MEASURE IT (FIG. 3–20)

These structures can be readily outlined in the standard horizontal BPD plane previously described.[5,8] The hypoechoic thalamus (T) is measured at the anterior tip of the ambient cistern. The basal nuclei (BN) and insula (I) can be measured as a whole from the edge of the thalamus to the echo of the

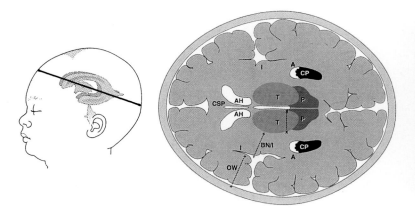
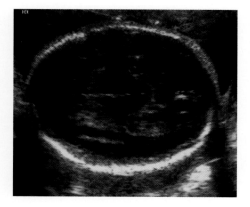

Figure 3–20.

cistern of the lateral sulcus. The opercular width (OW) of the temporal lobe corresponds sonographically to the distance between the inner surface of the temporal bone and the cistern of the lateral sulcus at the point of its invagination into the cerebral cortex.[51]

COMMENTS

The cerebral hemispheres buckle as their growth increases, creating the sulci and the gyri. The largest infolding corresponds to the developing lateral sulcus, where the caudal end of the cerebral hemispheres grows to form the operculum of the temporal lobe. With the described measurement method, the OW is overestimated in the second trimester because the gap that exists between the inner bone surface and the insular cortex is not taken into consideration. On the other hand, in the third trimester this measurement is underestimated because the distance between the cistern of the lateral sulcus and the calvarium does not represent exactly the full width of the developing temporal operculum. Nevertheless, by 35 postmenstrual weeks the OW has approximately doubled from its time of first appearance.[51]

By 18 postmenstrual weeks the basal nuclei and the insular cortex can be identified. Siedler and Filly[51] have proposed that with transabdominal sonography the basal nuclei appear as two zones of different echogenicity: (1) a echogenic curvilinear strip marginating the thalamus and posterolateral to the frontal horns that corresponds to the caudate and lentiform nuclei, and (2) a sonolucent band lateral to the previously described, corresponding to the external capsule, claustrum, and extreme capsule. The insular cortex is included when measuring this hypoechoic band.

The thalami, in the BPD plane, appear sonographically as two hypoechoic oval structures separated in the midline by the third ventricle. Their width increases from 7 $\pm$ 0.8 mm at 15 to 20 postmenstrual weeks to 9 $\pm$ 0.7 mm at 31 to 35 postmenstrual weeks, undergoing considerably less growth than the temporal operculum and the basal nuclei–insula (Table 3–37).

TABLE 3–37. MEASUREMENTS OF FETAL INTRACRANIAL STRUCTURES

Gestational Age (weeks)	Thalamus (mm)			Basal Nuclei–Insula (mm)			Temporal Operculum (mm)		
	Mean	*Range*	*SD*	*Mean*	*Range*	*SD*	*Mean*	*Range*	*SD*
15–20	7	6–9	0.8	6	5–7	0.7	6	5–7	0.9
21–25	8	6–9	0.7	7	6–11	1.2	9	7–11	1.0
26–30	8	8–9	0.4	9	8–12	1.2	11	10–13	0.6
31–35	9	8–10	0.7	11	9–14	1.1	13	11–15	0.7

After Siedler and Filly, 1987,[51] with permission.

Posterior Fossa: Cerebellum and Cerebellomedullary Cistern (Cisterna Magna)

DEFINITIONS

The cerebellum is a suprasegmental portion of the brain located within the cranial posterior fossa that receives input from virtually the entire nervous system, playing a key role in movement coordination.[69]

The cerebellomedullary cistern (CMC) corresponds to a portion of the subarachnoid space that bathes the cranial posterior fossa in CSF. It arcs around the cerebellum posteriorly, invaginating in the midline between the cerebellar hemispheres.[70]

HOW TO MEASURE IT (FIG. 3–21)

To evaluate the posterior fossa, a horizontal plane of the fetal head equal to that used for determination of the BPD must be obtained. Once the landmarks of the thalami (T) and the cavum septum pellucidum (CSP) are identified, a slight caudal rotation of the transducer will bring the characteristic butterfly-like appearance of the cerebellum into view. The transverse cerebellar diameter (TCD) can then be measured as the widest diameter across both hemispheres in an outer-to-outer fashion.[71]

The CMC depth is evaluated in the same plane and measured in the median plane from the posterior aspect of the cerebellum to the inner table of the occiput.

COMMENTS

The fetal cerebellum can be visualized sonographically as early as 10 to 11 postmenstrual weeks. It grows rapidly in the second trimester following a linear relationship with gestational age, so that during this period, measurements in millimeters equal approximately the gestational age in weeks. However, as pregnancy advances, the growth curve of the cerebellum tends to flatten, showing a slower rate of evolution (Tables 3–38 and 3–39).[71]

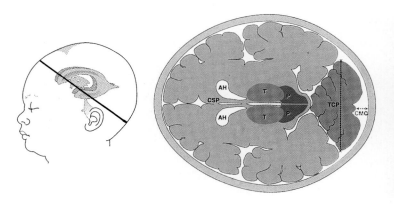
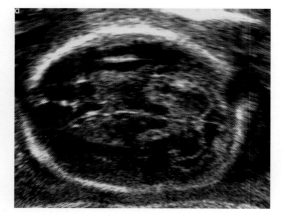

Figure 3–21.

TABLE 3–38. PREDICTED GESTATIONAL AGES FOR TRANSVERSE CEREBELLAR DIAMETERS OF 14 TO 56 mm

Cerebellar Diameter (mm)	Gestational Age (weeks)	Cerebellar Diameter (mm)	Gestational Age (weeks)
14	15.2	35	29.4
15	15.8	36	30.0
16	16.5	37	30.6
17	17.2	38	31.2
18	17.9	39	31.8
19	18.6	40	32.3
20	19.3	41	32.8
21	20.0	42	33.4
22	20.7	43	33.9
23	21.4	44	34.4
24	22.1	45	34.8
25	22.8	46	35.3
26	23.5	47	35.7
27	24.2	48	36.1
28	24.9	49	36.5
29	25.5	50	36.8
30	26.2	51	37.2
31	26.9	52	37.5
32	27.5	54	38.0
33	28.1	55	38.3
34	28.8	56	38.5

From Hill and colleagues, 1990,[76] with permission.

Because the cerebellum is located inside the posterior fossa and is surrounded by the dense, petrous ridges and the occipital bone, it should be able to withstand deformation by extrinsic pressure better than the parietal bone. Keeping this concept in mind, several authors[71–73] have proposed that the TCD, as opposed to the BPD, can better predict gestational age in cases in which variations of the fetal head shape, such as dolichocephaly and brachycephaly, have been described (e.g., breech presentation, oligohydramnios, twins, and uterine anomalies).

Intrauterine growth retardation remains a major cause of perinatal morbidity and mortality, affecting 4% to 8% of all deliveries in so-called developed countries.[74] In order to better evaluate fetal biometry, when intrauterine growth retardation is suspected, the TCD should also be used. Cabbad and associates[75] found that 22 out of 23 asymmetrically growth-impaired fetuses had a TCD lower than expected but within the normal range, suggesting that this measurement could be used to help estimate gestational age in these cases. On the other hand, Hill and colleagues[76] found, in a group of 116 diabetic and nondiabetic singleton gestations with an estimated fetal weight at or above the '90th percentile, that the TCD did not overestimate gestational age in the nondiabetic group, and overestimated age in the diabetic group by only 0.5 postmenstrual weeks, rendering it a useful tool for predicting age in this population. The TCD has also been used to evaluate fetal growth in twin gestations.[77] Dilmen and colleagues[78] have used the TCD/AC ratio obtained by transabdominal sonography to evaluate fetal growth. Ten of eleven fetuses with TCD/AC ratios exceeding 2 SD (0.1648) were found to have asymmetrical intrauterine growth retardation upon neonatal examination.

TABLE 3–39. NOMOGRAM OF THE TRANSVERSE CEREBELLAR DIAMETER ACCORDING TO PERCENTILE DISTRIBUTION

Gestational Age (weeks)	Cerebellar Diameter (mm)				
	10th Percentile	25th Percentile	50th Percentile	75th Percentile	90th Percentile
15	10	12	14	15	16
16	14	16	16	16	17
17	16	17	17	18	18
18	17	18	18	19	19
19	18	18	19	19	22
20	18	19	20	20	22
21	19	20	22	23	24
22	21	23	23	24	24
23	22	23	24	25	26
24	22	24	25	27	28
25	23	21.5	28	28	29
26	25	28	29	30	32
27	26	28.5	30	31	32
28	27	30	31	32	34
29	29	32	34	36	38
30	31	32	35	37	40
31	32	35	38	39	43
32	33	36	38	40	42
33	32	36	40	43	44
34	33	38	40	41	44
35	31	37	40.5	43	47
36	36	29	43	52	55
37	37	37	45	52	55
38	40	40	48.5	52	55
39	52	52	52	55	55

After Goldstein and colleagues, 1987,[71] with permission.

Since many congenital alterations of the cranial posterior fossa can modify the normal size of the CMC, its evaluation deserves special consideration when searching for infratentorial anomalies. The mean normal CMC depth has been reported to be 5 mm (range, 1 to 10 mm), with an SD of ±3 mm. The CMC can be enlarged in Dandy–Walker malformation as well as in posterior fossa arachnoid cysts. Joubert's syndrome should be also considered in the differential diagnosis of an enlarged CMC. In both conditions, the cerebellar hemispheres and fourth ventricles can be of normal size, the inferior and posterior vermian dysplasia is common to both disorders and, in both, the CMC communicates with the fourth ventricle. Joubert's syndrome, however, is associated with bilaterally enlarged echogenic kidneys, agenesis of the corpus callosum, occipital encephalocele, facial anomalies, and polydactily.[79] However, it is important to keep in mind that in the absence of other findings, e.g., hydrocephalus, shift of the midline, or dysgenesis of the cerebellar vermis, a prominent CMC is unlikely to be of clinical significance. On the contrary, in Arnold–Chiari malformation, the CMC is diminished in size, typically measuring 2 mm or less.[70] In this case the cerebellum can have a flattened, wedged appearance, giving the impression of the so-called "banana" sign.[80]

Frontal Lobe

DEFINITION

The frontal lobe corresponds to the portion of the cerebral hemisphere anterior to the central sulcus and an imaginary line drawn at the level of the lateral sulcus up to the circular sulcus of the insula.[68]

HOW TO MEASURE IT (FIG. 3–22)

Frontal lobe measurements are accomplished in the plane in which the BPD is measured, e.g., the horizontal plane. The frontal lobe distance (FLD) is measured between the anterior margin of the medial wall of the frontal horn of the lateral ventricles and the middle hyperechogenic frontal bone. The thalamic frontal lobe distance (TFD) is measured from the most posterior landmark of the thalami to the middle hyperechogenic frontal bone.

COMMENTS

Frontal lobe measurements (i.e., FLD and TFD) (Tables 3–40 and 3–41) can be used as an adjunct for the diagnosis of microcephaly, since several investigators agree that this entity is associated with a decreased size of the frontal fossa and flattening of the frontal bone, with other lobes of the brain remaining unchanged.[81,82] Goldstein and coworkers[29] reported on three cases of postnatally confirmed microcephaly in which the FLD and the TFD were below the 10th percentile. Although this is a small series, measuring the frontal lobe seems to be a logical suggestion in cases when microcephaly is suspected, since it adds only a few seconds to the scanning session. Frontal lobe measurements (especially the TFD) have also been used to aid in the antenatal midtrimester diagnosis of Down syndrome. Bahado-Singh and collaborators[83] found that among 19 fetuses with Down syndrome, 10 (52%) had a TFD below the 10th percentile for gestational age. It is possible that the combination of these measurements with other reported signs (e.g., enlarged nuchal fold, cardiovascular anomalies, hyperechogenic bowel, and hydronephrosis) could further enhance the ability of ultrasonography to diagnose this condition in utero.

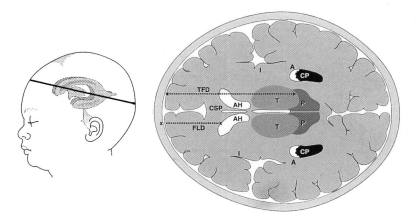

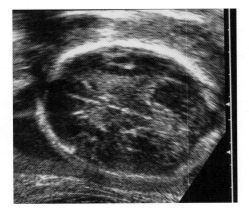

Figure 3–22.

TABLE 3–40 MEASUREMENTS OF THE FRONTAL LOBE DISTANCE

Gestational Age (weeks)	Mean ± 2 SD (cm)	Percentile				
		10th	25th	50th	75th	90th
16	1.4 ± 0.4	1.0	1.4	1.5	1.6	1.8
17	1.6 ± 0.2	1.5	1.6	1.6	1.8	1.8
18	1.6 ± 0.2	1.4	1.4	1.7	1.7	1.8
19	1.7 ± 0.2	1.4	1.5	1.8	1.9	1.9
20	1.7 ± 0.2	1.7	1.7	1.9	1.8	1.9
21	1.8 ± 0.4	1.4	1.5	2.0	2.0	2.1
22	1.8 ± 0.4	2.3	2.3	2.3	2.3	2.3
23	1.8 ± 0.4	1.8	1.9	2.1	2.2	2.3
24	1.9 ± 0.2	2.0	2.0	2.0	2.0	2.0
25	2.2 ± 0.4	2.0	2.0	2.3	2.4	2.5
26	2.3 ± 0.4	2.0	2.1	2.3	2.4	2.5
27	2.5 ± 0.6	2.5	2.5	2.7	3.1	3.2
28	2.8 ± 0.2	2.4	2.5	2.6	2.6	2.7
29	2.7 ± 0.2	2.7	2.7	2.8	2.8	2.8
30	2.8 ± 0.6	2.6	2.6	2.7	3.2	3.4
31	2.9 ± 0.4	2.7	2.7	2.8	3.0	3.0
32	3.0 ± 0.6	3.0	3.0	3.3	3.6	3.8
33	3.1 ± 0.6	2.5	2.6	3.2	3.4	3.4
34	3.2 ± 0.2	2.9	3.0	3.1	3.2	3.3
35	3.2 ± 0.4	3.2	3.4	3.5	3.7	4.0
36	3.2 ± 0.4	2.9	2.9	3.2	3.4	3.4
37	3.4 ± 0.4	3.1	3.2	3.4	3.6	3.8
38	3.5 ± 0.4	3.2	3.2	3.5	3.9	4.0
39	3.7 ± 0.6	3.5	3.5	3.7	4.2	4.3
40	4.0 ± 0.6	3.8	3.8	3.9	4.5	4.5

After Goldstein and colleagues, 1988,[29] with permission.

TABLE 3–41. MEASUREMENTS OF THALAMIC FRONTAL LOBE DISTANCE

Gestational Age (weeks)	Mean ± 2 SD (cm)	Percentile				
		10th	*25th*	*50th*	*75th*	*90th*
15	3.2 ± 0.4	3.2	3.2	3.2	3.2	3.2
16	3.2 ± 0.4	2.9	3.1	3.2	3.4	3.5
17	3.6 ± 0.6	3.2	3.4	3.5	3.8	4.5
18	3.7 ± 0.6	3.3	3.3	3.7	3.9	3.9
19	3.8 ± 0.4	3.5	3.5	3.7	3.9	4.0
20	4.1 ± 0.4	4.0	4.0	4.0	4.3	4.4
21	4.1 ± 0.4	3.9	3.9	4.1	4.4	4.5
22	4.6 ± 0.4	4.6	4.6	4.6	4.6	4.6
23	4.6 ± 0.4	4.6	4.6	4.6	4.6	4.6
24	4.7 ± 0.4	4.6	4.6	4.6	4.9	4.9
25	5.1 ± 0.6	4.7	4.8	5.2	5.3	5.4
26	5.2 ± 0.6	4.8	5.0	5.3	5.4	5.5
27	5.6 ± 0.8	5.3	5.6	5.6	6.8	7.2
28	5.7 ± 0.4	5.5	5.6	5.7	6.0	6.2
29	6.1 ± 0.4	6.0	6.0	6.1	6.4	6.4
30	6.2 ± 1.2	5.5	5.7	5.9	6.4	7.4
31	6.2 ± 0.8	6.1	6.1	6.1	6.2	6.2
32	6.4 ± 0.8	6.2	6.2	6.4	6.9	7.1
33	6.5 ± 0.6	5.9	6.0	6.3	6.5	6.6
34	6.7 ± 0.6	6.2	6.4	6.7	7.0	7.2
35	6.9 ± 0.6	6.6	6.7	7.1	7.2	7.3
36	7.0 ± 0.4	6.5	6.5	6.6	6.9	6.9
37	7.2 ± 0.6	6.2	6.4	6.7	7.0	7.1
38	7.3 ± 0.8	6.5	6.6	7.2	7.3	7.4
39	7.5 ± 0.8	7.1	7.0	7.4	7.7	7.8
40	7.7 ± 0.8	7.4	7.4	7.6	8.1	8.1

After Goldstein and colleagues, 1988,[29] with permission.

REFERENCES

1. O'Rahilly R, Müller F. Embryonic length and cerebral landmarks in staged human embryos. *Anat Rec.* 1984;209:265–271.
2. Robinson HP. Sonar measurement of fetal crown–rump length as means of assessing maturity in first trimester of pregnancy. *Br Med J.* 1973;4:28–31.
3. Robinson HO, Fleming JEE. A critical evaluation of sonar "crown–rump" length measurements. *Br J Obstet Gynaecol.* 1975;82:702–710.
4. Ott WJ. Accurate gestational dating: Revisited. *Am J Perinatol.* 1994;11:404–408.
5. Blaas HG, Eik-Nes SH, Berg S, Torp H. In vivi three-dimensional ultrasound reconstructions of embryos and early fetuses. *Lancet.* 1998;352:1182–1186.
6. Campbell S, Thoms A. Ultrasound measurement of the fetal head to abdomen circumference ratio in the assessment of growth retardation. *Br J Obstet Gynaecol.* 1977;84:165–174.
7. Hadlock FP, Deter RL, Harrist RB, et al. Fetal biparietal diameter: Rational choice of plane section for sonographic measurement. *AJR.* 1982;138:871–874.
8. Campbell S. An improved method of fetal cephalometry. *J Obstet Gynecol Br Commonw.* 1968;75:568–576.
9. Hadlock FP, Deter RL, Harrist RB, et al. Estimating fetal age: Computer assisted analysis of multiple fetal growth parameters. *Radiology.* 1984;152:497–501.
10. Gray DL, Songster GS, Parvin CA, et al. Cephalic index: A gestational age–dependent biometric parameter. *Obstet Gynecol.* 1989;74:600–603.
11. Wolfson RN, Zador IE, Halvorsen P, et al. Biparietal diameter in premature rupture of membranes: Errors in estimating gestational age. *J Clin Ultrasound.* 1983;11:371–374.
12. Hadlock FP, Deter RL, Carpenter RJ, et al. Estimating fetal age: Effect of head shape on BPD. *AJR.* 1981;137:83–85.
13. Hill LM, Breckle R, Gehrking WC. The variable effects of oligohydramnios on the biparietal diameter and the cephalic index. *J Ultrasound Med.* 1984;3:93–95.
14. Kasby CB, Poll V. The breech head and its ultrasound significance. *Br J Obstet Gynaecol.* 1982;89:106–110.
15. Gray DL, Songster GS, Parvin CA, et al. Cephalic index: A gestational age–dependent biometric parameter. *Obstet Gynecol.* 1989;74:600–603.
16. Ott WJ. The use of ultrasonic fetal head circumference for predicting expected date of confinement. *J Clin Ultrasound.* 1984;12:411–415.
17. Hadlock FP. Ultrasound determination of menstrual age. In: Callen PW, ed. *Ultrasonography in Obstetrics and Gynecology.* Philadelphia: WB Saunders; 1994: 94–95.
18. Hadlock FP, Deter RL, Harrist RB, et al. Fetal head circumference: Relation to menstrual age. *AJR.* 1982;138:649–653.
19. Hadlock FP, Deter RL, Carpenter RJ, et al. The effect of head shape on the accuracy in estimating fetal gestational age. *AJR.* 1981;137:83–85.
20. Hadlock FP, Harrist RB, Martinez-Poyer J. How accurate is the second trimester fetal dating? *J Ultrasound Med.* 1991;10:557–561.
21. Benson CB, Doubilet PM. Sonographic prediction of gestational age: Accuracy of second and third trimester fetal measurements. *AJR.* 1991;157:1275–1277.
22. Hill LM, Guzick D, Hixson J, et al. Composite assessment of gestational age: A comparison of institutionally derived and published regression equations. *Am J Obstet Gynecol.* 1992;166:551–555.
23. Hadlock FP, Harrist RB, Carpenter RJ, et al. Sonographic estimation of fetal weight. *Radiology.* 1984;150:535–540.
24. Benson CB, Boswell SB, Brown DL, et al. Improved prediction of intrauterine growth retardation with use of multiple parameters. *Radiology.* 1988;168:7–12.
25. Benson CB, Bellville JS, Lentini JF, et al. Intrauterine growth retardation: Diagnosis based on multiple parameters—A prospective study. *Radiology.* 1990; 177:499–502.
26. Romero R, Pilu G, Jeanty P, et al, eds. *Prenatal Diagnosis of Congenital Anomalies.* Norwalk, CT: Appleton & Lange; 1988:54–59.

27. Kurtz AB, Wapner RJ, Rubin CS, et al. Ultrasound criteria for in utero diagnosis of microcephaly. *J Clin Ultrasound.* 1980;8:11–16.

28. Chervenak FA, Jeanty P, Cantraine F, et al. The diagnosis of fetal microcephaly. *Am J Obstet Gynecol.* 1984;149:512–517.

29. Goldstein I, Reece EA, Pilu G, et al. Sonographic assessment of the fetal frontal lobe: A potential tool for prenatal diagnosis of microcephaly. *Am J Obstet Gynecol.* 1988;158:1057–1062.

30. Pilu G, Falco P, Milano V, Perolo A, Bovicelli L. Prenatal diagnosis of microcephaly assisted by vaginal sonography and power Doppler ultrasound. *Obstet Gynecol.* 1998;11:357–360.

31. Mayden KL, Tortora M, Berkowitz RL, et al. Orbital diameters: A new parameter for prenatal diagnosis and dating. *Am J Obstet Gynecol.* 1982;144:289–297.

32. Jeanty P, Dramaix-Wilmet M, Van Gansbeke D, et al. Fetal ocular biometry by ultrasound. *Radiology.* 1982;143:513–516.

33. Trout T, Budorick NE, Pretorius DH, et al. Significance of orbital measurements in the fetus. *J Ultrasound Med.* 1994;13:937–943.

34. Romero R, Pilu G, Jeanty P, et al, eds. *Prenatal Diagnosis of Congenital Anomalies.* Norwalk, CT: Appleton & Lange; 1988:81–97.

35. Birnholz JC. Ultrasonic fetal ophthalmology. *Early Hum Dev.* 1985;12:199–209.

36. Jeanty P, Dramaix-Wilmet M, Delbeke D, et al. Ultrasonic evaluation of fetal ventricular growth. *Neuroradiology.* 1981;21:127–131.

37. Johnson ML, Dunne MG, Mack LA, et al. Evaluation of fetal intracranial anatomy by static and real time ultrasound. *J Clin Ultrasound.* 1980;8:311–318.

38. Kurjak A. Ultrasound diagnosis of congenital malformations. In: de Viegler, ed. *Handbook of Clinical Ultrasound.* New York: Wiley; 1988:189–202.

39. Cardoza JD, Goldstein RB, Filly RA. Exclusion of fetal ventriculomegaly with a single measurement: The width of the lateral ventricular atrium. *Radiology.* 1988;169:711–714.

40. Hadlock FP, Deter RL, Park SK. Real-time sonography: Ventricular and vascular anatomy of the fetal brain in utero. *AJR.* 1981;136:133–137.

41. Goldstein I, Reece EA, Pilu G, et al. Sonographic evaluation of the normal developmental anatomy of the fetal cerebral ventricles. I: The frontal horn. *Obstet Gynecol.* 1988;72:588–592.

42. Denkhaus H, Winsberg F. Ultrasonic measurement of the fetal ventricular system. *Radiology.* 1979;131:781–787.

43. Jou HJ, Shyu MK, Wu SC, Chen SM, Su CH, Hsieh FJ. Ultrasound measurement of the fetal cavum septi pellucidi. *Ultrasound Obstet Gynecol.* 1998;12:419–421.

44. Mahony BS, Nyberg DA, Hirsch JH, et al. Mild idiopathic cerebral ventricular dilatation in utero: Sonographic evaluation. *Radiology.* 1988;169:715–721.

45. Filly RA, Cardoza JD, Goldstein RB, et al. Detection of fetal central nervous system anomalies: A practical level of effort for a routine sonogram. *Radiology.* 1989;172:403–408.

46. Farrell TA, Hertzberg BS, Kliewer MA, et al. Fetal lateral ventricles: Reassessment of normal values for atrial diameter at US. *Radiology.* 1994;193:409–411.

47. Chinn DH, Callen PW, Filly RA. The lateral cerebral ventricle in early second trimester. *Radiology.* 1983;148:529–531.

48. Hartung RW, Yiu-Chiu V. Demonstration of unilateral hydrocephalus in utero. *J Ultrasound Med.* 1983;2:369–71.

49. Pilu G, Reece EA, Goldstein I, et al. Sonographic evaluation of the normal developmental anatomy of the fetal cerebral ventricles: II. The atria. *Obstet Gynecol.* 1989;73:250–255.

50. Goldstein I, Reece EA, Pilu G, et al. Sonographic evaluation of the normal developmental anatomy of the fetal cerebral ventricles. IV: The posterior horn. *Am J Perinatol.* 1990;7:79–83.

51. Siedler DE, Filly RA. Relative growth of the higher fetal brain structures. *J Ultrasound Med.* 1987;6:573–576.

52. Callen PW, Hashimoto BE, Newton TH. Sonographic evaluation of cerebral cortical mantle thickness in the fetus and neonate with hydrocephalus. *J Ultrasound Med.* 1986;5:251–255.

53. Blaas HG, Eik-Nes SH, Kiserud T, et al. Early development of the forebrain and midbrain: A longitudinal study from 7 to 12 weeks of gestation. *Ultrasound Obstet Gynecol.* 1994;4:183–192.

54. Blaas HG, Eik-Nes SH, Kiserud T, et al. Early development of the hindbrain: A longitudinal ultrasound study from 7 to 12 weeks of gestation. *Ultrasound Obstet Gynecol.* 1995;5:151–160.

55. Achiron R, Achiron A. Transvaginal ultrasound assessment of the early fetal brain. *Ultrasound Obstet Gynecol.* 1991;164:497–503.

56. Timor-Tritsch IE, Monteagudo A, Warren WB. Transvaginal ultrasonographic definition of the central nervous system in the first and early second trimesters. *Am J Obstet Gynecol.* 1991;164:497–503.

57. Monteagudo A, Reuss ML, Timor-Tritsch IE. Imaging the fetal brain in the second and third trimesters using transvaginal sonography. *Obstet Gynecol.* 1991;77:27–32.

58. Monteagudo A, Timor-Tritsch IE, Moomjy M. In utero detection of ventriculomegaly during the second and third trimesters by transvaginal sonography. *Ultrasound Obstet Gynecol.* 1994;4:193–198.

59. Kushnir U, Shalev J, Bronshtein M, et al. Fetal intracranial anatomy in the first trimester of pregnancy: Transvaginal ultrasonographic evaluation. *Neuroradiology.* 1989;31:222–225.

60. Monteagudo A, Timor-Tritsch IE, Moomjy M. Nomograms of the fetal lateral ventricles using transvaginal sonography. *J Ultrasound Med.* 1993;5:265–269.

61. Poland RL, Slovis TL, Sharankaran S. Normal values for ventricular size determined by real time sonographic techniques. *Pediatr Radiol.* 1985;15:12–14.

62. Sauerbrei EE, Digney M, Harrison PB, et al. Ultrasonic evaluation of neonatal intracranial hemorrhage and its complications. *Radiology.* 1981;130:677–685.

63. Chin DH, Callen PW, Filly RA. The lateral cerebral ventricle in early second trimester. *Radiology.* 1983;148:529–531.

64. Monteagudo A, Tharakan T, Timor-Tritsch IE. Sonographic neuroembryology of the central nervous system. *J Assoc Acad Minority Physicians.* 1995;6:34–37.

65. Mallinger G, Zakut H. The corpus callosum: Normal fetal development as shown by transvaginal sonography. *AJR.* 1993;161:1041–1043.

66. Moore KL. ed. *The Developing Human: Clinically Oriented Embryology.* 4th ed. Philadelphia: WB Saunders; 1988:364–401.

67. O'Rahilly R, Müller F, eds. *The Embryonic Human Brain: An Atlas of Developmental Stages.* New York: Wiley–Liss; 1994:15–25.

68. Crosby EC, Humphrey T, Lauer EW, eds. *Correlative Anatomy of the Nervous System.* New York: Macmillan; 1962:343–345.

69. Martin JH. ed. *Neuroanatomy: Text and Atlas.* New York: Elsevier; 1989:240–266.

70. Mahony BS, Callen PW, Filly RA, et al. The fetal cisterna magna. *Radiology.* 1984;153:773–776.

71. Goldstein I, Reece EA, Pilu G, et al. Cerebellar measurements with ultrasonography in the evaluation of fetal growth and development. *Am J Obstet Gynecol.* 1987;156:1065–1069.

72. McLeary RD, Kuhns LR, Barr M. Ultrasonography of the fetal cerebellum. *Radiology.* 1984;151:439–442.

73. Hata K, Hata T, Daisaku S, et al. Ultrasonographic measurement of the fetal transverse cerebellum in utero. *Gynecol Obstet Invest.* 1989;28:111–112.

74. Creasy RK, Resnick R, eds. *Maternal–Fetal Medicine: Principles and Practice.* Philadelphia: WB Saunders; 1994:58–560.

75. Cabbad M, Kofinas A, Simin N, et al. Fetal weight-cerebellar diameter discordance as an indicator of asymmetrical fetal growth impairment. *J Reprod Med.* 1992;37:794–798.

76. Hill LM, Guzick D, Fries J, et al. The transverse cerebellar diameter in estimating gestational age in the large for gestational age fetus. *Obstet Gynecol.* 1990;75:981–985.

77. Shimizu T, Gaudette S, Nimrod C. Transverse cerebellar diameter in twin gestations. *Am J Obstet Gynecol.* 1992;167:1004–1008.

78. Dilmen G, Toppane MF, Turban NO, Ozturk M, Isik S. Tranverse cerebellar diameter/abdominal circumference index for assessing fetal growth.

79. Scanaill SN, Crowley P, Hogan M, Stuart B. Abnormal prenatal sonographic findings in the posterior cranial fossa: a case of Joubert's syndrome. *Ultrasound Obstet Gynecol.* 1999;13:71–74.

80. Nicolaides KH, Campbell S, Gabbe SG, et al. Ultrasound screening for spina bifida: Cranial and cerebellar signs. *Lancet.* 1986;2:72–74.

81. Devies H, Kizman BH. Microcephaly. *Arch Dis Child.* 1972;123:204–206.

82. Martin HP. Microcephaly and mental retardation. *Am J Dis Child.* 1970; 119:129–131.

83. Bahado-Singh RO, Wyse L, Dorr MA, et al. Fetuses with Down syndrome have disproportionately shortened frontal lobe dimensions on ultrasonographic examination. *Am J Obstet Gynecol.* 1992;167:1009– 1014.

CHAPTER FOUR

Fetal Neurosonography of Congenital Brain Anomalies

Ana Monteagudo
Ilan E. Timor-Tritsch

This chapter deals with the ultrasonographic evaluation and detection of neural tube defects (NTDs) and a variety of other malformations that affect the developing central nervous system (CNS). Anomalies dealing with the median structures (e.g., holoprosencephaly and agenesis of the corpus callosum etc.), are dealt with in Chapter 5.

A *malformation* is defined as any finding that deviates from the normal sonographic appearance of the prenatal brain. It is imperative that the health care provider is familiar with the normal sonographic appearance of the CNS at different ages, because the presence or absence of a structure may be deemed "normal" or "abnormal" depending on the age of the fetus. For example, the normal 8-week postmenstrual brain consists of a sonographically visible single ventricle with no apparent median structures; however, the same appearance of the brain at 10 postmenstrual weeks is consistent with holoprosencephaly.

When a malformation is encountered, the sonologist and/or sonographer is responsible not only for precisely describing the sonographic appearance, but also for looking for other associated malformations. This is crucial in order to counsel the patient and her family appropriately. All patients in whom a fetal malformation has been diagnosed should receive genetic counseling and further testing (e.g., karyotype analysis). Genetic counseling is important in that there are nonchromosomal syndromes with a high recurrence rate that feature a CNS malformation as part of their syndrome (e.g., Meckel–Gruber syndrome [MGS]).

NEURAL TUBE DEFECTS

Screening for Neural Tube Defects with α-Fetoprotein

In the United States as well as other countries all pregnant women are routinely offered screening with maternal serum α-fetoprotein (MSAFP) for NTDs at 16 to 18 postmenstrual weeks. Among low-risk women MSAFP screening results in the detection of 80% to 90% of cases of fetal open NTDs.[1] Limb and Holmes[2] published a report on the changes in prenatal detection and birth status of anencephaly between 1972 and 1990 in the Malformations Surveillance Program of Brigham and Women's Hospital in Boston. They found that during the 1970s, half of the infants with anencephaly were born alive at an average gestational age of 35.6 weeks, and few were diagnosed prenatally. Between 1988 and 1990, however, all affected fetuses were diagnosed either by prenatal ultrasonography or as a result of MSAFP and the average age at delivery was 18 postmenstrual weeks.

Maternal serum α-fetoprotein levels are expressed as multiples of the normal median. An abnormal value is one that exceeds 2.5 multiples of the median. Elevated MSAFP levels are associated with NTDs as well as a variety of other conditions (Table 4–1).

Prenatal sonography, when used by experienced operators, is a sensitive (97%) and specific (100%) tool for the diagnoses of neural tube defects in a targeted, at-risk population.[3] Reichler and associates,[4] in a retrospective study of 773 cases with elevated

TABLE 4–1. NON-NEURAL TUBE MALFORMATIONS ASSOCIATED WITH ELEVATED MATERNAL SERUM α-FETOPROTEIN

Fetal conditions
    Multiple pregnancy
    Intrauterine fetal death
    Wrong dates (i.e., pregnancy more advanced)
    Ventral wall defects: omphalocele or gastroschisis
    Renal: congenital nephrosis, bilateral renal agenesis, polycystic kidney or infantile
    Intestinal atresia
    Triploidy
    Congenital skin disorders: epidermolysis bullosa or aplasia cutis
    Teratoma: sacrococcygeal or pharyngeal
    Congenital cystic adenomatoid malformation type III
    Turner's syndrome with cystic hygroma
    Oligohydramnios
Placental conditions
    Hemangioma
Maternal conditions
    Maternal infection: parvovirus, cytomegalovirus, or hepatitis
    Maternal malignancy: hepatoma or ovarian teratoma
    Abdominal pregnancy
    Fetomaternal hemorrhage

MSAFP, evaluated the percentage of fetal anomalies detected. They found that there was a progressive increase in the incidence of fetal anomalies as a direct function of the level of MSAFP (Fig. 4–1).

To adequately assess a patient with an elevated MSAFP, it is important to review some of the basic information regarding this fetal protein. α-Fetoprotein (AFP) is a glycoprotein that is initially synthesized in the embryonic yolk sac and subsequently by the fetal liver and gastrointestinal tract. The molecule enters the amniotic fluid via fetal urination, gastrointestinal tract secretions, and transudation from exposed blood vessels.[5,6] It enters the maternal circulation by diffusion across either the placenta or the amnion.[7] In the normal pregnancy the highest concentration of AFP is found within the fetal serum (measured in milligrams), with the next highest value in the amniotic fluid (measured in micrograms), and the lowest concentration in the maternal serum (measured in nanograms) (Fig. 4–2). The mean concentration of AFP peaks at approximately 12 postmenstrual weeks in the fetal serum and then starts to decline. This peak occurs at approximately 14 postmenstrual weeks in the amniotic fluid. Maternal serum α-fetoprotein achieves its highest level at 32 postmenstrual weeks (Fig. 4–2).[5] To adequately assess MSAFP values, knowledge of the accurate fetal age is necessary. This is important to note, because even in the event of an open NTD the concentration of AFP in the amniotic fluid decreases with advancing age; such a decrease may place the value in the range of a normal, but much younger, fetus.

Neural tube defects can be categorized as *open* or *closed,* depending on whether they are covered by skin (Table 4–2).[5] In an open NTD the neural tissue is exposed and covered only by the thinnest of membranes; therefore, the lesion is directly in contact with the amniotic fluid. In these cases the AFP molecule freely diffuses across the lesion, which results in an abnormally increased level in the amniotic fluid, and hence in the maternal serum. Not all cases of NTDs are open lesions. For example, whereas all anencephalies are open defects, only 80% of spina bifida cases and 18% of cephaloceles are open NTDs.[5] In a closed neural tube lesion the defect is covered by skin or a thick membrane. In these cases, AFP cannot freely diffuse across the lesion into the amniotic fluid; therefore, the MSAFP level is within normal limits. Prenatal diagnosis in these cases cannot be made on the basis of serum or amniotic fluid AFP alone. An ultrasonographic examination should therefore be performed in a timely fashion.

Acetylcholinesterase, unlike AFP, is not a normal component of amniotic fluid. It is derived from neural tissue and is always present in amniotic fluid in the presence of an open NTD. Also, acetylcholinesterase may be present in cases of abdominal wall defects in which a nerve plexus is exposed to amniotic fluid. In addition, it is essential to know that acetylcholinesterase is normally found in fetal blood and may therefore be found in amniotic fluid which, at the time of amniocentesis, has been contaminated with fetal blood.[7,8]

Once an elevated MSAFP has been obtained, a sonogram to rule out an NTD as well as other conditions (see Table 4–1) should constitute the next step.

Neural tube defects result from failure of the neural tube to close during primary neurulation (Table 4–3). They are characterized by the presence of a cerebral, spinal, or combined cerebrospinal defect or dysraphia. Table 4–3 lists, in decreasing order of severity, the defects that arise as a result of primary neurulation. The occult dysraphic conditions affect the lower sacral and coccygeal areas of the spine. These lesions are covered by skin and may go undetected even for years after the birth of the infant. The important issue is that 4.1% of siblings of patients with these occult dysraphic conditions exhibit disorders of primary neurulation, such as meningocele or anencephaly.[9,10,11]

Risk of Recurrence

Most NTDs have a polygenic inheritance. In addition, several other factors, such as ethnicity, geographic

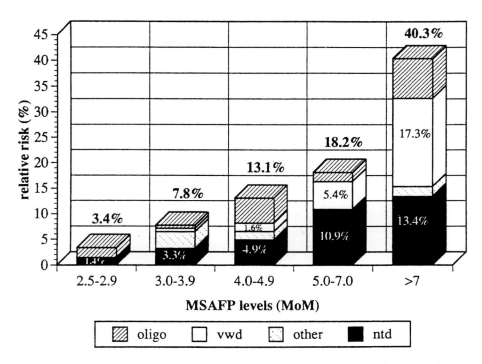

Figure 4–1. Anomalies and oligohydramnios distribution as a function of elevated maternal serum α-fetoprotein (MSAFP). Other, subchorionic bleeding, intraabdominal echogenicity, hydronephrosis, echogenic bowel, dilated kidney, and heart defect; NTD, neural tube defect; VWD, ventral wall defect; Oligo, oligohydramnios; MOM, multiples of the median. *(From Reichler and colleagues, 1994,[3] with permission.)*

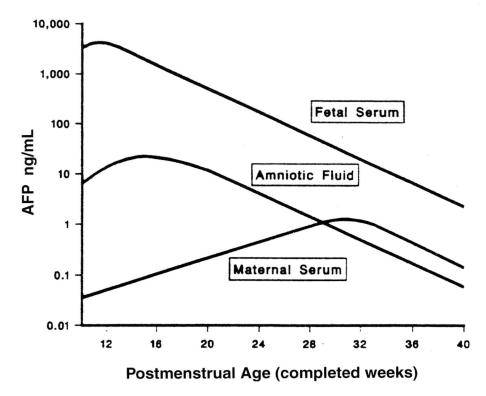

Figure 4–2. Mean concentrations of α-fetoprotein (AFP) in maternal serum, amniotic fluid, and fetal serum at various stages of pregnancy, α-Fetoprotein reaches peak concentrations in amniotic fluid and fetal serum early in pregnancy, with a steady decline thereafter. In contrast, AFP levels in maternal serum rise steadily until the third trimester. *(From Haddow, 1990,[4] with permission.)*

TABLE 4–2. CLASSIFICATION OF NEURAL TUBE DEFECTS

Location of Defect	Open	Closed
Cranial	Anencephaly	Cephalocele
Craniospinal	Craniorachischisis	Iniencephaly
Spinal	Meningomyelocele	Lumbosacral lesions

After Lemire, 1987,[54] with permission.

location, and nutritional (e.g., folate) deficiency, may play a significant role in the occurrence of NTDs. The incidence of NTDs in the United States is 1 to 2 per 1000 births, but this risk increases significantly if there is a family history of an NTD. If one of the parents has an NTD, the risk to the offspring is as high as 5%. If a previous sibling is affected, the recurrence risk is approximately 2%, and if two previous siblings are affected, this risk increases to 6% to 10%.[6]

Prevention of Neural Tube Defects

Approximately 95% of children with NTDs are born to couples with no family history of the disorder. A decrease in folate intake has been shown to be associated with an increased risk of NTDs.[12–15] In view of this association, the Centers for Disease Control and Prevention has recommended that all women of childbearing age should consume 0.4 mg of folic acid per day for prevention of NTDs.[16] It is important to note that not all NTDs will be eliminated with the use of folic acid. However, the use of 0.4 mg of folic acid will prevent the occurrence of more that 50% of NTDs when taken before conception and continued until about the 12th postmenstrual week of the pregnancy.[17,18] Therefore, it is important to continue to screen women for these defects. For women who have had a prior child with an NTD, the recommended dose of folic acid is 4 mg/d started at least 1 month before conception and continued for the first 12 weeks of pregnancy.[19] This regimen of folic acid in addition to the dietary intake as reported, by the Medical Research Council (MFC) Vitamin Study Group, resulted in a 72% reduction of recurrence of NTDs.[20,21] Doses of folic acid greater than 1 mg

TABLE 4–3. NEURAL TUBE DEFECTS: DEFECTS OF PRIMARY NEURULATION

Craniorachischisis totalis

Anencephaly

Myeloschisis

Encephalocele

Myelomeningocele and Arnold–Chiari malformation

After Volpe, 1995,[10] with permission.

must be taken under the supervision of a physician in order not to mask an underlying condition such pernicious anemia (vitamin B_{12} deficiency).

It is believed that folic acid works through a correction of a metabolic defect, caused by a mutation in the enzyme methyltetrahydrofolate reductase, that results in raised serum homocysteine.[22,23]

Anomalies of the Neural Tube

Anencephaly and Exencephaly

Anencephaly refers to a defect in which there is partial absence of the brain and overlying cranial vault. This is a lethal condition that more commonly affects female fetuses. Of all of the NTDs, this is the most common: the reported incidence is about 1 case per 1000 births.[2,24,25] It has been estimated that approximately 75% of the fetuses with anencephaly are stillborn. Most infants born alive with anencephaly die within the first 48 hours, and the remaining patients die within the first week of life,[26,27] although rare prolonged survivals up to 14 months have been reported.[28–30]

Palomaki et al[31] in a letter to the editor of the *New England Journal of Medicine* (*NEJM*) reported on a pilot study sponsored by New England Regional Genetics Group documenting the current use of prenatal screening and the effect of such screening on the baseline prevalence of open neural tube defects before the introduction of grain products fortified with folic acid and the use of folic acid (as described above). The overall rates of prevalence for open spina bifida and anencephaly were 6.4 per 10,000 (95% CI, 4.9 to 8.8) and 4.4/10,000 (95% CI, 3.1 to 6.0) respectively. At an AFP cutoff level of 2.0 MoM, 84% of the pregnancies in which open spina bifida was identified and 96% in which anencephaly was identified had positive results on the screening test. Eighty-one percent of the pregnancies in which open spina bifida had been identified and 92% of those with anencephaly were terminated. Several affected pregnancies were identified by ultrasonography or amniocentesis without serum screening. Overall, the prevalence of open spina bifida and anencephaly among births was reduced 51% and 79%, respectively, as a result of screening.

Anencephaly and related disorders are no longer theorized to be simple NTDs, but are complex developmental malformations that primarily affect the production of mesenchyme. This results in skeletal defects and imperfect fusion of the neural folds.[32,33]

The developmental sequence of events leading to anencephaly was first elucidated in experimental animals exposed to high doses of vitamin A. Subsequent studies in the human embryo have suggested that in humans the anomaly progresses in a similar fashion.[32–35] The three phases in the development of anencephaly are (1) *dysraphia,* or a failure of the neural groove to close in the rostral region (new evidence has suggested that the defect may occur as early as 18 to 20 postovulatory days, as a mesenchymal defect, far earlier than was previously believed); (2) *exencephaly,* or exposure of a well-developed and differentiated brain outside the skull during the embryonic period; and (3) disintegration of the exposed brain during the fetal period, resulting in *anencephaly* (Table 4–4).[9,32,34,35] It appears that early during development the generation of the brain and that of the skull are relatively independent of each other and that the brain of an anencephalic fetus attains a high degree of differentiation before it disintegrates.[35] Using prenatal sonography, the development of anencephaly from exencephaly has been observed and reported.[36] This degeneration of the brain tissue has been corroborated by findings of primitive neuronal cells in the amniotic fluid.[37]

Anencephaly is a historically important malformation in the field of ultrasonography because it was the first malformation reported using transabdominal sonography in a fetus at 17 postmenstrual weeks.[38] Almost 20 years later, it became the first

TABLE 4–4. THE THREE PHASES IN THE DEVELOPMENT OF ANENCEPHALY

Dysraphia
Exencephaly
Anencephaly

malformation reported using transvaginal sonography (TVS) in a fetus at 11 postmenstrual weeks, 5 days.[39]

Using TVS, the integrity of the skull can be assessed as early as the first trimester of pregnancy. This is because ossification of the vault begins and subsequently accelerates after 9 postmenstrual weeks.[40,41] Abnormal mineralization of the cranial bones can be sonographically determined early in the second trimester by assessing the degree of echogenicity of the bone.[42] Well-mineralized bone is highly echogenic. Absence of an echogenic outer border surrounding the fetal brain must raise suspicion of the presence of exencephaly (Figs. 4–3 through Fig. 4–9).

Exencephaly refers to a "transient" malformation in which the brain is exposed to amniotic fluid. Exencephaly is the second stage of the development of clinically apparent anencephaly in humans.[32,36,43–48] In exencephaly, a relatively large amount of well-developed brain is present in the absence of a fetal cranium. In exencephaly, significant portions of the cranium are missing, but there is preservation of the face and the bones of the base of the skull. Specific structures such as the ventricles and the choroid plexus are not apparent.[49] The first-trimester exencephalic fetus has an apparently wide fetal head, with sonolucent spaces

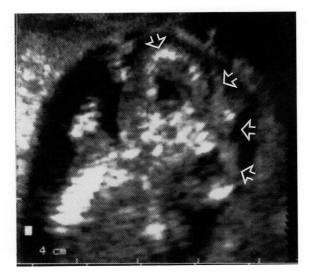
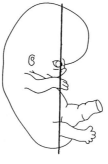

Figure 4–3. Exencephaly in an embryo of 9 postmenstrual weeks. The widened, flattened shape of the head is outlined by *open arrows.* Because of the resemblance of the head to Mickey Mouse, this condition has been termed Mickey Mouse-shaped head.

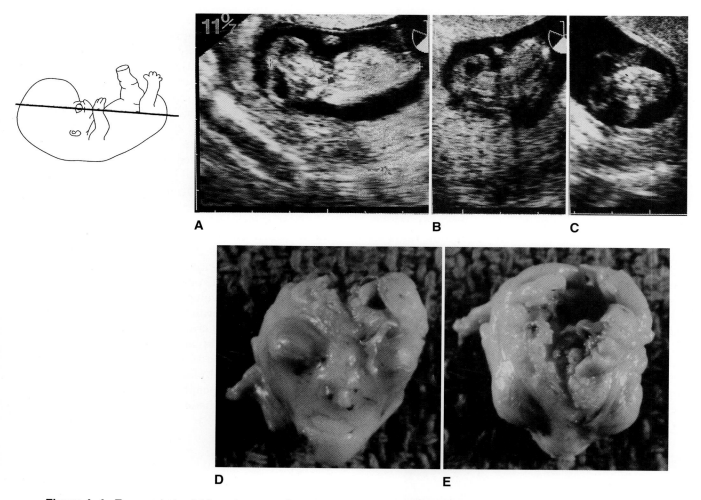

Figure 4–4. Exencephaly at 11 postmenstrual weeks (crown–rump length, 40 mm). **A–C.** Various views of the wide, flattened Mickey Mouse-shaped head. Some brain tissue is still present. **D, E.** The head of the aborted specimen. Note the large, bulging eyes, the protruding tongue, and the lack of brain tissue. This illustrates the natural progression of exencephaly to anencephaly.

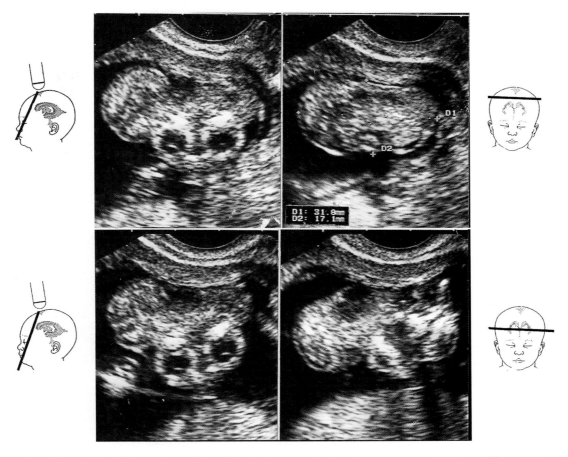

Figure 4–5. The Mickey Mouse shaped head is clearly seen in this picture composed of four different views of the fetal head in this 14 postmenstrual week's fetus with exencephaly. The exposed brain is disorganized and lacks any of the anatomic landmarks usually seen at this gestational age.

within the disintegrating brain. The outer shape of the head is bilobed; we and others have referred to this appearance of the fetal head as a "Mickey Mouse" head (Figs. 4–3 through 4–5.)[50,51] Exencephaly is rarely obseved in human infants because of the disintegration of the exposed brain that occurs during intrauterine life. Most cases of exencephaly diagnosed in utero have the typical anencephalic appearance at the time of delivery (Figs. 4–4, 4–6, and 4–12). Similar to anencephaly, exencephaly is a lethal malformation incompatible with postnatal life.

The anencephalic fetus is easy to detect using sonography, due to the severity of the malformation. This is especially true during the second and third trimesters (Figs. 4–7, and 4–10 through 4–14). During the first trimester the "typical anencephalic" phenotypic picture may not be sonographically apparent. Instead, an exencephalic fetus with an abnormally shaped head and some brain tissue may be imaged by sonography (Fig. 4–3 and 4–4).

Sepulveda[52] et al described the measurement of the crown–chin length and the ratio of the crown–chin to the crown–rump length (CRL) at 10–14 postmenstrual weeks as another tool to assist in the early recognition of anencephaly. Fetuses with anencephaly had a crown–chin length measurement below the 5th percentile in 77% of the cases and the ratio of the crown–chin to the CRL was below the 5th in 62% of the cases. Therefore, in well-dated pregnancies an abnormality in these measurements as well as an abnormal shape of the fetal head may enhance the early diagnosis of anencephaly.

Anencephaly is characterized by the symmetrical partial or total absence of the cranial vault above the orbits. In addition, variable degrees of disintegrating brain tissue may be present. The parts of the brain that are missing are the prosencephalon, the mesencephalon, and the rostral part of the rhombencephalon.[32] In a sagittal view of a fetus with anencephaly, the profile of the chin, lips, nose, and orbits appears relatively normal. However, superior to the

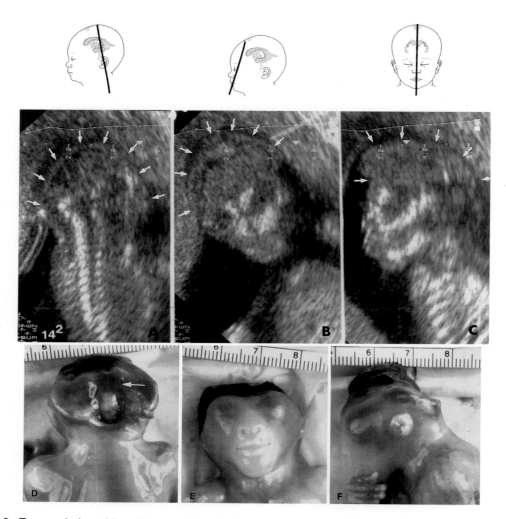

Figure 4–6. Exencephaly at 14 postmenstrual weeks, 2 days. **A.** Coronal section. The *arrows* outline the head. Note the absence of the fetal skull. **B.** Coronal section. The borders of the brain tissue are outlined by *arrows.* **C.** Image through the median plane. Note the flattened shape of the brain (outlined by *arrows*) with a small frontal bulge. **D–F.** Photographs of the aborted specimen corresponding to the sonographic images in **A–C,** respectively. The cerebrovasculosa, a loose, reddish tissue, is marked by the *arrow* in **D.**

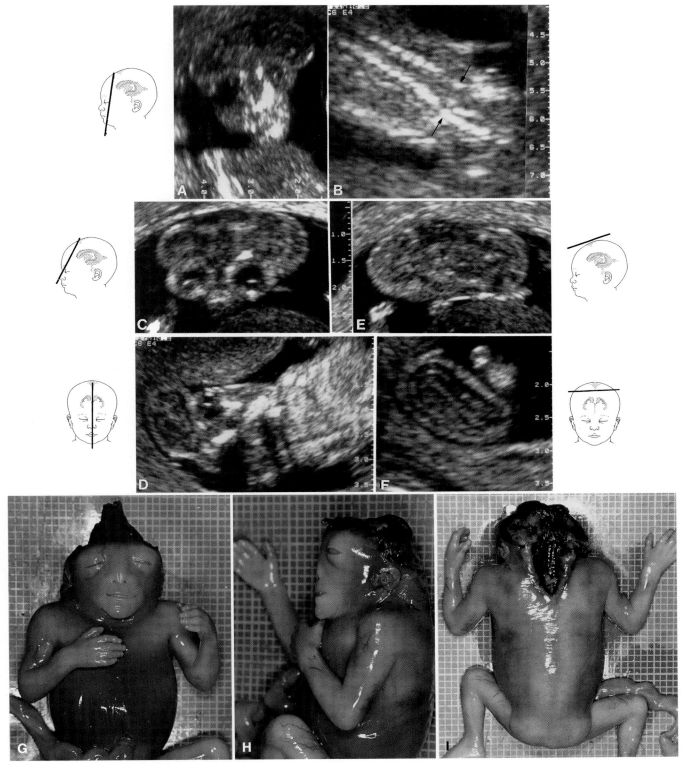

Figure 4–7. Exencephaly at 17 postmenstrual weeks. **A.** Coronal secton demonstrating the orbits and the brain tissue without the calvarium. **B.** The splayed upper part of the spinal column *(arrow)*. **C.** Coronal section highlighting the orbit with the lens pointing downward (strabismus). **D.** Median section showing the flat profile *(arrow)*. **E, F.** Horizontal sections of the brain. No hyperechoic bony structure is seen surrounding the brain tissue. **G–I.** Photographs of the aborted specimen from the front, side, and back, respectively. Note the resemblance of each specimen to the respective sonographic picture.

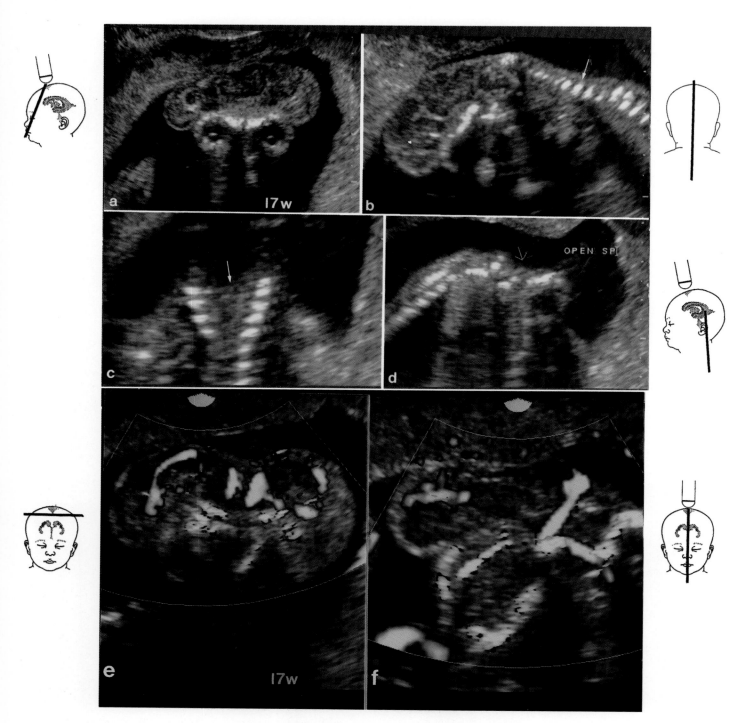

Figure 4–8. Exencephaly at 17 postmenstrual weeks. **A.** Coronal section. The exposed brain appears flattened and bulging over the sides of the fetal face. **B.** Median section. The abnormal profile of the head and face is apparent. The *arrow* points to a defect of the cervical area of the fetal spine. **C.** Coronal section of the cervical spine demonstrates an open neural tube defect with the vertebrae having the typical "U" shape seen in cases of open defects. **D.** The *arrow* points to the open spinal defect. **E, F.** Using color Doppler, the disorganized blood supply to the brain in this exencephalic fetus is evident.

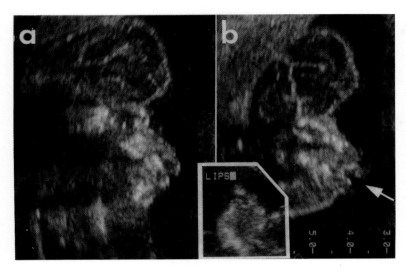

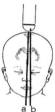

Figure 4–9. Exencephaly at 20 postmenstrual weeks. **A, B.** Median and sagittal sections. The profile of this fetus with exencephaly is very abnormal. In addition, to the exencephaly this fetus had a cleft lip *(arrow and inset).*

area of the orbital ridges, the forehead and the calvaria are obviously missing. A coronal view demonstrates the absence of the cranium above the prominent orbits with preservation of the base of the skull and the facial features (Figs. 4–10 and 4–11).[53] The prominent, bulging eyes give the anencephalic fetus its typical "frog's facies" (Figs. 4–7, 4–10 through 4–12, and 4–14B.) Several other abnormalities involving the eyes and the orbits of anencephalic fetuses have been described in pathological specimens such as coloboma, corneal dermoids, and anophthalmia.[54] In addition, it has been reported that although the eyes of the anencephalic fetus may appear normal, often they have no connection to the brain centrally. Using sonography, we have noted the lenses of the anencephalic fetus to have an apparent strabismus, with both lenses located in the lower lateral aspect of the orbits (Fig. 4–7 and 4–10 through 4–13). In most, if not all, cases of anencephaly, a soft, red, spongy vascular glial tissue simulating cerebral content is seen to protrude or be exposed at the site of the defect. This tissue is commonly referred to as the area cerebrovasculosa (Figs. 4–7 and 4–10 through 4–13).

Anencephaly can be further divided into two types, depending on the severity of the skull defect. (1) *Holoacrania* (*holos* is Greek for *entire*) is a condition in which most or all of the calvaria is missing to the level of the foramen magnum. This is the typical anencephaly that is easily recognized by sonography (Figs. 4–11, 4–12, and 4–14).[35,49,54] In addition, in holoacrania variable degrees of spinal rachischisis may be present (Figs. 4–7, 4–8, and 4–13). (2) In *meroacrania* (*meros* meaning "part") there is a partial or incomplete median cranial defect with ectopia of the brain. The foramen magnum is not involved and no cervical lordosis is present. Meroacrania may be confused with a cephalocele; however, meroacrania can be differentiated by the absence of skin covering the ectopic brain.[35,49,54]

Polyhydramnios, which complicates up to 50% of anencephalic pregnancies, usually develops during the second half of gestation. It is theorized that polyhydramnios results from decreased fetal swallowing.[43,49,55,56]

Other malformations can also be seen in anencephalic fetuses. However, due to the severity and lethality of this malformation, searching for other malformations does not alter the management or the prognosis for the fetus. Among the other associated malformations are hypoplastic or anomalous folding of the ears, subcutaneous clefts of the nose, cleft lip and/or cleft palate, diaphragmatic hernia, omphalocele, limb malformations, cardiac malformations, and hydronephrosis (Figs. 4–9 and 4–14).[54]

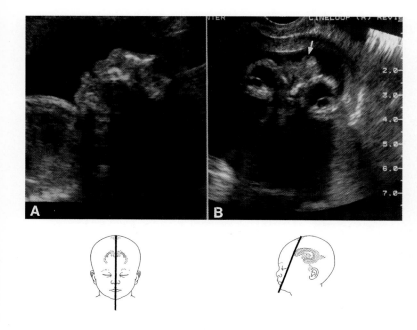

Figure 4–10. Anencephaly at 16 postmenstrual weeks. **A.** Profile showing the absence of the calvarium. **B.** Coronal picture of the orbits with strabismus of the lenses. The *arrow* indicates the cerebrovasculosa, the loose tissue on top of the orbits.

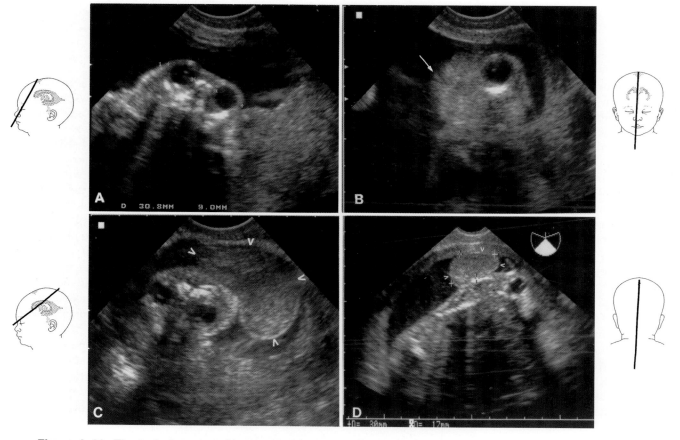

Figure 4–11. The typical sonographic appearance of anencephaly. **A.** The orbits with measurements of the outer and inner orbital diameters (30.8 and 9.0 mm, respectively). **B.** Paramedian image through the orbit, showing that there is no bony skull above the orbit. The large tongue is indicated by the *arrow*. **C.** Some brain tissue (area cerebrovasculosa) without covering bone (calvarium) was detected, highlighted by *arrowheads*. **D.** The same brain tissue (outlined by *arrowheads*) measuring 3 × 1.7 cm, seen on the median section.

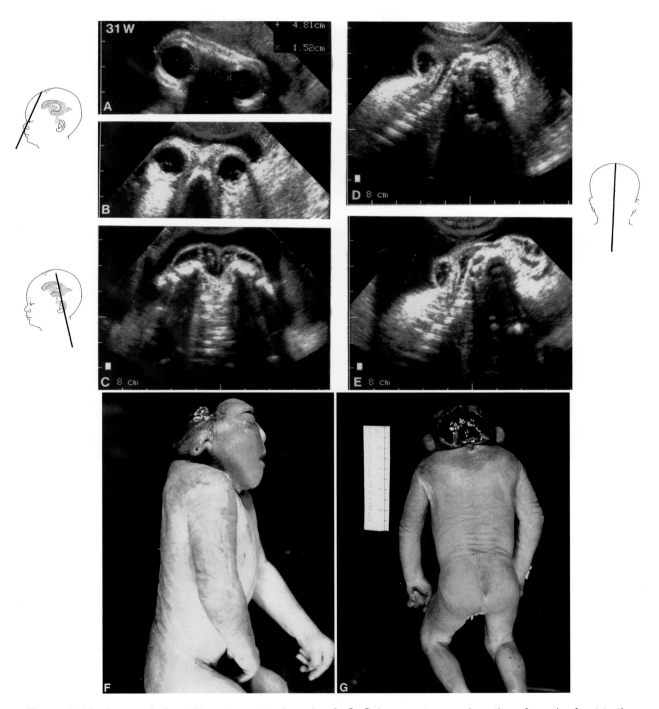

Figure 4–12. Anencephaly at 31 postmenstrual weeks. **A–C.** Subsequent coronal sections from the front to the back, showing the widely spaced orbits (hypertelorism), the lens in the dislocated position (strabismus), and the scant tissue at the base of the skull. **D, E.** Median views showing the upper end of the vertebral column covered by a small amount of tissue (cerebrovasculosa). **F, G.** Lateral and posterior views of the specimen after birth.

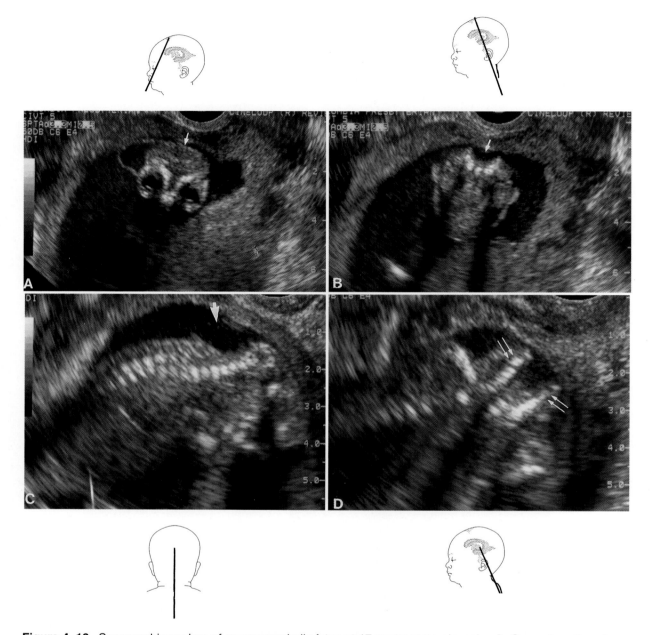

Figure 4–13. Sonographic workup of an exencephalic fetus at 17 postmenstrual weeks. **A.** Coronal section showing the orbits with the lenses exhibiting strabismus. Above the orbits some loose brain tissue is seen *(arrow)* covered by a thin membrane. **B.** Cross-section of the spina bifida *(arrow)*. **C.** Median section of the upper vertebral column, showing the defect encompassing at least five vertebrae *(arrow)*. **D.** An almost tangential image of the upper end of the vertebral column, showing the splaying of the vertebral column as it approaches the head *(double arrows)*.

Anencephaly or exencephaly may be a consequence of amniotic bands. This nonrecurring cause of anencephaly can be differentiated from the anencephaly occurring as a result of failure of the neural tube to close, in that the cranial lesion is asymmetrical and multiple amputations of the fingers or toes as well as defects of the abdominal wall may also be present. The key sonographic finding in making the diagnosis of amniotic band syndrome is the presence of a band between the fetal defect and the placenta.[48,57]

Craniorachischisis
Craniorachischisis refers to a defect in which the open cranial defect (anencephaly) is in continuity with the completely open spine (spinal dysraphia).

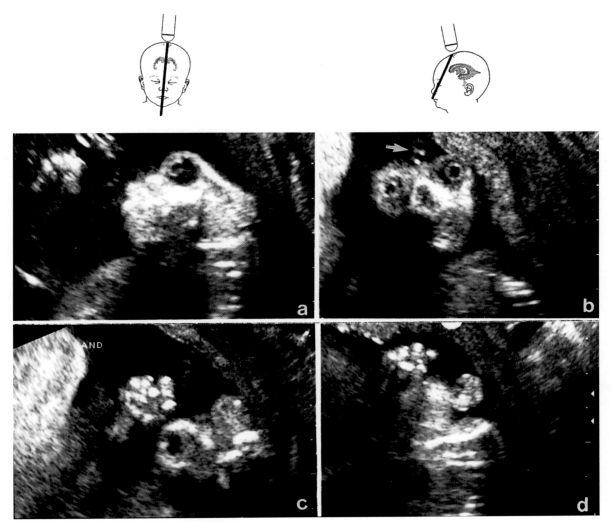

Figure 4–14. Anencephaly at 20 postmenstrual weeks. **A.** Median section depicting a relatively normal profile of the fetal head. However, the skull is totally missing. **B.** A coronal section of the face showing the fetal orbits with the lenses within. The arrow points to the two-vessel cord present in this fetus. **C** and **D** are two views of the hands of the fetus. Note that the hands are clenched with overlapping digits.

In this defect there is total failure of neurulation to occur, and it is believed to arise no later than 20 to 22 days after conception. Most of the fetuses affected with this extensive malformation are spontaneously aborted early in pregnancy.[10] Craniorachischisis is present in up to 10% of anencephalic fetuses.[49] Sonography demonstrates the anencephaly and the extensive spinal dysraphism (Figs. 4–10 and 4–13).

Iniencephaly

Iniencephaly is a complex and lethal malformation which has as its three main features (1) a defect in the occiput involving the foramen magnum; (2) retroflexion of the entire spine, which forces the fetus to look upward with its occiput directed toward the lumbar region; and (3) open spinal defects of variable degree.[58–63] The reported incidence of iniencephaly ranges from 1 to 6 per 10,000 births. As in anencephaly, most of the affected fetuses are female (90%). Most of the fetuses with this condition are stillborn. The malformation results from developmental arrest of the embryo no later than 24 days after conception. This results in persistence of the embryonic cervical retroflexion, which leads to failure of the neural groove to close in the area of the cervical spine or the upper thorax.[58,64,65] Iniencephaly has been divided into two types: (1) *iniencephalus clausus,* or the closed type; and (2) *iniencephalus apertus,* or the open type. In the latter, an occipital cephalocele protruding through the foramen magnum and an occipital bone defect are present (Fig. 4–15).[63]

Using TVS, iniencephaly has been diagnosed as early as 12.5 postmenstrual weeks (Fig. 4–16).[66] On the median plane the head appears large and held in retroflexion, the neck is not visualized, and the spine is usually lordotic. In cases of iniencephalus apertus, a posterior cephalocele is present in the occipital area (Fig. 4–15). On transverse views, the open spinal defect is present. On axial sections, the head circumference may be several standard deviations below the mean and consistent with microcephaly. In addition, a size–dates discrepancy in a well-dated pregnancy may be the first sign of an iniencephalic fetus (Fig. 4–16).

Other malformations occur in up to 84% of fetuses with iniencephaly. Many of these associated malformations can be diagnosed only beyond the first trimester. Among the associated anomalies are hydrocephaly, microcephaly, ventricular atresia, holoprosencephaly, polymicrogyria, agenesis of the cerebellar vermis, occipital encephalocele, anencephaly, diaphragmatic hernia, thoracic cage deformities, urinary tract anomalies, cleft lip and cleft palate, clubfoot, single umbilical artery, omphalocele (Fig. 4–16), and polyhydramnios.[58–60,64,67,68]

Cephalocele

Cephaloceles are cranial defects along bony sutures in which there is a herniation of the brain and/or the meninges. When the cephalocele sac contains brain tissue, these defects are termed *encephaloceles,* and if only cerebrospinal fluid (CSF) is present, they are termed *meningoceles.* The reported incidence ranges from 1 per 3500 to 1 per 5000 live births.[69] It is estimated that encephaloceles are approximately one tenth as common as meningocele.[70] Cephalocele may involve the occipital, frontal, temporal, and parietal regions of the fetal head (Table 4–5). The occurrence of the different types of cephaloceles reflects geographic variation. In Europe and North America between 66% and 89% of all cephaloceles are occipital, the balance being equally distributed among frontal and parietal cephaloceles. In Thailand and other countries of southern Asia, the frontal (sincipital) location is more common than the occipital.[25,53,56,70–74]

Occipital Cephalocele

Occipital cephaloceles occur more commonly in females than in males, in contrast to the parietal and sincipital cephaloceles, which are more prevalent in males.[70] The development of most severe cephaloceles takes place no later than 26 days after conception, at the time that the rostral neuroporc closes.[10]

Using TVS, occipital cephalocele has been diagnosed as early as 12 postmenstrual weeks (Fig. 4–17).[66] The sonographic appearance of an occipital cephalocele is that of a saclike structure adjacent to the fetal head (Figs. 4–18 through 4–20). The cephaloceles show a range in size not only of the skull defect but also of the cephalocele sac itself. The size of the cephalocele may range from a few millimeters to a mass exceeding the size of the normal cranial vault.[72] In infants the size distribution of the cephaloceles is as follows: 16% are greater than 20 cm, 14% are between 15 and 20 cm, 12% are 10 to 15 cm, 30% are between 5 and 10 cm, and 28% are less than 5 cm.[70] The head circumference and the biparietal diameter (BPD) may be significantly lower than expected for the fetal age. Microcephaly is reported to occur in 9% to 24% of the cases.[70] Closer inspection of the cranium reveals a defect through which the contents of the cephalocele sac communicate with the intracranial portion of the brain structures (Figs. 4–18 through 4–20). The sac may contain brain tissue (encephalocele [Figs. 4–18 through 4–20]) or may be sonolucent, containing only CSF (meningocele).[53,75,76] Meningoceles account for approximately 10% to 20% of the occipital lesions.[10] The brain tissue most often present in the encephalocele sac is the occipital lobe, which exhibits a normal gyral pattern (Fig. 4–18). Approximately half of the cephaloceles situated "low" in the cervical region contain the occipital lobes of the hemispheres, but almost all contain the cerebellum.[10]

Hydrocephaly may be present in 20% to 65% of the cases as a result of aqueductal stenosis or Chiari type III malformation. The corpus callosum is usually present, but may also be completely or partially missing. The septum pellucidum may be absent in up to 80% of the cases.[70] Other associated malformations that may be apparent include cerebellar dysplasia, spinal dysraphism, diastematomyelia, Klippel–Feil deformity, Dandy–Walker malformation, cleft palate, microphthalmos, tracheoesophageal fistula, and cardiac malformations.[56,70,75,77]

Early diagnosis of occipital cephalocele is possible. Fleming and colleagues[78] reported on the prenatal diagnosis of an occipital encephalocele using TVS at 12 postmenstrual weeks. It is important to note that some of the abnormalities associated with occipital cephaloceles (e.g., agenesis of the corpus callosum) may only become sonographically apparent later, during the late second or third trimester of pregnancy.

Cephaloceles usually occur as isolated lesions, but in a small percentage of the cases may be a part of a nonchromosomal or chromosomal syndrome (Table 4–6). Chromosomal abnormalities associated

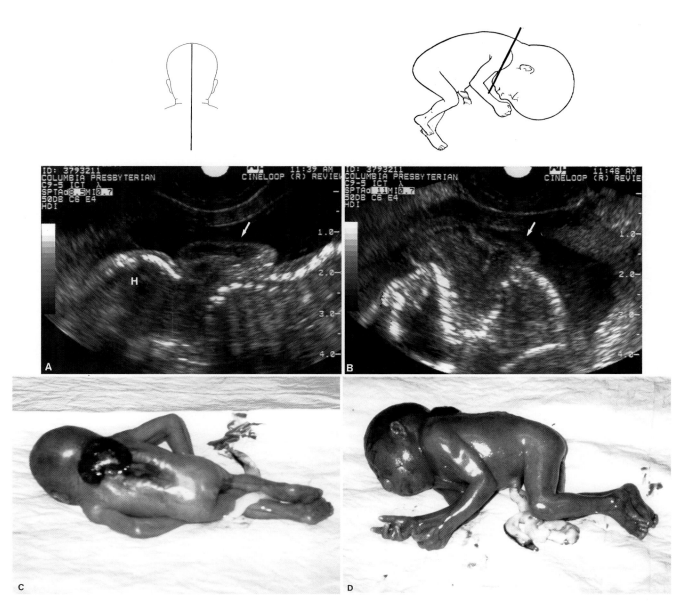

Figure 4–15. A fetus with iniencephaly at 22 postmenstrual weeks. **A.** Longitudinal median section. On the left deformation of the head is seen (H); to the right the distorted vertebral column is seen with severe kyphoscoliotic deformation. Bulging brain tissue (occipital meningomyelocele) is seen *(arrow)*. **B.** Transverse section with the open vertebral column (rachischisis) is seen with the bulging brain tissue *(arrow)*. **C, D.** The aborted specimen, demonstrating the absence of the neck (iniencephaly) and rachischisis with the myelomeningocele.

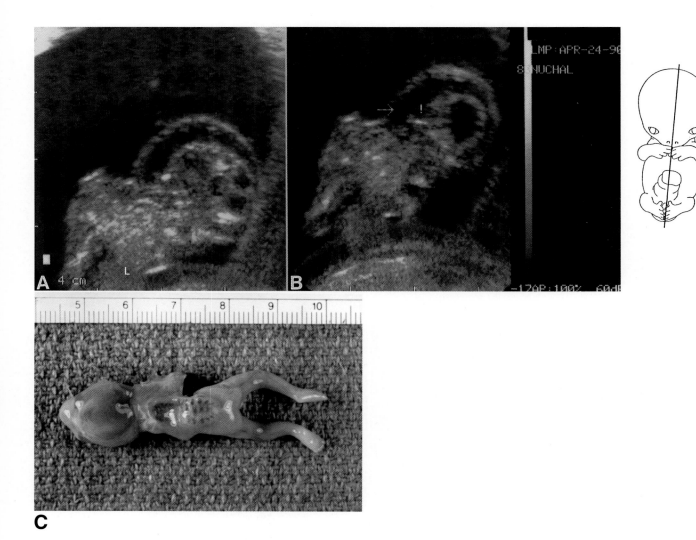

Figure 4–16. Iniencephaly at 12.5 postmenstrual weeks. **A.** Sonographic appearance in the median plane. Note the short body length due to the absence of the neck. Omphalocele was also present. L, Liver. **B.** Specimen from the side, showing the shortened neck. **C.** Dorsal view of the specimen, showing the total spinal rachischisis. *(From Bronshtein and colleagues, 1991,[66] with permission.)*

TABLE 4–5. CLASSIFICATION OF CEPHALOCELE ACCORDING TO THE SITE OF THE BONE DEFECT

Occipital
Anterior
  Sincipital
  Basal
Parietal

After Simpson DA and colleagues, 1984,[77] with permission.

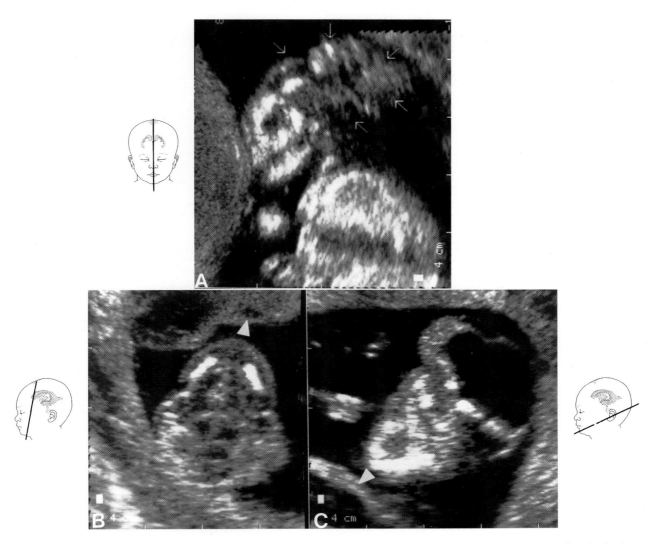

Figure 4–17. Occipital encephalocele at 12 postmenstrual weeks. **A.** Median section. Note the protruding brain tissue (outlined by *arrows*). **B.** Horizontal section. The *arrowhead* marks the anterior direction. **C.** Coronal section. Note the missing brain tissue and the sac of the cephalocele. (No specimen available since this was a selective fetal reduction of one of twins).

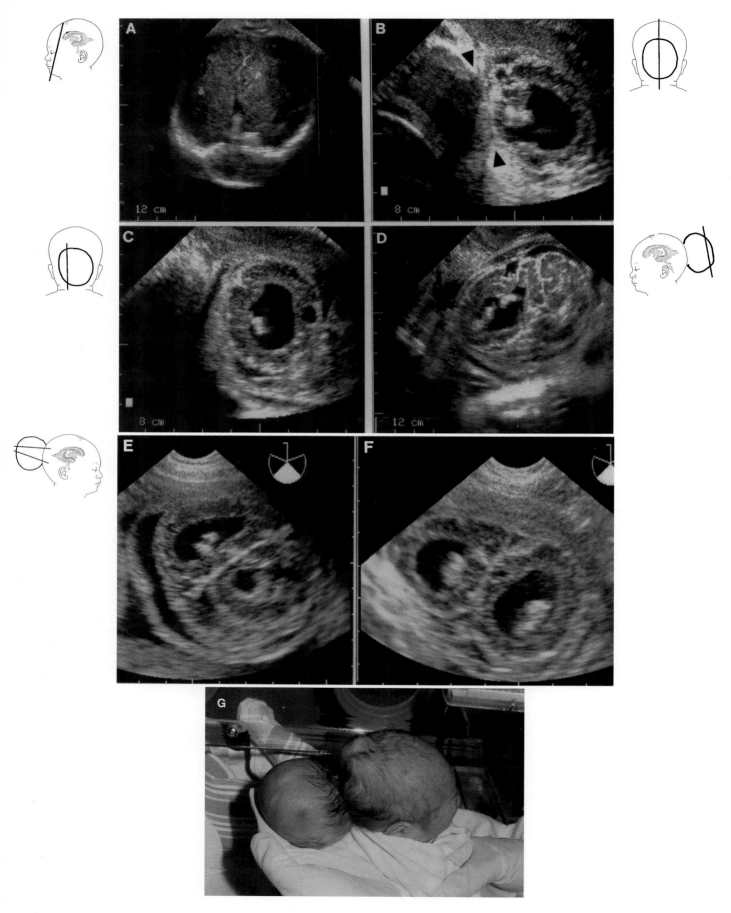

Figure 4–18. Occipital encephalocele in a fetus at 34 postmenstrual weeks. This patient presented for her first ultrasonographic examination at this gestational age. Microcephaly was also diagnosed (the biparietal diameter and the head circumference were consistent with 26 postmenstrual weeks). **A.** Frontal–2 section showing the longitudinal sulcus and apparently normal brain tissue. **B.** Median section depicting the large bony defect in the occipital region, marked by two *black arrowheads.* Brain tissue seems to protrude, "pulling" with it the posterior horn and the choroid plexus. **C, D.** Different sections of the encephalocele itself. **E, F.** Coronal sections, by definition, showing the longitudinal sulcus and the dilated occipital horns within the choroid plexus. **G.** A photograph of the neonate's head showing the large occipital encephalocele. During the clinical course the neonate was found to have a chromosome 13q deletion and was admitted to the hospital and discharged several times, but reached the age of 1½ years. Another anomaly included absence of the thumbs. Cranioplasty was performed, which was complicated by wound infection and worsening hydrocephaly. A drain was placed; however, the infant was admitted to the hospital several times because of a cerebrospinal fluid leak from the incision site. The infant has severe mental retardation and a seizure disorder. Computed tomographic studies showed that the encephalocele included the cerebellar hemispheres and a portion of the posterior horns (as diagnosed by the ultrasonographic images) and, in addition, has partial agenesis of the corpus callosum, the splenium being virtually absent.

with cephaloceles are trisomies 13 and 18; mosaic trisomy 20; deletion (13q), (2)(q21→q24); monosomy X; and duplication (6)(q21→qter), (7)(pter→p11), and (8)(q23→qter). We have encountered two fetuses with a large posterior encephalocele and a deletion of the short arm of chromosome 13 (13q) (Figs. 4–18 and 4–19). Besides having encephaloceles, these fetuses have skeletal malformations. The most remarkable of these is absence of the thumb.

Some of the nonchromosomal syndromes that feature a cephalocele are listed in Table 4–6. In these cases the karyotype is normal and the clues to the prenatal diagnosis are derived from sonographic findings. Therefore, it is imperative to perform a detailed targeted scan looking for other sonographic abnormalities. This is especially important if this is the first affected fetus. Of the nonchromosomal syndromes, Meckel–Gruber syndrome (MGS) is among the most common and is discussed below. Walker–Warburg syndrome is another relatively common entity that also features a cephalocele and is discussed later in the section dealing with lissencephaly.

Meckel–Gruber syndrome is a lethal autosomal recessive syndrome. Because of its 25% recurrence rate, it is important to distinguish this syndrome from sporadic occipital cephaloceles, which may carry only a 1% to 3% recurrence rate. Approximately 80% of the cases of MGS have an *occipital cephalocele.* The two other consistent findings in the typical triad of malformations are *bilateral renal cystic dysplasia* and *postaxial polydactyly* of both the hands and the feet.[70,73] The latter malformations have been reported to be present in 95% and 75% of the cases.[79]

To make the diagnosis of MGS, at least two of the three major signs must be present. Using sonography, the diagnosis of MGS can be made by the late first trimester or early second trimester. (Fig. 4–21).[80–82] The cystic dysplastic kidneys are the most consistent anomaly. The kidneys are enlarged up to 10 to 20 times over the normal size, are hyperechogenic, and contain multiple small cysts measuring between 2 and 5 mm.[73,83] As a result of the dysplastic kidneys, renal function is impaired and oligohydramnios is present. In addition, the fetal bladder is not imaged by ultrasonography. The size of the cephalocele may be variable. In one of our cases of MGS, the skull defect measured 2 mm (Fig. 4–22). Other sonographic findings are microcephaly, with a BPD and a head circumference lagging behind dates, and hydrocephaly.

Associated malformations that may present in MGS include renal agenesis, renal hypoplasia, ureteral duplication, cleft lip and cleft palate, micrognathia, microphthalmos, ambiguous genitalia, congenital hepatic fibrosis, talipes equinovarus, short-limb dwarfism, malformed tongue, intestinal malrotation, Dandy–Walker malformation, and congenital heart defects.[84,85] The heart defects include ventricular or atrial septal defect, aortic hypoplasia or coarctation, aortic valvular stenosis, and rotational anomalies.[73] Most fetuses with MGS either are stillborn or die within the first day of life due to the dysplastic kidneys, which result in oligohydramnios and, in turn, result in hypoplastic lungs, although prolonged survival up to 28 months has been reported.[86] Kaplan and coworkers[87] reported on a rare case of survival of a fetus with prenatally diagnosed Meckel's syndrome variant. In this case, the fetus had an occipital cephalocele and a unilateral multicystic kidney, the remaining kidney having normal renal function.

The prognosis for fetuses with a cephalocele depends on the location, size, and content of the lesion and on the concurrent intracranial as well as extracranial malformations (Table 4–7). The small

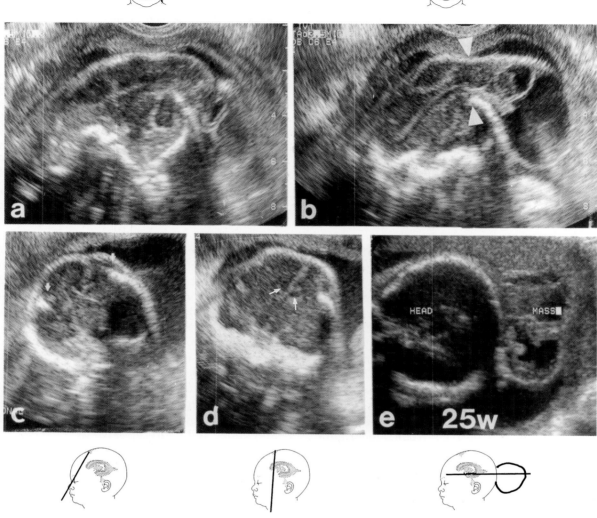

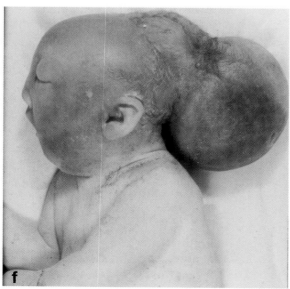

Figure 4–19. Sonographic images of an occipital encephalocele at 25 postmenstrual weeks. Delivery took place at 34.5 weeks. **A, B.** Median views showing the skull defect between the two *white arrows* and the bulging brain and cerebrospinal fluid within the sac. **C, D.** Frontal –1 and –2 views showing what appears to be normal symmetrical brain tissue. **D** shows the anterior horns *(small arrows).* **E.** Horizontal section of the defect and the herniated mass. The head demonstrated severe microcephaly for the gestational age. **F.** Specimen demonstrating severe microcephaly and the large posterior encephalocele. Chromosomal studies demonstrated a 13q deletion.

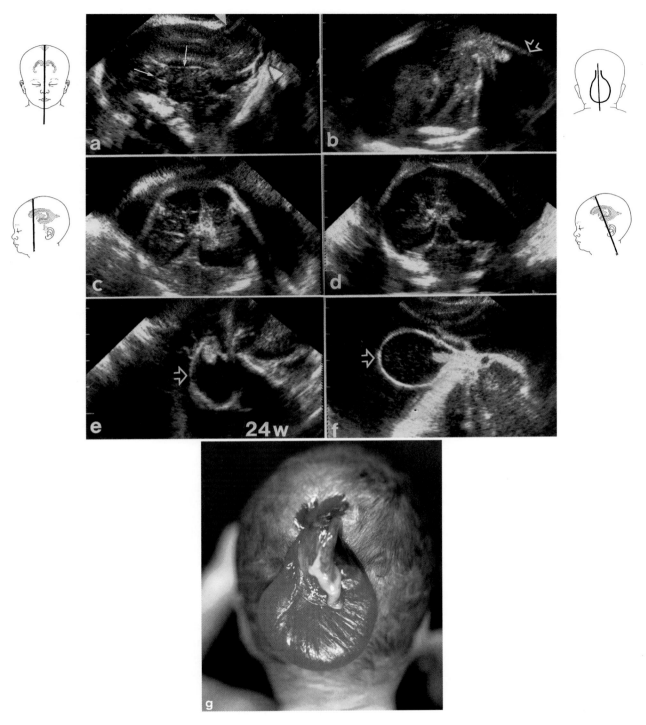

Figure 4–20. Occipital encephalocele. The pregnant patient presented at 24 postmenstral weeks for a dating ultrasonogram. The measurements revealed microcephaly and the occipital bulging structure. **A.** Median section of the brain, showing the bony lesion between the two *white arrowheads.* Note that the typical shape of the corpus callosum *(small arrows)* and of the small cavum septi pellucidi is seen. **B.** This view concentrates on the posterior herniated sac *(open arrow).* A very small, echogenic structure is seen bulging into the fluid. **C.** Midcoronal–1 section. Almost no anterior horns are seen on this section. **D.** Midcoronal–3 section. Very small lateral ventricles with an echogenic choroid plexus are seen. **E, F.** Targeted views of the posterior cephalocele *(open arrows).* Inside a small (0.5 cm), echogenic tissue is seen, which may correspond to the meninges or a very minute amount of brain tissue. **G.** Specimen showing the translucent thin membrane of the cephalocele bulging through the midline skull defect. In addition, this fetus had a single umbilical artery, dilated renal pelves, cardiomegaly with pericardial infusion, and an interventricular septal defect with a wide pulmonary artery.

TABLE 4–6. SYNDROMES WITH A CEPHALOCELE

Syndrome	Other Features Detectable With Prenatal Ultrasound
Apert	Craniosynostosis, short skull base, syndactyly hands and feet, megalencephaly, and encephalocele
Craniotelencephalic dysplasia	Craniosynostosis, frontal encephalocele at metopic region, microphthalmos, septo-optic dysplasia, agenesis of the corpus callosum, lissencephaly, and arhinencephaly
Cranium bifidum occultum	Occipital encephalocele
Dyssegmental dysplasia	Clefting, encephalocele, micromelia, and thick and bowed bones
Facioauriculovertebral	Face hypoplasia, cardiac and vertebral anomalies, and posterior cephalocele
Fried–Meckel-like	Lobar holoprosencephaly, large occipital encephalocele, microcephaly, and congenital heart disease
Frontofacionasaldysplasia	Cranium bifidum occultum, anterior cephalocele, and cleft lip and/or cleft palate
Frontonasal dysplasia	Hypertelorism, frontonasal encephalocele, and median cleft lip
Meckel–Gruber	Microcephaly, encephalocele, microphthalmos, cleft lip and cleft palate, cystic dysplastic kidneys, and polydactyly.
Oculoencephalohepatorenal	Micrognathia, postaxial polydactyly, cystic renal dysplasia, and meningoencephalocele
Phocomelia–encephalocele–urogenital anomalies	Bilateral radial aplasia, absent right thumb, fused pelvic kidney, dextroposed heart, hypoplastic lung, thin corpus callosum, and encephalocele
Robert's–SC–phocomelia	Microbrachycephaly, growth restriction, cleft lip and cleft palate, and frontal encephalocele
von Voss–Cherstvoy: limb defects–thrombocytopenia	Occipital encephalocele, absent corpus callosum, hypoplastic thumbs, and renal agenesis
Walker–Warburg	Lissencephaly type II, cerebellar malformations, vermis hypoplasia, microphthalmos, and posterior encephalocele
Warfarin embryopathy	Microphthalmos, cardiac anomalies, and occipital encephalocele

After Hunter AG. Brain and spinal cord. In: Stevenson RE, Hall JG, Goodman RM, eds. Human Malformations and Related Anomalies. *New York: Oxford University Press;* 1993;2:109–137. With permission.

defects can be corrected easily with surgery, but larger lesions are usually not compatible with life or may result in a neurologically impaired infant.[88] The reported survival rate for infants with posterior cephalocele ranges from 40% to 75%.[77,89–91] Mortality is most commonly due to the severity of the other associated malformation or the inability to repair the defect. Meningocele has a lower mortality rate, ranging from 10% to 25%.[92] Disabilities occur in those children who survive. Brown and Sheridan-Pereira[92] reported that 25% of the surviving infants with occipital cephalocele had severe long-term disabilities and 38% had mild handicaps. These disabilities occurred in their series regardless of defect size or the presence or absence of brain tissue in the cephalocele.

Anterior Cephalocele

Anterior or sincipital cephaloceles are frontonasal herniations of the brain and/or the meninges through a skull defect. Anterior cephaloceles always occur in the median plane of the cranium. The cephaloceles occur at the sites of the fontanelles (frontal and sphenoidal) or at the cribriform plate of the ethmoid, the foramen cecum, or the foramen magnum or through a suture line.[74,93,94] They are di-

vided into two main types: *sincipital defects* and *basal defects.* The sincipital cephaloceles are external lesions that occur near the root of the nose (glabella) and are subdivided into nasofrontal, nasoethmoidal, and naso-orbital types (Figs. 4–23 and 4–25). The basal cephaloceles are internal lesions that occur within the nose, the pharynx, or the orbit. These are further subdivided into five types: spheno-orbital, sphenomaxillary, transethmoidal, sphenoethmoidal, and sphenopharyngeal.[93–96]

The pathogenesis of anterior cephaloceles is unclear. Anterior cephaloceles occur quite early in development, at around 45 to 50 days of embryonic age. This is when the base of the occiput and the sphenoid body develop and assume their normal appearance.[97] Anterior cephaloceles, similarly to the occipital cephaloceles, may occur as a sporadic defect, associated with a chromosomal syndrome, or as part of a nonchromosomal developmental syndrome (Table 4–6). Syndromes with an associated anterior cephalocele include aberrant tissue band syndrome, frontonasal dysplasia, absent corpus callosum, clefting, craniostenosis, hypothalamic–pituitary dysfunction, meningocele, and Robert's–SC–phocomelia syndrome.[96,98,99]

The sonographic appearance of an anterior cephalocele is that of an irregularly shaped mass

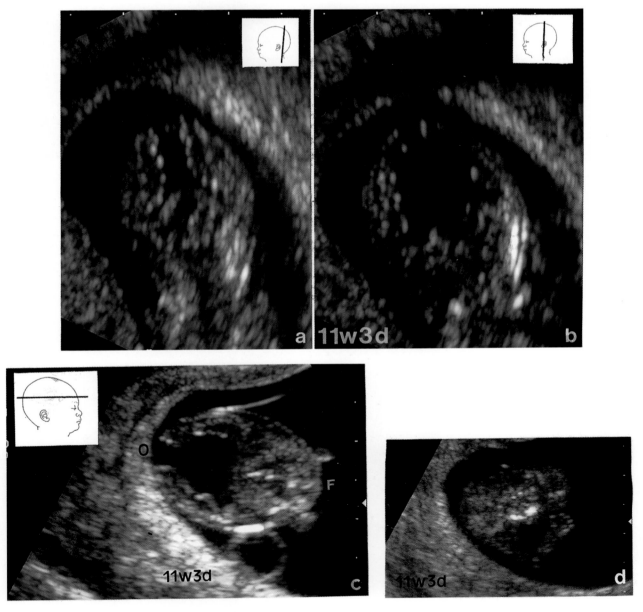

Figure 4–21. Meckel–Gruber syndrome (MGS) at 11 postmenstrual weeks, 3 days. This patient was at high risk for MGS since she had a previous infant with this syndrome. At the time of this scan, a posterior skull defect was seen as well as a large posterior fossa. There was no polydactyly (no polydactyly was present in her previous MGS infant). **A, B.** Posterior coronal sections showing a large sonolucent midline cystic area which freely connected with the amniotic cavity. **C.** Axial section showing the cranial defect and large cystic structure, which is completely filling the area of the posterior fossa. O, occipital; F, frontal. **D.** A view of the right arm and hand of the fetus showing five digits.

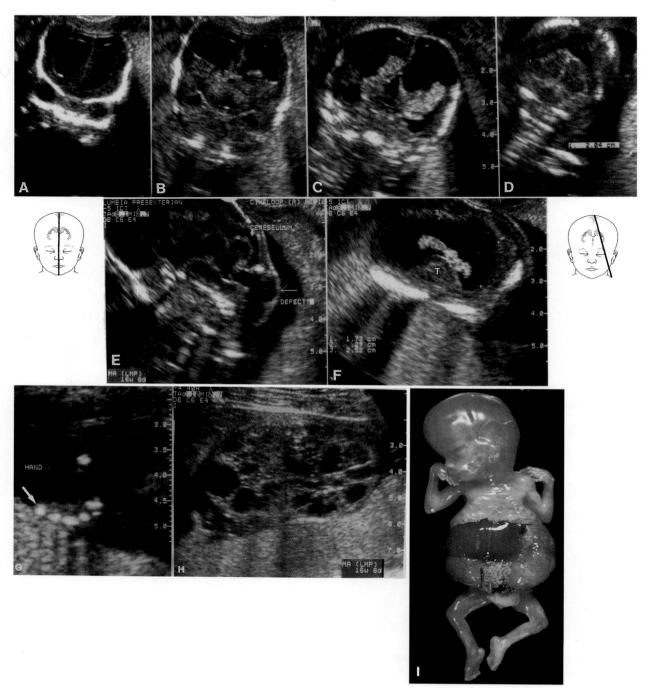

Figure 4–22. Meckel–Gruber syndrome at 16 postmenstrual weeks, 6 days. The systematic workup of the brain is shown in **A–F. A.** Frontal–2 section showing the enlarged anterior horns. **B.** Midcoronal–1 section. Severely dilated lateral ventricles are evident. **C.** Midcoronal–2 section. The dangling hyperechogenic choroid plexus is seen obeying gravity (the so-called dangling choroid plexus sign). The dilated third ventricle is also seen. **D.** Occipital–2 section showing the cerebellum. **E.** Median section. The *arrow* indicates a very small encephalocele. **F.** Oblique–1 section through the lateral ventricle; the anterior, posterior, and inferior horns are seen on the same section. The choroid plexus above the thalamus (T) is floating freely in the cerebrospinal fluid. **G.** The additional feature of this syndrome is postaxial polydactyly *(arrow)*. **H.** The enlarged multicystic kidneys. **I.** The aborted specimen, with the two large kidneys exposed.

TABLE 4–7. PROGNOSIS FOR FETUSES WITH A CEPHALOCELE

Prognosis Better	Prognosis Worse
Cranial meningocele	Cranial meningoencephalocele
Small nubbing of dysplastic glial or neuronal tissue in hernia	Larger portions of clearly recognizable brain in hernia
Cephalocele diameter <5 cm	Cephalocele diameter >5 cm
No associated anomalies	Concurrent microcephaly or holoprosencephaly
Normal ventricles	In utero ventricular enlargement

protruding from the fetal face (Figs. 4–23 through 4–25). Associated anomalies include ocular hypertelorism, nasal widening, cleft lip and/or cleft palate, median nasal fissure, spina bifida, agenesis of the corpus callosum, ventriculomegaly, and microcephaly.[74] The differential diagnosis of an anterior cephalocele includes teratoma, glioma, dermal sinus cyst, facial hemangioma, orbital duplication, and proboscis.

Anterior cephaloceles appear to carry a relatively better prognosis than other types of cephaloceles. Brown and Sheridan-Pereira[92] found that 42% of children with anterior cephaloceles were normal, 17% had mild handicaps, and 25% had severe handicaps. The primary morbidity in children with anterior defects is facial disfigurement, anosmia, and visual problems.[91,100] Surgical procedures for anterior cephalocele offer very limited improvement of the facial deformity, and many of the children who survive suffer cosmetic facial and eye deformities.[71,91,96,100,101]

Parietal Cephalocele
Parietal cephaloceles are located in the midline between the lambda and the bregma. The size, shape, position, and content of the cephalocele sac may be variable.[70] The cephalocele sac may contain parietal cortex. Using TVS, Cullen and colleagues[102] reported on the prenatal diagnosis of a parietal encephalocele at 17 postmenstrual weeks. Sonography demonstrates a midline skull defect with a protruding sac that may or may not contain brain tissue (Fig. 4–26). Other sonographic findings include microcephaly, which has been reported in about 20% of the cases[77] and ventriculomegaly, reported in 47% of in utero cases.[103] Associated malformations include agenesis of the corpus callosum, Dandy–Walker cyst, lobar holoprosencephaly,and Arnold–Chiari type II malformation.[70]

The prognosis for the infant with a parietal cephalocele is the following: approximately 33% will die, 40% will have marked mental retardation, 13% will be able to get an education, and 15% will develop normally.[103]

Spinal Dysraphism and Arnold–Chiari Type II Malformation
The main feature in spinal dysraphism is an open spine, with protrusion of the spinal contents through the bony defect. Myelocele and myelomeningocele develop similarly, but the term *myelocele* refers to a midline plaque of neural tissue (neural placode) that is flush with the surface and is not covered by skin. In contrast, the myelomeningocele is a bulging defect in which the elevated neural plate and meninges are contiguous laterally with the subcutaneous tissue.[104] Approximately 10% to 15% of spinal dysraphic defects are closed and normal skin covers the bony defect.

The incidence of myelomeningocele in the United States is 0.2 to 0.4 per 1000 live births. This number reflects a downward trend from the 1970s, when the incidence was reported to be 0.5 to 0.6 per 1000 live births.[105] Approximately 80% of the lesions occur in the lumbar, thoracolumbar, or lumbosacral areas of the spine, and the remainder are located in the cervical and sacral areas.[106] The onset of myelomeningocele is probably around the fourth week of gestation, at the time of closure of the posterior caudal neuropore. Transvaginal sonography can image the rudimentary neural tube by the seventh postmenstrual week. The vertebral column can be imaged by the ninth to 10th postmenstrual weeks, and using the median plane, the posterior fetal contour, including the covering skin, can be imaged well enough to detect major neural tube abnormalities.[107–109]

From late in the first trimester to early in the second, the fetal spine can be scanned in three planes (sagittal, coronal, and transverse). In a sagittal plane the vertebral column appears as two echogenic, parallel lines, flaring toward the upper cervical spine and converging toward the sacrum.[110] In a coronal plane it appears as two or three (depending on the depth of the scan) parallel bands of echoes corresponding to the body and one in each side of the posterior neural arch. In a transverse plane the intact vertebral arch is represented by a triangular configuration of three echoes, forming a closed circle around the neural canal.[111]

Prenatal diagnosis of spina bifida is possible before the 12th postmenstrual week by noting irregularities of the bony spine or a bulging within the posterior contour of the fetal back in sagittal view.[112] On transverse section the open spine has a U-shape,

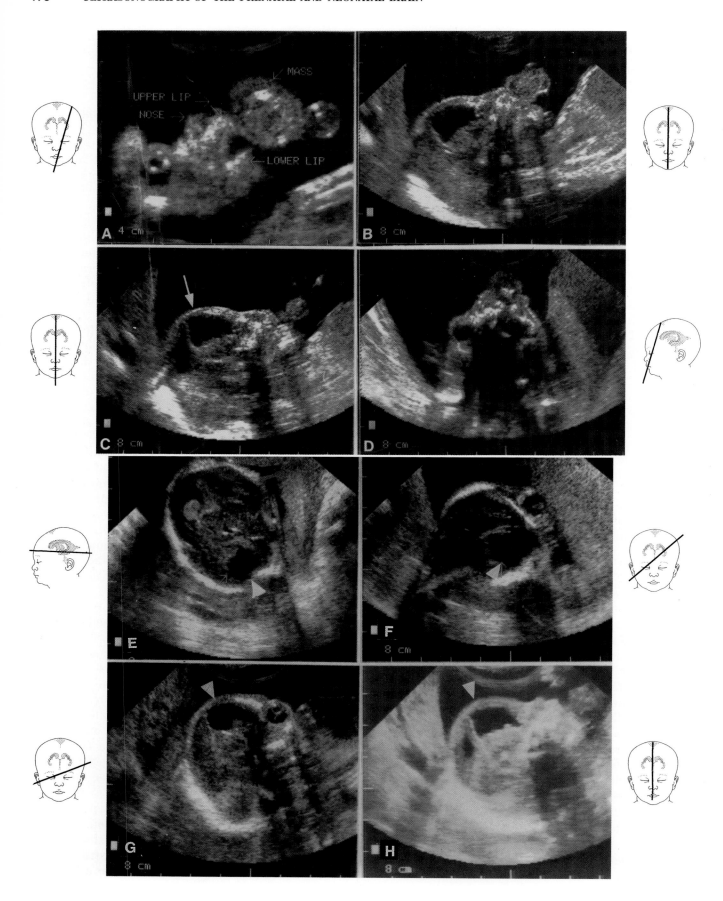

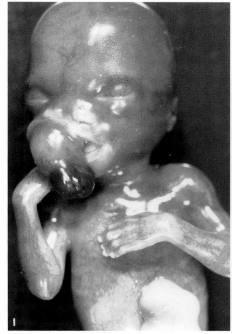

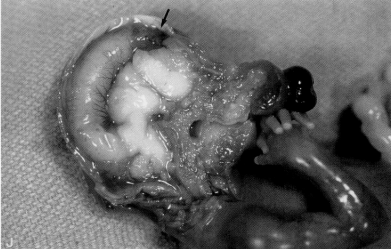

Figure 4–23. Anterior encephalocele at 13.5 postmenstrual weeks. **A.** Median section showing the eye, nose, upper and lower lips, and a lobulated mass protruding between the lips. **B, C.** Slightly and progressively lateral paramedian sections showing not only the lesion but also a quite sizable sonolucency in the area of the frontal lobes, probably "left behind" by the protruding mass, leaving that space vacant. **D.** Horizontal section of the lesion, showing the protruding mass between the two orbits. **E–H.** Horizontal paramedian and median sections of the lesion. These images were aimed at determining the location of the sonolucency in the skull. This was finally found to be in the area of the anterior horn, almost symmetrically between the two hemispheres *(arrowheads)*. **I.** Side view of the aborted specimen, showing the bulging cephalocele emerging through the mouth. **J.** Median transection of the head, demonstrating the origin of the lesion protruding from the anterior horn. The sonolucent space in the area of the frontal horn detected by ultrasonography is now clearly seen on this section *(black arrow)*. *(A–G from Monteagudo A and Timor-Tritsch IE, 1992,*[74] *with permission.)*

and on coronal section the affected bony segment shows a divergent configuration replacing the typical parallel lines of the normal vertebral arches (Figs. 4–27 through 4–32, 4–33A, and 4–34D). The diagnostic sensitivities for the prenatal sonographic detection of myelomeningocele are reported to be between 80% and 90%; these rates are even higher prior to knowledge of the MSAFP results.[3,113–115] Determining the site and extent of the spinal lesion is important because it correlates with the neurological outcome of the fetus. The higher and larger the lesion, the more severe the neurological dysfunction the neonate will have. The vertebral level can be assessed in a sagittal view of the spine by (1) counting up from the last ossified vertebral segment (S4 in the second trimester and S5 in the third), (2) assuming that the last rib corresponds to T12, and (3) assuming that the top of the iliac wing corresponds to L5 to S1[116] Using this method, Kollias and associates[116] reported that the pathology and in utero ul-

trasonographic assessment of the spinal level agreed in 64% of the cases and in an additional 14% it correlated to within one vertebra of the lesion. Recently, with the introduction of three-dimensional (3-D) ultrasonography the level of the spinal defect can be easier and better defined and the extent of the lesion can be more accurately determined (see Chapter 9).

After the 12th postmenstrual week there are well-established intracranial sonographic findings that can enhance the detection of spina bifida, namely, the "lemon" sign, the "banana" sign,[117,118] and hydrocephaly. The *"lemon" sign* refers to deformity of the frontal bone, and the *"banana" sign* refers to an abnormal shape of the flattened cerebellum, which obliterates the cisterna magna (Figs. 4–30B; 4–34A and C; 4–35). Blumenfeld's group[119] reported on the diagnosis of NTDs between 12 and 17 weeks using the "banana" and "lemon" signs. In one case followed serially from 10 weeks,

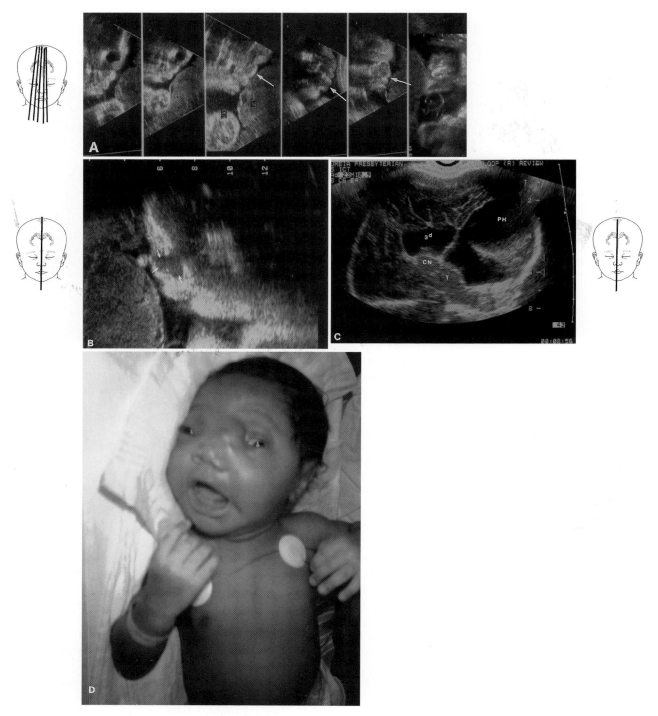

Figure 4–24. Anterior encephalocele in a fetus at 36 postmenstrual weeks. **A.** Serial sections in the sagittal plane, showing the profile and a bulging mass distorting the normal shape of the profile *(arrows).* **B.** Median section of the face, showing the sonolucent bulge *(arrows)* just behind the prominence of the nose. **C.** Median section of the brain, showing the typical sunburst appearance of the gyri above the space representing the third ventricle. This is typical of the sonographic image of agenesis of the corpus callosum. The posterior horn (PH) is widely dilated. CN, Caudate nucleus; T, thalamus. **D.** The neonate, clearly showing a distorted face, widely spaced eyes (hypertelorism), and a bulge in the midline or somewhat closer to the left eye. The slight distortion and slight displacement of the nose are evident.

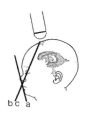

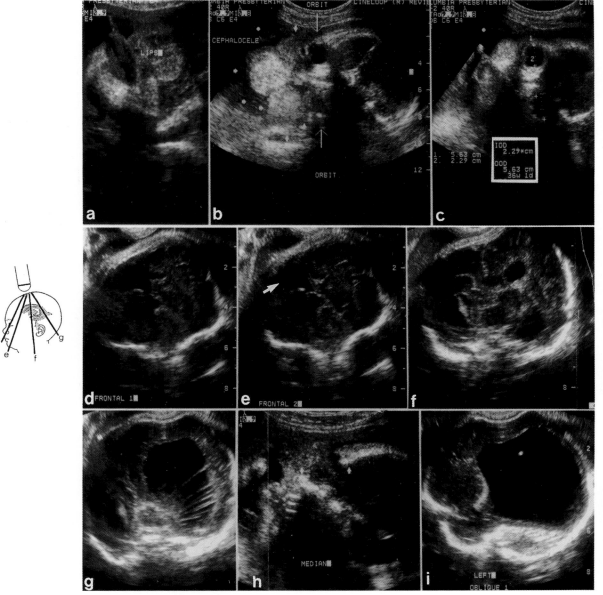

Figure 4–25. Anterior encephalocele at 35 postmenstrual weeks, 3 days. The patient was referred for a second opinion ultrasound because of a suspected large subarachnoid cyst, and microcephaly. **A, B,** and **C** are coronal sections of the fetal face. In **A,** the lips are seen to be intact. In **B** and **C,** hypertelorism is noted with a hyperechogenic mass protruding between the fetal orbits. IOD, inter orbital distance; OOD, outer orbital distance. **D–G** are serial coronal sections from anterior to posterior of the fetal brain. **D,** Frontal–1 section showing an irregular shape head and interhemispheric fissure. **E.** Frontal–2 section here a sonolucent structure is noted *(arrow).* **F** and **G** show that the hemispheres are not symmetrical and in **G** the ventricle is dilated and contains some adhesions. **H.** Median section showing the cranial defect *(arrow)* through which the brain tissue has herniated. **I.** Left Oblique–1 sections showing the unilateral hydrocephaly. *(Continued)*

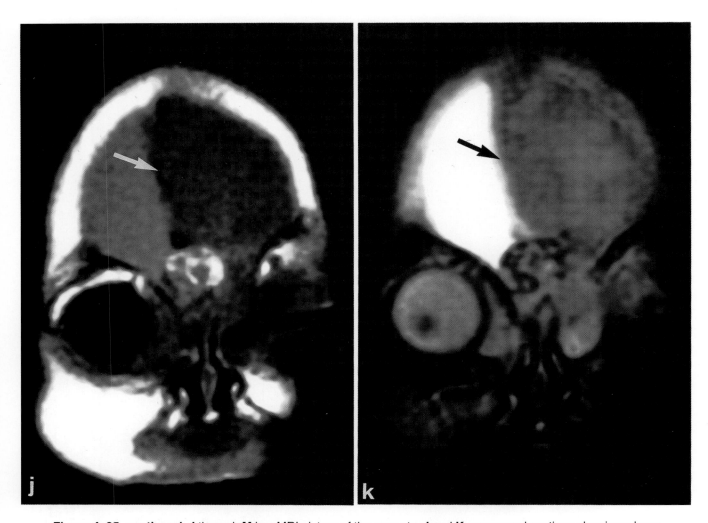

Figure 4–25. continued J through **M** is a MRI picture of the neonate. **J** and **K** are coronal sections showing a large left cystic area in addition to the encephalocele *(arrow).*

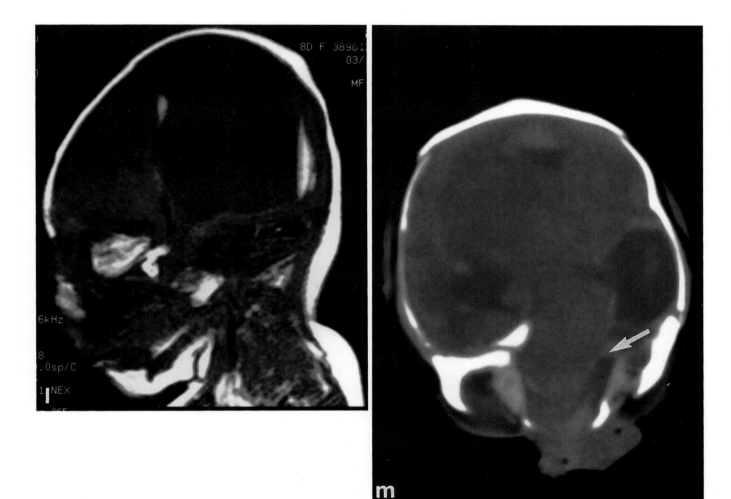

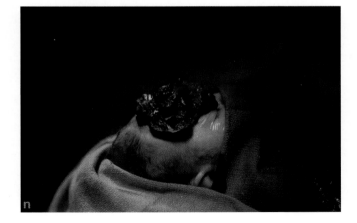

Figure 4–25. continued L. Sagittal section showing the unilateral hydrocephaly. **M.** Axial section showing the naso-ethmoidal skull defect *(arrow)* through which the brain is herniating. **N.** Picture of the neonate at the time of the surgical correction of the encephalocele. At birth, the neonate had multiple problems including severe anemia, seizures, tonic posturing, and abnormal tongue movements. A ventriculoperitoneal shunt was subsequently placed. By the eighth month of life the infant had had multiple hospital admissions and her problems included diabetes insipidus, epilepsy, and temperature instability.

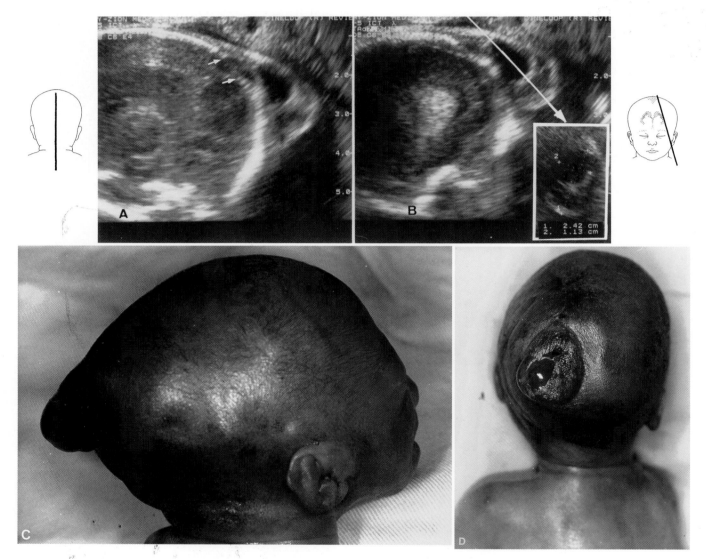

Figure 4–26. Parietal cephalocele at 22 postmenstrual weeks. **A.** The small (7-mm) bony defect lies between the *small white arrows*. Note that this is evident in the Oblique–1 sections. The brain tissue on all sections appeared normal. **B.** A slightly more lateral section showing the posterior horn with a hyperechogenic choroid plexus and the skull defect with the sonolucent meningocele. The inset picture was taken across the plane marked by the *white line*. The size of the lesion was 2.4 × 1.1 cm. **C, D.** Oblique and posterior views of the lesion. The patient refused further testing and requested termination of the pregnancy.

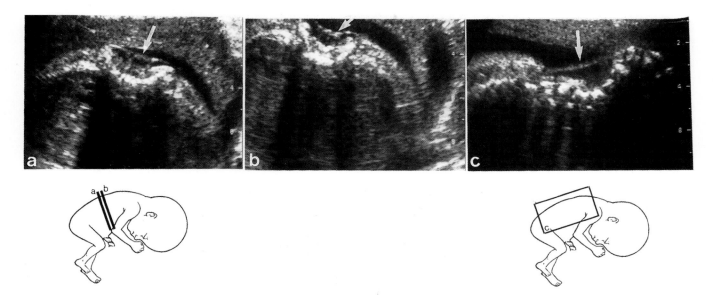

Figure 4–27. Transabdominal sonography shows a large lumbar sacral defect of a fetus at 28 postmenstrual weeks. **A, B.** Transverse sections through the spinal defect. Note that there is no skin covering the defect *(arrow)*. In addition, the vertebra has a "U" shape. **C.** Sagittal section showing the extent of the spinal leson. The skin contour is lost at the level of the defect *(arrow)* and the spine has an abnormal curvature (scoliosis).

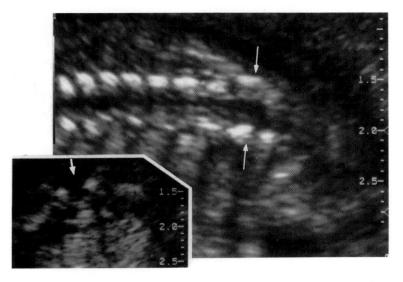

Figure 4–28. Spina bifida at 14 postmenstrual weeks and 3 days. Transvaginal sonography was used to image the spine of this fetus. This coronal section at the level of the defect *(arrows)* shows a divergent configuration of the spine. *Inset:* transverse section showing the typical "U" shape of the spine *(arrow)* in this case of open spina bifida.

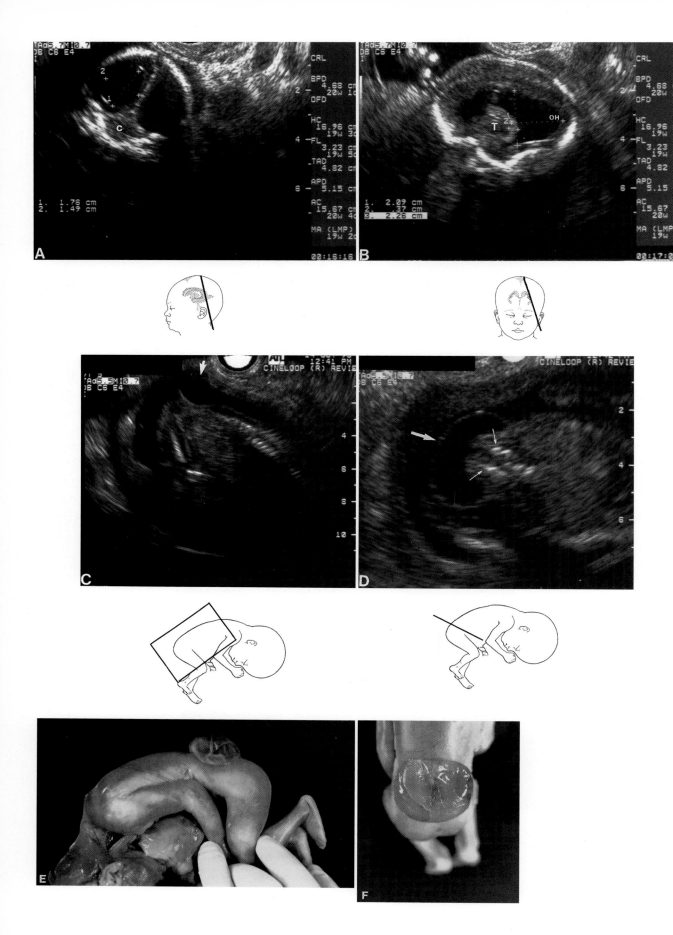

Figure 4–29. Arnold–Chiari type II malformation at 19 postmenstrual weeks. **A.** Occipital–1 section of the brain, demonstrating the dilatation of the posterior horns and the extremely thin cerebellum (C). **B.** Oblique–1 section showing the dilated ventricular system. Note the thin, hyperechoic choroid plexus above the thalamus (T). Note that the most dilated horn of the lateral ventricle is the posterior horn (OH). **C.** Median section of the vertebral column, showing the cystic appearance of the sacral meningocele *(white arrow)*. **D.** Transverse section of the lesion. The *white arrow* indicates the membranous coverage of the meningocele. Note the open vertebra *(small white arrow)*. **E.** View from the side of the aborted specimen. **F.** Dorsal view of the meningocele, through which the small opening of the spina bifida is apparent.

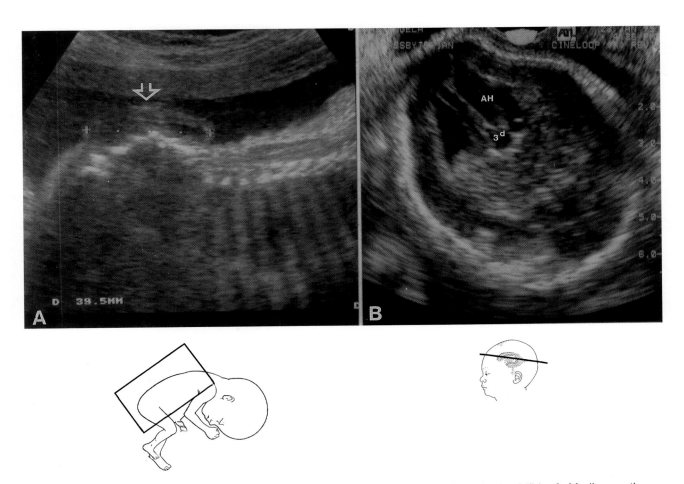

Figure 4–30. Arnold–Chiari type II malformation at 24 postmenstrual weeks. Sacral spina bifida. **A.** Median section of the lower spine, demonstrating the bulging membranes of the myelomeningocele, measuring 3.9 × 3.1 × 3.7 cm *(arrow)*. **B.** The "lemon sign" of the deformed bone at the temporal region is shown, as well as dilatation of the anterior horns (AH) and the third ventricle.

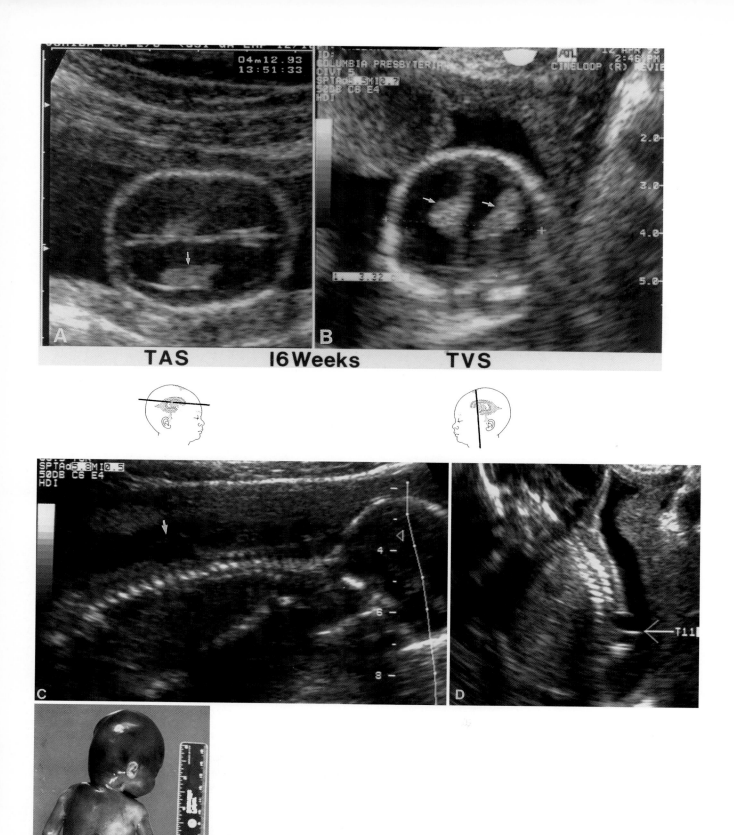

Figure 4–31. Arnold–Chiari type II malformation diagnosed at 16 postmenstrual weeks by both transabdominal and transvaginal sonography. Thoracic spina bifida. **A.** Horizontal transabdominal section of the brain, demonstrating the dilated lateral ventricles and the dangling choroid plexus *(arrow)*. **B.** Transvaginal scan in the Midcoronal–1 section, showing the dangling choroid plexus within the dilated ventricles *(arrow)*. **C.** Transabdominal scan with a 3.5-MHz probe, demonstrating the faint outlines of the myelomeningocele *(arrow)*. **D.** Transvaginal scan created with a 5-MHz probe, which easily images the lesion at the 11th thoracic vertebra *(arrow)*. **E.** The aborted fetus, with the lesion of the thoracic meningomyelocele and spina bifida.

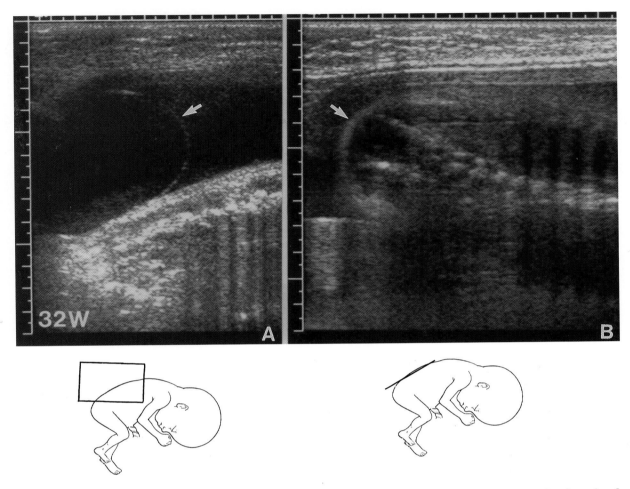

Figure 4–32. In a late registrant, a cystic spina bifida (meningocele) was detected at 32 postmenstrual weeks. **A.** Sagittal section of the meningocele *(arrow)*. **B.** Coronal section showing the spina bifida and the cystic meningocele *(arrow)*.

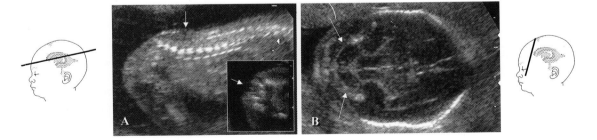

Figure 4–33. Open spina bifida at 17 postmenstrual weeks and 5 days. This patient presented with an elevated maternal serum alpha feto-protein. Transabdominal sonography showed a fetus with a lumbar sacral defect. **A.** Sagittal view of the fetal spine demonstrating the irregularity of the skin at the level of the spinal defect *(arrowhead). Inset:* transverse view of the spine demonstrating the open defect and the "U" shaped vertebrae. **B.** Axial view angled posteriorly to image the fetal cerebellum. Note that the cerebellum has a sickle or banana shape. In addition, the cisterna magna is not seen since the cerebellum has obliterated it as it herniates into the foramen magnum.

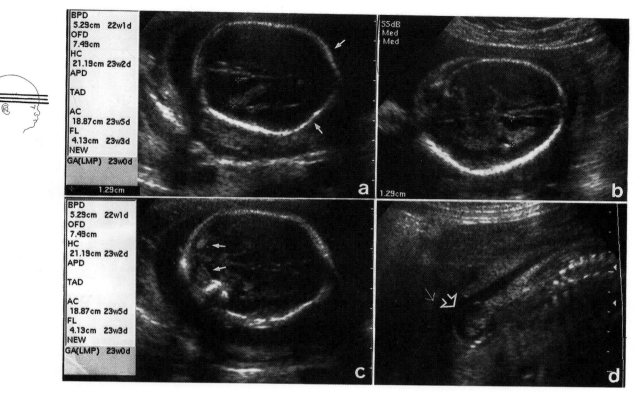

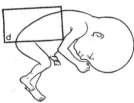

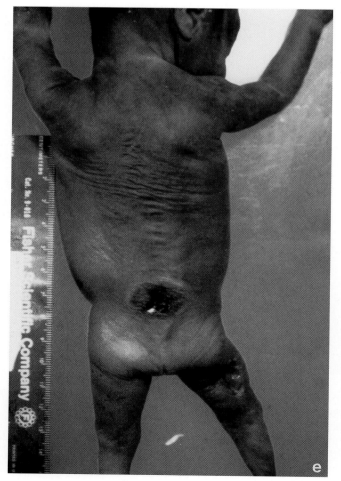

Figure 4–34. The work-up of a patient with an elevated maternal serum alpha feto-protein is shown. Biometry is consistent with 23 postmenstrual weeks. **A.** The fetal head shows a very subtle "lemon" sign *(arrows).* In addition, the lateral ventricles are dilated measuring 1.3 cm. **B.** Another view demonstrating the borderline dilation of the lateral ventricles. **C.** The posteriorly tilted axial view used to image the posterior fossa. The cerebellum *(arrows)* has the typical "banana" shape seen in cases of open spinal defects. Also, note that the cisterna magna is totally obliterated by the cerebellum. **D.** A sagittal section of the fetal spine showing a sacral meningocele *(arrowhead).* **E.** Pathology specimen demonstrating the defect that was imaged by ultrasound.

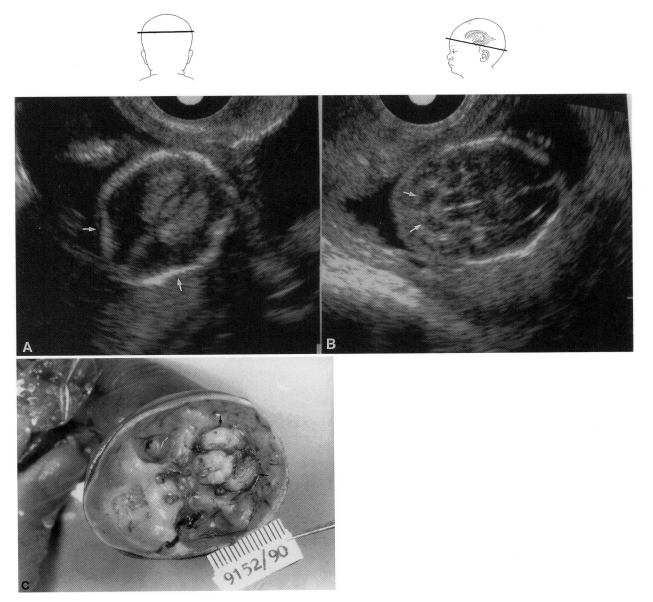

Figure 4–35. The "lemon" and "banana" signs at 15 postmenstrual weeks. **A.** Note the appearance of the frontal bones *(arrows)*. The typical lemon-shaped horizontal section of the skull is evident. **B.** The cerebellum *(arrows)* is impacted into the posterior fossa, which has obliterated the cisterna magna. **C.** The base of the skull in a specimen of comparable age. Note the impacted cerebellum *(arrows)*. The rest of the brain was removed. *(C is provided courtesy of M. Bronshtein, Al-Kol, Haifa, Israel.)*

the cerebellum initially appeared to be normal, but by 12 weeks there was a mild convexity of the cerebellum and by 14 weeks the typical "banana" and "lemon" signs were present. Although only a single report is currently available regarding the earliest appearance of these cranial findings, it seems that the "lemon" and "banana" signs may be imaged from 14 weeks on.

Therefore, from early in the second trimester these indirect cranial findings may be used to enhance the detection of open NTDs. Since these findings may be subtle at 14 to 15 weeks, a follow-up scan later in the second trimester may be indicated in cases at risk. The "lemon" sign is present in virtually all cases between 16 and 24 postmenstrual weeks, but after 24 weeks of gestation the "lemon" sign is a less reliable marker and is present in only 13% to 50% of the fetuses with spinal defects.[120–123] It is theorized that the loss of the "lemon" sign with advancing gestational age in fetuses with spina bifida is the result of maturation and strengthening of the fetal skull.[121,122] In contrast, cerebellar abnormalities with obliteration of the cisterna magna are present throughout gestation in 95% to 100% of the cases,[120,123–125] although after 24 weeks cerebellar absence is more commonly seen than the "banana" sign.[123] These indirect cranial findings in conjunction with a spinal defect are termed Arnold–Chiari type II malformation.

Arnold–Chiari type II malformation is present in almost every case of thoracolumbar (Figs. and 4–29 and 4–31), lumbar, and lumbosacral myelomeningocele (Figs. 4–27, 4–29, 4–30, and 4–32 through 4–34). The major features include (1) inferior displacement of the medulla and the fourth ventricle into the upper cervical canal, (2) elongation and thinning of the upper medulla and the lower pons and persistence of the embryonic flexures of these structures, (3) inferior displacement of the lower cerebellum through the foramen magnum (banana sign), and (4) a variety of bony defects of the foramen magnum, occiput, and upper cervical vertebrae.[10] Hydrocephaly probably results either from the hindbrain malformation that blocks the flow of CSF through the fourth ventricle or the posterior fossa or from aqueductal stenosis, which may be present in 40% to 75% of the cases.[10]

Associated brain abnormalities seen with myelomeningocele include hydrocephaly relative microcephaly, agenesis of the corpus callosum, and diastematomyelia. Other non-CNS anomalies include congenital scoliosis or kyphosis and hip deformities.[104,123]

Management of a pregnancy with myelomeningocele should include genetic counseling and karyotyping. Over the last few years there has been debate regarding the best method to deliver fetuses with spinal defects. Luthy and collaborators[126] published a retrospective review of 160 cases of myelomeningocele. The results showed that infants delivered by cesarean section before onset of labor had better motor function compared to infants delivered vaginally or by cesarean section after the onset of labor. In our institution, we electively perform cesarean section for all infants at 37 to 38 weeks' gestation after confirmation of lung maturity. This is especially important for those infants with hydrocephaly, because delaying the surgery may result in larger head size and worse neurological function as well as cosmetic results.

CONGENITAL HYDROCEPHALY

Hydrocephaly and *ventriculomegaly* are terms used almost interchangeably, and both refer to dilatation of the fetal lateral ventricles. *Hydrocephaly* is a dilatation of the lateral ventricles as a result of an increased amount of CSF, with an accompanying increase in intraventricular pressure and, subsequently, an increase in fetal head size. *Ventriculomegaly,* in contrast, refers to dilatation of the fetal lateral ventricles in the presence of normal fetal intraventricular pressures. The term *hydrocephalus* is incorrect, even though it is (mistakenly) used at times. The estimated incidence of hydrocephaly is 0.5 to 3 per 1000 live births. The incidence of isolated hydrocephaly is between 0.4 and 0.9 per 1000 live births.[113] Most cases of ventriculomegaly or hydrocephaly are bilateral, but unilateral hydrocephaly can, rarely, affect the fetus. Unilateral hydrocephaly usually occurs from obstruction of one of the interventricular foramina (of Monro) (Fig. 4–36).[114,115] Clinically, fetuses with hydrocephaly may present during a routine scan with dilated lateral ventricles or a size–dates discrepancy due to an increase in head circumference and/or BPD compared to their dates. The greater the discrepancy, the worse is the degree of hydrocephaly present.

The causes of hydrocephaly in the fetus are similar to those in the neonate. Hydrocephaly may be *noncommunicating* or *communicating* (Table 4–8). In noncommunicating hydrocephaly there is obstruction to the flow of CSF occurring within the intraventricular system, and the CSF cannot freely flow to the subarachnoid space. In communicating hydrocephaly the obstruction to the flow of CSF is extraventricular at the level of the subarachnoid space, i.e., the CSF can flow freely from the ventricles to the subarachnoid space. The CSF is produced by the choroid plexus, and its flow is unidirectional (see Chapter 2). In the neonate it is estimated that the choroid plexus produces approximately 650 mL of CSF per day.[131] The CSF circulates from the lateral ventricles to the third ventricle through the cerebral aqueduct (Sylvius), to the fourth ventricle, and finally through the median aperture (Magendie) or the lateral apertures (Luschka) into the basal cisterns, reaching the subarachnoid space, where it is absorbed by the arachnoid granulations (see Chapter 2).

Of the causes of hydrocephaly listed in Table 4–8, the most common are aqueductal stenosis, which accounts for approximately 33% to 43% of all cases; myelomeningocele with Arnold–Chiari mal-

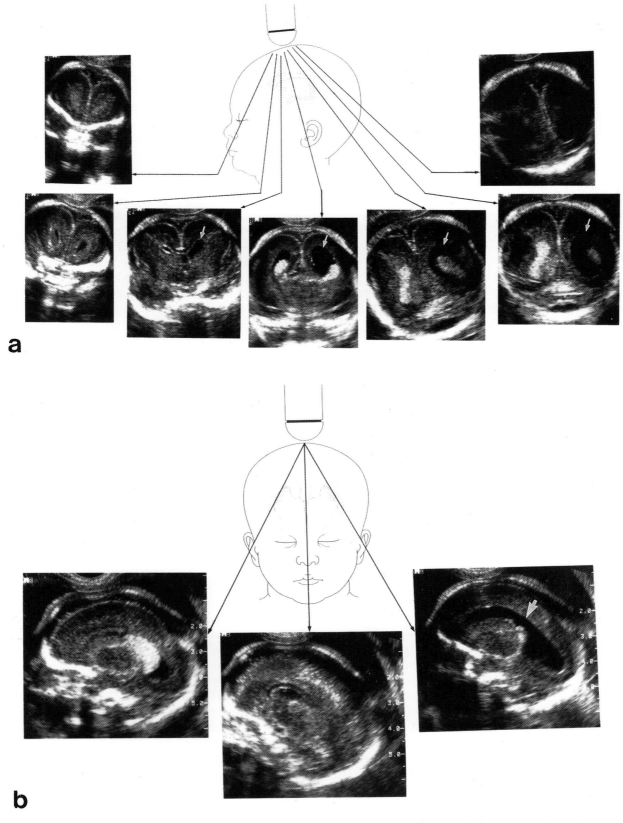

Figure 4–36. Unilateral ventriculomegaly is seen at 23 postmenstrual weeks. **A.** Serial coronal sections from anterior to posterior showing that the ventriculomegaly is confined to the left ventricle *(arrows)*. **B.** Median and right and left Oblique–1 sections demonstrating the normal right lateral ventricle and the dilated left ventricle *(arrow)*. This patient delivered at term a normal neonate.

TABLE 4–8. CONGENITAL HYDROCEPHALY

Noncommunicating hydrocephaly (intraventricular obstructive hydrocephaly)
  - Aqueductal stenosis
  - Dandy–Walker malformation
  - Masses

Communicating hydrocephaly (extraventricular obstructive hydrocephaly)
  - Arnold–Chiari malformation
  - Encephalocele
  - Leptomeningeal inflammation
  - Lissencephaly
  - Congenital absence of arachnoid granulations

Adapted from Milhorat, 1987,[136] with permission.

formation, which accounts for 28% (discussed previously); communicating hydrocephaly, with 22% to 38%; Dandy–Walker malformation, at 7% to 13% (see Chapter 6); and others, accounting for 6% to 10%. Other causes include agenesis of the corpus callosum (see Chapter 6), arachnoid cysts, and aneurysm of the vein of Galen.[10,132–134]

In aqueductal stenosis there is an obstruction to the flow of the CSF leaving the fourth ventricle. Aqueductal stenosis probably develops around 15 to 17 postmenstrual weeks of gestation, during the period of rapid elongation of the mesencephalon and evolution of the constriction of the aqueduct.[135] In approximately 70% of these cases, a lesion obstructing the flow through the cerebral aqueduct can be demonstrated. About 1% to 2% of all cases of aqueductal stenosis may be inherited as an X-linked disorder affecting males and transmitted through female carriers.[136,137] In addition, an autosomal recessive pattern of inheritance for aqueductal stenosis has also been described in families in which both males and females are affected.[136] The prenatal diagnosis of X-linked hydrocephaly has been made based on the presence of ventriculomegaly (lateral and third ventricles) in male fetuses and adducted thumb in a woman with a family history of two brothers with hydrocephaly. Adducted thumb(s) have been found in 44% of cases of X-linked hydrocephaly.[138] Early prenatal diagnosis of aqueductal stenosis may not be possible, because ventriculomegaly or hydrocephaly becomes evident later in pregnancy or in early infancy. Friedman and Santos-Ramos[135] described two cases of X-linked aqueductal stenosis in which the prenatal sonogram at 17 to 18 postmenstrual weeks was normal. In this case report ventriculomegaly became evident at 22 weeks and the increase in BPD was seen by 30 postmenstrual

weeks. X-linked hydrocephaly is severe, with a high rate of stillbirths and perinatal mortality, and survivors show significant neurological impairment.[139]

In one of our cases of X-linked hydrocephaly, the first scan at 21 postmenstrual weeks revealed severe hydrocephaly in a male fetus. The fourth ventricle was normal in size. The patient elected to terminate the pregnancy and pathology confirmed the diagnosis of hydrocephaly most likely as a result of aqueductal stenosis (Fig. 4–37 through 4–39). Subsequently, the patient became pregnant with a second male fetus. This fetus also had severe hydrocephaly diagnosed in utero at 22 postmenstrual weeks. The patient continued the pregnancy and delivered a live male infant at 36 weeks of gestation by cesarean section due to macrocephaly. The neonate shortly after birth required a ventriculoperitoneal shunt and was neurologically impaired.

In spite of our increasing understanding and advances in ultrasonography, the early diagnosis of in utero ventriculomegaly or hydrocephaly remains a diagnostic challenge. The reason for this is that in many cases hydrocephaly or ventriculomegaly does not become apparent until 16 to 18 postmenstrual weeks or later (Fig. 4–40). Early in the second trimester the size of the lateral ventricles in relation to the brain parenchyma is quite high, but as the fetus approaches term this ratio diminishes. At term the normal fetal lateral ventricle appears slitlike, while at 20 postmenstrual weeks of gestation its appearance is more "plump" but still within the normal limits for this age. Therefore, when assessing whether ventriculomegaly or hydrocephaly is present, fetal age must be taken into consideration.

Using sonography, the fetal lateral ventricles can be assessed in a *quantitative* as well as *qualitative* way (Figs. 4–37 through 4–45). Chapter 3 describes several measurements and includes widely accepted nomograms used to assess ventriculomegaly or hydrocephaly.[140–146] All of the commonly used nomograms of the fetal lateral ventricles were generated using measurements obtained transabdominally in the axial plane. The increasing acceptability and availability of TVS have allowed transfontanelle scanning of the fetal brain (see Chapter 2). Using TVS, the fetal brain can be assessed in a manner similar to that used for the preterm or term neonate. In this section, the qualitative and quantitative methods that can be used to assess the fetal brain when scanning transvaginally are described.[141,142,147–152]

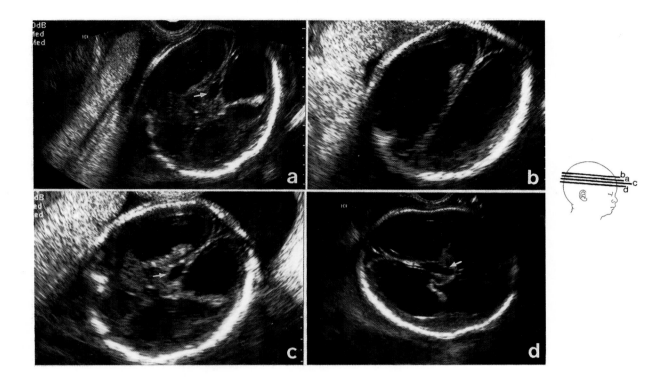

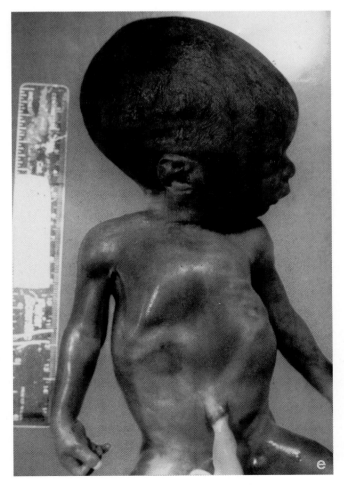

Figure 4–37. Sonographic work-up of a pregnancy at 21 post-menstrual weeks. **A–D** is a series of axial sections of the fetal head. **A, C.** There is bilateral hydrocephaly with a dangling choroid plexus. The third ventricle appears prominent *(arrow).* **B, D.** The lateral ventricles are dilated measuring 18 mm (the upper limit of normal is 10 cm). **E.** The pathological specimen demonstrates the large fetal head out of proportion to the body. Pathology confirmed the in utero diagnosis due to aqueductal stenosis.

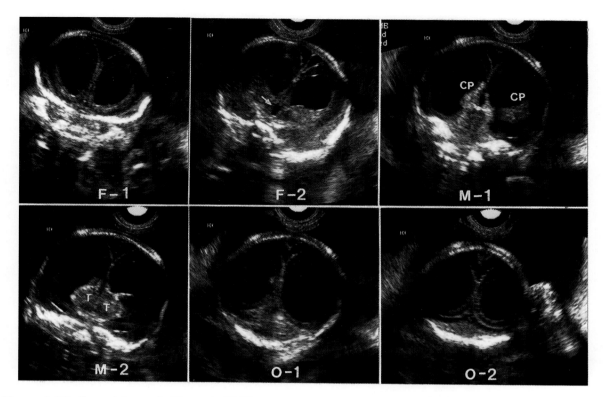

Figure 4–38. Same fetus as in Figure 4–37. These are a series of coronal sections from anterior to posterior. F–1: Frontal–1: showing the prominent anterior horns of the lateral ventricles. F–2: Frontal–2: The prominent ventricles have a tear-shape. The third ventricle is seen *(arrow)*. M–1: Midcoronal–1 showing the dysmorphic choroid plexus (CP) "dangling" in the large ventricular cavity. M–2: Mid-coronal–2; The dilated ventricles are seen as well as the third ventricle. O–1: Occipital–1: the occipital horns of the lateral ventricles are seen as large rounded sonolucent structures. O–2: Occipital–2: The most posterior coronal section depicting the dilated occiptal horns the lateral ventricles. Thalamus, T, third ventricle arrow.

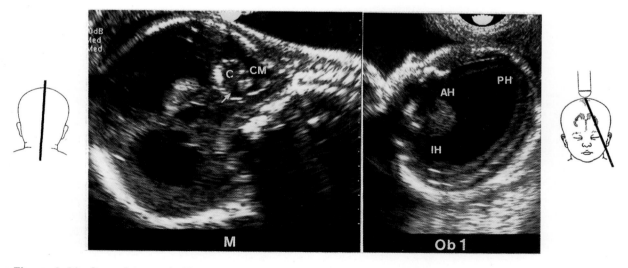

Figure 4–39. Same fetus as in Figure 4–37. These are sagittal images. M: Median section showing parts of the dilated ventricles, cisterna magna, cerebellum, (C) and fourth ventricle *(arrow)*. Ob–1: Oblique–1 is lateral to the previous section showing the anterior (AH), posterior (PH), and inferior horns (IH)) of the dilated lateral ventricle.

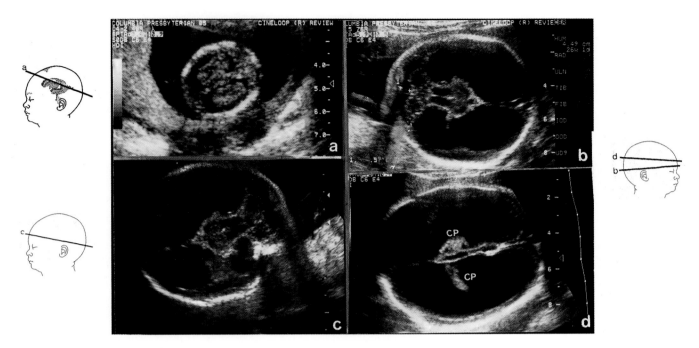

Figure 4–40. Transvaginal brain scan. **A.** The fetus at 15 postmenstrual weeks shows a normal appearing brain with the choroid plexus (CP) filling most of the lateral ventricle. **B–D.** The same fetus at 26 postmenstrual week, 1 day, demonstrating severe hydrocephaly. The BPD (not shown) is consistent with 29 postmenstrual weeks. **B, C.** The large lateral ventricles occupy most of the brain, only a thin rim of brain tissue is seen surrounding the large ventricles. The posterior fossa shows a relatively normal cerebellum, and cisterna magna, which measures 0.57 mm (normal). **D.** The large ventricles are seen to contain the thin and dysmorphic choroid plexus. The ventricles measured 26-mm; upper limit of normal is 10 mm.

Qualitative Methods to Assess the Lateral Ventricles

Qualitative methods for assessing the lateral ventricles include the following.

1. *The gestalt approach:* In this approach an experienced sonographer and/or sonologist can decide by looking only at the brain whether or not the ventricles are dilated.

2. *Looking for the suggestive changes in the shape of the lateral ventricles:* In the presence of dilated lateral ventricles, the anterior horns will already be imaged in the Frontal–1 section. Normally, in this section only the brain parenchyma is present (see Chapter 2). In the midcoronal sections there may be progressive rounding and bulging of the superior and lateral aspects of the frontal horns, with the inferior aspect resembling an inverted "teardrop," the rounded segment on top and the tapered end pointing toward the third ventricle (Fig. 4–38F-2).

On the right and left Oblique–1 planes all three components of the lateral ventricle (anterior, posterior, and inferior horns) can be imaged in the same plane (Figs. 4–39 Ob-1 and 4–42B, D). In the absence of ventriculomegaly or hydrocephaly, only the anterior and posterior horns should be imaged using the Oblique–1 plane.

3. *Using the shape of the choroid plexus:* In cases of ventriculomegaly or hydrocephaly, the choroid plexus thins, probably due to the increase in CSF pressure (Figs. 4–37, 4–40D, 4–41, and 4–42B, D). During real-time scanning the choroid plexus may be seen dangling or floating freely within the dilated ventricle.

4. *The obvious detection and the ability to measure the third ventricle:* The normal third ventricle is rarely imaged during scanning due to its narrowness (Figs. 4–37A,C; 4–38 M-2; 4–41D; and 4–43C).

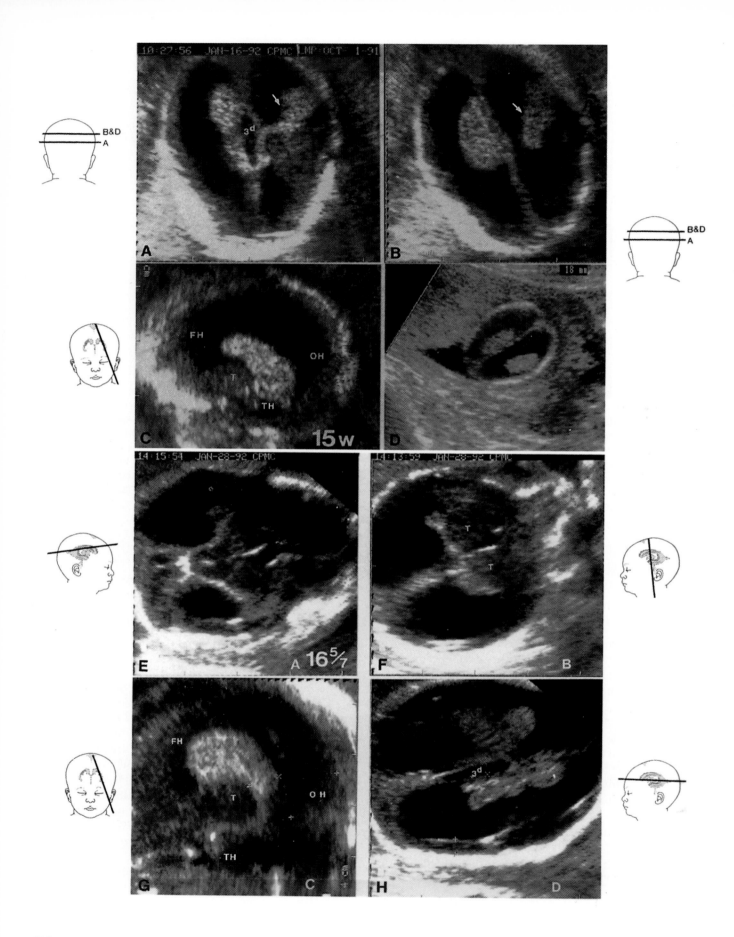

Figure 4–41. The evolution of obstructive hydrocephaly from 15 to almost 17 postmenstrual weeks. **A–D.** Scans at 15 postmenstrual weeks. **A.** Horizontal section showing the "dangling choroid plexus" *(arrow),* the dilated lateral ventricles, and the dilated third ventricle. **B.** Slightly higher horizontal section showing the dilated lateral ventricles and the dangling choroid plexus *(arrow).* **C.** Oblique–1 section through the lateral ventricle. The choroid plexus is not yet thin (a typical feature of advanced intracranial pressure). The anterior horn (FH), posterior horn (OH), and inferior horn (TH) are all seen on this section and seem to be dilated. **D.** Transabdominal ultrasonographic image, shown for comparison. **E–H.** Follow-up scans at almost 17 postmenstrual weeks. **E.** Horizontal section showing progress in the ventriculomegaly. **F.** Midcoronal–2 section demonstrating the dilated ventricles as well as the third ventricle (3d). T, Thalamus. **G.** Oblique–1 section similar to that seen in **C,** showing the progress in dilatation. T, Thalamus; FH, anterior horn; OH, posterior horn; TH, inferior horn. **H.** Horizontal section similar to that seen in **A,** showing the progress in dilatation. 3d, Third ventricle. The patient selected to terminate this pregnancy. The pathological examination confirmed the diagnosis.

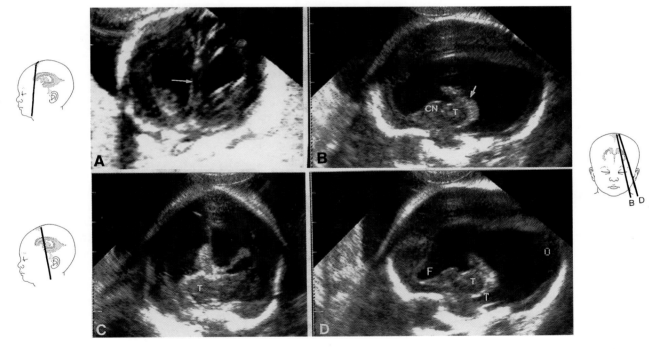

Figure 4–42. Typical sonographic images of hydrocephaly at 22 postmenstrual weeks. **A.** Frontal–2 section showing the dilated anterior horns and the cavum septi pellucidi *(small arrow).* **B.** Oblique–1 section showing the dangling choroid plexus *(arrow)* and, above, the caudate nucleus (CN) and the thalami (T). **C, D.** Oblique–1 sections demonstrating the dilated frontal anterior, posterior, and inferior horns (F, O, and T, respectively).

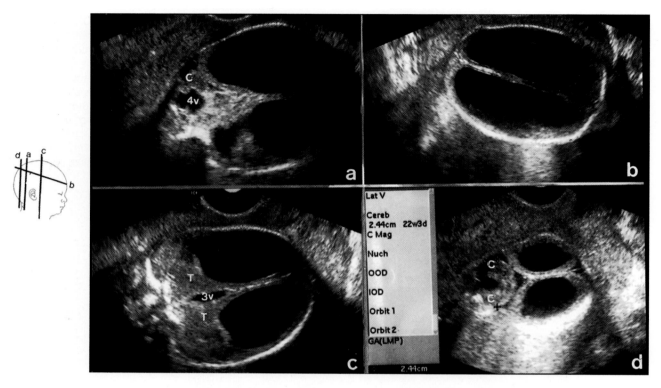

Figure 4–43. Severe hydrocephaly at 22 postmenstrual weeks, 3 days. **A.** The transvaginal brain scan revealed severe hydrocephaly and in addition the fourth ventricle (4V) was dilated and the cerebellar (C) bodies splayed apart (Dandy–Walker variant). **B.** An axial section showing severe hydrocephaly and no normal brain tissue. **C.** Midcoronal–2 section showing the large dilated ventricles. The dilated third ventricle (3V) is seen between the thalami (T). **D.** Is an Occipital–1 section showing the large and round posterior horns of the lateral ventricles. In addition, in the posterior fossa the cerebellar (C) bodies are splayed apart, although the pathology is not as evident as in **A.**

Quantitative Method to Assess the Lateral Ventricles

Obviously, the only objective and comparable method of detecting ventriculomegaly is to measure the size of the lateral ventricles using different scanning planes. This can be done using widely accepted nomograms generated transabdominally (a normal ventricular atrial measurement is ≤10 mm) or by recently developed and published nomograms of the fetal lateral ventricles obtained with TVS (see Chapter 3).[153,154] Nine nomograms were developed using 347 fetuses between 14 and 40 postmenstrual weeks. A total of seven measurements of the fetal lateral ventricles were used to generate the nomograms. In addition, two ratios were calculated using three of the seven measurements (see Table 3–1). The main difference between the transvaginal nomograms and those previously published in the literature is that in the former all of our measurements were obtained transvaginally using coronal and sagittal sections. Serial follow-up of 36 patients carrying fetuses with hydrocephaly was conducted.

As expected, nearly all parts of the lateral ventricles increased with progressing ventriculomegaly or hydrocephaly. The only exception was the thickness of the choroid plexus, which decreased as ventriculomegaly progressed.[153,154]

The earliest changes occurring in the size of the lateral ventricle during the development of ventriculomegaly or hydrocephaly are the following. (1) *Dilatation of the posterior horn* of the lateral ventricle occurs first, and the anterior horns are the last to increase in size.[149,155] This dilatation occurs in the direction of least resistance to increasing CSF pressures. In the posterior horn the increase in size can be detected in the up-and-down direction (on the Occipital–1 and Oblique–1 sections), in other words, toward the crown or base of the skull.[75,146,148,149] (2) There is *compression* or *thinning of the choroid plexus* as a result of increasing CSF pressure.[142,156–158] The normal choroid plexus usually fills the antrum of the lateral ventricle completely. Its normal appearance is fluffy, similar to that of cotton. In cases of ventriculomegaly, the choroid plexus

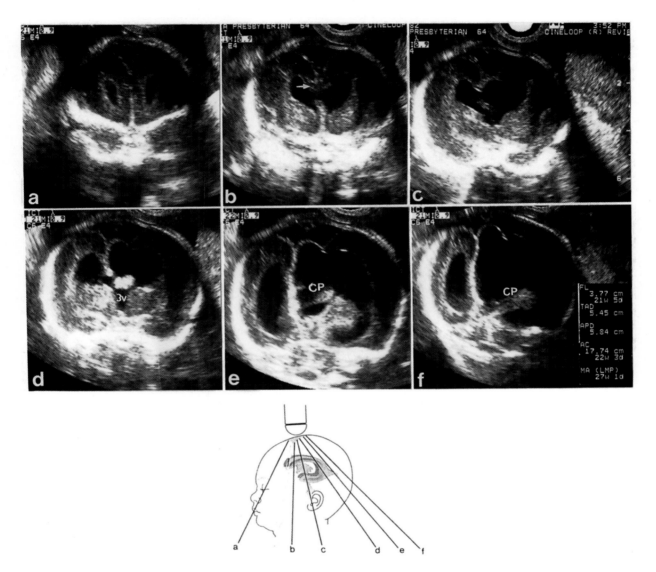

Figure 4–44. A transvaginal fetal neuroscan of a fetus showing size/dates discrepancy. By the last menstrual period this fetus was 27 postmenstrual weeks and 1 day, however, the femur length and abdominal circumference were consistent with 22 postmenstrual weeks. The BPD and HC could not be used to determine age due to the hydrocephaly. **A–F** are serial coronal sections. **A.** Frontal–1 section showing dilatation of the anterior horns of the lateral ventricle. **B.** Midcoronal–1 section showing the dilatation of the lateral ventricle as well as the genu of the corpus callosum *(arrow).* **C.** Midcoronal–2 showing a greater degree of dilatation of the lateral ventricle in the left side of the brain. **D.** Midcoronal–3, in this view the asymmetry between the two sides of the ventricular system is obvious. In addition, the third ventricle (3V) is dilated and the corpus callosum is no longer evident. **E.** Occipital–1 and **F.** Occipital–2 show the discrepancy between the right and the left ventricle. The choroid plexus (CP) is dysmorphic and under real-time sonography could be seen dangling freely in the large ventricular cavity.

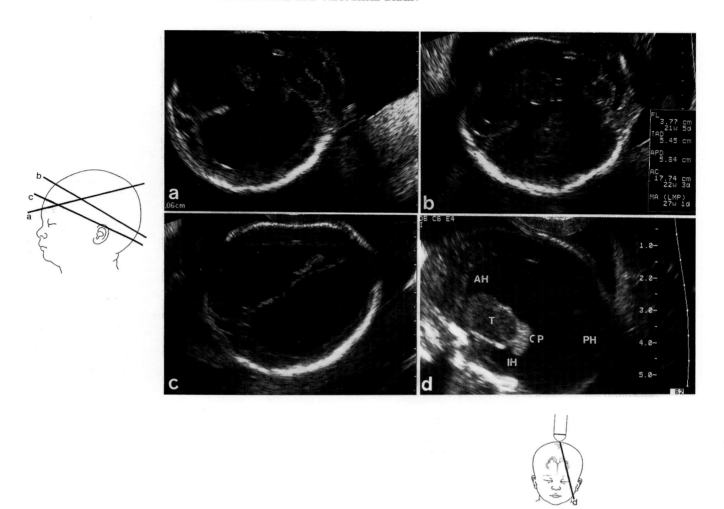

Figure 4–45. This is the same fetus as in figure 4–44. **A** and **B** are almost tilted posterior axial sections showing the discrepancy between the two ventricles. In addition, the cerebellum and the cisterna magna are clearly seen and appear normal. In **B**, the lateral ventricle seems to connect freely with the third ventricle. In this fetus only the genu of the corpus callosum was seen (Fig. 4–44B). This may be due to either partial agenesis of the corpus callosum or the increase intracranial pressure distorting the corpus callosum. **C.** Axial section showing the large ventricle. Note that both sides can be clearly seen and compared to each other, when scanning transabdominally, the near hemisphere is often obscured by artifact. **D.** Oblique–1 section showing the three horns of the lateral ventricle. The choroid plexus is thin and appears to be compressed against the thalamus. AH, anterior horn; PH, posterior horn; IH, inferior horn; T, thalamus; CP, choroid plexus.

is compressed and floats within the dilated ventricle (the dangling choroid plexus sign)[152] and in addition it is pulled by gravity toward the dependent part of the fetal head.

When scanning a fetus with suspected ventriculomegaly using TVS, the most practical and efficient section to obtain is a right or left paramedian section (right or left Oblique–1). In this section one can make qualitative observations of the lateral ventricle and the choroid plexus as well as perform measurements and plot the values on the described nomograms. Limiting the scan to only one view has

disadvantages, however. The main disadvantage is that TVS is not used to its full potential due to the significant number of intracranial and extracranial anomalies associated with hydrocephalus. In Chapter 9 the use of three-dimensional sonography of the fetal brain is discussed. In essence by obtaining a volume of the fetal brain transvaginally (or transabdominally) multiplanar imaging of the brain is possible. In addition, the volume can be saved and reviewed as many times as desired and if a section was not previously seen it is possible to obtain this new section even after the patient has left the office.

Prenatal diagnosis of hydrocephaly should trigger a careful search for associated anomalies. The prognosis for the fetus or neonate with hydrocephaly is closely related to the presence or absence of possible associated anomalies. Associated anomalies have been found in approximately 70% to 83% of cases presenting with fetal hydrocephaly.[159-163] Approximately 40% of these anomalies are intracranial (e.g., microcephaly or encephalocele) and 60% are extracranial (e.g., myelomeningocele or cardiac or renal anomalies).[159,164] Cardiac anomalies have been reported in approximately 20% of fetuses.[159,161] In the presence of anomalies, the prognosis for the fetus or neonate is poor, and developmental delay varying from mild to severe can be expected.[159] The mortality rate ranges from 60% to 74%, with an approximate survival rate of only 30%.[160-162,165-167] In addition, a relatively high percentage of chromosomal abnormalities (e.g., trisomies 13 and 18) have been reported in cases of fetal hydrocephaly ranging from as low as 4.2% to as high as 28.6%.[160,161,163,164]

Isolated ventriculomegaly has been reported to occur in 17% to 46% of fetuses with in utero hydrocephaly.[59,163,164] Gupta and colleagues[168] recently completed a detailed review of the English literature on cases of antenatally detected fetal ventriculomegaly. They found 21 reports with a total of 360 cases of apparently isolated fetal ventriculomegaly. Of these, 81 had additional anomalies at birth, of which 19 (23.5%) survived. Only 3 (15%) of the survivors were normal; the rest had mild to severe developmental delay. Of the 279 cases with isolated ventriculomegaly, 175 (63%) survived and postnatal evaluation was available. One hundred eleven (63%) were normal, the remainder having mild to severe mental and motor developmental delay. In the group with isolated ventriculomegaly, 9 (5%) had progressive ventriculomegaly; of these, 6 (67%) had a normal outcome.

Recently, increasing concern over the significance of mild or borderline cases of fetal ventriculomegaly has emerged.[169-177] Mild fetal lateral ventriculomegaly is defined as a width of the atrium of the lateral ventricle measuring between 10 to 15 mm, in an axial section of the brain, in the absence of other sonographically demonstrable malformations (Table 4-9).[173-177] However, in this group of fetuses, the incidence of other anomalies is lower than in the group of fetuses with obvious ventriculomegaly or hydrocephaly; thus, a search for subtle anomalies is warranted. Another important issue in this group of fetuses is that of the association with chromosomal abnormalities, especially trisomy 21. The calculated risk for trisomy 21 has been estimated at 3%.[172] Vergani and colleagues[177] recently

TABLE 4-9. DEFINITIONS OF MILD FETAL LATERAL VENTRICULOMEGALY (MFLVM)

Author	Year	Definition
Mahoney	1988 (169)	3 to 8 mm between CP and LV wall
Hudgins	1988 (162)	various degrees (+1 to +4) of above
Drugan	1989 (159)	LV/H ratio of ≤ 0.55
Goldstein	1990 (170)	10–15 mm
Bromley	1991 (171)	10–12 mm
Achiron	1993 (172)	10–15 mm
Patel	1994 (175)	10–15 mm

Concensus: MFLVM = 10 to 15 mm

published a paper dealing exclusively with mild fetal ventriculomegaly. They described 82 fetuses with mild fetal ventriculomegaly (lateral ventricle measuring between 10 to 15 mm). In 48 fetuses, this was an isolated finding and in 34, the finding was associated with other ultrasonographic findings or anomalies. Their results showed that of the 45 surviving euploid fetuses with isolated mild ventriculomegaly, neurologic follow-up was normal at a mean of 28 months. Male fetuses and those with a transverse atrial size, 12 mm had a good prognosis. *Ventricular atria ≥ 12 mm were more often associated with other anomalies and, when isolated, with abnormal postnatal neurodevelopment.* Aneuploidy (trisomy 21) was present in 2 cases of isolated mild ventricular dilatation; both of the cases were associated with advanced maternal age, and in seven cases associated with other anomalies. The authors concluded that mild fetal ventriculomegaly should trigger a targeted ultrasound examination, to look for markers of aneuploidy and other congenital anomalies (associated anomalies were present in 41% of the cases). In addition, imaging of the corpus callosum, fetal echocardiogram and serologic evaluation for congenital infections should be part of the work-up for these fetuses.

Subsequently, Pilu and colleagues[174] reported on 31 fetuses with isolated cerebral borderline ventriculomegaly and reviewed the literature. Of the 31 fetuses, two had chromosomal aneuploidy (trisomy 21 and 13) and three neurological complications (one infant developed shunt-dependent hydrocephaly, one lissencephaly, and one cerebral hemorrhage and periventricular leukomalacia). The review of the literature (including the 31 cases) revealed 234 cases. Abnormal outcome was documented in 22.8%; and perinatal death in 3.7%; chromosomal aberrations in 3.8% (mostly trisomy 21). In 8.6%, there were malformations undetected during the second-trimester sonogram and in 11.5%, there were neurological sequelae (mostly mild to moderate delay in cognitive and/or motor development). The risk of an abnormal neurological outcome was increased in females versus males, where the atrial width was ≥ 12 mm, and when the diagnosis was made in the second trimester versus later in gestation. Based on these cases and the literature review, Pilu and coworkers concluded that in most cases isolated borderline cerebral lateral ventriculomegaly has no consequence. However, this finding carries an increased risk of cerebral maldevelopment, delayed neurological development, and possibly, chromosomal aberrations. In addition, "normalization" of the lateral ventricular size has been reported. However, in view of the limited number of cases, it is hard to assess the percentage of fetuses with mild ventriculomegaly that have resolution of their lesion in utero.[171,172]

Polyhydramnios is present in approximately 30% of the cases of in utero hydrocephaly[178] and oligohydramnios may be present in 21% to 23% of such cases.[159,160] This high incidence of oligohydramnios is important because decreased amniotic fluid may impair or reduce the diagnostic quality of the transabdominal scan. In these cases TVS may provide additional information. Another option in cases of oligohydramnios is to perform an amnioinfusion and then proceed with the targeted scan.

The differential diagnosis of hydrocephaly is hydranencephaly or holoprosencephaly. The latter is discussed in Chapter 5.

Management of fetal hydrocephaly should include a careful targeted scan to look for associated anomalies both CNS and non-CNS, fetal echocardiogram, genetic counseling, and testing (for karyotype and fetal sex). In addition, other causes, such as infections (cytomegalovirus [CMV] and toxoplasmosis), must be ruled out.

Treatment of the fetus with hydrocephaly must wait until after delivery, when a shunt can be placed. The most common type of shunt is ventriculoperitoneal. In utero shunting procedures have been abandoned because no improvement over the expected natural history was shown. Between 1982 and 1985, 41 fetuses with isolated hydrocephaly were treated in utero.[179] Of these, 34 survived and 22 (65%) had varying degrees of neurological and physical handicaps. In utero shunting improved survival but not outcome. In addition, 22% had undetected associated malformations. Currently, a second look at this intrauterine procedure is taking place. Fetuses without other anomalies are considered for this therapy.

In conclusion, the most important prognostic factor for fetuses with in utero hydrocephaly is the presence or absence of associated anomalies.

CHOROID PLEXUS CYSTS

Choroid plexus cysts (CPCs) are fluid-filled cystic spaces present within the choroid plexus. These are a common finding during the second trimester, with a reported incidence of sonographically detected cysts of 0.95%, with a range of 0.18% to 3.6% of all fetuses scanned.[180–188] Choroid plexus cysts are usually asymptomatic and benign. They commonly resolve by the midtrimester (23 to 24 weeks) and have been associated with both a normal and an abnormal fetal karyotype.[189–194]

The choroid plexus is responsible for the production of CSF. The CPCs are thought to result from filling of the neuroepithelial folds with CSF. At 6 to 7 postmenstrual weeks the choroid plexus starts developing in the roof of the fourth ventricle, then in the lateral ventricle, and finally in the third ventricle, as fingerlike projections of neuroepithelium into the ventricles, creating choroidal villi. The choroid plexus grows rapidly, and by 9 postmenstrual weeks it fills 75% of the cavity of the lateral ventricle. Portions of the epithelium are pinched off and become either tubules or neuroepithelium-lined cysts within the choroidal matrix. By the 20th week the choroid plexus has achieved its adult appearance.[185,187]

The sonographic appearance of a CPC is that of a sonolucent structure within the hyperechogenic choroid plexus. The CPCs are usually small, measuring less than 10 mm, with a range of 3 to 20 mm. Their borders are well delineated and are located within the choroid plexus; they may be unilateral or bilateral and may contain debris or other small cystlike structures (Figs. 4–46 through 4–48).[186,187,189–191,195,196] Usually, CPCs are an isolated finding, but once a CPC is imaged, a targeted scan should be performed to look for other malformations. Malformations associated with CPCs include bowel containing omphalocele, congenital heart disease (e.g., ventricular septal defect or hypoplastic left heart), renal abnormalities (e.g., hydronephrosis or multicystic kidneys), nuchal thickening, cystic hygroma, cleft palate, micrognathia and hydrocephaly.[180,188,197] Most of these malformations are also associated with trisomies 18 and 21. In addition, CPCs have been reported in association with cri du chat (5p−) syndrome and mosaic trisomy 9.[188,198]

What is the best way to manage a pregnancy after a CPC has been diagnosed? In the literature there is a wide range of opinions regarding the need

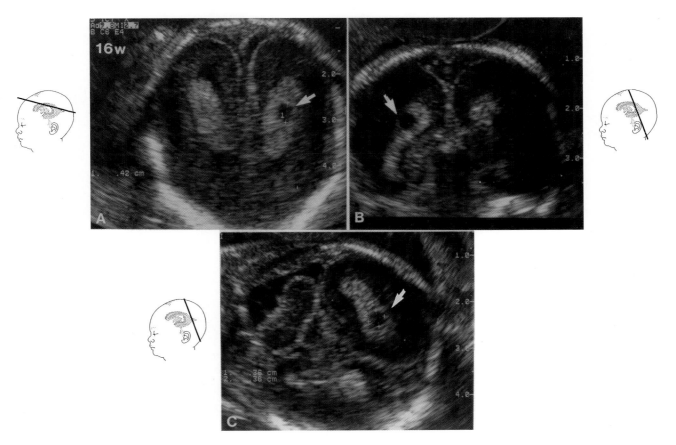

Figure 4–46. Routine structural evaluation at 16 postmenstrual weeks, revealing a unilateral choroid plexus cyst measuring 0.4 × 0.36 × 0.36 cm. The *white arrows* indicates the small choroid plexus cyst. **A.** Horizontal section. **B.** Midcoronal–3 section. **C.** Occipital–1 section.

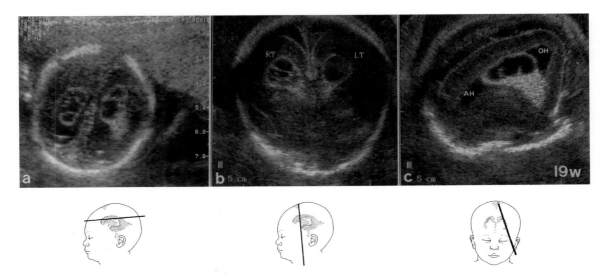

Figure 4–47. Three views of bilateral and septated choroid plexus cysts at 19 postmenstrual weeks. **A.** Horizontal section. **B.** Midcoronal–1 section. **C.** Oblique–1 section showing the normal anterior horn (AH) in the posterior horn (OH). The neonate was normal.

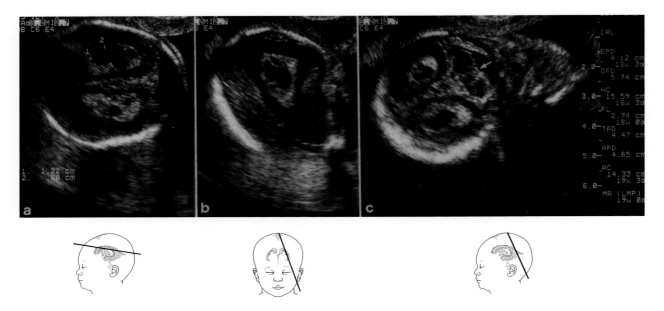

Figure 4–48. Three views of bilateral choroid plexus cysts at 19 postmenstrual weeks. **A.** Horizontal section, with the largest cyst measuring 1.2 × 2.6 cm. **B.** Occipital–2 section. **C.** Occipital–1 section depicting both posterior horns and the cerebellum with the normal vermis *(white arrow).* At 24 postmenstrual weeks, the choroid plexus on the left side was no longer apparent and all the lateral ventricle measurements were within normal limits. At 29 postmenstrual weeks, the left choroid plexus cyst disappeared. A repeat scan at 33 postmenstrual weeks showed normal brain anatomy. The neonate was normal.

for a fetal karyotype in the presence of CPC. In the presence of CPC and other malformations, there is general consensus that genetic counseling and testing are indicated, but there is disagreement regarding the need for fetal karyotyping in cases in which the CPC is an isolated finding. Some authors recommend that all patients should be offered genetic testing because the experience, equipment, or ability of all sonographers or sonologists may not be equal and some less experienced operators may miss an associated malformation.[181,182,187,191,194,197,199–201] Other authors believe that only in the presence of an associated congenital anomaly is genetic testing justified.[180,188,189] Kupferminc and coworkers[197] reported the risk of chromosomal abnormality in cases of isolated CPC to be 1 in 25. In their series among 98 cases of isolated CPC, four abnormal karyotypes were found among 75 women who elected to have amniocentesis. Of the four abnormal karyotypes, three were Down syndrome (trisomy 21) and one was trisomy 18. Gross and colleagues[188] subsequently reported on the risk of trisomy 18 in cases of isolated CPC. Using a meta-analysis and their own cases, they were able to calculate the risk of trisomy 18 in cases of isolated choroid plexus to be 1 in 374.

Five large series were identified from the literature dealing with the issue of the isolated choroid plexus cyst.[202–206] In Table 4–10, these five series are

summarized. A total of 55, 218 patients were screened and 764 choroid plexus cysts identified. The incidence of choroid plexus cyst(s) is 1.4% (range of 0.6% to 2.8%) and in 674 (88%) patients with choroid plexus cyst this was the only sonographic finding. Among the cases with isolated CPC and chromosomal aneuploidy all of these patients had additional high risk factors such as advance maternal age or abnormal maternal serum screening.

Snijders and coworkers[207] published on the association between fetal choroid plexus cysts (CPCs) and trisomy 18. In the 387 fetuses with CPCs, the incidence of trisomy 18 increased with maternal age. They concluded that if the cysts are apparently isolated, the risk for trisomy 18 is only marginally increased and maternal age should be the main factor in deciding whether or not to offer fetal karyotyping. If one additional abnormality is found, the maternal age-related risk is increased, so that even for a 20-year-old the risk for trisomy 18 is at least as high as the risk for trisomy 21 in a 35-year-old. Therefore, the option of karyotyping should be offered to the patient.

Sullivan and colleagues[206] had a group of 128 fetuses with choroid plexus cysts of which 51 patients had triple screen done. Results of the triple screen were normal in 32 patients. The choroid plexus cysts were isolated in 29 of the 32 patients,

TABLE 4-10. ISOLATED CHOROID PLEXUS CYST(S) (CPC) AND CHROMOSOMAL ANEUPLOIDY

Author/Year	Total Number of Patients Scanned	Number of CPC	Incidence (percent)	Isolated CPC	Isolated with Chromosomal Aneuploidy (percent)	Additional Sonographic Abnormalities	Chromosomal Aneuploidy in Patient with Additional Sonographic Findings (percent)
Geary 1997[202]	13,690	84	0.6	78	0	6	3 Trisomy 18
Sohn 1997[203]	4,326	41	0.94	40 (only 38 had amniocentesis)	0	1 (2 fetuses lost to follow up)	1 Trisomy 18
Reinsch 1997[204]	16,059	301	1.8	263	0	38[a]	3 (2 trisomy 18; 1 trisomy 21)
Morcos 1998[205]	7,617	210	2.8	181	1 (Trisomy 21)[b]	29	1 (trisomy 18)[b]
Sullivan 1999[206]	13,526	128	0.95	112[c]	4 (3 trisomy 18; 1 unbalanced translocation)[c]	16	12 (9 trisomy 18; 1 trisomy 21; 1 balanced translocation; 1 chromosomal inversion)
Total	55,218	764	1.4	674 (88%)	5 (0.74%)	90 (12%)	20 (22%)

[a] In addition to the CPC other risk factors included: other sonographic abnormalities, AMA, past obstetrical and family history.

[b] Patient reported to be at least 35 years of age.

[c] This group included 1 patient age 38 years who had trisomy 18; 6 patients with abnormal MSAFP; and 16 patients with abnormal triple screens.

and all 29 fetuses had normal karyotypes. The other 3 patients with normal triple screen results had additional fetal anomalies on ultrasonography. One fetus had normal chromosomes, and 2 had trisomy 18. The remaining 19 patients had abnormal triple-screen results. Among them, 16 fetuses had isolated choroid plexus cysts, 13 of whom were normal, 2 had trisomy 18, and 2 had a de novo unbalanced translocation. The remaining 3 fetuses had additional anomalies, and all 3 fetuses had trisomy 18. They concluded that (1) the triple screen is a useful adjunct to targeted ultrasonography in selecting patients with fetal choroid plexus cysts for amniocentesis; (2) a normal triple screen result in the absence of additional fetal anomalies on ultrasonography reliably exclude an underlying chromosomal abnormality, and amniocentesis is not indicated; and (3) if the triple screen result is abnormal, additional anomalies are seen on ultrasonography, or the mother is aged $\geq$ 35 years, then fetal karyotyping is recommended. In conclusion, once a choroid plexus cyst(s) is found during a routine scan, a detailed anatomic survey of the fetus should be performed. In addition, the maternal age and the results (if available) of the maternal serum screening should be reviewed. If the choroid plexus cyst(s) is a truly an isolated finding in a patient with no high risk factors no further work-up for this sonographic finding is necessary. However, if the choroid plexus cyst is present in either a patient who is 35 years of age or older, or in a younger patient with an abnormal triple screen, further genetic counseling and amniocentesis is suggested because of increased risk of chromosomal aneuploidy.

Digiovani and coworkers[208] followed 89 fetuses that had been diagnosed as having choroid plexus cyst(s). All fetuses underwent ultrasonographic detailed anatomy survey and fetal karyotyping and the neonatal outcomes and infant and early childhood developmental milestones were recorded. The children were followed subsequently, and developmental assessment was performed with a modified Denver II Developmental Screening Test. Three of the 61 women who underwent testing for fetal karyotype (4.9%) had abnormal karyotypes identified. All three karyotypes were trisomy 18, and all three trisomy 18 fetuses had additional sonographic abnormalities. All 28 women who chose not to undergo fetal karyotypic analysis delivered phenotypically normal infants. Infant and childhood developmental follow-up was performed on 76 children with cysts diagnosed prenatally. All 76 children were found to be developmentally normal by the Denver II Developmental Screening Test. The authors concluded that the finding of an isolated choroid plexus cysts is not associated with delayed infant and early childhood development or an increased risk of abnormal karyotype.

In conclusion, fetal karyotyping for CPCs should be offered to women carrying a fetus with other associated malformations, abnormal triple screen, or women over the age of 35. However, there is a still a small group of authors advocating fetal karyotyping for all fetuses with CPCs. This is due to the fact that the experience of all sonologists and/or sonographers may not be comparable and some fetuses with CPCs and other associated anomalies may be mistakenly labeled as having an isolated CPC.

DISORDERS OF NEURONAL PROLIFERATION, DIFFERENTIATION, AND HISTOGENESIS

Microcephaly

Microcephaly (micrencephaly) is defined as a fetal head size that falls at least 3 standard deviations (-3 SD) below the mean (see Chapter 3). The incidence of microcephaly based on observation at birth ranges from 1 in 6250 to 1 in 8500. The United States Collaborative Perinatal Project found an incidence of 1.6 per 1000 live births when infants were observed through the first year of life.[209] Isolated genetic microcephaly has been estimated to affect 1 in 25,000 to 1 in 50,000 live births.[210] Microcephaly is a disorder of neural proliferation and can be divided into two general types: *radial microbrain,* which appears to be related to a diminished number of proliferative units, and *microcephaly vera,* related to a diminished size of proliferation unit.[211] Radial microbrain is a rare lethal disorder (newborns die within the first month of life) in which the brain is extremely small, has normal gyral formation, no evidence of a destructive process, and no disturbance of cortical lamination. This type of microcephaly can be distinguished from anencephaly based on the presence of intact skull bones. Microcephaly vera is a heterogeneous group of disorders in which small brain size is the common denominator. It may occur as a result of a familial trait, which may be autosomal dominant (e.g., de Lange's syndrome), autosomal recessive (e.g., Smith–Lemli–Opitz syndrome), X-linked (e.g., Börjeson–Forssman–Lehmann syndrome), or part of a chromosomal syndrome (e.g., trisomies 18 and 21 or 5p− syndrome); may be due to a teratogenic factor such as irradiation, metabolic–toxic effects (e.g., fetal alcohol syndrome, cocaine, or hyperphenylalaninemia), or infections such as CMV, toxoplasmosis, and rubella; or may be sporadic.[211] In addition, an abnormality of the skull, such as craniosynostosis, in which there is precocious fusion of the sutures of the brain, may result in microcephaly.[209,212–218]

Using sonography, microcephaly can be diagnosed when the biometry of the fetal head lags behind the predicted mean for the gestational age (Figs. 4–18 through 4–20). Chervenak's group[213] found that microcephaly could be reliably diagnosed if the occipitofrontal diameter was less than 4 SD of the predicted mean, the head circumference (perimeter) was less than 5 SD, the head perimeter/abdominal perimeter ratio was smaller than 3 SD, and the femur length/head perimeter ratio was larger than 3 SD of the predicted mean. In addition, it is important to obtain serial ultrasound scans to establish the trend of growth or lack of it. Goldstein and colleagues[216] have suggested measurement of the frontal lobe as a potential tool for the prenatal diagnosis of microcephaly, in view of the fact that the anterior cranial fossa seems to be primarily involved in microcephaly. They obtained two measurements, frontal lobe distance and thalamic–frontal lobe distance (see Chapter 3), and found that in three cases of microcephaly diagnosed prenatally these measurements were 2 SD below the mean. Although they found that the parameters described by Chervenak and collaborators[213] were also reduced, adding this measurement can enhance the in utero diagnosis of microcephaly.

Recently, Persutte and colleagues[219] reported on the correlation of the fetal frontal lobe and the transcerebellar diameter. In their study, they measured the frontal lobe (posterior part of the cavum septi pellucidi to the inner calvarium [caval-calvarial distance (CCD)]) in an axial section at the same level as the BPD and transcerebellar diameter (TCD) in 221 patients. They found a correlation coefficient of 0.950 when comparing the two variables (P 0.0001). Using the 95th centile of this measurement, 8 of 12 (66%) abnormal fetuses (three with microcephaly, four with trisomy 21, and one with trisomy 18) were above this threshold. Only 12 (5.4%) of the 221 normal fetuses had a CCD/TCD ratio above the 95th centile. They concluded that this new technique may prove to be a useful tool in the in utero diagnosis of various conditions affecting the fetal brain.

Pilu and colleagues[220] reported on the prenatal diagnosis of microcephaly in two fetuses assisted by transvaginal sonography and color Doppler. In these two cases, transvaginal sonography revealed aberrant findings, including large subarachnoid spaces and a rudimentary shape of the lateral ventricles. In one of these fetuses, power Doppler ultrasound demonstrated a discrepancy in the size of the signals generated by the intracranial arteries branching from the internal carotids and those branching from the vertebral arteries, and this was interpreted as the consequence of a reduced blood supply to the undersized cerebral hemispheres. They suggest that evaluation of intracranial anatomy by transvaginal sonography and power Doppler examination of the cerebral vessels may be of value in the diagnosis of fetal microcephaly.

In cases of microcephaly, it is important to assess the brain structures and rule out associated brain anomalies. Microcephaly is commonly present in cases of lissencephaly, porencephaly, and holoprosencephaly. Other associated anomalies include agenesis of the corpus callosum and ventriculomegaly (hydrocephalus) secondary to brain atrophy.[209,216] Unfortunately, isolated microcephaly may not be diagnosed until late in the second trimester or early in the third, when the growth of the fetal head slows significantly.[214] Bromley and Benacerraf[221] recently published the results of a retrospective study based on seven fetuses with prenatally suspected microcephaly who had had a prenatal scan before 22 postmenstrual weeks. They found that only one of the seven fetuses had an abnormal BPD on the initial scan of 21 postmenstrual weeks. In the other six fetuses microcephaly was sonographically detected between 27 and 33 postmenstrual weeks. Therefore, they concluded that a single second-trimester biometry by BPD lacks sensitivity for the diagnosis of microcephaly and that serial sonograms may be helpful in the detection of head growth abnormalities.

The differential diagnosis of microcephaly is craniosynostosis. If the sagittal suture closes prematurely, the head becomes dolichocephalic, but if the coronal suture closes, the head becomes brachycephalic due to continued growth. Premature closure of the coronal and lambdoidal sutures results in the "kleeblattschädel deformity," in which the skull has an unusual cloverleaf shape.[222–224] Asymmetrical craniosynostosis, in which fusion of different sutures may occur, results in bizarre fetal head shapes.[222] The sonographic finding in craniosynostosis is an indentation of the cranial bone (Fig. 4–49). Craniosynostosis is associated with a variety of autosomal dominant (e.g., Crouzon's disease and Apert syndrome) and autosomal recessive conditions (e.g., Carpenter's and Antley–Bixler syndromes) and may be associated with mental retardation.[225]

The prognosis of a microcephalic infant is related to the severity of associated anomalies, the size of the head, and the nature of the microcephaly. Children with a head circumference between 2 and 3 SD below the mean are more likely to have learning disabilities with near-normal intelligence, but those with a head circumference of 3 SD or less are more likely to be developmentally delayed.[217] Data from the United States Collaborative Perinatal

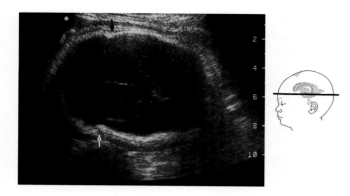

Figure 4–49. The horizontal section of the head at 36 post-menstrual weeks. Severe microcephaly was diagnosed as well as a bilateral indentation of the temporal bones at the level of the sutures. On other views the top of the cranium was slightly angulated or pointed. These sonographic findings were suggestive of craniosynostosis. The prenatal diagnosis was confirmed at birth.

Project found that children with microcephaly (−2 SD) at 1 year of age had a 50% chance of having an IQ below 80 at 4 years of age.[226]

Megalencephaly

Megalencephaly is defined as an occipitofrontal head circumference greater than 2 SD above the mean (Table 4–11).[221] The prevalence of megalencephaly is unknown, but the rates from autopsy series range from 1 in 1146 to 1 in 50,000.[218] The clinical features range from no apparent neurological deficit to severe seizures and developmental delay.[225] Conditions associated with megalencephaly include benign autosomal dominant megalencephaly, cerebral gigantism, Beckwith's syndrome, hemangiomatosis (Bannayan–Zonana syndrome), neurofibromatosis, and chromosomal syndromes (fragile X syndrome and Kleinfelter's syndrome), although the most common cause of megalencephaly is benign autosomal dominant megalencephaly not associated with anomalies.[225,228]

The prenatal diagnosis of benign megalencephaly can be made based on a prenatal sonogram showing a large fetal head and a family history of "large heads" (increased occipitofrontal diameter). In a case report by DeRosa and associates,[227] sonography demonstrated a large BPD and head circumference (greater than the 98th percentile) at 32 postmenstrual weeks' gestation. It is interesting to note that at 21 postmenstrual weeks the measurements of the BPD and the head circumference were within normal range.

A careful search of the intracranial anatomy must be performed to rule out any other conditions

TABLE 4–11. OCCIPITOFRONTAL DIAMETER

Week	Occipitofrontal Diameter (mm)		
	5th	**50th**	**95th**
10	7	14	21
11	11	18	25
12	16	23	30
13	20	27	34
14	24	31	38
15	29	36	43
16	33	40	47
17	37	44	51
18	41	48	55
19	46	53	60
20	50	57	64
21	54	61	68
22	58	65	72
23	62	69	76
24	65	72	79
25	69	76	83
26	73	80	87
27	76	83	90
28	80	87	94
29	83	90	97
30	86	93	100
31	89	96	103
32	92	99	106
33	95	102	108
34	97	104	111
35	99	106	113
36	102	109	116
37	104	111	118
38	105	112	119
39	107	114	121
40	108	115	122

or anomalies that may account for the increase in fetal head size before the diagnosis of benign megalencephaly can be made. The differential diagnosis includes any conditions that may increase the size of the fetal head, such as hydrocephaly, an intracranial tumor, or macrosomia. In addition, assessment of the fetal gender may help, since there is a male predominance in this condition.

No treatment is necessary because benign megalencephaly has a good outcome.

Unilateral megalencephaly is defined as a unilateral hypertrophy of the affected hemisphere, often associated with ipsilateral ventricular dilatation and a shift in the midline. The cerebellum and the brain stem, as well as hemihypertrophy of the body, may be present.[229]

Unilateral megalencephaly is a rare developmental malformation of the brain. The origin is unknown, but it is hypothesized to be the result of an insult to the germinal matrix between 8 and 16 postmenstrual weeks of gestation. The pathological findings include lissencephaly, polymicrogyria, and a thickened cortex with poor separation of the gray and white matter. The clinical syndrome in this condition includes progressive unilateral, intractable seizures associated with developmental delay, hemiplegia, and abnormal head growth.[230–232]

Prenatal diagnosis of unilateral megalencephaly was reported as early as 20 postmenstrual weeks.[231] The diagnosis was made based on the following sonographic features: asymmetry of the cerebral hemispheres with dilatation of the lateral ventricle in the affected side and a shift in the midline (Fig. 4–50). In addition, magnetic resonance imaging (MRI) of the fetal head confirmed the sonographic findings. The postmortem examination confirmed the in utero diagnosis. In this case the fetus also had a clenched left fist and abnormally long middle toes on both feet. Other findings associated with unilateral megalencephaly include progressive increases in the BPD, head circumference, and BPD/abdominal circumference ratio and focal areas of increased echogenicity in the affected hemisphere.[233,234] No karyotypic abnormalities have been described in association with this syndrome. The use of multiplanar imaging using three-dimensional sonography was reported as useful in the diagnosis of unilateral megalencephaly at 22 postmenstrual weeks, 1 day.[235]

The differential diagnosis includes intracranial tumors, chromosomal abnormalities, and intracranial hemorrhage. Unilateral megalencephaly should be part of the differential diagnosis of any condition that causes a shift in the midline. Treatment includes hemispherectomy of the affected hemisphere, usually before the age of 6 months.[230,232]

Schizencephaly

Schizencephaly is a rare congenital malformation in which bilateral and nearly symmetrical clefts are usually present in the cerebral hemispheres. The incidence of schizencephaly is unknown because since all cases appear to be sporadic and have normal chromosomes.[218] Two types of schizencephaly have been described.[236,237] *Type I* has small, symmetrical clefts in which the lips of the clefts are fused within a pia–ependymal seam that is continuous with the ependyma of the lateral ventricle. In *type II,* the lips of the clefts remain separated and the clefts are more extensive, extending from the ventricle to the surface of the brain.[236,238] The clefts may be unilateral or bilateral and symmetrical, are wedge shaped, and extend outward to the bones of the skull. Clinically affected children have seizures and developmental delay.[239] The pathogenesis of schizencephaly is not clear but it is believed to arise from an in utero insult. This insult may include ischemia, fetal hypotension, or toxic and/or infectious events occurring during the first trimester and leading to brain damage[240] (Fig. 4–51).

Sonographic findings include the presence of unilateral or bilateral, symmetrical brain clefts in the area of the lateral sulcus (Sylvius). The ventricles are dilated and freely communicate with the clefts. The midline structures are normal. Head size may be normocephalic or microcephalic.[241] Suche[242] performed color flow Doppler studies on three fetuses with schizencephaly. In two fetuses the internal carotid and middle cerebral artery waveforms

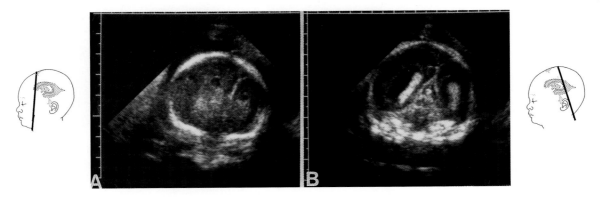

Figure 4–50. Unilateral megalencephaly at 20 postmenstrual weeks. **A.** Frontal–2 section showing the asymmetry between the two cerebral hemispheres. Note that the ipsilateral ventricle of the hemisphere with the megalencephaly is dilated. **B.** Occipital–1 section showing the discrepancy in size between the two hemispheres. This asymmetry is more evident on the lateral ventricle of the hemisphere with the megalencephaly. *(Courtesy of Isabelle A. Wilkins, MD.)*

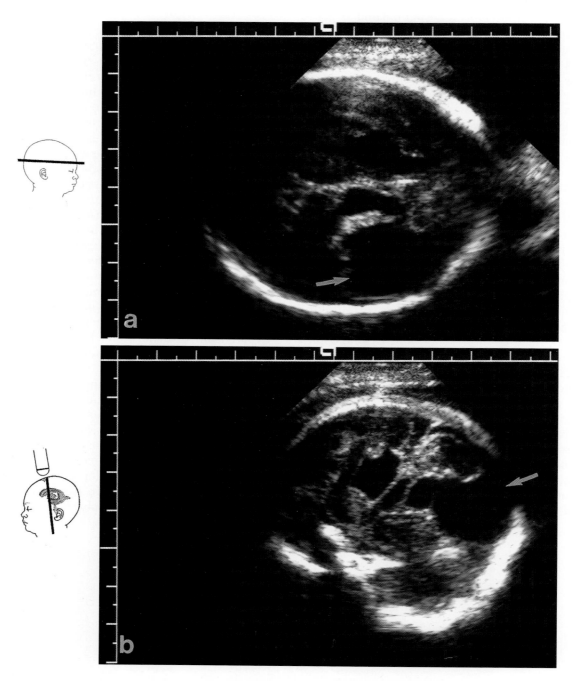

Figure 4–51. Transabdominal brain scan of a 16-year-old woman at 30 postmenstrual weeks with cytomegalo virus infection (CMV). **A.** Axial section showing a large unilateral brain defect extending to the cranium *(arrow)*. **B.** Mid-coronal–1 section showing dilatation of the lateral ventricle. The cavum septi pellucidi is prominent. The large defect which communicates with the right lateral ventricle extends all the way to the cranium *(arrow)*. This is consistent with type II schizencephaly.

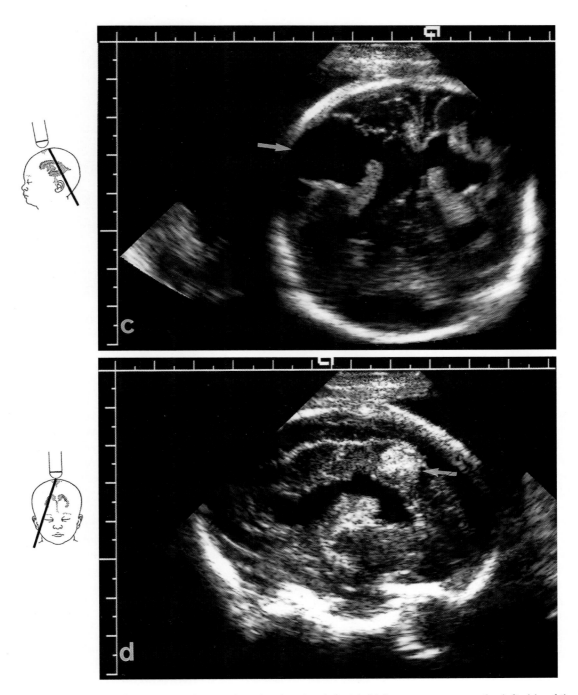

Figure 4–51. continued C. Midcoronal–3 section showing the defect (which now appears on the left side of the image), which freely communicates with the lateral ventricle. There is some degree of hydrocephaly. The periventricular area has a "moth eaten" appearance and is slightly hyperechoic consistent with CMV in utero infection (*arrow, cleft*). **D** and **E** are Oblique–1 sections showing the right and left ventricle. Note that there is moderate dilatation of the lateral ventricle. In addition, hyperechoic material (calcifications) are present both around the periventricular area as well as in the brain parenchyma (*arrow* calcifications). *(Courtesy of Paula Woletz RDMS, New Jersey.)*

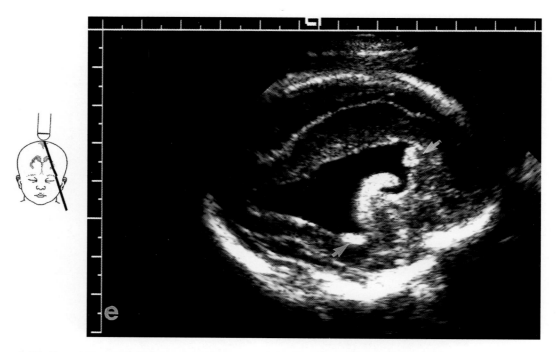

Figure 4–51. D and **E** are Oblique–1 sections showing the right and left ventricle. Note that there is moderate dilatation of the lateral ventricle. In addition, hyperechoic material (calcifications) are present both around the periventricular area as well as in the brain parenchyma (*arrow* calcifications). *(Courtesy of Paula Woletz RDMS, New Jersey.)*

(pulsatility index) were normal, and in the third fetus the right middle cerebral artery was persistently occluded. This lends support to the belief that schizencephaly results from occlusion of the middle cerebral artery, with subsequent recanalization of the vessel.[243]

The differential diagnosis includes holoprosencephaly, bilateral arachnoid cysts, and hydranencephaly. In holoprosencephaly there is a single ventricle with no midline structures and the thalami are fused (see Chapter 5). Arachnoid cysts can be differentiated from schizencephaly because they do not communicate with the lateral ventricles. Associated findings include ventriculomegaly, polymicrogyria, heterotopia, agenesis of the corpus callosum, and absent cavum septi pellucidi (septo-optic dysplasia).[237,238,244,245] Septo-optic dysplasia and schizencephaly often occur together, and both have been associated with absence of the septum pellucidum in 75% to 100% of these patients.[239,246–248]

Barkovich and coworkers[240] retrospectively reviewed the clinical records and MRI scans of 20 patients with schizencephaly. The results showed that the size and location of the clefts are very important in determination of the prognosis. In cases of bilateral schizencephaly and in those with large or medium unilateral schizencephaly, there is a very poor prognosis for intellectual development. Patients with bilateral clefts also have a poor prognosis in terms of development of speech. Patients with unilateral closed-lip or small open-lip schizencephaly have a good prognosis for intellectual development.

Lissencephaly and Pachygyria

Lissencephaly, or agyria (smooth brain), is a rare developmental anomaly of the brain characterized by a lack of gyral development with or without pachygyria.[249] *Pachygyria (macrogyria)* refers to the presence of a few gyri wider and thicker than those of the normal brain.[250]

Lissencephaly has been divided into two general types.[251] *Type I* is characterized by microcephaly and facial dysmorphism, and *type II* is characterized by hydrocephaly, ocular anomalies (retinal dysplasia), and muscular dysplasia.

Lissencephaly is a neuronal migrational disorder. Neuronal migration begins in the sixth postmenstrual week of gestation. In lissencephaly type I the formation of the neocortex is severely affected. This results in the classical four-layered cortex (consisting, from the inside to the outside, of heterotopic nonmigrated neurons, a cell-sparse layer, components of layers III, V, and VI combined, and a molecular layer[252]) found in lissencephaly and on the outside there is agyria. According to Sidman and Rakio,[253] the neuronal migration is disturbed in lissencephaly between the 11th and 13th postmenstrual weeks of gestation. In pachygyria the presumed disturbance occurs after the 13th week but before completion of the neuronal migration. Pachygyria and lissencephaly (agyria) are usually found in the same brain.[254] In lissencephaly type II migration defects involve all of the major pathways, beginning no later than 6 postmenstrual weeks, and are associated with a spectrum of defects not clearly attributed to a defect in migration.[255]

The most common clinical syndrome associated with lissencephaly type I is Miller–Dierker syndrome. Other clinical syndromes with lissencephaly type I include Norman–Roberts syndrome (autosomal recessive) and isolated lissencephaly sequence.[255] In Miller–Dierker syndrome there is microcephaly, bitemporal hollowing, micrognathia, a high forehead, anteverted nares, low-set ears, and a prominent occiput. In addition, 20% to 25% of these patients have cardiac abnormalities, 70% of the males have genital anomalies, 70% have a sacral dimple, 65% to 70% have palmar creases, and 40% to 45% have clinodactyly. A chromosomal abnormality of a deletion in the region of chromosome 17p13.3 has been detected in most cases with this syndrome.[225,255–257]

There are two syndromes characterized by lissencephaly type II: Walker–Warburg syndrome (WWS) and Fukuyama congenital muscular dystrophy.[225,256] Walker–Warburg syndrome was known in the past as HARD±E syndrome (Hydrocephaly, Agyria, and Retinal Dysplasia, with or without Encephalocele). All cases of WWS have lissencephaly type II, cerebellar malformation, retinal malformation, and congenital muscular dystrophy; 95% have ventricular dilatation; and 84% have macrocephaly. Fifty percent have a Dandy–Walker cyst and 25% to 50% have a posterior encephalocele. In addition, there may be cleft lip and/or cleft palate.[225,256–260] The origin of WWS is a lethal autosomal recessive syndrome.

The primary sonographic finding in lissencephaly syndrome is absence of the gyri with a smooth brain. Associated intracranial findings include mildly dilated lateral ventricles with colpocephaly (dilatation of the atria and the occipital horns); rarely, hydrocephaly microcephaly; hypoplasia or absence of the corpus callosum; Dandy–Walker malformation; and cephalocele. In addition, micromelia, clubfoot, polydactyly, duodenal atresia, micrognathia, omphalocele, hepatosplenomegaly, and cardiac and renal anomalies may be present. Polyhydramnios is a common

feature, most likely a result of impaired swallowing. Fetal movements are decreased, probably the result of the brain abnormality.

Intrauterine growth restriction (IUGR) may be present in up to 50% of the cases.[261–263] Using MRI, in utero diagnosis of lissencephaly has been made by observing the smooth surface of the cortex, the large lateral sulcus (of Sylvius), and dilatation of the lateral ventricles.[264,265] In utero diagnosis of WWS has been made based on the presence of dilated ventricles, posterior encephalocele, and Dandy–Walker cyst in a family with a prior affected infant.[263] Differentiating in utero between the two major types of lissencephaly may be difficult.

Prenatal diagnosis of lissencephaly without a previous history of an affected child probably cannot be reliably made until 26 to 28 weeks' gestation, when the normal gyri and sulci become well defined, since up to this time the normal fetal brain has a smooth appearance. Transvaginal sonography allows the gyri and the sulci to be reliably and easily imaged (see Chapter 2). The diagnosis may be suspected earlier in cases in which polyhydramnios, agenesis of the corpus callosum, IUGR, cardiac malformation, and microcephaly are present. Prenatal diagnosis in families with a previously affected infant with Miller–Dierker syndrome can be made by either chorionic villi sampling or early amniocentesis.

Management of a pregnancy in which any of these anomalies are present should include genetic counseling and testing to search for the chromosome deletion. All children with this type of migrational disorder are severely neurologically impaired. The prognosis for the fetus with lissencephaly is very poor. In Miller–Dierker syndrome the neurological findings include early hypotonia, followed by hypertonia, seizures, and severe mental retardation. This is a lethal abnormality and survival usually extends to 18 months. Infants with WWS are severely mentally retarded and have severe hypotonia and seizures. Similarly to Miller–Dierker syndrome, WWS is also a lethal abnormality, with survival up to 5 postnatal months.[256]

ARACHNOID CYSTS

Arachnoid cysts, similarly to CPCs, are collections of CSF. They are usually benign, congenital, space-occupying lesions. The cyst wall is lined with collagen and cells of the arachnoid matter. In the arachnoid cyst the CSF is located within the layers of the arachnoid membrane, which may or may not communicate with the subarachnoid space. Arachnoid cysts account for 1% of all intracranial masses in children.[266] They usually occur as sporadic and single lesions, but may appear in siblings, may be bilateral and symmetrical, or may arise in multiple sites. The left side of the brain is more commonly affected. Males are more commonly affected than females.[267–270] The clinical manifestations are related to the size of the cyst and its location: small cysts are usual, incidental findings; however, a larger cyst may cause seizures, headaches, and focal neurological signs.[271] Approximately 60% to 80% of arachnoid cysts are symptomatic. In infants there may be increased head circumference and calvarial asymmetry.[270] Arachnoid cysts are usually supratentorial. Between 50% and 65% are located in the middle cranial fossa, 5% to 10% are in the suprasellar cistern, 5% to 10% are in the quadrigeminal cistern, 5% spread along the convexities, and only 5% to 10% are located in the posterior fossa at the level of the cerebellopontile angle and the cisterna magna.[272]

The arachnoid cysts can be further divided into open-necked and narrow-necked arachnoid cysts. The open-neck arachnoid cysts have free access to CSF into their interiors and those with narrow-neck trap CSF within them. Postanally the open-necked cysts are frequent incidental findings, although rarely may present with hemorrhage after minor trauma. They are often associated with agenesis of associated parts of the brain (tip of the temporal lobe or corpus callosum). The narrow-necked arachnoid cysts postanally are identified because they cause obstructive hydrocephaly as they increase in size.[273] Bannister and colleagues[273] published a paper dealing with the outcome of prenatally diagnosed arachnoid cysts. In their study, 15 arachnoid cyst were identified in utero: five were identified at or before 20; four between 21 to 30 and 6 at or later than 31 postmenstrual weeks. Thirteen of the cysts were in the supratentorial compartment and two in

the posterior fossa. Seven of the supratentorial cysts lay in the interhemispheric fissure and the remaining five were in front of, below or behind the third ventricle. Four pregnancies were terminated and 11 continued to term. Of these 11 pregnancies, one fetus with a posterior fossa cyst developed hydrocephaly and delivered at 36 postmenstrual weeks for a ventriculoperitoneal shunt to be inserted. The infant is moderate mentally retarded. Of the other ten pregnancies that went to term, two children had syndromes (Pallister–Hall and Aicardi syndrome) and one was lost to follow-up. The other seven children were reported to be developing normal. They assumed that these children that were developing normally most likely had open-necked arachnoid cysts.

Arachnoid cysts are either primary or acquired. Primary cysts may arise from an abnormal developmental process of the leptomeningeal formation. Acquired or secondary arachnoid cysts may be the result of CSF entrapment within arachnoid adhesions following in utero hemorrhage, infection, or trauma.[274–278]

The sonographic appearance is that of a sonolucent cystic mass with thin, smooth walls, and therefore these cysts are easily spotted (Figs. 4–52 through 4–59). Arachnoid cysts do not communicate with the lateral ventricles.[274,275] Hydrocephaly may be present and is the result of a mass effect from a large arachnoid cyst, secondary to obstruction of flow of the CSF. Arachnoid cysts in the posterior fossa must be differentiated from Dandy–Walker malformation. This can be done by identifying the normally formed fourth ventricle and the vallecula.[272] In one of our cases (Fig. 4–58), the first ultrasonographic scan at 15.5 postmenstrual weeks was completely normal; however, at 28 postmenstrual weeks a cyst of the posterior fossa was imaged and at 31 postmenstrual

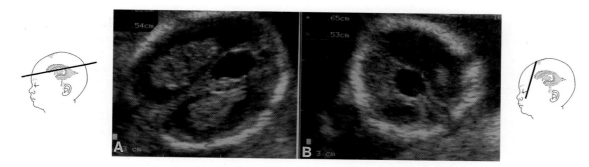

Figure 4–52. Arachnoid cyst at 16 postmenstrual weeks. **A.** Horizontal image showing the 0.7 × 0.54 cm cystic structure between the frontal lobes of the hemispheres. **B.** Midcoronal–2 section localizing the cyst between the hemispheres in the longitudinal sulcus. The exact location of this arachnoid cyst was in the suprachiasmatic area. In spite of counseling, the patient requested termination of the pregnancy. *(Courtesy of Z. Leiborici, Haifa, Israel.)*

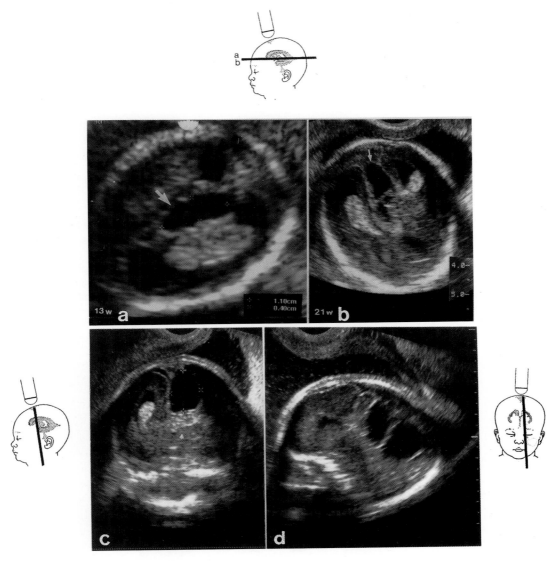

Figure 4–53. Arachnoid cyst. **A.** Transvaginal sonography at 13 postmenstrual weeks of gestation revealed a sonolucent cystic structure measuring 1.1 × 0.4 cm in the fetal head. After extensive counseling, the patient decided to continue the pregnancy. **B.** At 21 postmenstrual weeks, it became obvious that this cyst was side-by-side with the falx cerebri (arachnoid cysts, which do not straddle the falx cerebri, have better neonatal outcomes). **C.** Coronal and **D.** sagittal view of the same cyst at 26 weeks showing the corpus callosum and the location of the cyst, which remained on one-side of the falx.

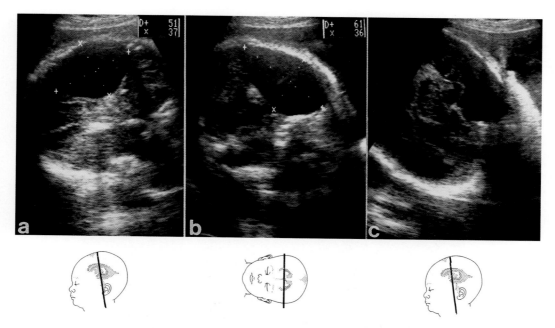

Figure 4–54. Three sections of the brain at midtrimester, showing a right temporal sonolucency of 5.1 × 6.1 × 3.6 cm. **A.** Midcoronal–2 section. **B.** Midcoronal–3 section. **C.** Horizontal section. The fetus was delivered at 36 weeks for placenta abruptio and had good Apgar scores. Magnetic resonance imaging and ultrasonography confirmed the presence of an arachnoid cyst. At 1 month of age, the cyst was removed surgically. At 36 months of age, the infant was developing normally and had no sequelae. The patient since delivered a second, normal child. *(Courtesy of Harley B. Friedenson, MD, and Terri L. Flander, RN, RDMS, Friedenson Women's Clinic, Brooklyn Center, Minnesota.)*

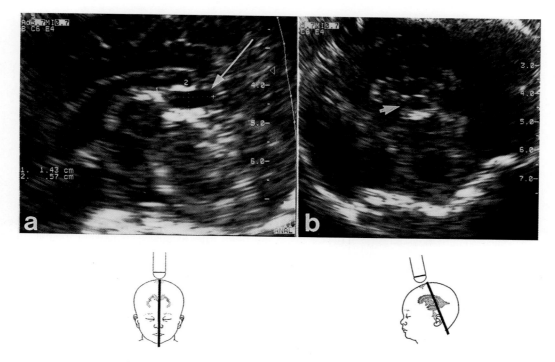

Figure 4–55. Small quadrigeminal plate arachnoid cyst at 35 postmenstrual weeks. **A.** median section showing the corpus callosum and a 1.4 × 0.5 cm sonolucent cystic structure in the quadrigeminal cistern. *(arrow).* **B.** Shows the cyst *(arrow)* below the cavum septum pellucidum in a Midcoronal–3 section.

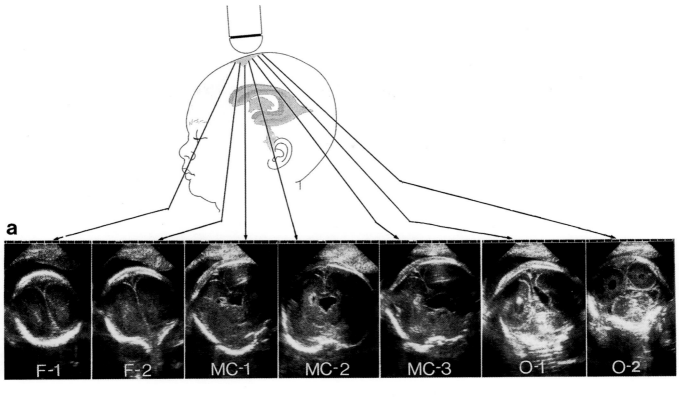

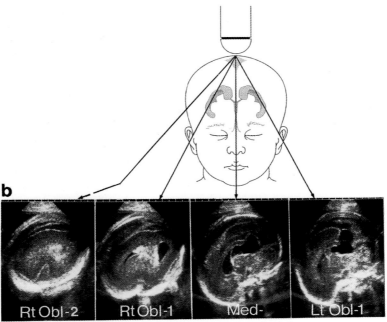

Figure 4–56. Transvaginal brain study of a 25 postmenstrual weeks fetus showing a quadrigeminal plate cistern arachnoid cyst. **A.** Serial coronal sections from Frontal–1 to Occipital–2 (F–1 to O–2). Frontal–1 (F–1) and Frontal–2 (F–2) section showing the parynchyma of the frontal lobes. Midcoronal–1 through Midcoronal–3 (MC–1 through MC–3) shows the midline sonolucent cyst. In Occipital–1 (O–1), the cyst can be seen slightly impinging on the posterior lobe of the brain. **B.** Median (Med) and right and left Oblique (Rt. And Lf. Obl) sections showing the extend and the exact location of the cyst. Right Oblique–1 and –2 (Rt Obl–1 and –2) shows the normal right cerebral hemispheres. Note that there is no dilatation of the lateral ventricles. Median (Med) section the arachnoid cyst is seen below the splenium (tail) of the corpus callosum extending almost to the cranium. Left Oblique–1 (Lt. Obl–1) more of the cyst is seen in this section the cyst extends all the way to the surface of the fetal brain. Note that this fetus has a normal corpus callosum, therefore, long-term prognosis for this fetus is good.

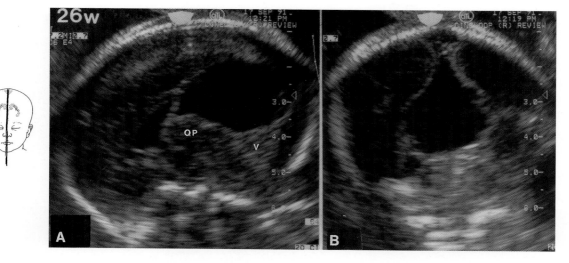

Figure 4–57. Images of a large quadrigeminal plate arachnoid cyst at 26 postmenstrual weeks. **A.** Median section showing the displacement of the quadrigeminal plate (QP) and the vermis of the cerebellum (V). **B.** Midcoronal–3 section showing the symmetrical position of the cyst displacing the hemispheres.

weeks it appeared similar to Dandy–Walker malformation. Postnatal MRI and computed tomographic scans confirmed the diagnosis of a posterior fossa arachnoid cyst (Fig. 4–58).

The differential diagnosis of an arachnoid cyst includes epidermoid tumors, porencephalic cysts, open-lip schizencephaly, and cystic neoplasm or vein of Galen malformation.[272,278] All of these are sonolucent fluid cyst–like masses, except for the neoplasms, which can be heterogeneous, can be associated with hydrocephaly, and may cause a mass effect. Porencephalic cysts communicate with the ventricles and the subarachnoid space and are located in the brain parenchyma; the great cerebral vein (vein of Galen) malformations have turbulent flow, which is evident on color Doppler studies. The sonolucent structure of the dilated great cerebral vein does not communicate with the ventricles or the subarachnoid space and is located in the area of the quadrigeminal plate cistern. For the sake of distinction, cystic neoplasms may communicate with the ventricles and are located in the brain parenchyma.[278]

The arachnoid cysts can be isolated lesions or may be associated with other CNS malformations, such as agenesis of the corpus callosum, absent septum pellucidum, deficient cerebellar lobulation, Arnold–Chiari type I malformation, and arteriovenous malformation. Non-CNS malformations associated with arachnoid cyst are tetralogy of Fallot, sacrococcygeal tumor, and neurofibromatosis type I.[277–281] In addition, arachnoid cysts may be part of a chromosomal and a nonchromosomal syndromes

such as distichiasis–lymphedema and Mohr syndrome and have also been associated with trisomy 18, triploidy, unbalanced translocations, and a partial trisomy 12q24.31.[218,282–284]

The natural history of arachnoid cysts is poorly understood, however some are known to increase in size in utero specially during the third trimester, may cause hydrocephaly as a result of a mass effect while others resolve in utero.[278,285] Elbers and coworkers[282] reported on a case of presumed arachnoid cyst that was initially diagnosed at 18.5 weeks of gestation, developed a hematoma at 28 weeks, and had virtually resolved by 32 weeks of gestation.

Isolated arachnoid cysts in general have a good prognosis. Once an arachnoid cyst is diagnosed in utero, a careful brain study is indicated to rule-out other brain anomalies and to determine its exact location. Arachnoid cysts which are interhemispheric, and straddles the falx cerebri, are associated with agenesis of the corpus callosum and secondary obstruction of interhemispheric foramina (Monro) with uni- or bilateral ventriculomegaly and have a worse prognosis for the fetus/neonate. However, those arachnoid cysts which are side-by-side with falx, and have an intact falx cerebri have a better prognosis (Fig. 4–53). In addition, a fetal karyotype is warranted in all these cases.

Treatment of arachnoid cysts includes primary postnatal ventriculoperitoneal and cystoperitoneal shunting and resection of the outer wall and shunting of the cyst, as well as resection of the inner wall to allow communication with the arachnoid space.[286] A report dealing with the long-term prognosis of

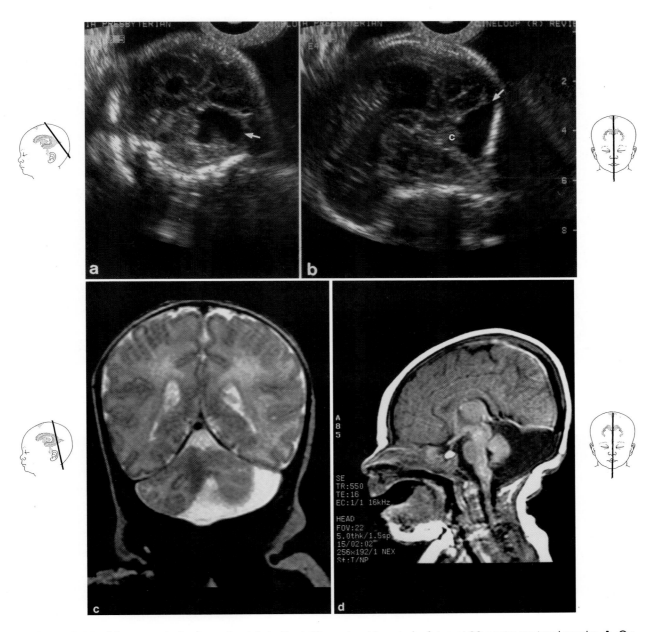

Figure 4–58. A large posterior fossa (mainly to the left) arachnoid cyst of a fetus at 28 postmenstrual weeks. **A.** Occipital–1 section showing the cystic structure marked by the *white arrow.* **B.** Median section showing the normal appearing midline structures as well as the sonolucent structure *(white arrow)* displacing the cerebellum (C). The lesion was followed up until delivery. **C, D.** Magnetic resonance images of the neonate. **C.** Coronal image of the posterior fossa, showing what appeared to be a cerebellar arachnoid cyst displacing both lobes of the cerebellum. **D.** Median image of the brain, clearly showing the cystic structure in the posterior fossa, with displacement of the cerebellum, the midbrain of the cerebellum, and midbrain structures. The diagnosis of arachnoid cyst was reached because there was minimal deformity of the vermis, which is contrary to the diagnosis of Dandy–Walker cyst. The fourth ventricle is of normal size but slightly pushed by the increasing cerebrospinal fluid pressure. The lateral and third ventricles were of appropriate size. There was no evidence of hemorrhage.

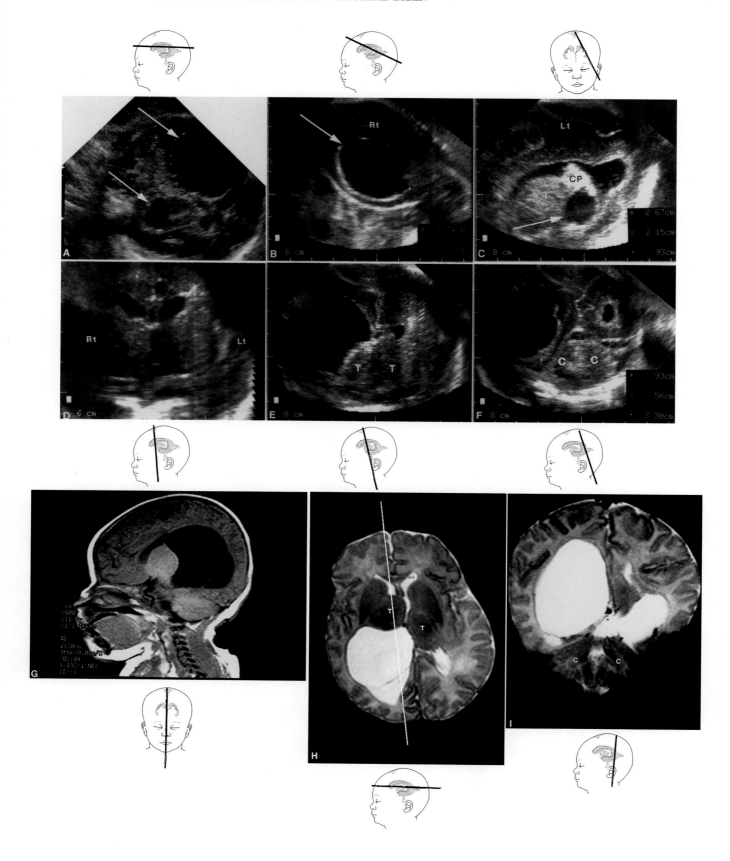

Figure 4–59. Bilateral cysts at 32 postmenstrual weeks. The working diagnosis based on the ultrasonographic images was bilateral choroid plexus cysts. **A.** Horizontal section. The cysts are marked by *arrows;* the right is larger than the left. **B.** Posterior-angled horizontal section. The *arrow* indicates the larger, right-sided cyst. **C.** Left Oblique–1 section. Note the slightly dilated posterior horn and the smaller cyst *(arrow)* below the choroid plexus. **D.** Midcoronal–1 section. Note that the anterior horns are slightly dilated. **E.** Midcoronal–2 section. The cyst on the right side is shown. T, Thalamus. **F.** Occipital–1 section. The larger, right-sided cyst is seen extending posteriorly even on this section. C, cerebellum. The neonate was born at term. Magnetic resonance images suggested the diagnosis of an arachnoid cyst, rather than a cyst arising from the choroid plexus. **G.** Slightly right paramedian section. Note the thin wall of the cysts in the right lateral ventricle. This plane was obtained along the *white line* transecting the brain in **H. H.** Horizontal section. Note that the anterior horns (AH) are not dilated and that the right thalamus (T) is pushed slightly forward. **I.** Coronal section through the two cystic structures and the cerebellum (C).

more than 60 children treated for arachnoid cysts showed that 64% experienced complete recovery, 15% had a slight deficit, 13% had severe postoperative deterioration, and 8% died.[287] The outcome of the children was dependent on the location of the cyst: of the children with temporal cysts, 93% had full recovery or minimal deficit and none died, while 64% of patients with cysts in other locations did well and 16% died. Intrauterine management of arachnoid cyst was also performed (see Chapter 19).

In summary, when managing a fetus with an arachnoid cyst, the exact location and the effect on the brain structures in its immediate vicinity should be determined. This should be followed by a targeted scan and a fetal echocardiogram. In addition, when faced with this anomaly, as in the case of any anomaly, genetic counseling should be conducted and genetic testing should be offered to the patient.

CONGENITAL VASCULAR MALFORMATIONS: ANEURYSM OF THE GREAT CEREBRAL VEIN

Aneurysm of the great cerebral vein (of Galen) is rare, but it is probably the most representative prenatal venous malformation of the brain. The great cerebral vein is one of the deep cerebral veins; it curves under the splenium of the corpus callosum and unites with the inferior sagittal sinus to form the straight sinus (see Chapter 2). Approximately 40% to 50% of cases have a neonatal presentation.[288–291] No data are available regarding the percentage of these neonatal cases that can be or are diagnosed prenatally. Approximately 95% of the neonates present with high-output cardiac failure, and the other 5% present with hydrocephalus, subarachnoid hemorrhage, or intraventricular hemorrhage.[291]

Using neonatal angiography, the great cerebral vein malformation has been classified into four types,[290,292,293] however, in general terms, there are two basic types. In the first type a single or multiple arteries drain directly into enlarged deep venous structures of the "Galenic system." In the second type, which is the most common, there is a single or multiple direct arteriovenous fistulae between the choroidal or quadrigeminal arteries and a median venous sac. This sac (although considered by most to represent the dilated great cerebral vein is actually a persistent median prosencephalic vein of Markowski, a transient fetal structure that normally disappears by the 11th postmenstrual week of gestation.[289,291,294,295]

The sonographic appearance of the malformation in the coronal plane is that of a well-defined, round, midline sonolucent mass. In a median plane the malformation appears as a large, well-defined, supratentorial, nonpulsatile tubular structure running from the splenium of the corpus callosum, in the area of the quadrigeminal plate cistern superior and posterior to the thalamus, above the cerebellum and extending all the way to the bony cranium (Fig. 4–60). Using color Doppler sonography, the structure fills with bright color due to the turbulent flow within the dilated vessel.[296–298] In addition, macrocephaly and hydrocephaly may also be present. Hydrocephaly is believed to be the result of compression at the level of the quadrigeminal plate and the cerebral aqueduct by the aneurysmal mass.[291,299] In the literature, in the prenatally detected cases of great cerebral vein malformation, the diagnosis was made in the third trimester of pregnancy.[296] It is not clear when these malformations develop, but they seem to become apparent only in the third trimester.

Other sonographic findings reported with great cerebral vein aneurysm include cardiomegaly, pericardial effusion, dilated neck and head veins with turbulent flow, hepatomegaly, ascites, hydrops, and polyhydramnios.[296,300,301] In addition, Ballantyne syndrome, which includes fetal edema, maternal edema, and placentomegaly, has also been reported in association with this malformation.[297]

The morbidity and mortality rates of great cerebral vein malformation are dependent on the age at presentation. The neonate with severe congestive

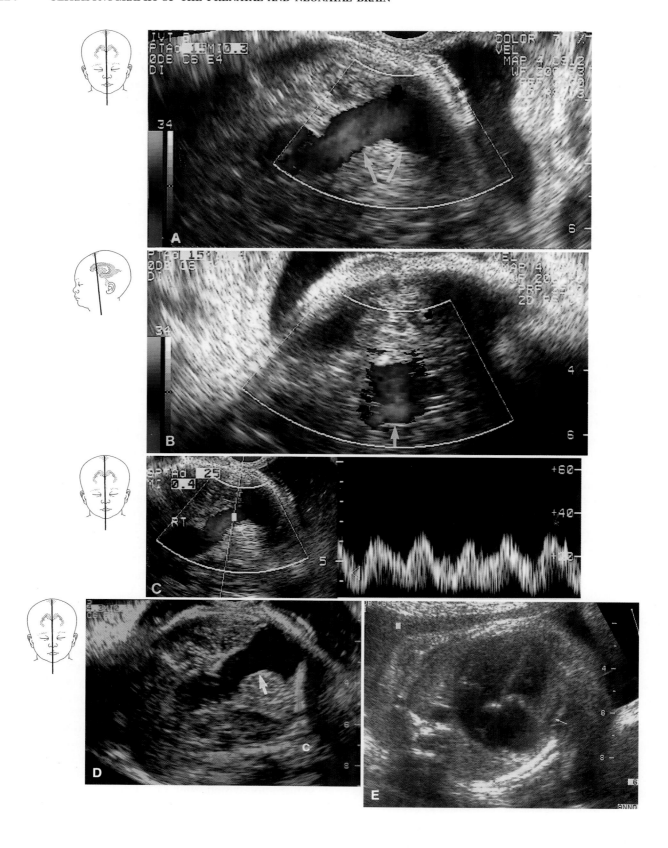

Figure 4–60. Aneurysm of the vein of Galen at 33 postmenstrual weeks. **A–C.** Color-coded Doppler images of the lesion *(arrows)*. **A.** Median plane. **B.** Midcoronal–1 plane. **C.** In the median plane note the wide (about 1.2-cm) structure above the cerebellum (C), with flow toward the posterior pole of the brain. The Doppler evaluation showed pulsatile venous flow. **D.** Gray-scale image in the median plane. **E.** Four-chamber view of the heart, showing relative cardiomegaly (heart-to-chest diameter ratio, 0.65; normal, 0.45 to 0.5) and a very small amount of pericardial effusion *(arrow)*. There was no arteriovenous valve regurgitation, but the heart had hyperdynamic motion consistent with cerebral arteriovenous malformation. There was no dilatation of the vessels in the neck of the fetus. Three attempts at embolization were made after delivery, but the neonate died during the final attempt.

heart failure experiences high morbidity and mortality. Development of high-output failure in utero or before 3 months of life, demonstrating the above-described sonographic findings, is usually lethal despite medical and surgical treatments.[302–304] The outcome of untreated cases or those treated prior to the development of embolization techniques was reported as follows: 84% died early in infancy, approximately 13% survived with neurological impairment, and only 3% were normal at follow-up.[289] Current neurosurgical treatment aims at eliminating the high flow through the malformation; this may be accomplished by arterial embolization of a liquid adhesive agent or microcoils, or by venous embolization using a transtorcular approach with placement of metal coils.[290,305–310] Using embolization techniques, 30% to 45% of infants survive and are neurologically normal, but the mortality rate still ranges from 8% to 33%.[290,310] In the cases presented in Fig. 4–60, the neonate underwent three embolization procedures and died shortly thereafter as a result of a complication.

INFECTIONS AFFECTING THE CENTRAL NERVOUS SYSTEM

The fetus may become infected with a variety of organisms through transplacental passage or as a result of an ascending infection. Among the most common agents are those that encompass the TORCH syndrome (toxoplasmosis, rubella, cytomegalovirus, and herpes). Cytomegalovirus is the first and toxoplasmosis is the second most common cause of congenital CNS infection. Other organisms that less commonly infect the developing fetus include varicella–zoster.

Cytomegalovirus

Cytomegalovirus (CMV) infection is the most common infection affecting the developing human fetus. It is estimated that approximately 3000 to 4000 infants are born yearly with symptomatic disease and an additional 30,000 to 40,000 have asymptomatic diseases.[311] A study[312] from the congenital CMV

Disease Registry revealed that the most common clinical signs among infected children were hepatosplenomegaly and petechiae. In 55% of the children, severe permanent neurological sequelae were found, including intracranial calcifications in 43%, microcephaly in 27%, chorioretinitis in 15%, and seizures in 10%. Fetal infection can result from a primary maternal infection, reinfection, or reactivation of a latent infection. In contrast to the situation with toxoplasmosis, in utero transmission can occur even in the presence of maternal antibodies to CMV. Primary maternal infection is usually asymptomatic, or the patient may experience a mononucleosis-like syndrome.[313] Diagnosis of a primary disease during pregnancy is made by documentation of seroconversion or the presence of CMV-specific IgM antibodies.[314] Primary infection during the pregnancy results in a 30% to 40% risk of intrauterine transmission. The gestational age of the fetus has no influence on the rate of transmission, but a primary infection early in pregnancy carries a worse prognosis for the fetus.[131]

The intracranial sonographic findings include microcephaly, hydrocephaly, intracranial calcifications, cerebellar hypoplasia, large cisterna magna, lissencephaly, paraventricular cysts, and ischemic destructive lesions such as porencephaly, hydranencephaly, and polymicrogyria (Fig. 4–51, and 4–61 through 4–63).[315–323] The hallmark sonographic findings in affected fetuses are bilateral periventricular hyperechogenicities (calcifications).[324,325] These "calcifications," or hyperechoic foci, although they can be highly reflective, may not cast an acoustic shadow.[326] The periventricular calcifications are thought to be the result of a necrotizing inflammation of the periventricular area of the lateral ventricles, with subsequent calcification (Fig. 4–61 through 4–63).

A recent report[327] described ring-like areas of periventricular lucency as probably the earliest sonographic findings of congenital CMV prior to the development of subependymal calcifications. The investigators suggested that these lucencies, or hypoechoic areas, may be related to cellular necrosis with

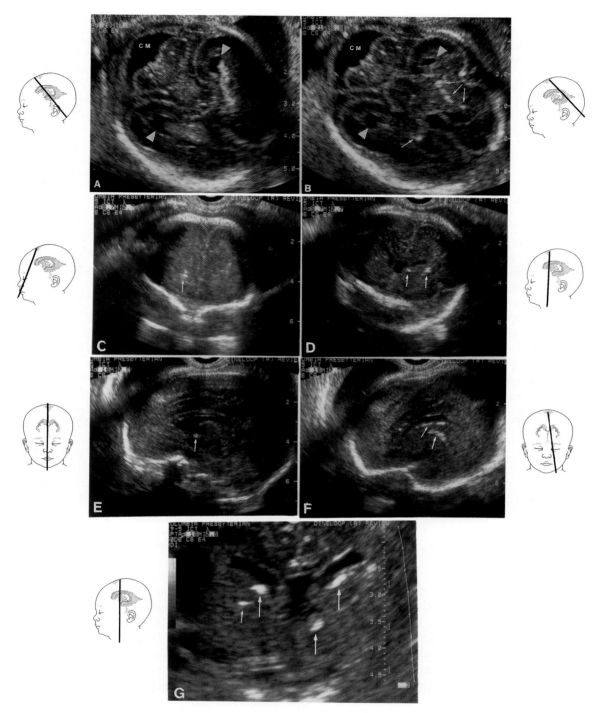

Figure 4–61. Neurosonography of a fetus with cytomegalovirus infection at 20 postmenstrual weeks. **A, B.** Two successive horizontal sections are shown. A prominent cisterna magna is evident (CM). At this gestational age no particular pathology was seen; however, the inferior horns (arrowheads) seem somehow widened. **C.** Frontal–2 section showing one or two hyperechoic foci (arrow), probably consistent with the typical calcifications. **D.** Midcoronal–1 section. The lateral ventricular system and the cavum septi pellucidi seem normal; however, there are two or three small, hyperechoic foci (arrows). **E.** Median section with one hyperechoic focus (arrow). **F.** Oblique–1 paramedian section. The ventricle seems to be outlined by hyperechoic borders (arrows). Some hyperechogenicity is seen in the area of the thalamus. **G.** A close-up view of the ventricular system and the thalami on a Midcoronal–1 section, clearly showing the hyperechoic foci typical of cytomegalovirus infection (arrows).

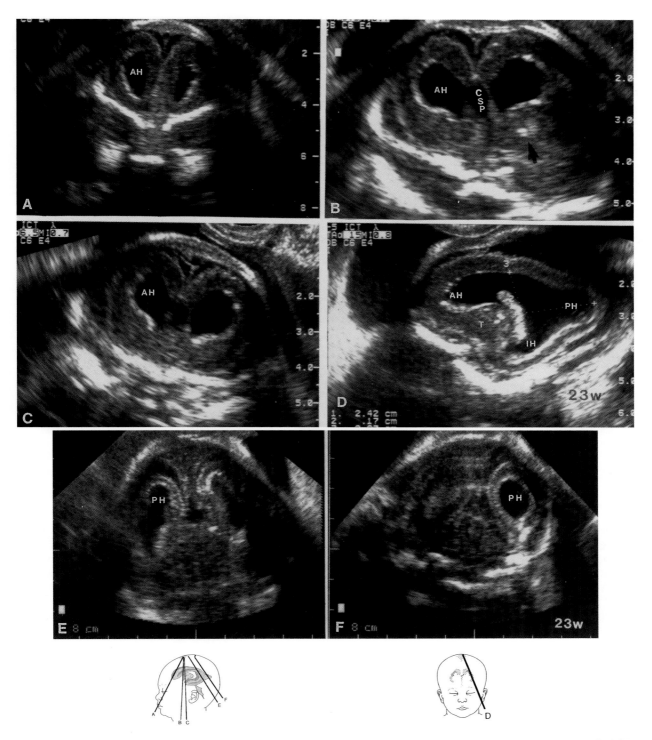

Figure 4–62. Fetus with a cytomegalovirus infection at 23 postmenstrual weeks. **A.** Frontal–2 section. **B, C.** Mid-coronal–1 sections. All three demonstrated the hyperechoic coating of the ependyma lining the anterior horns (AH). The cavum septi pellucidi is slightly dilated (CSP). **D.** Oblique–1 (paramedian) section of the lateral ventricle. Note that on this section not only the anterior horn (AH) and the posterior horn (PH) but also the inferior horn (IH) is seen. This is due to the extreme dilatation of the ventricular system. The flattened, hyperechoic choroid plexus is seen on top of the thalamus (T). **E.** Occipital–1 section. **F.** Occipital–2 sections show the dilated posterior horns (PH). Note that the Occipital–2 section should not contain the tip of the posterior horns; however, due to its extreme dilatation, it "pushes through" and appears on this section.

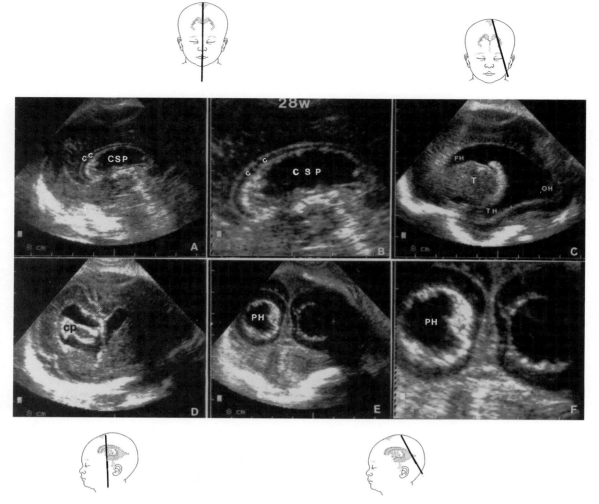

Figure 4–63. The lateral ventricles of a fetal brain infected with cytomegalovirus are shown at 28 postmenstrual weeks. **A, B.** Median sections of the dilated cavum septi pellucidi (CSP), above which the thin corpus callosum (CC) is evident. T, Thalamus. **C.** Paramedian or Oblique–1 section showing the dilated anterior horns (FH), the posterior horns (OH), and the inferior horn (TH). The hyperechoic choroid plexus is on top of the thalamus (T). **D.** Midcoronal–3 section highlighting the dilated lateral ventricles with a hyperechoic choroid plexus (CP). **E, F.** Images of the dilated posterior horns (PH) on Occipital–1 section. Note that on all of the images the ventricular system is lined with an extremely hyperechoic structure of different thickness. This is typical of cytomegalovirus infection. The neonate was tested and the diagnosis was confirmed.

inflammatory edema and/or local blood effusion, which may result from a direct cytopathic effect of CMV on the neuroblasts or on the regional vasculature. Subsequently, the effusions are cleared by the reticuloendothelial system and replaced with glial scarring and dystrophic calcification. The end result is the typical pattern of bilateral periventricular calcifications seen with CMV infection.

In addition, calcifications can be seen in the brain parenchyma, thalami, and basal ganglia. Estroff and colleagues[328] first reported on branching linear echogenic areas in the thalami of a fetus with CMV.

In neonates branching linear echogenic areas in the thalami and the basal ganglia have been reported in association with CMV infection. These branching echogenic structures correspond to arteries in the basal ganglia and the thalamus (Fig. 4–61).[328–329]

Other findings associated with CMV infection include paraventricular cysts and intraventricular synechiae, which represent fetal ventriculitis.[330] Paraventricular cysts are believed to occur as a result of a mechanism similar to that of the calcifications in which there is focal subependymal necrosis and glial reaction.[331] Ischemia of the fetal subependyma with subsequent necrosis and calcification is another proposed mechanism for the damage seen in cases of CMV. This ischemic mechanism may account for the association of CMV with other ischemic destructive lesions, such as porencephaly, hydranencephaly, and polymicrogyria.[320,327,332] In addition, the affinity of CMV to the metabolically active subependymal areas also causes a "predilection" for the germinal matrix area.[333]

In summary, different theories have been proposed in the literature regarding the mechanism of brain injury in cases of in utero CMV. The two more prevalent theories have been recently summarized[334]: (1) due to the special affinity of CMV for the immature cells of the germinal matrix, injury to this zone results in loss of periventricular brain tissue and abnormalities of the cerebral cortex; and (2) placentitis and secondary chronic perfusion insufficiency result in ischemia with subsequent necrosis and calcification.

Intracranial calcifications can be imaged from the second trimester on. The differential diagnosis of intracranial calcifications includes other infectious agents, intracranial teratomas, tuberous sclerosis, Sturge–Weber syndrome, and sagittal or transverse sinus thrombosis.[325,335–337] In addition, linear areas of echogenicity in the basal ganglia and the thalamus have also been associated with trisomies 13 and 21 as well as other injuries to the developing brain.[329,338]

Other non-CNS sonographic findings in fetuses with CMV infection include IUGR (with a reported frequency of 21% to 50%, fetal hepatosplenomegaly, liver calcifications (Fig. 4–64), fetal ascites, and cardiac malformations.[322,339–341]

The prognosis for the infant relates to the severity of the intracranial abnormalities. Affected fe-

tuses are usually born prematurely, and the neonate may exhibit hepatosplenomegaly, jaundice, thrombocytopenia, and chorioretinitis. Approximately 95% of the infants with microcephaly and intracranial calcifications either die or exhibit major neurological sequelae such as developmental delay, seizures, deafness, and motor deficits. Infants with "milder" neurological signs have a better prognosis.[342,343] Those with microcephaly alone have a better neurological outcome comparable to that for patients with only systemic signs of CMV infection.[343,344] It has been found that approximately 50% of infants with systemic signs and no neurological deficits are normal and 16% exhibit major neurological sequelae or die.[342,343]

Prenatal diagnosis of fetal CMV infection relies on a combination of diagnostic tests: sonography may identify fetuses with intracranial calcifications, hydrocephaly, microcephaly, ascites, and IUGR. Tests based on examining the amniotic fluid for either viral culture or a polymerase chain reaction to amplify CMV DNA are reliable for the diagnosis. In a recent publication 12 of 13 cases of affected fetuses were identified using either amniotic fluid culture or polymerase chain reaction for CMV DNA; furthermore, this was compared to their sensitivity in identifying CMV IgM antibody in fetal blood, which was only 69%.[345] This study as well as others concluded that, at present, amniotic fluid studies appear to be the best way to diagnose CMV in utero. In addition, it has been suggested that in cases in which CMV infection was suspected, serial amniocentesis may be necessary before the definitive diagnosis can be reached.

At present, no drug therapy is available to treat fetal CMV infection. Prevention of a primary disease during pregnancy or just prior to conception seems to be the most effective method to avoid fetal CMV.

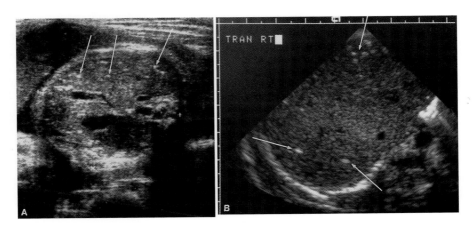

Figure 4–64. The prenatal and postnatal images of the liver, showing the typical hyperechoic lesions of cytomegalovirus *(arrows)*. **A.** The fetal liver. **B.** The neonatal liver.

Toxoplasmosis

Toxoplasmosis is the result of a transplacental infection with the parasite *Toxoplasma gondii.* In humans the most common source of infection is exposure to the domesticated cat or the ingestion or handling of contaminated meat. The reported incidence of congenital toxoplasmosis ranges from 0.5 to 2.0 per 1000 live births.[346-348] In the immunocompetent adult the infection is mild and symptoms, if they do occur, are similar to a mononucleosis-like syndrome.[349] The clinical features of congenital toxoplasmosis include premature delivery, seizures, meningoencephalitis, microcephaly, hydrocephalus, intracranial calcifications, chorioretinitis, hepatosplenomegaly, anemia, petechiae, hyperbilirubinemia, and pneumonitis.[343]

In the life cycle of the parasite, the cat or other animals play an essential role. Within the gastrointestinal tract of the cat, the sexual cycle of the parasite takes place and oocysts are produced, which are then excreted in the feces. Women may become exposed while cleaning the litter box of an infected cat or by handling soil or meat that has been contaminated. The oocytes are then ingested, with subsequent circulation of the parasite in the blood (tachyzoites). The tachyzoites penetrate into tissues, such as muscle and brain, and can be transmitted across the placenta. Fetal infection occurs when the mother has a primary active infection with toxoplasmosis and has circulating tachyzoites. The placenta then becomes infected, and after a lag period there is a subsequent hematogenous spread to the fetus.[350,351]

The risk of fetal infection depends on when during the pregnancy the primary maternal infection took place. The overall risk of transmission to the fetus is approximately 40%.[352] The severity of the disease is also dependent on when in gestation the primary maternal infection takes place. If maternal infection took place during the first and second trimesters, only approximately 20% to 25% of the fetuses will become infected. However, if maternal infection occurred in the third trimester, the risk of fetal infection increases to 65%.[349,353,354] In contrast, the severity of the disease *decreases* with increasing gestational age at the time of infection, the most severe cases of infection developing when the infection occurred early in gestation. The risk of severe manifestation is 75% if infection ensued in the first trimester versus 0% if it occurred in the third trimester.[355] The diagnosis of primary disease is made based on documentation of seroconversion, a marked increase in antibody titers, or the presence of toxoplasmosis-specific IgM. Rarely, a latent infection in an immunocompromised mother may result in a fetal infection.[349]

The intracranial sonographic findings of fetal toxoplasmosis include intracranial calcifications (Fig. 4–65), hydrocephaly, microcephaly, brain atrophy, and hydranencephaly.[356] Hohlfeld and coworkers[357] reported on 89 cases of fetal toxoplasmosis, in 34 of which the pregnancy was electively terminated. In this subgroup the most common brain sonographic finding was hydrocephaly, which was present in 74%, followed by intracranial calcifications, present in 18%. The hydrocephaly was bilateral and symmetrical, evolved very rapidly, and did not result in an increase in BPD.

The intracranial calcifications in fetal toxoplasmosis are multifocal and present in many areas of the brain, such as the basal ganglia, periventricular area, white matter, and cerebral cortex, unlike CMV infection, which has a predilection for the periventricular area of the brain (Fig. 4–65).[356,358] The toxoplasmosis lesions in the brain start as vasculitis, subsequently followed by necrosis and cellular infiltration in the cortex, meninges, white matter, basal ganglia, brain stem, and spinal cord. The necrosis is followed by calcification.[359]

The differential diagnosis of the intracranial calcifications is from other infectious and noninfectious causes, such as CMV, tuberous sclerosis, teratoma, and transverse or sagittal thrombosis.[325,335-337]

Other sonographic findings reported in cases of fetal toxoplasmosis include a thickened placenta

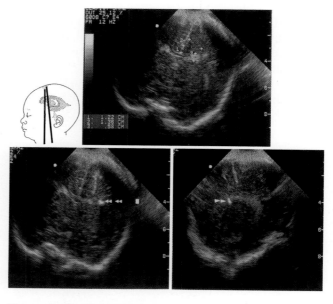

Figure 4–65. Three sections of the fetal brain, demonstrating apparently normal anatomy; however, note several hyperechoic foci in the thalamic area *(arrows).* These are "calcifications" in the nuclei of the midbrain, typical of toxoplasmosis. The diagnosis was confirmed by laboratory tests.

with hyperechoic areas, liver echogenicities, hepatomegaly, ascites, and pericardial or pleural effusion.[357,360,361]

Prenatal diagnosis of fetal toxoplasmosis has relied on sonography, to look for intracranial calcifications and hydrocephaly; amniocentesis, to obtain amniotic fluid for tissue culture, and inoculation of mice; and fetal blood sampling, for the determination of toxoplasmosis-specific IgM. A recent report[362] demonstrated that prenatal diagnosis of toxoplasmosis using a polymerase chain reaction test performed on amniotic fluid is a rapid (results within 24 hours), safe, and accurate means of diagnosing fetal toxoplasmosis. This report went on to state that prenatal diagnosis should not be attempted until at least 4 weeks after the acute disease in the mother, because testing too soon may result in a false-negative test result. In addition, it was suggested that prenatal diagnosis is not warranted if maternal infection occurred within the first 2 weeks of pregnancy, due to the slight risk of infection to the fetus.

Fetal therapy in cases of toxoplasmosis includes treatment of the mother with spiramycin in cases of primary infection during the pregnancy. It is important to start the treatment quickly, before fetal infection can occur. This may be possible, since there is a lag period between the onset of maternal infection and the fetal infection. Once fetal infection has been confirmed (see above), a combination of pyrimethamine, sulfadiazine, and folinic acid is recommended. In the literature there appears to be proof of benefit with this treatment, although pregnancies with severely affected fetuses are more likely to be electively terminated.[350,363–366]

The prognosis for the affected neonate with toxoplasmosis relates to the severity of the neuropathology, which correlates with the clinical syndrome. Only 9% of neonates with severe neurological features are normal on follow-up. The remaining patients suffer from mental retardation, seizures, spastic motor deficits, and severe visual impairment.[353]

Rubella

Congenital rubella syndrome is now a rarity due to the widespread use of immunization. The reported incidence is less than 1 per 1 million live births.[367,368] The clinical syndrome is characterized by cataracts, glaucoma, chorioretinitis, microphthalmus, cardiac malformations, microcephaly, and deafness. Primary maternal disease can be asymptomatic. Maternal viremia results in infection of the placenta, with subsequent infection of the fetus. Infection can occur at any time during pregnancy, but first-trimester infection results in more severely af-

fected infants. Congenital rubella lesions are found in 50% of fetuses affected at 1 month of gestation, 22% of those infected in the second month of gestation, and 7% of those infected between the third and fifth months.[356,369]

Findings include microcephaly, subependymal cysts in the caudate nucleus and striothalamic regions, and echogenic foci in the basal ganglia. The echogenic foci may represent mineralizing vasculitis.[333,370]

Prognosis of the neonate relates to the clinical features. Of those fetuses symptomatic at birth, very few are free of neurological deficits. In a group of 100 infants with congenital rubella syndrome, 81% had microcephaly, 47% had severe neuromotor deficits, 72% had hearing loss, 78% had ocular manifestations, and only 9% appeared to be free of deficits at 18 months of age.[371]

INTRACRANIAL TUMORS

Intracranial tumors occurring during fetal life are rare. Tumors that develop or are diagnosed within the first 2 months after birth represented 0.5% to 1.5% of all tumors detected during childhood.[372] Of the congenital brain tumors, the most common are teratomas, tumors of neuroepithelial tissue or mesenchymal tissues, craniopharyngiomas, and hemangioblastoma (Figs. 4–66 through 4–68).[372,373] Among these tumors, teratomas account for one third to one half of all neonatal tumors.[374] Clinically, the neonate may present with a large head circumference, hydrocephaly, irritability, seizures, or vomiting, among other symptoms. The overall prognosis is poor. Wakai and collaborators[372] found that the 1-year survival rate in infants with congenital intracranial tumors symptomatic at birth is 7%, the rate in those infants with probable congenital tumors symptomatic within the first week is 33.3%, and in those infants with possible congenital tumors that became symptomatic within the first few months of life the rate is 18%.

Teratomas

Teratomas are derived from the three embryonic layers; their pathogenesis is unclear and they are usually histologically benign. In fetuses approximately two thirds of intracranial teratomas are supratentorial.

Prenatal diagnosis of fetal intracranial teratoma has been reported.[375–385] The sonographic appearance of the fetal intracranial teratoma is that of an irregular solid, cystic echogenic mass with calcifications distorting the normal appearance of the fetal brain. Midline structures may not be identifiable.

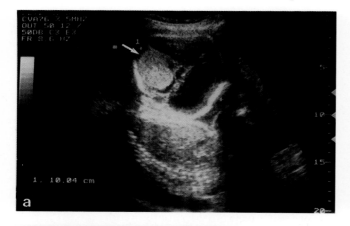

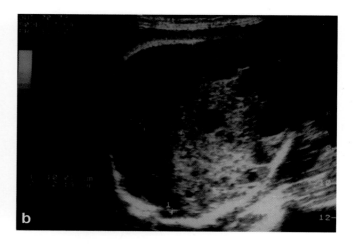

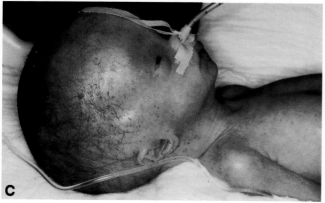

Figure 4–66. This is a fetal intracranial teratoma diagnosed prenatally at 28 postmenstrual weeks. **A.** The tumor *(arrow)* originated in the area of the sella turcica and occupied most of the left hemisphere displacing the right hemispheric structures. **B.** The head circumference of the fetus was 37 cm and the BPD was 11 cm. **C.** The neonate expired shortly after birth. The pathological report was consistent with a teratoma with neuroepithelial structures. *(Courtesy of Dr. Péter, Bödecs, Györ, Hungary).*

Other CNS findings include hydrocephaly, and increased BPD and head circumference may be present (Fig. 4–66). Kuller's group[385] reported on a case in which there was severe distortion of the fetal facies, probably as a result of the tumor. In their case the fetus had hypertelorism, a rudimentary left eye, asymmetrical orbits, and a large cleft lip and cleft palate. Polyhydramnios has been reported in over 50% of the cases. In addition, fetal hydrops with high-output cardiac failure has been described.[386] The differential diagnosis of intracranial teratomas includes hydrocephalus, hydranencephaly, porencephaly, and holoprosencephaly.

The prognosis for the neonate with an intracranial teratoma is extremely poor, with a perinatal mortality rate approaching 100%. Neonatal death usually occurs within the first few days of life,[387] although rare prolonged survivals have been described.[383,384,388] Ferreira and associates[384] reported a prolonged survival of up to 18 months. In utero diagnosis was made on the basis of ventriculomegaly, large echogenic mass with calcifications, and distortion of the normal architecture of the brain. Although the infant had survived to 18 months at the time of the case report, the neurological condition of the infant was described as compatible with quadri-

paresis with truncal hypotonia, hyperreflexia, and cortical blindness with hyperreflexia. In addition, the infant was reported as severely developmentally delayed and profoundly retarded. In contrast, Ulreich and colleagues[388] also reported prolonged survival of an infant with an intracranial teratoma diagnosed in utero. At the time of the case report, the child was 3½ years old, had had the tumor resected at 7 days of life, and neurologically was reported as having little neurological deficit (complete third nerve palsy or difficulty with speech development). In the latter case there was no ventriculomegaly, the brain lesion was well demarcated, and normal anatomic structures were identified within the head at the time of the in utero diagnosis. In summary, the prognosis for the neonate with an intracranial teratoma seems to depend on the size of the tumor, the extent of normal brain destruction, and the degree of hydrocephaly. Large tumors with little, if any, normal brain tissue and severe hydrocephaly carry a poor prognosis for the fetus or neonate.

Fetus-in-fetu

An extremely rare congenital condition *fetus-in-fetu* has been described as presenting as a mass. The mass may be present intracranially, intraabdomi-

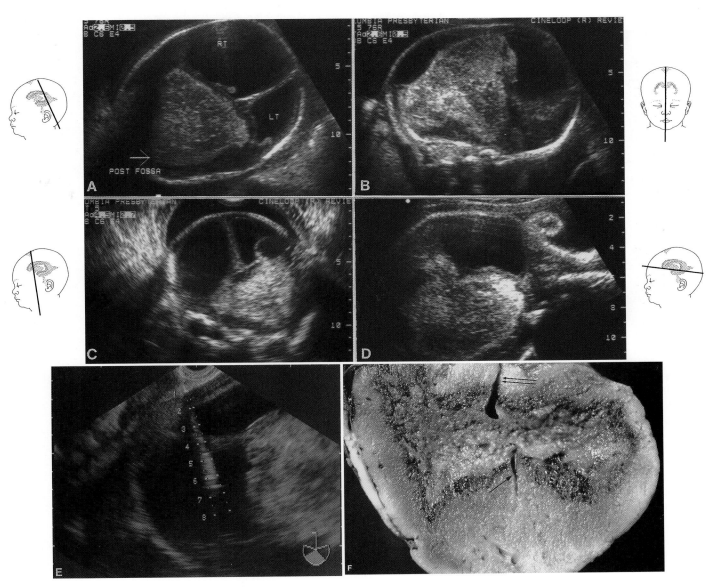

Figure 4–67. Four views of the brain of a fetus at 34 postmenstrual weeks having a tumor of the brain. **A.** Midcoronal–3, almost Occipital–1, section, showing the dilated right and left lateral ventricles, the thin and dangling hyperechoic choroid plexus, and the extremely thin posterior fossa *(arrow).* **B.** Median section showing the extent of the tumor in the midline, above and behind which the dilated ventricles are seen. **C.** Midcoronal–1 section. **D.** Horizontal section. After the diagnosis of the space-occupying lesion in the brain, causing severe obstructive hydrocephalus, it was decided that the patient's labor would be induced. Cephalocentesis, to decrease the size of the head by draining cerebrospinal fluid, was performed. **E.** The needle is seen in the fluid at a depth of 6.5 cm. The head circumference decreased from 40 cm to enable vaginal birth, which was achieved after inducing labor. **F.** The stillborn neonate was examined by the pathologist. The *arrow* indicates the third ventricle, and the *double arrow* indicates the longitudinal sulcus. Histological examination of the tumor revealed a glioblastoma. *(Courtesy of Susan Stavgaitis, MD, PhD, Division of Neuropathology Columbia–Presbyterian Medical Center, New York.)*

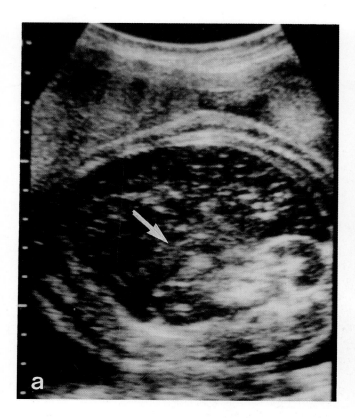

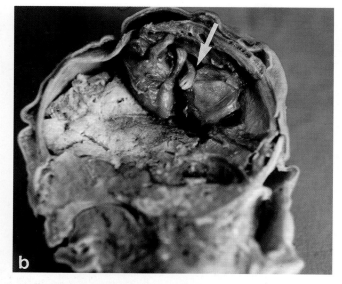

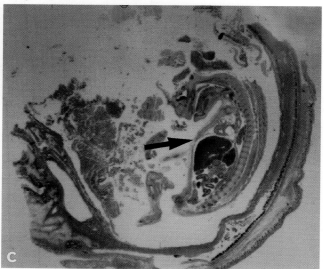

Figure 4–68. A very rare case of a true intracranial fetus-in-fetu that presented at 17 weeks with an intracranial mass. Upon closer inspection, the mass had the sonographic appearance of a fetus. **A.** Transabdominal scan at 17 weeks showing intracranial mass *(arrow)*. Patient elected to terminate the pregnancy. **B.** Picture of the gross specimen showing the well-formed fetus *(arrow)* within the cranial cavity pushing the brain to one side. **C.** Histology demonstrated a well-formed fetal vertebral column. *(Courtesy of Prof. A. Ianniruberto, Italy.)*

nally, retroperitoneally or in the scrotum. The exact relationship between teratome and fetus-in-fetus is controversial.[389–394] Some feel that this might in fact be two edges of the same entity, namely a teratoma.[390] However, it has been stated that to distinguish between fetus-in-fetus from a teratoma the vertebral column must be present.[395]

Choroid Plexus Papilloma

Choroid plexus papilloma is a rare, benign tumor of the choroid plexus.[396,397] The tumor may occur anywhere the choroid plexus is present, but most commonly is unilateral and located in the atria of the lateral ventricle. Polyhydramnios and communicating hydrocephaly are usually present. *Hydrocephaly* may result from an overproduction of CSF by the choroid plexus or an obstruction to the flow caused by the mass.[398–401] The sonographic appearance is that of a large, lobulated, highly echogenic mass within the lateral ventricle. Transvaginal sonography can further characterize the mass as well as demonstrate the papillary nature of the tumor (Fig. 4–69).

PORENCEPHALY, HYDRANENCEPHALY AND PERIVENTRICULAR LEUKOMALACIA

Porencephaly and *hydranencephaly* refer to partial or subtotal defects of the cerebral hemispheres resulting from a fetal or neonatal insult such as ischemia, hemorrhage, infection, or trauma occurring between the second trimester and the early postna-

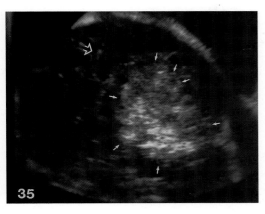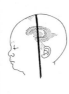

Figure 4–69. Midcoronal–2 section of the fetal brain at 35 postmenstrual weeks. A large, hyperechoic, lobulated mass *(small arrows)* within the left lateral ventricle is seen. The falx *(open arrow)* is displaced to the right. One week later, progressing obstructive ventriculomegaly was seen in both lateral ventricles. A stillborn infant was delivered, and autopsy was declined by the family. By its appearance, location, and fast growth, the presumptive diagnosis of choroid plexus tumor was made. *(From Monteagudo and colleagues, Transvaginal sonography of the fetal brain. In: Timor-Tritsch IE, Rottem S (eds). Transvaginal Sonography. New York: Chapman & Hall, 1991, pp 393–425).*

tal period.[402] Volpe[402] uses the term *porencephaly* in cases in which a single unilateral cavity is present within the hemisphere which may or may not communicate with the ventricles and *hydranencephaly* when there are massive bilateral lesions, in which most of the cerebral hemispheres has been reduced to a CSF-filled sac. Most of the cases are sporadic. As previously mentioned, the pathogenesis of hydranencephaly and porencephaly results from insults to the brain as early as the second trimester. There are several factors determining the propensity of the immature brain to undergo dissolution and, eventually, cavitation: (1) the high water content of the unmyelinated brain, (2) the relative paucity of myelinated fibers, and (3) deficient glial response. The first two factors result in dissolution of the brain, while the latter is responsible for cavitation.[402]

The sonographic findings of porencephaly and hydranencephaly include a normocephalic or macrocephaly fetus with a large, fluid-filled intracranial cavity. Several reports on the in utero evolution of hydranencephaly resulting from an intracranial hemorrhage exist in the literature.[403,404] The usual presentation is the finding of a bright, homogeneous, hyperechoic mass, most consistent with an intracranial hemorrhage. As the cases are followed prospectively with serial sonography, the echo-dense mass becomes more sonolucent with the development of the hydranencephaly. No cerebral cortex is present,

but there is partial preservation of portions of the occipital lobe. The falx cerebri is usually intact. The midbrain and the basal ganglia are variably preserved. The brain stem and the cerebellum are usually intact.[403] Polyhydramnios is usually present.

The differential diagnosis of hydranencephaly is massive hydrocephaly or alobar holoprosencephaly. Holoprosencephaly can be differentiated from hydranencephaly in that the thalami are never fused in hydranencephaly. In hydrocephaly all parts of the ventricular system become dilated, but in hydranencephaly the third ventricle is present and visible but is not enlarged.[405] Belfar and collaborators[406] have reported on a case of evolving hydranencephaly in which the differential diagnosis included a fetal teratoma. In their case the sonographic appearance was that of abnormal conglomeration of disorganized tissue replacing both cerebral hemispheres. Hydranencephaly has been associated with several syndromes (e.g., familial hydranencephaly [autosomal recessive]) and with trisomy 13.[218]

The sonographic appearance of porencephaly is that of a cystic lesion that communicates with the lateral ventricle (Fig. 4–70). The ipsilateral ventricle is dilated. The porencephalic cyst never causes a mass effect, which helps differentiate it from arachnoid and interhemispheric cysts.[405] A recent report[407] documented a prenatally detected case of porencephaly at 28 weeks following inadvertent penetration of the fetal skull during an amniocentesis unguided by continuous ultrasonography at 16 weeks. Initially, the head ultrasonographic examination was normal, but at 28 weeks at left-sided ventriculomegaly and an anechoic mass in the area of the lateral ventricle were noted and confirmed at birth by computed tomography and MRI studies.

The prognosis for children with hydranencephaly is poor.

Periventricular leukomalacia (PVL) is an ischemic lesion of the periventricular white matter. This is a relatively frequent finding in brain scans of premature infants. However, is very rarely seen during a fetal brain scan. Clinically, in neonates, the most common presentation of PVL is spastic diplegia, which is common form of cerebral palsy with nonprogressive but permanent impairment of movement and posture. In addition these infants may have prominent intellectual deficits.[408,409] Periventricular leukomalacia has been reported in fetuses.[410–413] The most common location of periventricular leukomalacia is in the optic radiation at the trigone of the lateral ventricle and/or in the cerebral white matter just lateral to the anterior horns (Figs. 4–71 through 4–73) (see also Chapter 16).

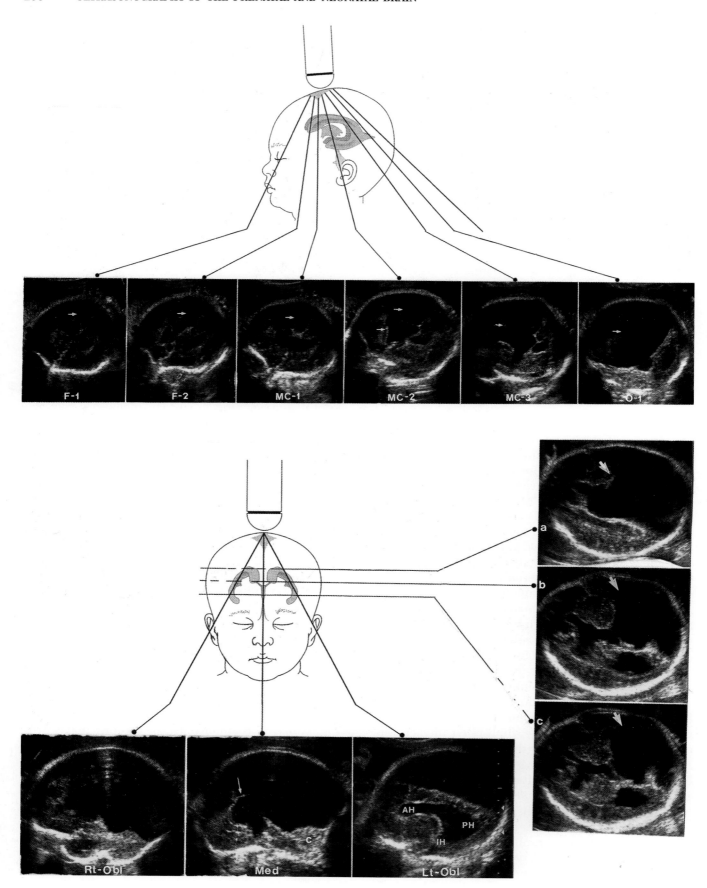

Figure 4–70. Porencephalic cyst at 32 postmenstrual weeks. **A.** Serial coronal sections from Frontal–1 to Occipital–1. Frontal–1 and Frontal–2 (F–1 and F–2): shows minimal dilatation of the lateral ventricles. To the left of the interhemispheric fissure and just below the cranial vault, a sonolucent cystic (porencephalic cyst) structure is imaged. Midcoronal–1, –2, and –3 (MC–1, MC–2, and MC–3) shows that the cyst extends all the way to the to the lateral ventricles and in MC–3 is seen to be continuous with the cavity of the lateral ventricles. Please note that no midline structures namely the corpus callosum and the cavum septum pellucidi are seen. Occipital–1 just almost no normal brain present in the left hemisphere and there is hydrocephaly of the right lateral ventricle. **B.** Consists of a Median (Med) and right and left oblique–1 (Rt–1 and Lt–1) sections as well as a series of axial sections. The left Oblique–1 (Lt Obl–1) shows the extent of the destruction of the brain. Essentially most of this left hemisphere is now part of the porencephalic cyst. Median (Med) section demonstrates that most of the corpus callosum has been destroyed, however, there seems to be a small part of genu of the corpus callosum present *(arrow)*. Note that the porencephalic cyst extends all the way to the tentorium of the cerebellum. Right Oblique–1 (Rt Obl–1) shows the right ventricle with mild to moderate hydrocephaly. Axial sections a–c. *a* axial section above the level of the lateral ventricles showing the cyst which extends to the cranial vault. *b* and *c* also shows the lateral ventricle as well as the missing cavum septi pellucidi. The dilated right ventricle is seen *(arrow)*. After the delivery of this very affected infant, the mother was diagnosed as having sickle cell disease as well as being HIV positive.

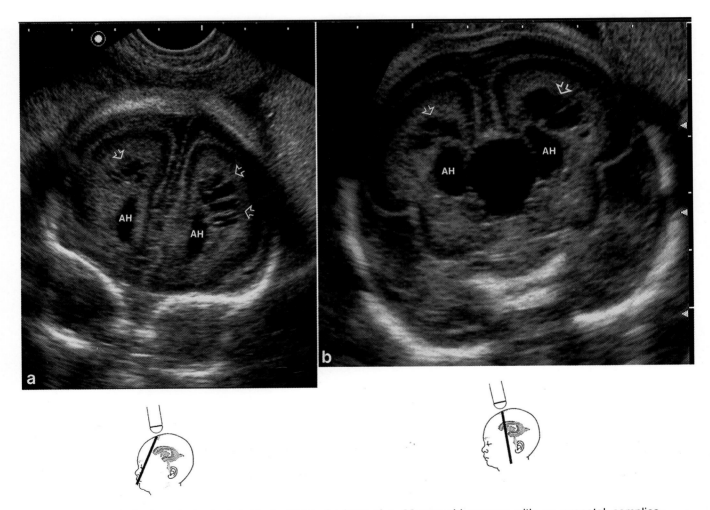

Figure 4–71. Periventricular leukomalacia (PVL) of a fetus of a 33-year-old woman with no prenatal complications. **A** through **D.** Transvaginal brain scans of the fetus at 27 postmenstrual weeks, 1 day. **A** is a Frontal–2 (F–2) showing the anterior horns (AH) of the lateral ventricles. Lateral to the anterior horns there is a cystic lesion noted *(arrows)*. This cystic area is consistent with PVL. **B.** Midcoronal–1 (MC–1) sections showing the cavum septi pellucidi as well as the anterior horns and the area of the PVL *(arrows)*.

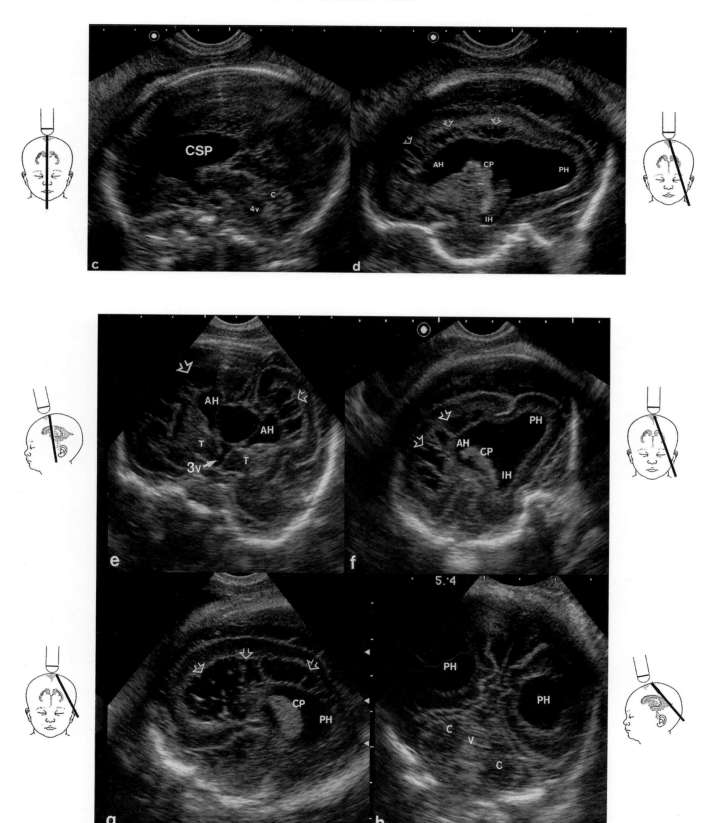

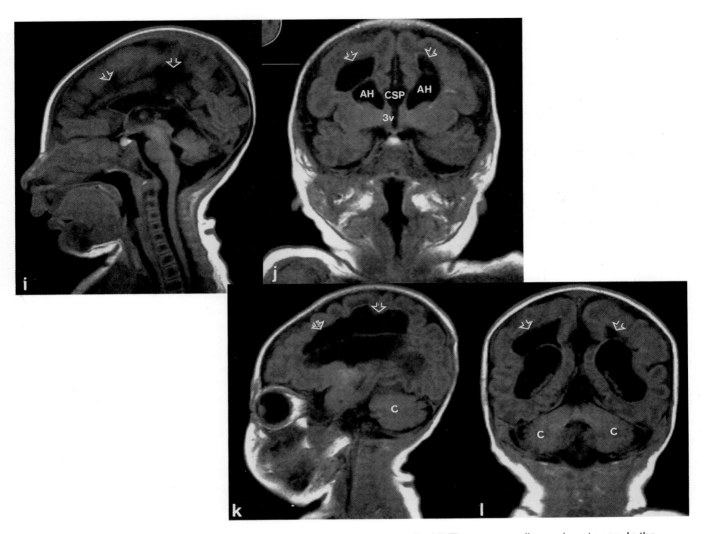

Figure 4–71. C. Median section showing a prominent cavum septi pellucidi. The corpus callosum is not seen. In the posterior fossa the fourth ventricle is seen as a triangular structure in front of the cerebellum. **D.** Oblique–1 (obl–1) section showing mild to moderate dilatation of the lateral ventricle. In addition superior to the ventricle in the periventricular area the extent of the periventricular leukomalacia is seen as a cystic area. **E** through **H** is the same fetus at 29 postmenstrual weeks, 5 days. **E.** Midcoronal–2 (MC–2) section showing the PVL *(arrows)* lateral to the anterior horns. The third ventricle is seen and appears to be dilated. **F.** Oblique–1 (Obl–1) section showing the three parts of the lateral ventricle. The choroid plexus appears to be dysmorphic and under real-time sonography, it was found to be freely dangling within the ventricular cavity. The extent of the area of periventricular leukomalacia (PVL) is seen paralleling the upper surface of the lateral ventricle. **G** is slightly more lateral than the section shown on **F.** The region of the PVL is seen extending superior from the anterior horns reaching almost to the tip of the posterior horns. **H.** Occipital–1 (O–1) section showing the normal round sonolucent appearance of the posterior horns of the lateral ventricle. The cerebellum and vermis are seen in the posterior fossa. The patient underwent a cesarean section at 38 weeks for a 2524 grams female fetus with Apgar scores of 8 (1 minute) and 9 (5 minutes). **I** through **L** are images of the neonatal MRI. **G** is a median section showing the area of PVL *(arrow).* **H** is a coronal section. The area of PVL *(arrow)* is seen lateral to the anterior horns of the lateral ventricle. Note how well the fetal scan shown on **E** compares to this MRI picture. **I** is a parasagittal image comparable to **F** demonstrating the extent of the PVL *(arrow).* **J** is a posterior coronal section comparable to **E.** The posterior horns with the area of PVL *(arrow)* is seen superior and lateral to these horns. In the posterior fossa the cerebellum is seen. At the time of this writing, the infant is 10 months old and cannot sit down by herself. She has no seizures and takes no medications. However, she receives daily physical therapy. AH, anterior horn; PH, posterior horn; IH, inferior horn; C, cerebellum; V, vermis; 4V, fourth ventricle; CSP, cavum septi pellucidi; 3V, third ventricle; T, thalamus. *(Courtesy of Professor Ritsuko Pooh, Japan)*

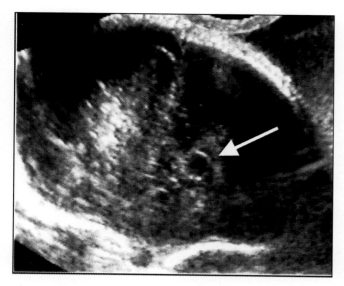

Figure 4–72. Coronal view of a fetus at 30 postmenstrual weeks with a cystic brain lesion. The arrow points to a small cystic area in the region of the caudate nucleus. This most likely represents an area of ischemia, possibly periventricular leukomalacia. This was the only ultrasound finding in this fetus. A week later the fetus expired in utero. The postmortem examination was not demonstrative due to maceration of the fetus. However, the mother was diagnosed as having homocystinuria *(Courtesy of Professor Gad Malinger, Israel).*

IN UTERO INTRACRANIAL HEMORRHAGE

Subdural hematomas, periventricular, and cerebellar hemorrhages have been diagnosed in utero. These entities, although commonly diagnosed in the preterm neonate (see Chapter 12), rarely occur in utero. Possible causes of in utero intracranial hemorrhage described in the literature include trauma, hypoxia, infection, congenital vascular defects, blood dyscrasia, ingestion of drugs, maternal complications of pregnancy (pre-eclampsia, abruptio placenta, and seizure), thrombosis of the umbilical cord, umbilical cord entanglement, and alloimmune thrombocytopenia.[410,414–420] Hydrocephaly is commonly associated with intracranial hemorrhage.[421] Hydrocephaly results from blockage of the CSF and/or obliterative arachnoiditis. Nonimmune hydrops has also been reported with in utero intracranial hemorrhage as a result of fetal anemia due to significant intracranial blood loss.[422]

Periventricular Hemorrhage

The incidence of periventricular hemorrhage in utero is unknown. Papile and coworkers[423] classified intracranial hemorrhage of the neonate into four grades (see Chapter 12). These grades can be applied equally to the fetus. *Grade I* is a germinal ma-

trix hemorrhage or a hemorrhage that is confined to the subependymal area of the brain. *Grade II* is an intraventricular hemorrhage, but there is no associated hydrocephalus. *Grade III* is an intraventricular hemorrhage with ventricular dilatation. *Grade IV* is an intraventricular hemorrhage with parenchymal hemorrhage and hydrocephaly. The sonographic appearance of the blood is brightly echogenic; therefore, whether the blood is located within the ventricle or the brain parenchyma, the hemorrhage can be diagnosed in utero (Figs. 4–74 through 4–77).

The end result of intraparenchymal hemorrhage is porencephaly. The size of the original hemorrhage correlates with the size of the porencephalic cyst. Grant[424] has described the progression of an intraparenchymal hemorrhage to a porencephalic cyst. The initial sonographic appearance of an intraparenchymal hemorrhage is homogeneous and brightly echogenic. Over a period of a few days to 2 weeks, the inner portions of the hematoma become hypoechoic (during the process of liquefaction), while the outer border remains echogenic and becomes sharply demarcated from the surrounding parenchyma. Subsequently, the clot undergoes retraction and becomes progressively smaller. As the clot retracts, the developing porencephalic cyst becomes evident (Fig. 4–74 and 4–75).

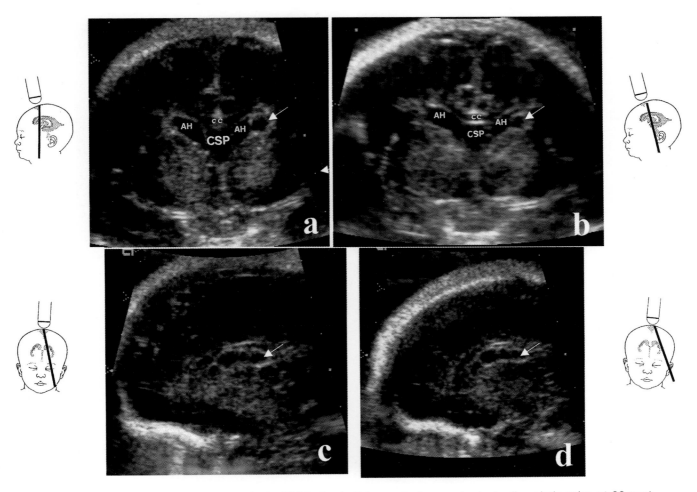

Figure 4–73. Periventricular leukomalacia (PVL) of twin B in a set of monochorionic diamniotic twins at 32 post-menstrual weeks. **A.** Midcoronal–1 (MC–1) showing a small cystic area consistent with PVL lateral to the anterior horn of the lateral ventricle *(arrow)* **B.** Midcoronal–2 (MC–2) is slightly more posterior coronal section showing the area of the PVL *(arrow)*. **C** and **D** are two views of Oblique–1 (Obl–1) sections showing the extent of the PVL *(arrows)*. This area is just above the lateral ventricle at the level of the germinal matrix region. AH, anterior horn; CSP, cavum septi pellucidi; CC, corpus callosum.

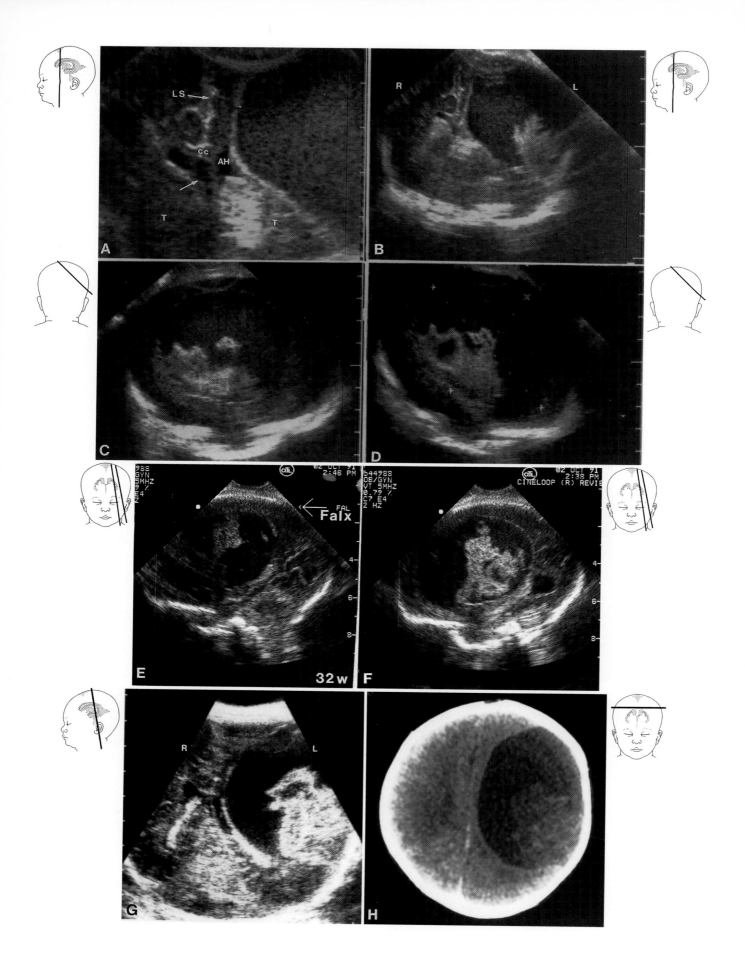

Figure 4–74. Fetus with a left-sided intraparenchymal hemorrhage resulting from alloimmune thrombocytopenia (32 postmenstrual weeks). **A.** Midcoronal–1 section. The normal longitudinal sulcus (LS), corpus callosum (CC), anterior horns (AH), and cavum septi pellucidi *(small arrow)* are shown. On the left side of the brain, a large structure is shown to slightly distort the left anterior horn. Its consistency is of low-level echogenicity, probably an old hemorrhage. Below it, the hyperechoic structure is seen around the area of the thalamus (T), which may be consistent with a recent hemorrhage. **B.** Panoramic picture of the same lesion, shown situated in the left hemisphere. **C, D.** Additional views of the encapsulated hemorrhage, having liquid and partly slightly hyperechoic structures (clots?). **E, F.** Sections in the sagittal plane, showing the anteriorly located lesion. A cesarean section was performed, and the neonatal sonogram confirmed the diagnosis **(G).** A computed tomogram was also performed **(H),** showing the same size and location of the hemorrhage. The infant died 48 hours after delivery.

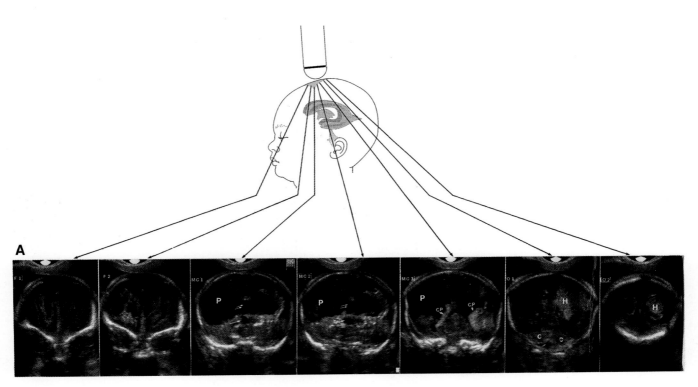

Figure 4–75. Brain neuroscan of a fetus at 23 postmenstrual weeks and 1 day. **A.** Serial coronal sections showing a porencephalic (P) cyst most likely the result of a previous intracranial hemorrhage undergoing resolution. The *double arrows* point to the cavum septi pellucidi and the *single arrow* to the third ventricle. In O–1 and O–2 (Occipital–1 and Occipital–2), a hyperechoic area is seen. This represents a recent hemorrhage (H).

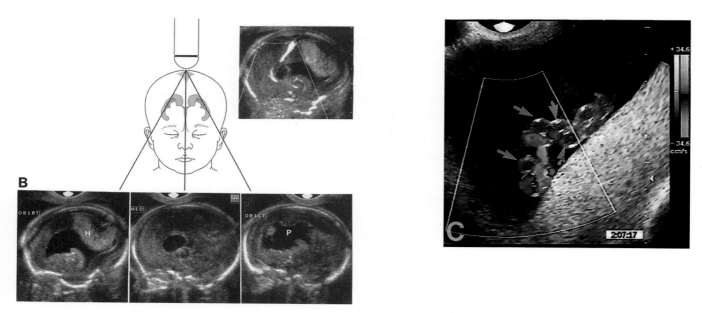

Figure 4–75. B. Serial sagittal sections. OB–1RT is right Oblique–1 in which the extent of the intraparenchymeal hemorrhage can be appreciated. Med is a median section showing a prominent cavum septi pellucidi. OB–1 LT is a left Oblique–1 showing the porencephalic cyst. **C.** Color Doppler of the umbilical cord demonstrates one vessel with no flow most likely the result of thrombosis.

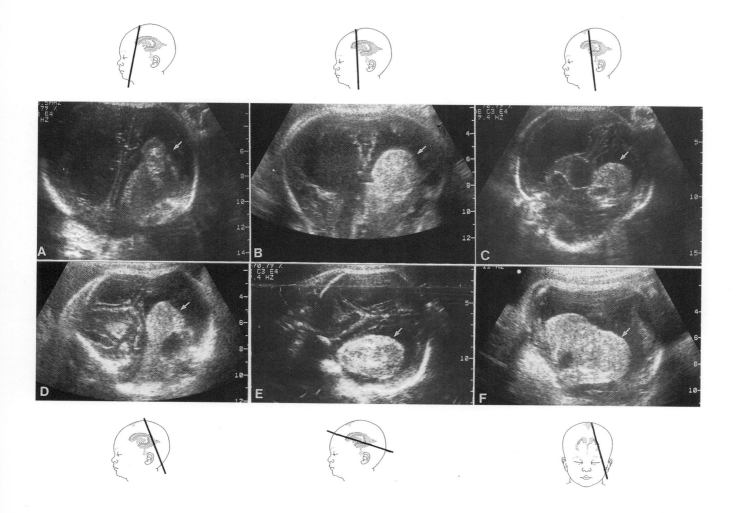

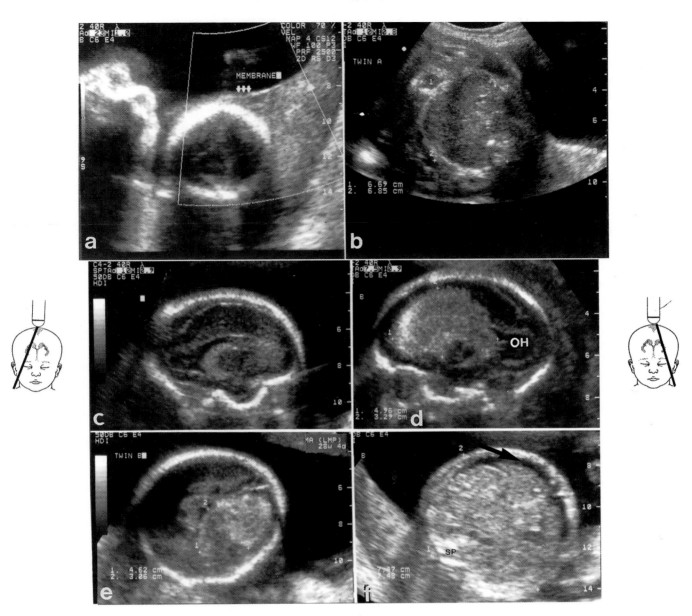

Figure 4–77. Monochorionic-diamniotic twin pregnancy at 28 postmenstrual weeks and 4 days with twin-to-twin transfusion syndrome. Twin A **(A** and **B)** the donor twin had severe oligohydramnios. Twin B **(C** through **F)** the recipient twin with polyhydramnios, ascites, and intracranial hemorrhage. **C.** Right Oblique–1 (Obl–1) showing a normal configuration of the right lateral ventricle with no hydrocephaly. **D.** Left Oblique–1 (Olb–1) section showing a large hyperechoic area measuring 4.9 × 3.3. cm. This hyperechoic area represents a large intracranial hemorrhage. The posterior horns (OH) appear normal. **E.** Axial section demonstrating the intracranial hemorrhage (between the calipers), which measures 4.6 × 3.1 cm and involves most of the right hemispheres of the fetal brain. **F.** Transverse view of the fetal abdomen showing the ascites *(arrow).* This pregnancy was delivered by emergency cesarean section and immediately after birth, twin B died. Sp, spine.

Figure 4–76. Transabdominal sonographic views of an intraventricular hemorrhage within the left lateral ventricle of a fetus at 36 postmenstrual weeks in one of a pair of monochorionic, diamniotic twins. **A.** Frontal–2 section showing the bilateral ventriculomegaly and the left-sided intraventricular hyperechoic clot. **B.** Midcoronal–1 section showing the dilated ventricles and the hyperechoic clot *(arrow).* **C.** Midcoronal–2 through the thalamus and the dilated third ventricle. **D.** Occipital–1 section showing dilated ventricles, with the clot on the left side above the tentorium and the normal-appearing posterior fossa. **E.** Horizontal section highlighting the clot. **F.** Left Oblique–1 section through the entire clot. The fetus died in the uterus several days later.

The outcome of fetal periventricular hemorrhage is unknown. Achiron and associates[410] reported on five cases of intracranial hemorrhage diagnosed in utero. Of the five affected fetuses, one was stillborn and two died after birth. Two were reported to be developing normally at 12 and 18 months of life, respectively. In the neonate the neurodevelopmental delay is related to the severity of the hemorrhage, but even in cases with grades III and IV, approximately 45% have a normal outcome.[424]

Cerebellar Hemorrhage

Prenatal diagnosis of cerebellar hemorrhage has been reported.[415,425] The incidence of this condition is unknown, but in preterm infants the problem has been reported to occur in up to 21% of neonates at autopsy.[426] The sonographic appearance is that of a large, echogenic mass in the area of the cerebellum. In fetuses, as in neonates, blood appears highly echogenic; the echogenicity is comparable to that of the normal choroid plexus. In addition, ventriculomegaly or frank hydrocephaly has also been present in the reported cases.

The differential diagnosis of a cerebellar hemorrhage is from a tumor, although blood, regardless of the site, always retains its highly echogenic appearance.

The prognosis for the fetus with a significant cerebellar hemorrhage appears to be dismal. In the case reported by Jennette's group,[415] the infant died at age 46 hours, despite supportive treatment, and in the case reported by Hadi and collaborators[375] the infant died at the age of 18 hours.

Subdural Hemorrhage

In the neonate, the incidence of subdural hemorrhage has been reported to range between 3% and 18%. Most of these subdural hematomas in the neonate are related to trauma during the perinatal period.[427] In fetuses it is a rare condition with an unknown frequency, although it has been reported using prenatal sonography. Fetal subdural hematomas have been reported to occur as a result of trauma (e.g., the result of a motor vehicle accident), maternal drug ingestion (e.g., warfarin), maternal medical complication of pregnancy (e.g., pancreatitis), a coagulation factor deficiency (e.g., factor X), or unknown etiology.[427–432]

The sonographic appearance is that of extracerebral fluid collection with compression of the cortical surfaces. Ben-Chetrit and associates[427] performed Doppler velocimetry studies on a patient with a fetal subdural hematoma and found that the middle cerebral artery had a high-resistance pattern with reverse end-diastolic flow. Other sonographic findings described with fetal subdural hematoma include hydrocephaly, polyhydramnios, and fetal hydrops.

The outcome for neonates with in utero diagnosis of subdural hematoma has ranged from in utero fetal death to survival with no gross neurodevelopmental abnormalities.[427–431]

SUMMARY

We believe that a meaningful brain scan of the fetus must be an integral part of a targeted structural evaluation in every case. To achieve this "diagnostic-quality" neuroscan of the fetal brain, it is no longer enough to use the customary axial plane permissible by transabdominal sonography, but the added planes afforded by transvaginal transfontanelle scanning are useful to effectively complement the abdominal scan.

There is greater pressure at this time for a better, faster, and more accurate diagnosis using modern machines operated by better-trained and skillful operators. The time when a simple four-chamber view for the heart anomaly workup was sufficient is long gone. The right and left outflow tracts, aortic arch, crossing of the great vessels, and inflows feeding the atria can, are, and should be scanned to minimize missed pathology. Similarly, the time of the gold standard axial "BPD plane" offering a glimpse into the fetal brain is gone, and this practice should be abandoned.

Additional sections in the sagittal and coronal planes, using a high-frequency transvaginal probe, should be added to the axial scan, in order to be able to call such an evaluation a fetal neuroscan. Optimally, this should take place between 15 and 22 postmenstrual weeks to enable the performance of a transvaginal scan, since at this age fetuses easily change their presenting part, at times even doing so during the scanning session.

Finding brain anomalies and correctly diagnosing them has two major prerequisites: to look for them and to understand them. Prenatal detection of brain pathology will enable meaningful counseling and, at times, early and successful management of the patient and the fetus.

Finally, serious consideration should be given to a relatively new imaging modality of the fetal brain namely three dimensional sonography. This scanning technique is currently being actively researched and literature supporting its use is being generated (see Chapter 9). We feel that three-dimensional neuro imaging will become widely used in the not-so-far future.

REFERENCES

1. Richards DS, Seeds JW, Katz VL, et al. Elevated maternal serum alpha-protein with a normal ultrasound: Is amniocentesis always appropriate? A review of 26,069 screened patients. *Obstet Gynecol.* 1988;1:203–207.
2. Limb J, Holmes LB. Anencephaly: Changes in prenatal detection and birth status, 1972 through 1990. *Am J Obstet Gynecol.* 1994;170:1333–1338.
3. Lennon CA, Gray DL. Sensitivity and specificity of ultrasound for the detection of neural tube and ventral wall defects in a high-risk population. *Obstet Gynecol.* 1999;94:562–566.
4. Reichler A, Hume RF, Drugan A, et al. Risk of anomalies as a function of level of elevated maternal serum α-fetoprotein. *Am J Obstet Gynecol.* 1994;171:1052–1055.
5. Haddow JE. Prenatal screening for open neural tube defects, Down's syndrome, and other major fetal disorders. *Semin Perinatol.* 1990;14:488–503.
6. American College of Obstetricians and Gynecologists (ACOG). *Alpha-fetoprotein.* Washington, DC: ACOG; 1991. ACOG technical bulletin 154.
7. Bock JL. Current issues in maternal serum alpha-fetoprotein screening. *Am J Clin Pathol.* 1992;97:541–554.
8. Burton BK. Elevated maternal serum alpha-fetoprotein (MSAFP): Interpretation and follow-up. *Clin Obstet Gynecol.* 1988;31:293–305.
9. O'Rahilly R, Müller F. *The Embryonic Human Brain: An Atlas of Developmental Stages.* New York: Wiley–Liss; 1994.
10. Volpe JJ. *Neuronal Proliferation, Migration, Organization and Myelination* (3rd ed) Philadelphia; WB Saunders *Neurology of the Newborn* 1995:3–42.
11. Carter CO, Evans KA, Till K. Spinal dysraphism: Genetic relation to neural tube malformations. *J Med Genet.* 1976;13:343–350.
12. American Academy of Pediatrics. Committee on Genetics. Folic acid for the prevention of neural tube defects. *Pediatrics.* 1999;104:325–327.
13. Bower C, Stanley FJ. Dietary folate as a risk factor for neural tube defects: Evidence from a case control study in western Australia. *Med J Aust.* 1989;150:163–169.
14. Werler MM, Shapiro S, Mitchell AA. Periconceptional folic acid exposure and risk of occurrent neural tube defects. *JAMA.* 1993;269:1257–1261.
15. Milunsky A, Jick H, Jick SS, et al. Multivitamin/folic acid supplementation in early pregnancy reduces the prevalence of neural tube defects. *JAMA.* 1989;262:2847–2852.
16. Centers for Disease Control. Recommendations for the use of folic acid to reduce the number of cases of spina bifida and other neural tube defects. *MMWR.* 1992;42:34.
17. American Academy of Pediatrics. Committee on Genetics. Folic acid for the prevention of neural tube defects. *Pediatrics* 1999;104:325–327.
18. Centers for Disease Control and Prevention. Recommendations for the use of folic acid to reduce the number of cases of spina bifida and other neural tube defects. *MMWR.* 1992;41:1–8.
19. MRC Vitamin Study research group. Prevention of neural tube defects: Results of the Medical Research Council Vitamin Study. *Lancet.* 1991;338:131.
20. American Academy of Pediatrics. Committee on Genetics. Folic acid for the prevention of neural tube defects. *Pediatrics* 1999;104:325–327.
21. MRC Vitamin Study Research Group. Prevention of neural tube defects: results of the Medical Research Council vitamin study. *Lancet.* 1991;338:131–137.
22. Kadir RA, Sabin C, Whitlow B, Brockbank E, Economides D. Neural tube defects and periconceptional folic acid in England and Wales: Retrospective study. *BMJ.* 1999;319(7202):92–93.
23. Bekkers RL, Eskes TK. Periconceptional folic acid intake in Nijmegen, Netherlands [letter] [see comments]. *Lancet.* 1999;353(9149):292.
24. Cunningham ME, Walls WJ. Ultrasound in the evaluation of anencephaly. *Radiology.* 1976;118:165–167.
25. Icenogle DA, Kaplan AM. A review of congenital neurologic malformations. *Clin Pediatr.* 1981;9:565–576.
26. Pomerance J, Morrison A, Williams R, et al. Anencephalic infants: Life expectancy and organ donation. *J Perinatol.* 1989;9:33–37.
27. Baird PA, Sadovnick AD. Survival in infants with anencephaly. *Clin Pediatr.* 1984;23:268–271.
28. McAbee G, Sherman J, Canas JA, et al. Prolonged survival of two anencephalic infants. *Am J Perinatol.* 1993;19:175–177.
29. Brackbill Y. The role of the cortex in orienting: Orienting reflex in an anencephalic human infant. *Dev Psychol.* 1971;5:195–201.
30. Gianelli DM. Anencephalic heart donor creates new ethics debate. *Am Med News.* 1987;3:47–49.
31. Palomaki GE, Williams JR, Haddow JE. Prenatal screening for open neural-tube defects in Maine [letter]. *N Engl J Med.* 1999;340:1049–1050.
32. O'Rahilly R, Müller F. The nervous system. In: *Human Embryology & Teratology.* New York: Wiley–Liss; 1992.
33. Marin-Padilla M. Cephalic axial skeletal–neural dysraphia disorders: Embryology and pathology. *Can J Neurol Sci.* 1991;18:153–169.
34. Müller F, O'Rahilly R. Cerebral dysraphia (future anencephaly) in a human twin embryo at stage 13. *Teratology.* 1984;30:167–177.
35. Müller F, O'Rahilly R. Development of anencephaly and its variants. *Am J Anat.* 1991;190:193–218.
36. Bronshtein M, Ornoy A. Acrania: Anencephaly resulting from secondary degeneration of a closed neural tube: Two cases in the same family. *J Clin Ultrasound.* 1991;19:230–234.
37. Timor-Tritsch IE, Greenbaum E, Monteagudo A, Baxi L. Exencephaly–anencephaly sequence: Proof by ultrasound imaging and amniotic fluid cytology. J. Matern Fetal Med 1996;5(4):182–185.

38. Campbell S, Johnstone FD, Holt EM, et al. Anencephalus: Early ultrasonic diagnosis and active management. *Lancet*. 1972;2:1226.

39. Rottem S, Bronshtein M, Thaler I, et al. First trimester transvaginal sonographic diagnosis of fetal anomalies. *Lancet*. 1989;1:444–445.

40. Inman VT, de CM, Saunders JB. The ossification of the human frontal bone. *J Anat*. 1937;71:383–394.

41. Kennedy KA, Flick KJ, Thurmond AS. First-trimester diagnosis of exencephaly. *Am J Obstet Gynecol*. 1990;162:461–463.

42. Bronshtein M, Weiner Z. Anencephaly in a fetus with osteogenesis imperfecta: Early diagnosis by transvaginal sonography. *Prenat Diagn*. 1991;12:831–834.

43. Moore KL. *The Developing Human: Clinically Oriented Embryology*. Philadelphia: WB Saunders; 1988: 364–401.

44. Vergani P, Ghidini A, Sirtori M, et al. Antenatal diagnosis of fetal acrania. *J Ultrasound Med*. 1987;6: 715–717.

45. Cox GG, Rosenthal SJ, Holpsapple JW. Exencephaly: Sonography findings and radiologic–pathologic correlation. *Radiology*. 1985;155:755–756.

46. Granchrow D, Ornoy A. Possible evidence for secondary degeneration of central nervous system in the pathogenesis of anencephaly and brain dysraphia: A study in young human fetuses. *Virchows Arch*. 1979; 384:285–294.

47. Padmanabhan R. Is exencephaly the forerunner of anencephaly? An experimental study on the effect of prolonged gestation on the exencephaly induced after neural tube closure in the rat. *Acta Anat*. 1991; 141:182–192.

48. Casellas M, Ferrer M, Rovira M, et al. Prenatal diagnosis of exencephaly. *Prenat Diagn*. 1991;13: 417–422.

49. Salamanca A, Gonzalez-Gomez F, Padilla MS, et al. Prenatal ultrasound semiography of anencephaly: Sonographic–pathological correlations. *Ultrasound Obstet Gynecol*. 1992;2:95–100.

50. Nishi T, Nakano R. First-trimester diagnosis of exencephaly by transvaginal ultrasonography. *J Ultrasound Med*. 1994;13:149.

51. Chatzipapas IK, Whitlow BJ, Economides DL. The "Mickey Mouse" sign and the diagnosis of anencephaly in early pregnancy. *Ultrasound Obstet Gynecol*. 1999;13:196–199.

52. Sepulveda W, Sebire NJ, Fung TY, Pipi E, Nicolaides KH. Crown–chin length in normal and anencephalic fetuses at 10 to 14 weeks' gestation. *Am J Obstet Gynecol*. 1997;176:852–855.

53. Hidalgo H, Bowie J, Rosenberg ER, et al. In utero sonographic diagnosis of fetal cerebral anomalies. *AJR*. 1982;139:143–148.

54. Lemire RJ. Anencephaly. In: Myrianthopoulos NC, ed. *Handbook of Clinical Neurology*. Amsterdam: Elsevier; 1987;6:71–95.

55. Johnson A, Losure TA, Weiner S. Early diagnosis of fetal anencephaly. *J Clin Ultrasound*. 1985;13:503.

56. Pretorius DH, Reuss PD, Rumack CM, et al. Diagnosis of brain neuropathology in utero. *Neuroradiology*. 1986;28:386–397.

57. Mahoney BS, Filly R, Callen PW, et al. The amniotic band syndrome: Antenatal sonographic diagnosis and potential pitfall. *Am J Obstet Gynecol*. 1985;152: 63–68.

58. Foderaro AE, Abu-Yousef MM, Benda JA, et al. Antenatal ultrasound diagnosis of iniencephaly. *J Clin Ultrasound*. 1987;15:550–554.

59. Shoham (Schwatz) Z, Caspi B, Chemke J, et al. Iniencephaly: Prenatal ultrasonographic diagnosis—A case report. *J Perinat Med*. 1988;16:139–143.

60. Lemire RJ, Beckwith JB, Shepard TH. Iniencephaly and anencephaly with spinal retroflexion. A comparative study of eight human specimens. *Birth Defects Orig Artic Ser*. 1987;23:27–36.

61. Nishimura H, Okamoto N. Iniencephaly. In: Vinken PJ, Bruyn GW, eds. *Handbook of Clinical Neurology*. Amsterdam: Elsevier/North-Holland Publishing; 1976;30:257–268.

62. Rodriguez MM, Reik RA, Carreno TD, et al. Cluster of iniencephaly in Miami. *Pediatr Pathol*. 1991;11: 211–221.

63. Aleksic SN, Budzilovich GN. Iniencephaly. In: Myrianthopoulos NC, ed. *Handbook of Clinical Neurology*. Amsterdam: Elsevier; 1987;6:129–136.

64. Romero R, Pilu G, Jeanty P, et al. *Prenatal Diagnosis of Congenital Anomalies*. Norwalk, CT: Appleton & Lange; 1988:65–67.

65. Aleksic S, Budzilovich G, Greco MA, et al. Iniencephaly: Neuropathologic study. *Clin Neuropathol*. 1983;2:55–61.

66. Bronshtein M, Timor-Tritsch IE, Rottem S. Early detection of fetal anomalies. In: Timor-Tritsch IE, Rottem S, eds. *Transvaginal Sonography*. New York: Chapman & Hall; 1991;327–371.

67. David TJ, Nixon A. Congenital malformations associated with anencephaly and iniencephaly. *J Med Genet*. 1976;13:263–265.

68. Dogan MM, Ekici E, Yapar EG, Soysal ME, Soysal SK, Gokmen O. Iniencephaly: Sonographic-pathologic correlation of 19 cases. *J Perina Med*. 1996;24: 501–511.

69. Harley EH. Pediatric nasal masses. *Ear–Nose–Throat J*. 1991;70:28–32.

70. Naidich TP, Altman NR, Braffman BH, et al. Cephaloceles and related malformations. *Am J Neuroradiol*. 1992;13:655–690.

71. Chervenak FA, Isaacson G, Mahoney MJ, et al. Diagnosis and management of fetal cephalocele. *Obstet Gynecol*. 1984;64:86–90.

72. McLaurin RL. Encephalocele and cranium bifidum. In: Myrianthopoulos NC, ed. *Handbook of Clinical Neurology*. Amsterdam: Elsevier; 1987;6:97–111.

73. Nyberg DA, Hallesy D, Mahony BS, et al. Meckel–Gruber syndrome. Importance of prenatal diagnosis. *J Ultrasound Med*. 1990;9:691–696.

74. Monteagudo A, Timor-Tritsch IE. Cephalocele, anterior. *Fetus*. 1992;2(4):1–4.

75. Fiske EC, Filly RA. Ultrasound evaluation of the ab-

normal fetal neural axis. *Radiol Clin North Am.* 1982;20:285–296.

76. Nyberg DA, Mahony BS, Pretorius DH. *Diagnostic Ultrasound of Fetal Anomalies: Text and Atlas.* Chicago: Year Book Medical Publishers; 1990:83–202.

77. Simpson DA, David DJ, White J. Cephalocele: Treatment, outcome and antenatal diagnosis. *Neurosurgery.* 1984;15:14–21.

78. Fleming AD, Vintzileos AM, Scorza WE. Prenatal diagnosis of occipital encephalocele with transvaginal sonography. *J Ultrasound Med.* 1991;10:285–286.

79. Moerman Ph, Verbeken E, Fryns JP, et al. The Meckel syndrome. Pathological and cytogenetic observations in eight cases. *Hum Genet.* 1982;62:240.

80. Pachi A, Giancotti A, Torcia F, et al. Meckel–Gruber syndrome: Ultrasonographic diagnosis at 13 weeks' gestational age in an at-risk case. *Prenat Diagn.* 1989;9:187–190.

81. Sepulveda W, Sebire NJ, Souka A, Snijders RJ, Nicolaides KH. Diagnosis of the Meckel–Gruber syndrome at eleven to fourteen weeks' gestation. *Am J Obstet Gynecol.* 1997;176:316–319.

82. Braithwaite JM, Economides DL. First-trimester diagnosis of Meckel–Gruber syndrome by transabdominal sonography in a low-risk case. *Prenat Diagn.* 1995;15:1168–1170.

83. Andersen VM. Meckel syndrome: Morphologic considerations. *Birth Defects Orig Artic Ser.* 1982;18(3B):145.

84. Vernekar JA, Mishra GK, Pinto RGW, et al. Antenatal ultrasonic diagnosis of Meckel–Gruber syndrome (a case report with review of literature). *Australas Radio.* 1991;35:186–188.

85. Herriot R, Hallam LA, Gray ES. Dandy–Walker malformation in the Meckel syndrome. *Am J Med Genet.* 1991;39:207–210.

86. Ramadani HM, Nasrat HA. Prenatal diagnosis of recurrent Meckel syndrome. *Int J Gynecol Obstet.* 1992;39:327–332.

87. Kaplan M, Ben-Neriah Z, Achiron R. Survival in an infant with a prenatally diagnosed Meckel syndrome variant. *Am J Perinatol.* 1993;10:172–174.

88. Sarnat HB, Mueller DL. Fetal neurology. In: Eden RD, Boehm FH, Haire M, eds. *Assessment and Care of the Fetus: Physiological, Clinical, and Medicolegal Principles.* Norwalk, CT: Appleton & Lange; 1990:43–67.

89. Lorber J. The prognosis of occipital encephalocele. *Dev Med Child Neurol.* 1967;9(suppl b):75–86.

90. Lorber J, Schofield JK, The prognosis of occipital encephalocele. *Z Kinderchir.* 1979;28:347–351.

91. Mealey J, Dzenitis AJ, Hockey AA. The prognosis of encephaloceles. *J Neurosurg.* 1970;32:209–218.

92. Brown MS, Sheridan-Pereira M. Outlook for the child with a cephalocele. *Pediatrics.* 1992;90:914–919.

93. Mood GF. Congenital anterior herniations of brain. *Ann Otorhinolaryngol.* 1938;47:391–401.

94. Whatmore WJ. Sincipital encephalomeningoceles. *Br J Surg.* 1973;60:261–279.

95. Warkany J, Lemire RJ, Cohen MM. *Mental Retardation and Congenital Malformations of the Central Nervous System.* Chicago: Year Book Medical Publishers; 1981:158–175.

96. Cohen MM, Lemire RJ. Syndromes with cephaloceles. *Teratology.* 1982;25:161–172.

97. Rapport RL, Dunn RC, Alhady F. Anterior encephalocele. *J Neurosurg.* 1981;54:213–219.

98. Diebler C, Dulac O. Cephalocele: Clinical and neuroradiological appearance. *Neuroradiology.* 1983;25:199–216.

99. Jones KL. *Smith's Recognizable Patterns of Human Malformation.* 4th ed. Philadelphia: WB Saunders; 1988.

100. Suwanwela C. Hongsprabhas C. Fronto-ethmoidal encephalomeningocele. *J Neurosurg.* 1966;25:172–182.

101. Lipschitz R, Beck JM, Froman C. An assessment of the treatment of encephalomeningoceles. *East Afr Med J.* 1969;43:609–619.

102. Cullen MT, Athanassiadis AP, Romero R. Prenatal diagnosis of anterior parietal encephalocele with transvaginal sonography. *Obstet Gynecol.* 1990;75:489–491.

103. Yokota A, Kajiwara H, Kohchi M, et al. Parietal cephalocele: Clinical importance of its atretic form and associated malformations. *J Neurosurg.* 1988;69:545–551.

104. Osborn AG. *Diagnostic Neuroradiology: Normal Anatomy and Congenital Anomalies of the Spine and Spinal Cord.* St. Louis: Mosby–Year Book: 1994:799–807.

105. Yen IH, Khoury MJ, Erickson JD, et al. The changing epidemiology of neural tube defects—United States, 1968–1989. *Am J Dis Child.* 1992;146:857–861.

106. Welch K, Winston KR. Spina bifida. In: Myrianthopoulos NC, ed. *Handbook of Clinical Neurology.* Amsterdam: Elsevier; 1987;6:477–508.

107. Timor-Tritsch IE, Monteagudo A, Peisner DB. High-frequency transvaginal sonographic examination for the potential malformation assessment of the 9-week to 14-week fetus. *J Clin Ultrasound.* 1992;20:231–238.

108. Birnholz J. Smaller parts scanning of the fetus. *Radiol Clin North Am.* 1992;30:977–991.

109. Rottem S, Bronshtein M, Thaler I, et al. First trimester transvaginal sonographic diagnosis of fetal anomalies. *Lancet.* 1989;1:444–445.

110. Campbell S. Early prenatal diagnosis of neural tube defects by ultrasound. *Clin Obstet Gynecol.* 1977;20:351–359.

111. Sarnat HB, Mueller DL. Fetal neurology. In: Eden RD, Boehm FH, Haire M, eds. *Assessment and Care of the Fetus: Physiological, Clinical, and Medicolegal Principles.* Norwalk, CT: Appleton & Lange; 1990:43–67.

112. Baxi L, Warren W, Collins MH, et al. Early detection of caudal regression syndrome with transvaginal scanning. *Obstet Gynecol.* 1990;74:486–489.

113. Main DM, Mennuti MT. Neural tube defects: Issues in prenatal diagnosis and counseling. *Obstet Gynecol.* 1986;67:1–16.

114. Thornton JG, Lilford RJ, Newcomb RG. Tables for estimation of individual risks of fetal neural tube and ventral wall defects, incorporating prior probability, maternal serum alpha-fetoprotein levels, and ultrasonographic examination results. *Am J Obstet Gynecol.* 1991;164:154–160.

115. Hogge WA, Thiagarajah S, Fergunson JE, et al. The role of ultrasonography and amniocentesis in the evaluation of pregnancies at risk of neural tube defects. *Am J Obstet Gynecol.* 1989;161:520–524.

116. Kollias SS, Goldstein RB, Cogen PH, et al. Prenatally detected myelomeningocele: Sonographic accuracy in estimation of the spinal level. *Radiology.* 1992;185:109–112.

117. Nicolaides KH, Gabbe SG, Guidetti R, et al. Ultrasound screening for spina bifida: Cranial and cerebellar signs. *Lancet.* 1986;1:71–74.

118. Campbell J, Gilbert WM, Nicolaides KH, et al. Ultrasound screening for spina bifida: Cranial and cerebellar signs in a high risk population. *Obstet Gynecol.* 1987;70:247–250.

119. Blumenfeld Z, Siegler E, Bronshtein M. The early diagnosis of neural tube defects. *Prenat Diagn.* 1993;13:863–871.

120. Thiagarajah S, Henke J, Hogge WA, et al. Early diagnosis of spina bifida: The value of cranial ultrasound markers. *Obstet Gynecol.* 1990;76:54–57.

121. Nyberg DA, Mack LA, Hirsch J, et al. Abnormalities of fetal cranial contour in sonographic detection of spina bifida: Evaluation of the "lemon" sign. *Radiology.* 1988;167:387–392.

122. Penso C, Redline RW, Benacerraf BR. A sonographic sign which predicts which fetuses with hydrocephalus have an associated neural tube defect. *J Ultrasound Med.* 1987;6:307–311.

123. Van den Hof MC, Nicolaides KH, Campbell J, et al. Evaluation of the lemon and banana signs in one hundred thirty fetuses with open spina bifida. *Am J Obstet Gynecol.* 1990;162:322–327.

124. Goldstein RB, Podrasky AE, Filly RA, et al. Effacement of the fetal cisterna magna in association with myelomeningocele. *Radiology.* 1989;172:409–413.

125. Pilu G, Romero R, Reece A, et al. Subnormal cerebellum in fetuses with spina bifida. *Am J Obstet Gynecol.* 1988;158:1052–1056.

126. Luthy DA, Wardinsky T, Shurtleff DB, et al. Cesarean section before the onset of labor and subsequent motor function in infants with myelomeningocele diagnosed antenatally. *N Engl J Med.* 1991;324:662–666.

127. Habib Z. Genetics and genetic counselling in neonatal hydrocephalus. *Obstet Gynecol Surv.* 1981;36:529.

128. Patten RM, Mack LA, Finberg HJ. Unilateral hydrocephalus: Prenatal sonographic diagnosis. *AJR.* 1991;156:359–363.

129. Chari R, Bhargava R, Hammond I, et al. Antenatal unilateral hydrocephalus. *Can Assoc Radiol J.* 1993;44:57–59.

130. Senat MV, Bernard JP, Schwarzler P, Britten J, Ville Y. Prenatal diagnosis and follow-up of 14 cases of unilateral ventriculomegaly. *Ultrasound Obstet Gynecol.* 1999;14:327–332.

131. Freeman JN, Brann AW Jr. Central nervous system disturbances. In: Behrman R, ed. *Neonatal Perinatal Medicine.* 2nd ed. St. Louis: CV Mosby; 1977;9–15.

132. Mealy J Jr, Gilmor RL, Bubb MP. The prognosis of hydrocephalus overt at birth. *J Neurosurg.* 1973;39:348–355.

133. McCollough DC, Balzer-Martin LA. Current prognosis in overt neonatal hydrocephalus. *J Neurosurg.* 1982;57:378–383.

134. Burton BK. Recurrence risks for congenital hydrocephalus. *Clin Genet.* 1979;16:47.

135. Friedman JM, Santos-Ramos R. Natural history of X-linked aqueductal stenosis in the second and third trimesters of pregnancy. *Am J Obstet Gynecol.* 1984;150:104–106.

136. Milhorat TH. Hydrocephaly. In: Myrianthopoulos NC, ed. *Handbook of Clinical Neurology.* Amsterdam: Elsevier; 1987;6:285–300.

137. Bickers DS, Adams RD. Hereditary stenosis of the aqueduct of Sylvius as a cause of congenital hydrocephalus. *Brain.* 1949;72:246–262.

138. Brocard O, Ragage C, Vilbert M, et al. Prenatal diagnosis of X-linked hydrocephalus. *J Clin Ultrasound.* 1993;21:211–214.

139. Hunter AG. Brain: Hydrocephalus. In: Stevenson RE, Hall JG, Goodman RM, eds. *Human Malformations and Related Anomalies.* New York: Oxford University Press; 1993;2:62–73.

140. Jeanty P, Dramaix-Wilmet M, Delbeke D, et al. Ultrasonic evaluation of fetal ventricular growth. *Neuroradiology.* 1981;21:127–131.

141. Pretorius DH, Drose JA, Manco-Johnson ML. Fetal lateral ventricular ratio determination during the second trimester. *J Ultrasound Med.* 1986;5:121–124.

142. Cardoza JD, Goldstein RB, Filly RA. Exclusion of fetal ventriculomegaly with a single measurement of the width of the lateral ventricular atrium. *Radiology.* 1988;169:711–714.

143. Pilu G, Reece EA, Goldstein I, et al. Sonographic evaluation of the normal developmental anatomy of the fetal cerebral ventricles: II. The atria. *Obstet Gynecol.* 1989;73:250–255.

144. Siedler DE, Filly RA. Relative growth of higher fetal brain structures. *J Ultrasound Med.* 1987;6:573–576.

145. Denkhaus H, Winsberg F. Ultrasonic measurement of the fetal ventricular system. *Radiology.* 1979;131:781–787.

146. Johnson ML, Dunne MG, Mack LA, et al. Evaluation of fetal intracranial anatomy by static and real-time ultrasound. *J Clin Ultrasound.* 1980;8:311–318.

147. Rumack CM, Johnson ML. Real-time ultrasound evaluation of the neonatal brain. *Clin Diagn Ultrasound.* 1982;10:179.

148. Shackelford GD. Neurosonography of hydrocephalus in infants. *Neuroradiology.* 1986;28:452–462.

149. Naidich TP, Schott LH, Baron RL. Computed tomography in evaluation of hydrocephalus. *Radiol Clin North Am.* 1982;20:143–167.

150. Naidich TP, Epstein F, Lin JP, et al. Evaluation of pediatric hydrocephalus by computed tomography. *Radiology.* 1976;119:337–345.

151. Edwards MK, Brown DL. Hydrocephalus and shunt function. *Semin Ultrasound.* 1982;3:242.

152. Cardoza JD, Filly RA, Podrasky AE. The dangling choroid plexus: A sonographic observation of value in excluding ventriculomegaly. *AJR.* 1988;151:767–770.

153. Monteagudo A, Timor-Tritsch IE, Moomjy M. Nomograms of the fetal lateral ventricles using transvaginal sonography. *J Ultrasound Med.* 1993;5:265–269.

154. Monteagudo A, Timor-Tritsch IE, Moomjy M. In utero detection of ventriculomegaly during the second and third trimesters by transvaginal sonography. *Ultrasound Obstet Gynecol.* 1994;4:193–198.

155. Epstein F, Naidich T, Kricheff I, et al. Role of computerized axial tomography in diagnosis, treatment and follow-up of hydrocephalus. *Child's Brain.* 1977;3:91–100.

156. Benacerraf BR, Birnholz JC. The diagnosis of fetal hydrocephalus prior to 22 weeks. *J Clin Ultrasound.* 1987;15:531–536.

157. Bronshtein M, Ben-Shlomo I. Choroid plexus dysmorphism: A sonographic sign of fetal hydrocephalus. *J Clin Ultrasound.* 1991;19:547–553.

158. Chinn DH, Callen PW, Filly RA. The lateral cerebral ventricle in early second trimester. *Radiology.* 1983;148:529–531.

159. Drugan A, Krause B, Canady A, et al. The natural history of prenatally diagnosed cerebral ventriculomegaly. *JAMA.* 1989;261:1785–1788.

160. Pretorius DH, Davis K, Manco-Johnson ML, et al. Clinical course of fetal hydrocephalus: 40 cases. *AJR.* 1985;144:827–831.

161. Nyberg AD, Mack LA, Hirsch J, et al. Fetal hydrocephalus: Sonographic detection and clinical significance of associated anomalies. *Radiology.* 1987;163:187–191.

162. Hudgins RJ, Edwards MSB, Goldstein R, et al. Natural history of fetal ventriculomegaly. *Pediatrics.* 1988;82:692–697.

163. Chervenak FA, Berkowitz RL, Tortora M, et al. The management of fetal hydrocephalus. *Am J Obstet Gynecol.* 1985;151:933–942.

164. Glick PL, Harrison MR, Nakayama KD, et al. Management of ventriculomegaly in the fetus. *J Pediatr.* 1984;105:97–105.

165. Chervenak FA, Duncan C, Ment LR, et al. Outcome of fetal ventriculomegaly. *Lancet.* 1984;2:179–181.

166. Serlo W, Kirkinen O, Jouppila P, et al. Prognostic signs in fetal hydrocephalus. *Child's Nerv Syst.* 1986;2:93–97.

167. Cochrane DD, Miles ST, Nimrod C, et al. Intrauterine hydrocephalus and ventriculomegaly: Associated anomalies and fetal outcome. *Can J Neurol Sci.* 1985;12:51–59.

168. Gupta JK, Bryce FC, Lilford RJ. Management of apparently isolated fetal ventriculomegaly. *Obstet Gynecol Surv.* 1994;49:716–721.

169. Mahony BS, Nyberg DA, Hirsch JH, et al. Mild idiopathic lateral cerebral ventricular dilatation in utero: Sonographic evaluation. *Radiology.* 1988;169:715–721.

170. Goldstein RB, LaPidus AS, Filly RA, et al. Mild lateral cerebral dilation in utero: Clinical significance and prognosis. *Radiology.* 1990;176:237–242.

171. Bromley B, Frigoletto FD, Benacerraf BR. Mild fetal lateral cerebral ventriculomegaly: Clinical course and outcome. *Am J Obstet Gynecol.* 1991;164:863–867.

172. Achiron R, Schimmel M, Achiron A, et al. Fetal mild idiopathic lateral ventriculomegaly: Is there a correlation with fetal trisomy? *Ultrasound Obstet Gynecol.* 1993;3:89–92.

173. Bromley B, Frigoletto FD, Jr., Benacerraf BR. Mild fetal lateral cerebral ventriculomegaly: clinical course and outcome. *Am J Obstet Gynecol.* 1991;164:863–867.

174. Pilu G, Falco P, Gabrielli S, Perolo A, Sandri F, Bovicelli L. The clinical significance of fetal isolated cerebral borderline ventriculomegaly: Report of 31 cases and review of the literature. *Ultrasound Obstet Gynecol.* 1999;14:320–326.

175. Patel MD, Filly AL, Hersh DR, Goldstein RB. Isolated mild fetal cerebral ventriculomegaly: Clinical course and outcome. *Radiology.* 1994;192:759–764.

176. Goldstein RB, La Pidus AS, Filly RA, Cardoza J. Mild lateral cerebral ventricular dilatation in utero: Clinical significance and prognosis. *Radiology.* 1990;176:237–242.

177. Vergani P, Locatelli A, Strobelt N, et al. Clinical outcome of mild fetal ventriculomegaly [see comments]. *Am J Obstet Gynecol.* 1998;178:218–222.

178. Vintzileos AM, Ingardia CJ, Nochimson DJ. Congenital hydrocephalus: A review and protocol for perinatal management. *Obstet Gynecol.* 1983;62:539–549.

179. Pinckert TL, Golbus MS. Fetal surgery. *Clin Perinatol.* 1988;15:943–953.

180. Nadel AS, Bromley BS, Frigoletto FD, et al. Isolated choroid plexus cysts in the second-trimester fetus: Is amniocentesis really indicated? *Radiology.* 1992;185:545–548.

181. Gabrielli S, Reece EA, Pilu G, et al. The clinical significance of prenatally diagnosed choroid plexus cysts. *Am J Obstet Gynecol.* 1989;160:1207–1210.

182. Achiron R, Barkai G, Katznelson B, et al. Fetal lateral ventricle choroid plexus cysts: The dilemma of amniocentesis. *Obstet Gynecol.* 1991;78:815–818.

183. Chinn DH, Miller EI, Worthy LM, et al. Sonographically detected fetal choroid plexus cysts: Frequency and association with aneuploidy. *J Ultrasound Med.* 1991;10:255–258.

184. Clark SL, DeVore GR, Sabey PL. Prenatal diagnosis of cysts of the fetal choroid plexus. *Obstet Gynecol.* 1988;72:585–587.

185. Chan L, Hixson JL, Laifer SA, et al. A sonographic and karyotypic study of second-trimester fetal choroid plexus cysts. *Obstet Gynecol.* 1989;73:703–706.

186. De Roos TR, Harris RD, Sargent SK, et al. Fetal choroid plexus cysts: Prevalence, clinical significance, and sonographic appearance. *AJR.* 1988;151:1179–1181.

187. Chitkara U, Cogswell C, Norton K, et al. Choroid plexus cysts in the fetus: A benign anatomic variant or pathologic entity? *Obstet Gynecol.* 1988;72:185–189.

188. Gross SJ, Shulman LP, Tolley EA, et al. Isolated fetal choroid plexus cysts and trisomy 18: A review and meta-analysis. *Am J Obstet Gynecol.* 1995;172:83–87.

189. Benacerraf BR, Harlow B, Frigoletto FD. Are choroid plexus cysts an indication for second-trimester amniocentesis? *Am J Obstet Gynecol.* 1990;162:1001–1006.

190. Benacerraf BR, Laboda A. Cyst of the fetal choroid plexus: A normal variant? *Am J Obstet Gynecol.* 1989;160:319–321.

191. Hertzberg BS, Kay HH, Bowie JD. Fetal choroid plexus lesions. Relationship of antenatal sonographic appearance to clinical outcome. *J Ultrasound Med.* 1989;8:77–82.

192. Farhood AI, Morris JH, Bieber FR. Transient cysts of the fetal choroid plexus: Morphology and histogenesis. *Am J Med Genet.* 1987;27:977–982.

193. Nicolaides KH, Rodeck CH, Godsen CM. Rapid karyotyping in nonlethal fetal malformations. *Lancet.* 1986;1:283–286.

194. Fitzsimmons J, Wilson D, Pascoe-Mason J, et al. Choroid plexus cysts in fetuses with trisomy 18. *Obstet Gynecol.* 1989;73:257–260.

195. Chudleigh P, Pearce JM, Campbell S. The prenatal diagnosis of transient cysts of the fetal choroid plexus. *Prenat Diagn.* 1984;4:135–137.

196. Benacerraf BR. Asymptomatic cysts of the fetal choroid plexus in the second trimester. *J Ultrasound Med.* 1987;6:475–478.

197. Kupferminc MJ, Tamura RK, Sabbagha RE, et al. Isolated choroid plexus cyst(s): An indication for amniocentesis. *Am J Obstet Gynecol.* 1994;171:1068–1071.

198. Sarno AP, Polzin WJ, Kalish VB. Fetal choroid plexus cyst in association with cri du chat (5p–) syndrome. *Am J Obstet Gynecol.* 1993;169:1614–1615.

199. Porto M, Murata Y, Warneke LA, et al. Fetal choroid plexus cysts: An independent risk factor for chromosomal anomalies. *J Clin Ultrasound.* 1993;21:103–108.

200. Perpignano MC, Cohen HL, Klein VR, et al. Fetal choroid plexus cysts: Beware the smaller cyst. *Radiology.* 1992;182:715–717.

201. Platt LD, Carlson DE, Medearis AL, et al. Fetal choroid plexus in the second trimester of pregnancy: A cause for concern. *Am J Obstet Gynecol.* 1991;164:1652–1656.

202. Geary M, Patel S, Lamont R. Isolated choroid plexus cysts and association with fetal aneuploidy in an un-selected population. *Ultrasound Obstet Gynecol.* 1997;10:171–173.

203. Sohn C, Gast AS, Krapfl E. Isolated fetal choroid plexus cysts: Not an indication for genetic diagnosis? *Fetal Diagn Ther.* 1997;12:255–259.

204. Reinsch RC. Choroid plexus cysts—Association with trisomy: Prospective review of 16,059 patients. *Am J Obstet Gynecol.* 1997;176:1381–1383.

205. Morcos CL, Platt LD, Carlson DE, Gregory KD, Greene NH, Korst LM. The isolated choroid plexus cyst [see comments]. *Obstet Gynecol.* 1998;92:232–236.

206. Sullivan A, Giudice T, Vavelidis F, Thiagarajah S. Choroid plexus cysts: Is biochemical testing a valuable adjunct to targeted ultrasonography? *Am J Obstet Gynecol.* 1999;181:260–265.

207. Snijders RJ. Isolated choroid plexus cysts: Should we offer karyotyping? [comment] [see comments]. *Ultrasound Obstet Gynecol.* 1996;8:223–224.

208. Digiovanni LM, Quinlan MP, Verp MS. Choroid plexus cysts: Infant and early childhood developmental outcome. *Obstet Gynecol.* 1997;90:191–194.

209. Chervenak FA, Jeanty P, Cantrine F, et al. The diagnosis of fetal microcephaly. *Am J Obstet Gynecol.* 1984;49:512–517.

210. Konai T, Kishimoto K, Ozaki Y. Genetic study of microcephaly based on Japanese material. *Am J Hum Genet.* 1955;7:51–65.

211. Volpe JJ. In: *Neurology of the Newborn: Neuronal Proliferation, Migration, Organization and Myelination.* Philadelphia: WB Saunders; 1995;45–49.

212. Jones KL. *Smith's Recognizable Patterns of Human Malformation.* 4th ed. Philadelphia: WB Saunders; 1988.

213. Chervenak FA, Rosenberg J, Brightman F, et al. A prospective study of the accuracy of ultrasound in predicting fetal microcephaly. *Obstet Gynecol.* 1987;69:908–910.

214. Tolmie JL, McNay M, Stepheson JBP, et al. Microcephaly: Genetic counseling and antenatal diagnosis after birth of an affected child. *Am J Med Genet.* 1987;27:583–594.

215. Bauman ML. Neuroembryology—Clinical aspects. *Semin Perinatol.* 1987;11:74–84.

216. Goldstein I, Reece EA, Pilu G, et al. Sonographic assessment of the fetal frontal lobe: A potential tool for prenatal diagnosis of microcephaly. *Am J Obstet Gynecol.* 1988;1158:1057–1062.

217. Haslam RH. Microcephaly. In: Myrianthopoulos NC, ed. *Handbook of Clinical Neurology.* Amsterdam: Elsevier; 1987;6:267–284.

218. Hunter AG. Brain. In: Stevenson RE, Hall JG, Goodman RM, eds. *Human Malformations and Related Anomalies.* New York: Oxford University Press; 1993;2:2–19.

219. Persutte WH, Coury A, Hobbins JC. Correlation of fetal frontal lobe and transcerebellar diameter measurements: The utility of a new prenatal sonographic technique. *Ultrasound Obstet Gynecol.* 1997;10:94–97.

220. Pilu G, Falco P, Milano V, Perolo A, Bovicelli L. Prenatal diagnosis of microcephaly assisted by vaginal sonography and power Doppler. *Ultrasound Obstet Gynecol.* 1998;11:357–360.

221. Bromley B, Benacerraf BR. Difficulties in the prenatal diagnosis of microcephaly. *J Ultrasound Med.* 1995;14:303–305.

222. Meilstrup JW, Botti JJ, MacKay DR, et al. Prenatal sonographic appearance of asymmetric craniosynostosis: A case report. *J Ultrasound Med.* 1995;14:307–310.

223. Stamm ER, Pretorius DH, Rumack CM, et al. Kleeblattschädel anomaly. In utero sonographic appearance. *J Ultrasound Med.* 1987;6:319–324.

224. Witt PD, Hardesty RA, Zuppan C, et al. Fetal kleeblattschädel cranium: Morphologic, radiologic, and histologic analysis. *Cleft Palate–Craniofac J.* 1992;29:363–368.

225. Volpe JJ. In: *Neurology of the Newborn: Neuronal Proliferation, Migration, Organization and Myelination.* 3rd ed. Philadelphia: WB Saunders; 1995:97–98.

226. Nelson KB, Deutschberger J. Head size at one year as a predictor of four year IQ. *Dev Med Child Neurol.* 1970;12:487–495.

227. DeRosa R, Lenke RR, Kurczynski TW, et al. In utero diagnosis of benign fetal macrocephaly. *Am J Obstet Gynecol.* 1989;161:690–692.

228. DeMyer W. Megalencephaly: Types, clinical syndromes, and management. *Pediatr Neurol.* 1987;2:321–328.

229. Rugel A, Palldini G, Zappella M. Unilateral megalencephaly with nerve cell hypertrophy. An anatomical and quantitative histochemical study. *Brain Res.* 1986;9:103.

230. King M, Stephenson JB, Zievogel M, et al. Hemimegalencephaly—A case for hemispherectomy? *Neuropediatrics.* 1985;16:46–55.

231. Ramirez M, Wilkins I, Kramer L, et al. Prenatal diagnosis of unilateral megalencephaly by real-time ultrasonography. *Am J Obstet Gynecol.* 1994;170:1384–1385.

232. Barkovich JA, Chuang SH, Norman D. MR of neuronal migration anomalies. *Am J Radiol.* 1988;150:179–187.

233. Babyn P, Chuang S, Daneman A, et al. Sonographic recognition of unilateral megalencephaly. *J Ultrasound Med.* 1992;11:563–566.

234. Sandri F, Pilu G, Dallacas P, et al. Sonography of unilateral megalencephaly in the fetus and newborn infant. *Am J Perinatol.* 1991;8:18–20.

235. Hafner E, Bock W, Zoder G, Schuchter K, Rosen A, Plattner M. Prenatal diagnosis of unilateral megalencephaly by 2D and 3D ultrasound: A case report. *Prenat Diagn.* 1999;19:159–162.

236. Page LK, Brown SB, Gargano FP, et al. Schizencephaly: A clinical study and review. *Child's Brain.* 1975;1:348.

237. Yakovlev PI, Wadsworth RC. Schizencephalies: A study of the congenital clefts in the cerebral mantle II. Clefts with hydrocephalus and lips separated. *J Neuropathol Exp Neurol.* 1946;5:169–206.

238. Komarniski CA, Cyr DR, Mack LA, et al. Prenatal diagnosis of schizencephaly. *J Ultrasound Med.* 1990;9:305–307.

239. Barkovich AJ, Norman D. MR imaging of schizencephaly. *AJR.* 1988;150:1391–1396.

240. Barkovich AJ, Kjos BO. Schizencephaly: Correlation of clinical findings with MR characteristics. *Am J Neuroradiol.* 1992;13:85–94.

241. Robinson RG. Agenesis and anomalies of other brain structures. In: Myrianthopoulos NC, ed. *Handbook of Clinical Neurology.* Amsterdam: Elsevier; 1987;6:197–210.

242. Sauchet IB. Schizencephaly: Antenatal and postnatal assessment with color-flow Doppler imaging. *Can Assoc Radiol J.* 1994;45:193–200.

243. Messer J, Haddad J, Casanova R. Transcranial Doppler evaluation of cerebral infarction in the neonate. *Neuropediatrics.* 1990;22:147–151.

244. Klingensmith WC III, Cioffi-Reagan DT. Schizencephaly: Diagnosis and progression in utero. *Radiology.* 1986;159:617–618.

245. Lithuania M, Passamonti U, Cordone MS, et al. Schizencephaly: Prenatal diagnosis by computed sonography and magnetic resonance imaging. *Prenat Diagn.* 1989;9:649–655.

246. Osborn RE, Byrd SE, Naidich TP, et al. 1988 MR imaging of neuronal migrational disorders. *Am J Neuroradiol.* 1988;9:1101–1106.

247. Miller GM, Stears JC, Guggenheim MA, et al. Schizencephaly: A clinical and CT study. *Neurology.* 1984;34:997–1001.

248. Zimmerman RA, Bilaniuk LT, Grossman RI. Computed tomography in migratory disorders of human brain development. *Neuroradiology.* 1983;25:257–263.

249. Dobyns WB, Kirkpatrick JB, Hittner HM, et al. Syndromes with Lissencephaly. II: Walker–Warburg and cerebro-oculo-muscular syndrome and a new syndrome with type II lissencephaly. *Am J Med Genet.* 1985;22:157–195.

250. Banna M, Malabarey T. Lissencephaly and pachygyria. *J Can Assoc Radiol.* 1989;40:156–158.

251. Dobyns WB, Greenberg F. Syndromes with lissencephaly type I: Miller–Dierker and Norman–Roberts syndromes and isolated lissencephaly. *Am J Med Genet.* 1984;18:509–526.

252. Stewart RM, Richman DP, Caviness VS. Lissencephaly and pachygyria: An architectonic and topographical analysis. *Acta Neuropathol.* 1975;31:1–12.

253. Sidman RL, Rakie P. Neuronal migration, with special reference to developing human brain: A review. *Brain Res.* 1973;62:1–35.

254. Rijk-van Andel JF, Arts WFM, Barth PG, et al. Diagnostic features and clinical signs of 21 patients with lissencephaly type I. *Dev Med Child Neurol.* 1990;32:707–717.

255. Dobyns WB. Developmental aspects of lissencephaly and the lissencephaly syndromes. *Birth Defects Orig Artic Ser.* 1987;23(1):225–241.

256. Byrd SE, Osborn RE, Bohan TP, et al. The CT and MR evaluation of migrational disorders of the brain. *Pediatr Radiol.* 1989;19:151–156.

257. Chitayat D, Toi A, Babul R, et al. Omphalocele in Miller–Dieker syndrome: Expanding the phenotype. *Am J Med Genet.* 1997;69:293–298.

258. Jones KL. Warburg syndrome (HARD ± E syndrome). In: *Smith's Recognizable Patterns of Human Malformation.* 4th ed. Philadelphia: WB Saunders; 1988:158–159.

259. Dobyns WB, Pagon RA, Armstrong D, et al. Diagnostic criteria for Walker–Warburg syndrome. *Am J Med Genet.* 1989;32:195–210.

260. Gasser B, Lindner V, Dreyfus M, et al. Prenatal diagnosis of Walker–Warburg syndrome in three sibs. *Am J Med Genet.* 1998;76:107–110.

261. Farrell SA, Toi A, Leadman M, et al. Prenatal diagnosis of retinal detachment in Walker–Warburg syndrome. *Am J Med Genet.* 1987;28:619–624.

262. Crowe C, Jassani M, Dickerman L. The prenatal diagnosis of the Walker–Warburg syndrome. *Prenat Diagn.* 1986;6:177–185.

263. Maynor CH, Hertzberg BS, Ellington KS. Antenatal sonographic features of Walker–Warburg syndrome. Value of endovaginal sonography. *J Ultrasound Med.* 1992;11:301–303.

264. Saltzman DH, Krauss CM, Goldman JM, et al. Prenatal diagnosis of lissencephaly. *Prenat Diagn.* 1991;11:139–143.

265. Okamura K, Murotsuki J, Sakai T, et al. Prenatal diagnosis of lissencephaly by magnetic resonance image. *Fetal Diagn Ther.* 1993;8:56–59.

266. Nyberg DA, Pretorius DH. Cerebral malformations. In: Nyberg DA, Mahoney BS, Pretorius DH, eds. *Diagnostic Ultrasound of Fetal Anomalies: Text and Atlas.* Chicago: Mosby–Year Book; 1990:83–145.

267. Handa J, Okomato K, Sato M. Arachnoid cyst of the middle cranial fossa: Report of bilateral cysts in siblings. *Surg Neurol.* 1981;16:127–130.

268. Galassi E, Tognetti F, Gaist G, et al. CT scan and metrizamide CT cisternography in arachnoid cysts of the middle cranial fossa: Classification and pathophysiological aspects. *Surg Neurol.* 1982;17:363–369.

269. Sato K, Shimoji T, Yaguchi K, et al. Middle fossa arachnoid cyst: Clinical neuroradiological and surgical features. *Child's Brain.* 1983;10:301–316.

270. Naidich TP, McLone DG, Radkowski MA. Intracranial arachnoid cysts. *Pediatr Neurosci.* 1985–1986; 12:112–122.

271. Robertson SJ, Wolper SM, Runge VM. MR imaging of middle cranial fossa arachnoid cysts: Temporal lobe agenesis syndrome revisited. *Am J Neuroradiol.* 1989;10:1007–1010.

272. Osborn AG. Miscellaneous tumors, cysts and metastases. In: *Diagnostic Neuroradiology.* St. Louis: Mosby–Year Book; 1994:639–642.

273. Bannister CM, Russell SA, Rimmer S, Mowle DH. Fetal arachnoid cysts: Their site, progress, prognosis and differential diagnosis. *Eur J Pediatr Surg.* 1999;(9 Suppl) 1:27–28.

274. Chuang S, Harwood-Nash D. Tumors and cysts. *Neuroradiology.* 1986;28:463–475.

275. Banna M. Arachnoid cysts on computed tomography. *AJR.* 1976;127:979–982.

276. Robinson RG. Congenital cysts of the brain: Arachnoid malformations. *Prog Neurol Surg.* 1971;4: 133–174.

277. Menezes AH, Bell WE, Perret GE. Arachnoid cysts in children. *Arch Neurol.* 1980;37:168–172.

278. Langer B, Haddad J, Favre R, et al. Fetal arachnoid cysts: Report of two cases. *Ultrasound Obstet Gynecol.* 1994;4:68–72.

279. Galassi E, Tognetti E, Frank F, et al. Infratentorial arachnoid cysts. *J Neurosurg.* 1985;63:210–217.

280. Pascual-Catroviejo I, Roche MC, Bermejo AM, et al. Primary intracranial arachnoidal cysts. *Child's Nerv Syst.* 1991;7:257–263.

281. Jones RBC, Warnock TH, Nayanar V, et al. Suprasellar arachnoid cysts: Management by cyst wall resection. *Neurosurgery.* 1989;25:554–561.

282. Elbers SE, Furness ME. Resolution of presumed arachnoid cyst in utero [see comments]. Ultrasound Obstet Gynecol, 1999;14(5):353–5.

283. Pilu G, Pilu A, Falco P, Perolo A, Sandri F, Cocchi G, Aucora G, Bovicelli L. Differential diagnosis and outcome of fetal intracranial hypoechoic lesions: Report of 21 cases. *Ultrasound Obstet Gynecol.* 1997; 9:229–236.

284. Hogge WA, Schnatterly P, Ferguson JE. 2nd Early prenatal diagnosis of an infratentorial arachnoid cyst: Association with an unbalanced translocation. *Prenat Diagn.* 1995;15:186–188.

285. Rafferty PG, Britton J, Penna L, Ville Y. Prenatal diagnosis of a large fetal arachnoid cyst. *Ultrasound Obstet Gynecol.* 1998;12:358–261.

286. Marinov M, Undjian S, Wetzka P. An evaluation of the surgical treatment of intracranial cysts in children. *Child's Nerv Syst.* 1989;5:177–183.

287. Richard KE, Dahl K, Sanker P. Long-term followup of children and juveniles with arachnoid cysts. *Child's Nerv Syst.* 1989;5:184–187.

288. Wisoff JH, Berenstein A, Choi IS, et al. Management of vein of Galen vascular malformation. In: Marlin AE, ed. *Concepts in Pediatric Neurosurgery.* Basel: Karger; 1990;137–155.

289. Hoffman HJ, Chuang S, Hendrick B, et al. Aneurysms of the vein of Galen. Experience at The Hospital for Sick Children, Toronto. *J Neurosurg.* 1982;57:316–322.

290. Lylyk P, Vinuela F, Dion JE, et al. Therapeutic alternatives for vein of Galen vascular malformations. *J Neurosurg.* 1993;78:438–445.

291. Volpe JJ. Brain tumors and vein of Galen malformation. In: *Neurology of the Newborn: Neuronal Proliferation, Migration, Organization and Myelination.* 3rd ed. Philadelphia: WB Saunders; 1995:802–806.

292. Yasargil MG. *Microneurosurgery.* New York: Thieme Medical Publishers; 1988:3.

293. Yasargil MG, Antic J, Laciga R, et al. Arteriovenous malformations of vein of Galen: Microsurgical treatment. *Surg Neurol.* 1976;6:195–200.

294. Raybaud CA, Strother CM, Hald JK. Aneurysms of the vein of Galen: Embryonic considerations and anatomical features relating to the pathogenesis of the malformation. *Neuroradiology.* 1989;31:109–128.

295. Osborn AG. Intracranial vascular malformations. In: *Diagnostic Neuroradiology.* St. Louis: Mosby–Year Book; 1994:320–324.

296. Vintzileos AM, Eisenfeld LI, Campbell WA, et al. Prenatal ultrasonic diagnosis of arteriovenous malformation of the vein of Galen. *Am J Perinatol.* 1986;3:209–211.

297. Ordorica SA, Marks F, Frieden FJ, et al. Aneurysm of the vein of Galen: A new cause for Ballantyne syndrome. *Am J Obstet Gynecol.* 1990;162:1166–1167.

298. Rodemyer CR, Smith WL. Diagnosis of a vein of Galen aneurysm by ultrasound. *J Clin Ultrasound.* 1982;10:297–298.

299. Diebler C, Dulac O, Dominque R, et al. Aneurysms of the vein of Galen in infants ages 2 to 15 months. Diagnosis and natural evolution. *Neuroradiology.* 1981;21:185–197.

300. Reiter AA, Huhta JC, Carpenter RJ, et al. Prenatal diagnosis of arteriovenous malformation of the vein of Galen. *J Clin Ultrasound.* 1986;14:623–628.

301. Hirsch JH, Cyr D, Eberhardt H, et al. Ultrasonographic diagnosis of an aneurysm of the vein of Galen in utero by duplex scanning. *J Ultrasound Med.* 1983;2:231–233.

302. Babcock DS. Sonography of congenital malformations of the brain. *Neuroradiology.* 1986;28:428–439.

303. Mendelsohn DB, Hertzanu Y, Butterworth A. In utero diagnosis of vein of Galen aneurysm by ultrasound. *Neuroradiology.* 1984;26:417–418.

304. Watson DG, Smith RR, Brann AW. Arteriovenous malformation of the vein of Galen. *Am J Dis Child.* 1976;130:520–525.

305. Wisoff JH, Berenstein A, Choi IS, et al. Mangement of vein of Galen malformation. In: Marlin AE, ed. *Concepts in Pediatric Neurosurgery.* Basel: Karger; 1990;137–155.

306. McCord FB, Shields MD, McNeil A, et al. Cerebral arteriovenous malformation in a neonate: Treatment by embolization. *Arch Dis Child.* 1987;1273–1275.

307. King WAS, Wackym PA, Vinuela F, et al. Management of vein of Galen aneurysm. Combined surgical and endovascular approach. *Child's Nerv Syst.* 1989;5:208–211.

308. Miller VS, Roach ES. Embolization and radiosurgical treatment of cerebral arteriovenous malformations. *Int Pediatr.* 1992;7:173–180.

309. Yamashita Y, Abe T, Ohara N, et al. Successful treatment of neonatal aneurysmal dilatation of the vein of Galen: The role of prenatal diagnosis and trans-arterial embolization. *Neuroradiology.* 1992;34:457–459.

310. Lasjaunias P, Garcia MR, Rodesh G, et al. Vein of Galen malformation. Endovascular management of 43 cases. *Child's Nerv Syst.* 1991;7:360–367.

311. Yow MD. Congenital cytomegalovirus disease: A NOW problem. *J Infect Dis.* 1989;159:163–167.

312. Dobbins JG, Stewart JA, Demmler GJ. Surveillance of congenital cytomegalovirus disease, 1990–1991.

Collaborating Registry Group. *MMWR CDC Surveill Summ.* 1992;41:35–39.

313. Stagno S, Pass RF, Cloud G, et al. Primary cytomegalovirus infection in pregnancy. *JAMA.* 1986;256:1904–1908.

314. Griffiths PD, Stagno S, Pass RF, et al. Cytomegalovirus infection during pregnancy: Specific IgM antibodies as a marker of recent primary infection. *J Infect Dis.* 1982;145:647–653.

315. Mittlemann-Handwerker S, Pardes JG, Post RC, et al. Fetal ventriculomegaly and brain atrophy in a woman with intrauterine cytomegalovirus infection. A case report. *J Reprod Med.* 1986;11:1061–1064.

316. Ceballos R, Ch'ien LT, Whitley RJ, et al. Cerebellar hypoplasia in an infant with congenital cytomegalovirus infection. *Pediatrics.* 1976;57:155–157.

317. Shackelford GD, Fulling KH, Glasies CM. Cysts of the subependedymal germinal matrix: Sonographic demonstration with pathologic correlation. *Radiology.* 1983;149:117–121.

318. Butt W, Mackay RJ, de Crespingy LC, et al. Intracranial lesions of congenital cytomegalovirus infection detected by ultrasound scanning. *Pediatrics.* 1984;73:611–614.

319. Marques-Dias MJM, van Rijckevorsel GH, Landriue P, et al. Prenatal cytomegalovirus disease and cerebral microgyria: Evidence for perfusion failure, not disturbance of histogenesis, as a major cause of fetal cytomegalovirus encephalopathy. *Neuropediatrics.* 1984;15:18–24.

320. Friede RL, Mikolasek J. Postencephalic porencephaly, hydranencephaly or polymicrogyria. A review. *Acta Neuropathol.* 1978;43:161–168.

321. Perlman JM, Argyle C. Lethal cytomegalovirus infection in preterm infants: Clinical radiological, and neuropathological findings. *Ann Neurol.* 1992;31:64–68.

322. Drose JA, Dennis MA, Thickman D. Infection in utero: US findings in 19 cases. *Radiology.* 1991;178:369–374.

323. Twickler DM, Pearlman J, Maberry MC. Congenital cytomegalovirus infection presenting as cerebral ventriculomegaly on antenatal sonography. *Am J Perinatol.* 1993;10:404–406.

324. Graham D, Guide SM, Saunders RC. Sonographic features of in-utero periventricular calcification due to cytomegalovirus infection. *J Ultrasound Med.* 1982;1:171–172.

325. Ghidini A, Sirtori M, Vergani P, et al. Fetal intracranial calcifications. *Am J Obstet Gynecol.* 1989;160:86–87.

326. Fakhry J, Khoury A. Fetal intracranial calcifications. The importance of periventricular hyperechoic foci without shadowing. *J Ultrasound Med.* 1991;10:51–54.

327. Tassin GB, Maklad NF, Stewart RR, et al. Cytomegalic inclusion disease: Intrauterine sonographic diagnosis using findings involving the brain. *Am J Neuroradiol.* 1991;12:117–122.

328. Estroff JA, Parad RB, Teele RL, et al. Echogenic vessels in the fetal thalami and basal ganglia associated

with cytomegalovirus infection. *J Ultrasound Med.* 1992;11:686–688.

329. Teele RL, Hernaz-Schulman M, Sotrel A. Echogenic vasculature in the basal ganglia of neonates: A sonographic sign of vasculopathy. *Radiology.* 1988;169:423–427.

330. Achiron R, Pinchas-Hamiel O, Lipitz S, et al. Prenatal ultrasonographic diagnosis of fetal cerebral ventriculitis associated with asymptomatic maternal cytomegalovirus infection. *Prenat Diagn.* 1994;14:523–526.

331. Shaw CM, Alvord EC. Subependymal germinolysis. *Arch Neurol.* 1974;31:374–381.

332. Marques-Dias MJM, van Rijckevorsel GH, Landriue P, et al. Prenatal cytomegalovirus disease and cerebral microgyria: Evidence for perfusion failure, not disturbance of histogenesis, as a major cause of fetal cytomegalovirus encephalopathy. *Neuropediatrics.* 1984;15:18–24.

333. Osborn AG. Infections of the brain and its linings. In: *Diagnostic Neuroradiology.* St. Louis: Mosby–Year Book; 1994;673–715.

334. Barkovich AJ, Lindan CE. Congenital cytomegalovirus infection of the brain: Imaging analysis and embryologic considerations. *Am J Neuroradiol.* 1994;15:703–715.

335. Lebowitz RL. Tuberous sclerosis. *Soc Pediatr Urol Newsl.* 1984:109–110.

336. Han BK, Babcock DS, Oestreich AE. Sonography of brain tumors in infants. *Am J Radiol.* 1984;143:31–36.

337. Grant EG, Williams AL, Schellinger D, et al. Intracranial calcification in the infant and neonate: Evaluation by sonography and CT. *Radiology.* 1985;157:63–68.

338. Hughes P, Weinberger E, Shaw DW. Linear areas of echogenicity in the thalami and basal ganglia of neonates: An expanded association. Work in progress. *Radiology.* 1991;179:103–105.

339. Eliezer S, Ester F, Ehud W, et al. Fetal splenomegaly, ultrasound diagnosis of cytomegalovirus infection: A case report. *J Clin Ultrasound.* 1984;12:520–521.

340. Shackelford GD, Kirks DR. Neonatal hepatic calcification secondary to transplacental infection. *Radiology.* 1977;122:753–757.

341. Binder ND, Buckmaster JW, Benda GI. Outcome for fetuses with ascites and cytomegalovirus infection. *Pediatrics.* 1988;82:100–103.

342. MacDonald H, Tobin HO. Congenital cytomegalovirus infection: A collaborative study on epidemiological, clinical, and laboratory findings. *Dev Med Child Neurol.* 1978;20:471–482.

343. Volpe JJ. Viral, protozoan, and related intracranial infections. In: *Neurology of the Newborn: Neuronal Proliferation, Migration, Organization and Myelination.* 3rd ed. Philadelphia: WB Saunders; 1995; 675–729.

344. Bale JF, Blackman JA, Sato Y. Outcome in children with symptomatic congenital cytomegalovirus infection. *J Child Neurol.* 1989;5:131–136.

345. Donner C, Liesnard C, Content J, et al. Prenatal diagnosis of 52 pregnancies at risk for congenital cy-

tomegalovirus infection. *Obstet Gynecol.* 1993;82:481–486.

346. Gordon N. Toxoplasmosis: A preventable cause of brain damage. *Dev Med Child Neurol.* 1993;35:567–573. Review.

347. Stagno S. Congenital toxoplasmosis. *Am J Dis Child.* 1980;134:635–637.

348. Walpole IR, Hodgen N, Bower C. Congenital toxoplasmosis: A large survey in western Australia. *Med J Aust.* 1991;154:720–724.

349. Lee RV. Parasites and pregnancy: The problems of malaria and toxoplasmosis. *Clin Perinatol.* 1988;15:351–363.

350. Matsui D. Prevention, diagnosis, and treatment of fetal toxoplasmosis. *Clin Perinatol.* 1994;21:675–689.

351. Stray-Pedersen B. Treatment of toxoplasmosis in the pregnant mother and newborn child. *Scand J Infect Dis.* 1992;84(suppl):23–31.

352. Peckham CS, Logan S. Screening for toxoplasmosis during pregnancy. *Arch Dis Child.* 1993;68(special issue 1):3–5.

353. Desmonts G, Couvreur J. Toxoplasmosis in pregnancy and its transmission to the fetus. *Bull NY Acad Med.* 1974;50:146–159.

354. Desmonts G, Couvreur J. Congenital toxoplasmosis. A prospective study of 378 pregnancies. *N Engl J Med.* 1974;290:1110–1116.

355. Carter AO, Frank JW. Congenital toxoplasmosis: Epidemiological features and control. *Can Med Assoc J.* 1986;135:618–623.

356. Becker LE. Infections of the developing brain. *Am J Neuroradiol.* 1992;13:537–549.

357. Hohlfeld P, Mac Aleese J, Capella-Pavlovski M, et al. Fetal toxoplasmosis: Ultrasonographic signs. *Ultrasound Obstet Gynecol.* 1991;1:241–244.

358. Fitz CR. Inflammatory diseases of the brain in childhood. *Am J Neuroradiol.* 1992;13:551–557.

359. Gordon N. Toxoplasmosis: A preventable cause of brain damage. *Dev Med Child Neurol.* 1993;35:567–573.

360. Blaakaer J. Ultrasonic diagnosis of fetal ascites and toxoplasmosis. *Acta Obstet Gynecol Scand.* 1986;65:653–654.

361. Vanhaesebrouck P, De Wit M, Smets K, et al. Congenital toxoplasmosis presenting as massive neonatal ascites. *Helv Paediatr Acta.* 1988;43:97–101.

362. Hohlfeld P, Daffos F, Costa JM, et al. Prenatal diagnosis of congenital toxoplasmosis with polymerase-chain-reaction test on amniotic fluid. *N Engl J Med.* 1994;331:605–609.

363. Couvreur J. Prophylaxis of congenital toxoplasmosis: Effects of spiramycin on placental infection. *J Antimicrob Chemother.* 1988;22(suppl B):193–200.

364. Daffos F, Forestier F, Capella-Pavlovsky M, et al. Prenatal management of 746 pregnancies at risk for congenital toxoplasmosis. *N Engl J Med.* 1988;318:271–275.

365. Couvreur J, Thulliez PH, Daffos F, et al. In utero treatment of toxoplasmic fetopathy with the combination pyrimethamine–sulfadiazine. *Fetal Daign Ther.* 1993;8:45–50.

366. Georgiev VS. Management of toxoplasmosis. *Drugs.* 1994;48(2):178–188.

367. Freij BJ, Sever JL. Chronic Infections. In: Neonatology: Pathophysiology and management of the newborn. Avery GB, Fletcher MA, MacDonald MG eds. Philadelphia: JB Lippincott; 1994, pp 1029–1081.

368. Preblud SR, Alford CA. Rubella. In: Diseases of the fetus and neonate. Remington JS, Klein JO, eds. WB Saunders; 1990; pp. 196–240.

369. Fucillo DA, Sever JL. Viral teratology. *Bacteriol Rev.* 1973;37:19–31.

370. Yamashita Y, Matsuishi T, Murkmi Y, et al. Neuroimaging findings (ultrasonography, CT, MRI) in 3 infants with congenital rubella syndrome. *Pediatr Radiol.* 1991;21:547–549.

371. Desmond MM, Wilson GS, Melnick JL. Congenital rubella encephalitides. Course and early sequelae. *J Pediatr.* 1967;71:311–331.

372. Wakai S, Arai T, Nagai M. Congenital brain tumors. *Surg Neurol.* 1984;21:597–609.

373. Sherer DM, Onyeije CI. Prenatal ultrasonographic diagnosis of fetal intracranial tumors: A review. *Am J Perinatol.* 1998;15:319–328.

374. Kwoon T, Jeanty P. Cystic teratoma. *Fetus.* 1990; 1:7–9.

375. DeVore G, Hobbins J. Diagnosis of structural abnormalities in the fetus. *J Clin Ultrasound.* 1980;8: 247–249.

376. Hoff NR, Mackay IM. Prenatal ultrasound diagnosis of intracranial teratoma. *Clin Perinatol.* 1979;6: 293–319.

377. Crade M. Ultrasonic demonstration in utero of an intracranial teratoma. *JAMA.* 1982;247:1173.

378. Kirkinen P, Suramo I, Jouppila P, et al. Combined use of ultrasound and computed tomography in the evaluation of fetal intracranial abnormality. *J Perinat Med.* 1982;10:257–265.

379. Paes BA, DeSa DJ, Hunter DJ, et al. Benign intracranial teratoma—Prenatal diagnosis influencing early delivery. *Am J Obstet Gynecol.* 1982;143: 600–601.

380. Lipman SP, Pretorius DH, Rumack CM, et al. Fetal intracranial teratoma. US diagnosis of three cases and a review of the literature. *Radiology.* 1985; 157:491–494.

381. Richard SR. Ultrasonic diagnosis of intracranial teratoma in utero: A case report and literature review. *J Reprod Med.* 1987;32:73–75.

382. Ferreira O, Morvan J, Cleophax JP. Prenatal diagnosis of intracranial teratoma. A case report. *J Gynecol Obstet Biol Reprod.* 1988;17:1075–1080.

383. Dolkart LA. Balcom RJ, Eisenger G. Intracranial teratoma: Prolonged neonatal survival after prenatal diagnosis. *Am J Obstet Gynecol.* 1990;162:768–769.

384. Ferreira J, Eviatar L. Schnieider S, et al. Prenatal diagnosis of intracranial teratoma. Prolonged survival after resection of a malignant teratoma diagnosed prenatally by ultrasound: A case report and literature review. *Pediatr Neurosurg.* 1993;19:84–88.

385. Kuller JA, Laifer SA, Martin JG, et al. Unusual presentations of fetal teratoma. *J Perinatol.* 1991; 11:294–296.

386. Sherer DM, Abramowicz JS, Eggers PC, et al. Prenatal ultrasonographic diagnosis of intracranial teratoma and massive craniomegaly with associated high-output cardiac failure. *Am J Obstet Gynecol.* 1993;168:97–99.

387. ten Broeke EDM, Verdonk GW, Roumen FJME. Prenatal ultrasound diagnosis of an intracranial teratoma influencing management: Case report and review of the literature. *Eur J Obstet Gynecol Reprod Biol.* 1992;45:210–214.

388. Ulreich S, Hanieh A, Furness ME. Positive outcome of fetal intracranial teratoma. *J Ultrasound Med.* 1993;3:163–165.

389. Afshar F, King TT, Berry CL. Intraventricular fetus-in-fetu. Case report. *J Neurosurg.* 1982;56:845–849.

390. Goldstein I, Jakobi P, Groisman G, Itskovitz-Eldor J. Intracranial fetus-in-fetu. *Am J Obstet Gynecol.* 1996;175:1389–1390.

391. Hung CF, Lam MS. Intracranial fetus in fetu: Report of a case. *J Formos Med Assoc.* 1993;92:920–922.

392. Wakai S. [On the origin of intracranial teratomas]. *No To Shinkei* 1989;41:947–953.

393. Yang ST, Leow SW. Intracranial fetus-in-fetu: CT diagnosis. *AJNR Am J Neuroradiol.* 1992;13:1326–1329.

394. Yasuda Y, Mitomori T, Matsuura A, Tanimura T. Fetus-in-fetu: Report of a case. *Teratology.* 1985;31:337–344.

395. Willis RA. *The Borderline of Embryology and Pathology.* London: Butterworth, 1985:147.

396. Gradin WC, Taylon C, Fruin AH. Choroid plexus papilloma of the third ventricle: Case report and review of the literature. *Neurosurgery.* 1983;12:217–220.

397. Hawkins JC. Treatment of choroid plexus papilloma in children: A brief analysis of twenty years' experience. *Neurosurgery.* 1980;6:380.

398. Milhorat TH, Hammock MK, Davis DA, et al. Choroid plexus papilloma I. Proof of cerebrospinal fluid overproduction. *Child's Brain.* 1976;2:273–289.

399. Eisenberg HM, McComb JG, Lorenzo AV. Cerebrospinal fluid over production and hydrocephalus associated with choroid plexus papilloma. *J Neurosurg.* 1974;40:381–385.

400. Smith WL, Menezes A, Franken EA. Cranial ultrasound in the diagnosis of malignant brain tumors. *J Clin Ultrasound.* 1983;11:97–100.

401. Cappe IP, Lam AH. Ultrasound diagnosis of choroid plexus papilloma. *J Clin Ultrasound.* 1985;13:121–123.

402. Volpe JJ. Hypoxic–ischemic encephalopathy, neuropathology, and pathogenesis. In: *Neurology of the Newborn: Neuronal Proliferation, Migration, Organization and Myelination.* Philadelphia: WB Saunders; 1995:299–307.

403. Greene MF, Benacerraf B, Crawford JM. Hydranencephaly: US appearance during in utero evolution. *Radiology.* 1985;156:779–780.

404. Edmondson SR, Hallak M, Carpenter RJ, et al. Evolution of hydranencephaly following intracerebral hemorrhage. *Obstet Gynecol.* 1992;79:870–871.

405. Filly RA. Ultrasound evaluation of the fetal neural axis. In: Callen PW, ed. *Ultrasonography in Obstetrics and Gynecology.* Philadelphia: WB Saunders; 1994:189–234.

406. Belfar HL, Kuller JA, Hill LM, et al. Evolving fetal hydranencephaly mimicking intracranial neoplasm. *J Ultrasound Med.* 1991;10:231–233.

407. Eller KM, Kuller JA. Porencephaly secondary to fetal trauma during amniocentesis. *Obstet Gynecol.* 1995;85:865–867.

408. Banker B. Periventricular leukomalacia. *Arch Neurol.* 1962;7:32–50.

409. Grunnet ML. Periventricular leukomalacia complex. *Arch Pathol Lab Med.* 1979;103:6–10.

410. Achiron R, Pinchas OH, Reichman B, et al. Fetal intracranial haemorrhage: Clinical significance of in utero ultrasonographic diagnosis [see comments]. *Br J Obstet Gynaecol.* 1993;100:995–999.

411. Fukuda Y, Yasumizu T, Ohta S, Tsurugi Y, Hoshi K. Prenatal confirmation of periventricular leukomalacia in a surviving monochorionic diamniotic twin after death of the other fetus: A case report [In Process Citation]. *Tohoku J Exp Med* 2000;190:61–64.

412. Saito K, Ohtsu Y, Amano K, Nishijima M. Perinatal outcome and management of single fetal death in twin pregnancy: A case series and review. *J Perinat Med.* 1999;27:473–477.

413. Truwit CL, Barkovich AJ, Koch TK, Ferriero DM. Cerebral palsy: MR findings in 40 patients [see comments]. *AJNR Am J Neuroradiol.* 1992;13:67–78.

414. Zalneraitis EL, Young RSK, Krishnamoorthy KS. Intracranial hemorrhage in utero as a complication of isoimmune thrombocytopenia. *J Pediatr.* 1979;95:611–614.

415. Jennette RJ, Daily WJR, Tarby TJ, et al. Prenatal diagnosis of intracerebellar hemorrhage: Case report. *Am J Obstet Gynecol.* 1990;162:1472–1475.

416. Portman M, Brouillette RT. Fetal intracranial haemorrhage complicating amniocentesis. *Am J Obstet Gynecol.* 1982;144:731–735.

417. Lustig-Gillman I, Young BK, Silverman F, et al. Fetal intraventricular hemorrhage: Sonographic diagnosis and clinical implications. *J Clin Ultrasound.* 1983;11:277–280.

418. Burrows RF, Caco CC, Kelton JG. Neonatal alloimmune thrombocytopenia: Spontaneous in utero intracranial hemorrhage. *Am J Hematol.* 1988;28:98–102.

419. Fogarty K, Cohen HL, Haller JO. Sonography of fetal intracranial hemorrhage: Unusual causes and a review of the literature. *J Clin Ultrasound.* 1989;17:366–370.

420. Knuppel RA, Salvatore DLD, Agarwal R, et al. Documented fetal brain damage resulting from a motor vehicle accident. *J Ultrasound Med.* 1994;13:402–404.

421. Jackson JC, Blumhagen JD. Congenital hydrocephalus due to prenatal intracranial hemorrhage. *Pediatrics.* 1983;72:344–346.

422. Coulson CC, Kuller JA, Sweeney WJ. Nonimmune hydrops and hydrocephalus secondary to fetal intracranial hemorrage. *Am J Perinatol.* 1994;11:253–254.

423. Papile LA, Burstein J, Burstein R, et al. Incidence and evolution of subependymal and intraventricular hemorrhage: A study of infants with birth weights less than 1,500 gm. *J Pediatrics.* 1978;92:529–534.

424. Grant EG. Neurosonography: Germinal matrix–related hemorrhage. In: Grant EG, ed. *Neurosonography of the Pre-term Neonate.* New York: Springer-Verlag; 1986:31–68.

425. Haidi HA, Finley J. Mallette JQ, et al. Prenatal diagnosis of cerebellar hemorrhage: Medicolegal implications. *Am J Obstet Gynecol.* 1994;170:1392–1395.

426. Martin R, Roessman U, Fanaroff A. Massive intracerebellar hemorrhage in low birth weight infants. *J Pediatr.* 1976;89:290–293.

427. Ben-Chetrit A, Anteby E, Zacut D, et al. Increased middle cerebral artery blood flow impedance in fetal subdural hematoma. *Ultrasound Obstet Gynecol.* 1991;1:357–358.

428. Kawabata I, Iami A, Tamaya T. Antenatal subdural hemorrhage causing fetal death before labor. *Int J Gynecol Obstet.* 1993;43:57–60.

429. Gunn TR, Mok PM, Becroft DMO. Subdural hemorrhage in utero. *Pediatrics.* 1985;76:605–609.

430. Hanigan WC, Ali MB, Cusak TJ, et al. Diagnosis of subdural hemorrhage in utero. *J Neurosurg.* 1985;63:977–979.

431. Demir RH, Gleicher N, Myers SA. Atraumatic antepartum subdural hematoma causing fetal death. *Am J Obstet Gynecol.* 1989;160:619–620.

432. de Sousa CD, Clark T, Bradshaw A. Antenatally diagnosed subdural haemorrhage in congenital factor X deficiency. *Arch Dis Child.* 1988;63:1168–1170.

CHAPTER
FIVE

Median Anomalies of the Brain

Gianluigi Pilu,
Antonella Perolo,
Pietro Falco,
Antonella Visentin

Median (sometimes erroneously called midline) anomalies of the brain include a heterogenous group of conditions with similarities in the etiology and pathogenetic mechanisms. Table 5–1 reports the classification originally proposed by De Myer[1] and later revised by Fitz,[2] that distinguishes two main categories: disorders of closure and disorders of diverticulation. Disorders of closure include mostly neural tube defects, which are considered elsewhere in this book. Disorders of diverticulation include a series of conditions that are thought to derive from failure of cleavage of the cerebral hemispheres and/or formation of the midline structures. The ontogenesis of the cerebral median plane is frequently referred to as the process of *ventral induction.* It takes place between the seventh week of amhenorrea and midgestation, and is embryologically related to the development of the midface.[3] Disorders of cerebral diverticulation are indeed often a part of malformative sequences that include typical craniofacial malformations.[4]

This chapter covers intracranial abnormalities in the median plane, namely holoprosencephaly, septo-optic dysplasia, agenesis of corpus callosum, and Dandy–Walker malformation (Fig. 5–1). The rational for grouping these conditions together is mostly clinical and is two-fold: first, these disorders are very frequently found in association, and are therefore most likely related embryologically and/or etiologically. Second, the approach to the sonographic diagnosis in the antenatal period requires a similar approach. Indeed, these anomalies result in complex rearrangements of the cerebral architecture. A meticulous scanning technique and the use of nonroutinary views of the fetal brain, such as those obtained in coronal and sagittal planes, are frequently necessary for a specific recognition.

HOLOPROSENCEPHALY

Holoprosencephaly is rarely found at birth. An incidence of 1 in 16,000 neonates is commonly quoted.[5] However, this condition is probably associated with a high intrauterine fatality rate and it is likely that the obstetric sonographers and sonologists will encounter it more frequently than expected from epidemiologic surveys at birth. This concept is supported by one study on voluntary terminations of pregnancies in the first and second trimester in which holoprosencephaly was found in 1 of 250 conceptuses,[6] and by a considerable number of reports on cases diagnosed antenatally with ultrasound published in the last few years. Although the most severe forms of holoprosencephaly are probably associated with early pregnancy loss, it is also very likely that the minor forms will not be recognized at birth, thus escaping epidemiologic surveys.

The etiology is heterogeneous. In most cases, the anomaly is isolated and sporadic. In other cases, chromosomal abnormalities have been found, as well as other congenital anatomical deformities such as anencephaly, encephalocele, and DiGeorge and Meckel syndrome. Several familial cases suggest

TABLE 5–1. CLASSIFICATION OF MEDIAN ANOMALIES OF THE BRAIN AFTER DEMYER[1] AND FITZ[2]

Disorders of diverticulation
  Holoprosencephaly
    Lobar
    Semilobar
    Alobar
Disorders of closure
  Facial clefts
  Cranioschisis
  Corpus callosum
    Agenesis
    Lipoma
  Chiari malformation
  Dandy–Walker malformation

mendelian etiology with autosomal dominant transmission.[5] An overall recurrence risk of 6% is frequently quoted.[7] This, however, reflects mostly the experience with the severe varieties of this condition.

It has been postulated that the pathogenesis of holoprosencephaly depends on failure of embryologic induction of the precordal mesenchyma, which is responsible for the differentiation of both forebrain and median facial structures. Holoprosencephaly indeed fits the definition of a malformative sequence, featuring both cerebral and facial anomalies. Although a continuum of malformations is found in these cases, a widely accepted classification recognizes three major varieties: the alobar, semilobar, and lobar type (Fig. 5–2).[5] In the *alobar* variety,

the most severe one, the longitudial (interhemispheric) fissure and the falx cerebrii are totally absent; there is a single primitive ventricle; the undivided thalami appear fused on the median plane; and there is absence of the third ventricle, neurohypophysis, olfactory bulbs, and tracts. The term arhinencephaly is frequently used as a synonym of holoprosencephaly. In the *semilobar* variety, the two cerebral hemispheres are partially separated posteriorly but there is still a single ventricular cavity. In both the alobar and semilobar forms, the roof of the ventricular cavity, the *tela choroidea,* normally enfolded within the brain, may balloon out between the cerebral convexity and the skull to form a cyst of variable size. This is commonly referred to as the dorsal sac.

With *lobar holoprosencephaly,* the anatomical derangement is much more subtle. In pathologic studies, this condition is usually described as a brain almost completely divided into two distinct hemispheres, with the only exception of a variable degree of fusion at the level of the cyngulate gyrus and frontal horns of lateral ventricles. The septum pellucidum is always absent. The olfactory bulbs and tracts and the corpus callosum may be absent, hypoplastic, or normal.[5] An interesting aspect of lobar holoprosencephaly that has been recently described in studies employing magnetic resonance imaging is the fusion of the fornices, which are seen as a solid fasicle running in the midline in the upper portion of the third ventricle.[8,9]

Pleomorphic facial anomalies are a part of the holoprosencephalic sequence. According to the classification suggested by DeMyer and coworkers,[4,10] five categories can be recognized.

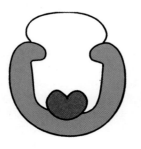

Alobar holoprosencephaly

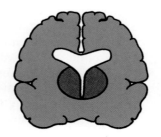

Lobar holoprosencephaly

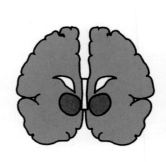

Agenesis of corpus callosum

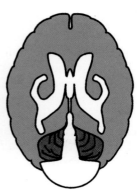

Dandy–Walker malformation

Figure 5–1. Schematic representation of midline brain anomalies

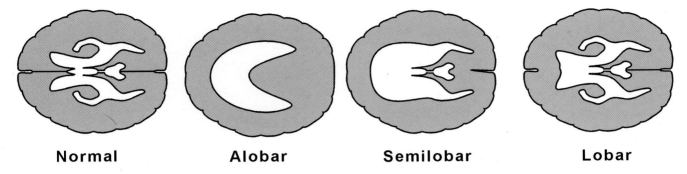

Normal   **Alobar**   **Semilobar**   **Lobar**

Figure 5–2. Schematic representation of holoprosencephaly. In the alobar type, total failure of division of the cerebral hemispheres is found and a single primitive ventricle is present. In semilobar holoprosencephaly, there is one single ventricular cavity but there is incipient separation of the hemispheres in the occipital area and partial development of occipital and temporal horns. In the lobar variety, there is almost complete separation of both cerebral hemispheres and lateral ventricles except for the frontal area.

1. *Cyclopia,* which features a single eye or partially divided eyes in a single orbit and the absence of the nose (arhinia) with a proboscis that usually emerges above the orbit (see Figs. 6-23, and 6-24, Chapter 6).
2. *Ethmocephaly,* which is characterized by extreme hypothelorism, arhinia, and a proboscis emerging above the orbits.
3. *Cebocephaly,* which is characterized by extreme hypothelorism and a proboscis-like nose (see Figs. 6-25 and 6-26, Chapter 6).
4. *A face with median cleft lip* that also has features of hypothelorism and a very flattened or absent nose;
5. *A face with a median philtrum–premaxilla anlage and flat nose.* This condition involves the presence of bilateral cleft lip/palate, hypothelorism, and a flat nose.

Cyclopia and etmocephaly are invariably associated with alobar holoprosencephaly. Cebocephaly and median cleft lip face may be found in either the alobar or semilobar variety. The face with median philtrum–premaxilla anlage is indicative of either semilobar or lobar varieties. It should be stressed that infants with any kind of holoprosencephaly may have a normal face.[5]

Holoprosencephaly reflects a very early derangement of embryogenesis. As such, it is very frequently associated with other malformations. Apart from facial anomalies that are considered a part of the malformative sequence, holoprosencephaly has a striking association with two other conditions: chromosomal aberrations and Dandy–Walker malformation.[5,7] Among chromosomal aberrations, trisomy 13 is typical. It has been estimated that over 60% of infants with trisomy 13 have holoprosencephaly; conversely, holoprosencephaly is associated with trisomy 13 in about 20% of cases. We have found that fetal holoprosencephaly is also frequently found with triploidy.[11] All varieties of holoprosencephaly are often associated with microcephaly and less frequently, with macrocephaly, which is invariably due to internal obstructive hydrocephalus.

Several cases of sonographic antenatal diagnosis of alobar holoprosencephaly have been reported in the literature. A variety of findings has been described.[12–16] In our experience, the most valuable clue to the diagnosis is the demonstration of the single primitive ventricle (Fig. 5–3). When present, the dorsal sac can be recognized (Fig. 5–4), as well as facial anomalies such as cyclopia, hypothelorism, anophtalmia, arhinia, a proboscis, and median cleft lip.[17,18] Demonstration of facial anomalies strengthens the diagnosis of holoprosencephaly based on central nervous system findings. Conversely, should any of the mentioned facial features be unexpectedly encountered, a careful examination of the intracranial contents is recommended.

By using high frequency transvaginal transducers, diverticulation of the forebrain can be demonstrated as early as the 7th week of amhenorrea.[19] Indeed, by using this approach a diagnosis of the alobar variety can be easily made at the onset of the second trimester,[20] and may be possible as early as the 10th week of amhenorrea (Fig. 5–5).

Antenatal diagnosis of semilobar holoprosencephaly has been reported in a limited number of cases.[21] The ultrasonic findings were very similar to the ones described in cases of alobar holoprosencephaly. The diagnosis of the semilobar variety is suggested by the presence of well developed occipital horns.[22,23]

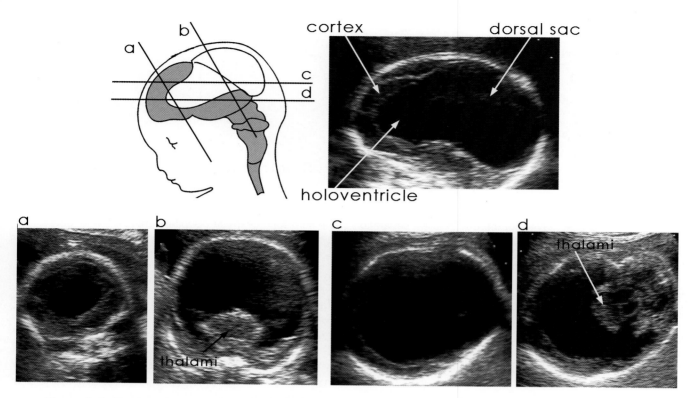

Figure 5–3. Sonography of alobar holoprosencephaly in the midtrimester. A median view reveals the anterior pancaked cortex, and the cavity of the holoventricle widely communicating posteriorly with the large dorsal sac. The different appearance in coronal and axial scanning planes is demonstrated in a through d.

Although lobar holoprosencephaly is amenable to antenatal identification, a specific diagnosis is difficult. The typical case will present with some degree of enlargement of lateral ventricles, absence of the septum pellucidum, and a wide communication between the frontal horns and the inferior third ventricle (Fig. 5–6). The major problem resides in the differential diagnosis between lobar holoprosencephaly and other hydrocephalic conditions associated with secondary disruption of the septum pellucidum. An important clue is the demonstration of a flat roof of frontal horns in a midcoronal view of the brain.[24,25] However, this approach does carry some subjectivity, and is certainly hampered in cases with gross ventricular enlargement. In some cases of lobar holoprosencephaly, the fornices have an abnormal configuration and are seen in the midline as a thick fasicle running from the anterior to the posterior commissure (Fig. 5–6).[7,8] In the midcoronal scan, the abnormal fornices result in a peculiar image: a small round structure is seen in the midportion of the third ventricle. Demonstration of this finding allows a specific diagnosis on objective grounds.

Both alobar and semilobar holoprosencephaly are associated with a dismal prognosis. When these conditions are identified in utero, termination of pregnancy should be offered prior to viability. Conservative management is strongly recommended in continuing pregnancies.[14]

The prognosis of lobar holoprosencephaly is uncertain. The available clinical data are limited. It has been reported that affected individuals may have a normal life span, but mental retardation and neurologic sequelae are common.[5,26] Dysplasia of the cerebral acqueduct (Sylvius) is presumably present in many cases, leading to obstructive hydrocephaly.[26] The only available antenatal series includes five infants that were followed up after birth, and all had very abnormal developmental quotients.[25] This series may be biased by the inclusion of fetuses with severe hydrocephaly and other associated anomalies.

Evaluation of the karyotype should always be offered, as this information has a major impact on the formulation of the recurrence risk for future pregnancies.

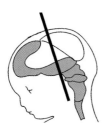

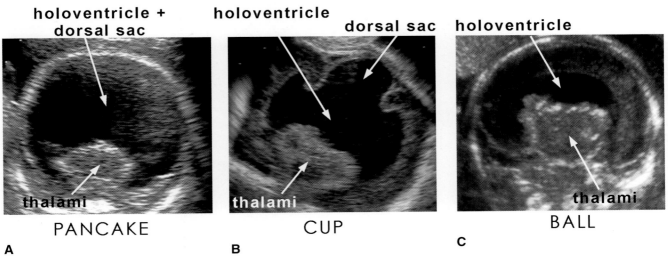

Figure 5–4. Varieties of alobar holoprosencephaly in the coronal plane. **A.** In the "pancake variety", only a thin rim of cortex is found and there is ample communication between the holoventricle and the dorsal sac. **B.** In the "cup" variety, the cortex is partially enfolded forming a ridge between the cavity of the holoventricle and the superior dorsal sac. In the "ball" variety, the cortex is completely enfolded and no dorsal sac is found. The pancake and cup varieties are more frequently associated with hydrocephalus and macrocephaly. **C.** The ball variety is more frequently found with microcephaly. *(Courtesy of Ana Monteagudo and Ilan E. Timor-Tritsch.)*

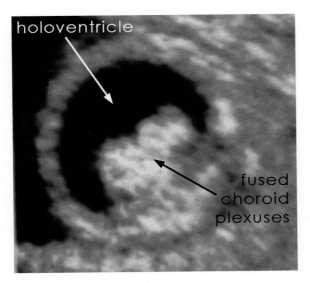

Figure 5–5. In this transvaginal sonography of an embryo at 11 post-menstrual weeks reveals profound derangement from the normal intracranial architecture. The midline echo is absent, most of the intracranial cavity is occupied by a single fluid-filled cavity—the holoventricle—and the glomi of choroid plexuses of lateral ventricles are incompletely divided. These findings are compatible with alobar holoprosencephaly. *(Courtesy of Ana Monteagudo and Ilan E. Timor-Tritsch.)*

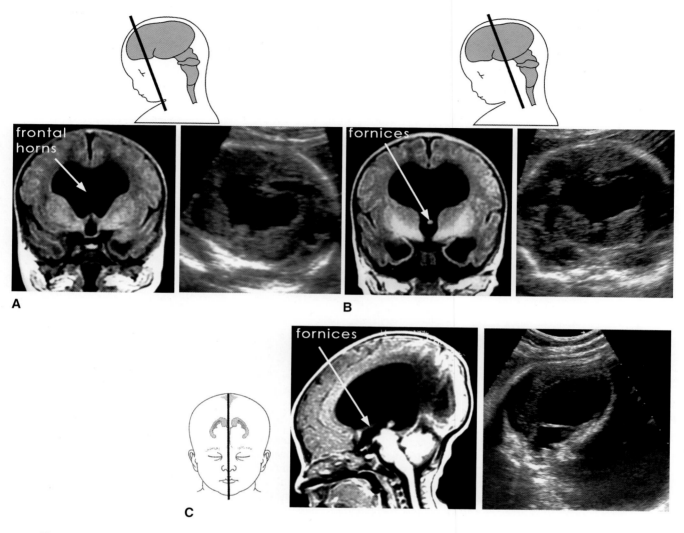

Figure 5–6. A combination of scanning planes obtained with postnatal MRI and prenatal ultrasound in a case with lobar holoprosencephaly. **A** and **B.** The coronal planes demonstrate the fusion of the frontal horns, which have a typically flat roof and communicate inferiorly with the cavity of the third ventricle *(arrow)*. In between the cavities of lateral ventricles and third ventricle, the fused fornices are seen in the coronal and in the median plane **(C)** as well.

Septo-Optic Dysplasia

Septo-optic dysplasia (de Morsier syndrome) is a rare cerebral anomaly of unknown etiology that features an absence of the septum pellucidum and optic disk hypoplasia. Affected individuals have visual impairment and pituitary–hypothalamic axis dysfunction. Occasional findings include ventriculomegaly, mental retardation, hemiparesis, and craniofacial anomalies such as hypothelorism and clefting.[27,28]

Postnatal[29] and prenatal sonographic findings[30] in septo-optic dysplasia are virtually identical to those of lobar holoprosencephaly (Fig. 5–7). A definitive diagnosis of this condition is possible after birth by demonstrating optic tract hypoplasia,[28] but this does not seem possible at present. It has been sug-gested that fetal blood sampling could be helpful in such cases, by demonstrating signs of hypopitu-itarism,[25] but this approach is untested thus far.

Agenesis of the Corpus Callosum

Agenesis of the corpus callosum (ACC) is an anom-aly of uncertain prevalence and clinical significance. The incidence varies in different studies, depending upon the population investigated and the method of ascertainment. Estimates of 0.3% to 0.7% in the general population[31] and 2% to 3% in the develop-mentally disabled[32,33] are usually quoted.

The available literature suggests a heteroge-nous etiology. Genetic factors are probably predomi-nant. Autosomal dominant, autosomal recessive,

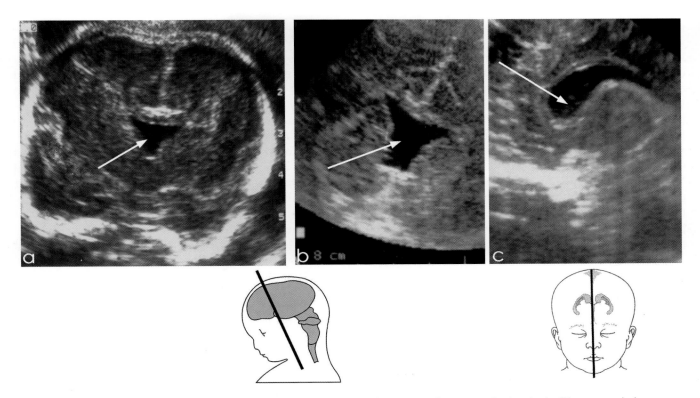

Figure 5–7. Prenatal (a) and postnatal (b and c) sonograms in a case of septo-optic dysplasia. The coronal views demonstrate the absence of the septum pellucidum and the typical square-shaped appearance of the fused frontal horns. In a sagittal view, a thin hypoplastic corpus callosum is seen arching above the fused cavity of frontal horns. *(Courtesy of Ana Monteagudo and Ilan E. Timor-Tritsch.)*

and sex-linked transmission have all been documented.[34,35] Agenesis of the corpus callosum is also a part of mendelian syndromes (Table 5–2), including Walker–Warburg syndrome[36]; Andermann's syndrome[37], acrocallosal syndrome[38]; F.G. syndrome[39]; and Fryns syndrome.[40] Callosal agenesis is also found in two conditions with sex-linked dominant etiology and lethality in males: the orofaciodigital type I syndrome[41] and Aicardi syndrome.[42] Frontonasal dysplasia or median cleft face syndrome is also frequently associated with ACC. This condition is usually a sporadic disease, but a few familial cases consistent with an autosomal dominant transmission have been described.[43] A high frequency of ACC has been documented in infants with inborn errors of metabolism.[44] Various teratogens have also been implicated as a possible cause of ACC, including alcohol, valproate, cocaine and the rubella and influenza viruses.

The corpus callosum is the largest commissure connecting the cerebral hemispheres. It is a broad plate of dense myelinated fibers located deep in the longitudinal fissure. These fibers are two way inter-

TABLE 5–2. SYNDROMES FEATURING AGENESIS OF THE CORPUS CALLOSUM

Acrocallosal syndrome (AR)
Apert syndrome (AR)
Aicardi syndrome (X-linked dominant)
Andermann syndrome (AR)
Callosogenital dysplasia (AR)
Cerebro-oculo-facio-skeletal (COFS) syndrome (AR)
Neu–Laxova syndrome (AR)
FG syndrome (X-linked recessive)
Frontonasal dysplasia (sporadic/AD)
Hydrolethalus (AR, X-linked dominant)
Lens dysplasia (X-linked recessive)
Oculo-cerebro-cutaneous syndrome (Delleman syndrome) (unknown)
Oro-facio-digital syndrome type I (X-linked dominant)
Shapiro syndrome (X-linked recessive)
Fetal alcohol syndrome
Chromosomal aberrations
Metabolic disorders

AR, autosomal recessive; AD, autosomal dominant.
Modified from Blum et al. Genet Counsel. 1992; 38:115.

connections between regions of the cortex in all lobes with corresponding regions of the opposite hemispheres. It derives from the conmissural plate, an embryologic structure formed by the fusion of the lateral margins of the groove that separates the primitive telencephalic vesicles. Development of the corpus callosum is a late event in cerebral ontogenesis that takes place between 12 and 18 postmenstrual weeks. The corpus callosum is in close anatomic and embryologic relationship with the underlying septum pellucidum. Although there is no a priori evidence to suggest that the development of the septum pellucidum cannot proceed independently of the corpus callosum, most observers claim that there can be no septum pellucidum without a corpus callosum.[3]

Agenesis of the corpus callosum may be either complete or partial. In the latter case, also referred to as dysgenesis of the corpus callosum, the posterior portion (splenium and body) is missing to varying degrees. Agenesis of the corpus callosum is typically associated with significant distorsion of the intracranial architecture. The lateral ventricles tend to be larger than normal, particularly at the level of the atria and occipital horns. It has been postulated that the absence of the posterior portion of the corpus callosum results in distortion of the array of white matter tracts in the occipital lobes leading to posterior expansion of the ventricles.[45] Such ventricular enlargement tends to be stable and is not usually associated with intracranial hypertension. The anterior horns are usually normal in size but are more separated than normal from the midline. The third ventricle is often superiorly elongated, reaching the area normally occupied by the corpus callosum. Absence of the corpus callosum also results in abnormal induction of medial cerebral convolutions, determining a radiate arrangement of cerebral sulci around the roof of the third ventricle, extending through the zone normally occupied by the cyngulate gyrus. The modification of the arterial vascular supply in infants with agenesis of the corpus callosum has been investigated in depth with both angiography[46] and transfontanellar sonography[47] and are relevant for antenatal diagnosis. Under normal conditions, a branch of the anterior callosal artery runs along the superior surface of the corpus callosum, describing a semicircular loop (see Chapter 2). When the corpus callosum is absent, the loop of the pericallosal artery is lost and branches of the anterior cerebral artery are seen ascending linearly with a radiate arrangement.

The high frequency of associated malformations suggest that agenesis of the corpus callosum is frequently a part of a widespread developmental disturbance. In a review of the literature, associated central nervous system anomalies, including microcephaly, abnormal convolutional patterns, neural tube defects, Dandy–Walker malformation and aplasia or hypoplasia of the pyramidal tracts, were found in 85% of the cases. Systemic anomalies including a variety of musculoskeletal, cardiovascular, genitourinary, and gastrointestinal malformations were found in 62% of cases.[48] In the largest antenatal series, anatomic anomalies were present in 50% of cases. The anomaly most frequently encountered was Dandy–Walker malformation. Cardiovascular anomalies mainly included conotruncal malformations such as tetralogy of Fallot and double outlet right ventricle.[49]

Intracranial lipomas are also occasionally found in association with agenesis of the corpus callosum. Conversely, they are associated in 50% of cases with complete or partial agenesis of the corpus callosum.[50]

An abnormal karyotype is found in 20% of affected fetuses.[49] In a review of the pediatric literature about agenesis of the corpus callosum and chromosomal aberrations, trisomy 18 was found in 30% of cases; a form of trisomy 8 and trisomy 13 in 20% each; and a variety of different conditions in the remaining.[51] It has been postulated that chromosomes 8, 13, and 18 have a direct influence on the development of the corpus callosum.

The corpus callosum is a thin band of white matter, and its sonographic demonstration requires adequate angles of insonation. Only sagittal and coronal scans of the fetal brain usually allow a clear visualization. Such views require a meticulous scanning technique but can be obtained with standard transabdominal ultrasound in most fetuses in breech or transverse lie.[52] In fetuses in vertex presentation, transvaginal sonography is the technique of choice.[53]

Fetal agenesis of the corpus callosum is associated with elusive findings. The diagnosis of this condition is a challenge even for expert sonologists, particularly prior to 20 weeks. Development of the corpus callosum is a late event in cerebral ontogenesis that takes place between 12 and 18 postmenstrual weeks of gestation. Prior to 18 postmenstrual weeks, the diagnosis is probably impossible in most cases. In routine examinations performed after this time, failure to visualize the cavum septum pellucidum and/or an increased atrial width should alert to the possibility of agenesis of the corpus callosum. Once a suspicion has been formulated, direct demonstration of the absence of the corpus callosum is possible by coronal and sagittal scans (Fig. 5–8). These views are at times difficult to obtain, in particular in vertex fetuses. However, transvaginal sonography is of great advantage in such cases.

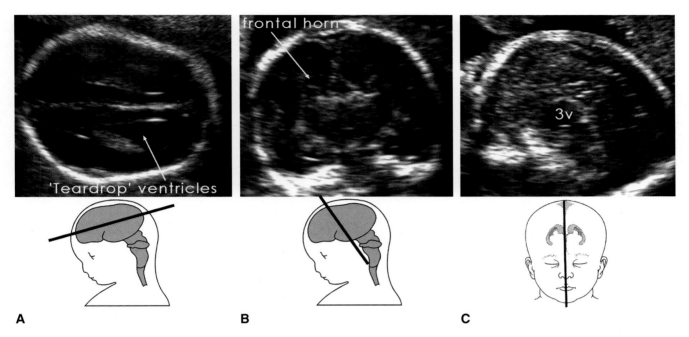

Figure 5–8. Typical presentation of complete agenesis of the corpus callosum in the midtrimester. **A.** An axial plane demonstrates absence of the cavum septi pellucidi, and lateral ventricles with a teardrop shape and a borderline internal diameter. **B** and **C.** The coronal plane and median plane demonstrates absence of both the cavum septi pellucidi and corpus callosum. 3v, Third ventricle.

Imaging by Doppler techniques, the anterior cerebral artery is ascending vertically without forming the loop of the pericallosal artery. This sonographic image strengthens the diagnosis (Fig. 5–9).[47,54–61] Upward displacement of the third ventricle, which is also frequently enlarged, can be identified by demonstrating that this structure reaches superiorly the level of lateral ventricles in either a coronal or axial scan. As mentioned previously, intracranial lipomas are frequently associated with agenesis of the corpus callosum. Demonstration of a brightly echogenic mass in the area of the corpus callosum should, therefore, raise the suspicion of a callosal anomaly. It is worth noting that lipomas are usually not demonstrable in the second trimester and tend to appear only in late gestation.[49,50] Agenesis of the corpus callosum may also be associated with interhemispheric (arachnoid) cysts (Fig. 5–10).

The available evidence suggests that the elusive findings associated with agenesis of corpus callosum can be identified in most cases by targeted examinations. The sensitivity of nontargeted examinations is unknown, but it is probably very low (Fig. 5–11). In a routine survey of fetal anatomy, failure to visualize the cavum septi pellucidi later than 18 postmenstrual weeks of gestation should raise the suspicion of fetal ACC.[49] The observation that the ventricular atria and posterior horns (colpocephaly)

are abnormally large in ACC has a practical value. Routine sonography of the fetal brain is usually performed with axial scans[62] that do not allow the demonstration of the corpus callosum itself. The final diagnosis is established if one can obtain a median plane on which the absence of the corpus callosum can directly be observed. However, enlargement of the atria of lateral ventricles is readily appreciated with the customary axial views. With this regard, it is worth noting that ACC has been found in 3% of all fetuses with ventriculomegaly[62] and in almost 10% of those with mild ventriculomegaly.[63] Unfortunately, the proportion of fetuses with ACC that have an abnormal atrial width remains uncertain.

A distinction should be made between complete and partial ACC. Complete ACC is commonly regarded as a malformation, deriving from faulty embryogenesis, whereas partial ACC may represent both a true malformation and a disruptive event occurring at any time during pregnancy. Partial agenesis of the corpus callosum has been recognized antenatally in two cases.[49,60] Both fetuses had an unequivocal "teardrop" configuration of lateral ventricles. The natural history of partial ACC is nevertheless uncertain, and the cerebral findings associated with it are probably more subtle than with the complete form. It is expected that antenatal diagnosis will not be possible in all cases.

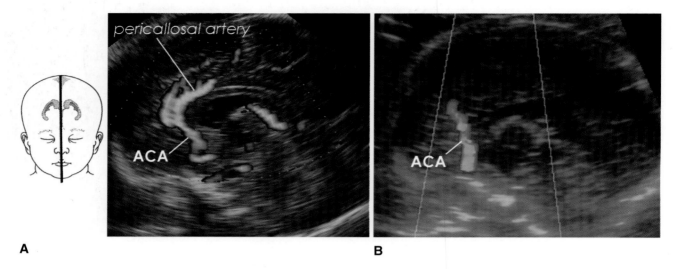

A   B

Figure 5–9. Color Doppler of the anterior cerebral circulation in the midtrimester. In a normal fetus **(A),** the pericallosal artery is seen arising from the anterior cerebral artery (ACA) and looping over the corpus callosum. In a fetus with agenesis of the corpus callosum **(B),** the pericallosal artery is absent and the anterior carotid artery ascends vertically.

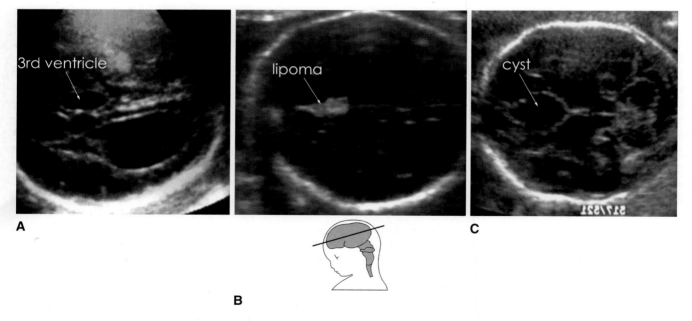

A   C

B

Figure 5–10. Different presentations of agenesis of the corpus callosum. **A.** Enlargement and upward displacement of the third ventricle result in the presence of a cystic structure between the hemispheres (the position normally occupied by the cavum septum pellucidi). **B.** An echogenic mass suggest the presence of a lipoma. **C.** A large interhemispheric cyst is present.

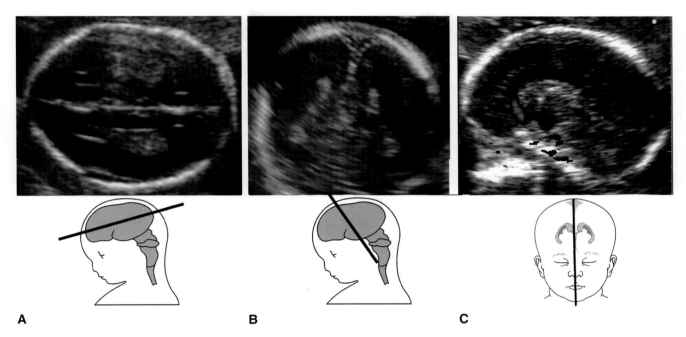

Figure 5–11. In this case of complete agenesis of the corpus callosum, the indirect sign of absence of the cavum septi pellucidi, that is, the colpocephaly was the only abnormal finding in the axial planes **(A)**. **B.** A midcoronal plane was not useful because it appears normal. **C.** On the median plane using Doppler flow study only the incipent portion of one pericallosid artery is seen.

Agenesis of the corpus callosum is associated with an excess of both cerebral and noncerebral anomalies as well as with a high risk of chromosomal aberrations.[49] Antenatal identification of this condition dictates the need of a careful survey of the entire fetal anatomy, including echocardiography and karyotype.

Counselling couples in which isolated ACC is unexpectedly encountered at antenatal sonography in the absence of associated anomalies is a difficult task. Pediatric series are mainly based on investigation of symptomatic individuals and are, therefore, presumably biased. Many authorities believe that ACC in itself has little consequence on neurologic development, which will be revealed only by specific tests.[64] However, no specific risk figures are available at present. A total of 30 infants with a prenatal diagnosis of isolated agenesis of the corpus callosum (that is, no other malformations demonstrable at sonography and a normal karyotype) and a postnatal follow-up ranging between a few months to 11 years have been reported thus far. A normal or borderline development was present in 26, or 87%.[65,66] In all cases with severe handicap, other anomalies were present (ethmoidal cephalocele in one case, CHARGE association in another one, and Aicardi syndrome in two). Although it is acknowledged that the number of cases and the duration of

follow-up are limited, these results are worth noting. The diagnosis of isolated ACC in the fetus does raise concerns about the possibility of association with either genetic syndromes, inborn errors of metabolism, or anatomic anomalies unpredictable by antenatal testing. However, the available experience suggest that callosal agenesis is compatible with a normal or borderline postnatal development in most cases. As some genetic conditions associated with ACC, such as Aicardi syndrome, have sex-linked dominant etiology, it has been proposed that documentation of a male karyotype is reassuring.[66] It should be remembered that ACC is a unique condition that, even in the presence of a normal intelligence, is associated with peculiar neurologic findings and subtle cognitive deficits. The interested reader is referred to specific works on this subject.[67–71] A possible relationship between ACC and psychotic disorders has also been hypothesized.[72]

Some intracranial findings have been found in excess in fetuses with a poor outcome, and may have therefore prognostic value (albeit the experience thus far is limited). In our series, upward displacement of the third ventricle and a distended longitudial (interhemispheric) fissure were most frequently associated with neurologic impairment, associated anomalies, or both.[49] This is perhaps not surprising when one considers that these findings probably indicate a more severe derangement of cerebral development. Interestingly enough, no correlation was found between the degree of ventricular enlargement and the outcome.[49]

In continuing pregnancies, the diagnosis of fetal isolated ACC does not require any modification of standard obstetric management. In our experience, failure to progress in labor requiring cesarean delivery occurred on several occasions, and this may be somehow related to the high frequency of macrocrania in infants with callosal agenesis.[49]

DANDY–WALKER MALFORMATION AND VARIANTS

The Dandy–Walker malformation has an estimated incidence of about 1 in 30,000 births, and is found in 4% to 12% of all cases of infantile hydrocephalus.[73] It is a severe anomaly, with associated malformation in 50% to 70% of cases and a poor neurodevelopmental outcome in 50% to 70% of survivors.

Genetic factors have a major role in the etiology of this condition. Dandy–Walker malformation may occur as a part of mendelian disorders, such as Meckel syndrome and Walker–Warburg syndrome. It has been found in chromosomal aberrations, such as 45,X, 6p−, and triploidy. In the absence of a recognizable syndrome, the empiric recurrence risk is 1% to 5%. In rare cases, the disease is inherited as an autosomal recessive trait. Joubert syndrome, a cerebral anomaly similar to Dandy–Walker malformation, is also transmitted as an autosomal recessive trait.[74] Environmental factors, including viral infections, alcohol use, and diabetes, have also been suggested to play a role in the genesis of Dandy–Walker malformation, but the evidence in uncertain.

The term Dandy–Walker malformation was originally introduced to indicate the association of (1) ventriculomegaly of variable degree, (2) a large cerebello-medullar cistern (cisterna magna), and (3) a defect in the cerebellar vermis through which the "cyst" communicates with the fourth ventricle.[75,76] Following the introduction of computed tomography, variations of the classic Dandy–Walker malformation have been described, and the term *Dandy–Walker complex* was introduced to indicate a spectrum of anomalies that were originally classified as follows.

1. Classic Dandy–Walker malformation: enlarged posterior fossa, complete or partial agenesis of the cerebellar vermis, and elevated tentorium.
2. Dandy–Walker variant: variable hypoplasia of the cerebellar vermis with or without enlargement of the cerebello-medullar cistern.
3. Megacisterna magna: enlarged cerebello-medullar cistern with integrity of both cerebellar vermis and fourth ventricle.

This classification has been challenged after the introduction of magnetic resonance imaging. The axial scans traditionally employed in computed tomography scans do not have the capability of assessing clearly the status of the cerebellar vermis and may both underestimate and overestimate the size of a defect. The excellent resolution in the sagittal planes made possible by magnetic resonance has allowed demonstration that the classification based on computed tomography is inadequate to describe the anatomic derangement encountered in the Dandy–Walker complex. Some degree of vermian dysgenesis can be found in all cases, even with megacisterna magna, whereas classic Dandy–Walker malformation and Dandy–Walker variant have so many similarities that a clear-cut distinction is often impossible.[77]

Sonographic antenatal diagnosis of the Dandy–Walker complex. It is achieved most frequently with the use of axial planes and obviously suffers the same limitations as computed tomography. The classic type of Dandy–Walker malformation, with a greatly enlarged posterior fossa, splayed cerebellar hemispheres, and a large vermian defect, is easily recognized since midgestation (Fig. 5–12).[78,79] It has indeed been reported as early as 14 postmenstrual weeks by using transvaginal sonography.[80] Much less certain is the identification of minor variants (Fig. 5–13). It has been suggested that a cerebello medullar cistern with a depth greater than 10 mm is suggestive of megacisterna magna,[81] and that a communication between the fourth ventricle and this cistern is indicative of the Dandy–Walker variant.[82] Caution is warranted when making these diagnoses. In the early second trimester, the sonographic appearance of the normal cerebellar development can resemble pathology: the relatively large fourth ventricle and the incompletely formed inferior cerebellar vermis may give the false impression of a vermian defect. It is imprudent to make such a diagnosis at this gestational age.[83,84] A follow-up scan at 18 postmenstrual weeks or later is recommended. Even at this time, however, a scanning angle that is too steep may create the impression of an excessively sized cistern and even of a vermian defect. The origin for this artifact remains unclear, but it is probably conjured up by the very high resolution of modern ultrasound equipment, demonstrating a layer of

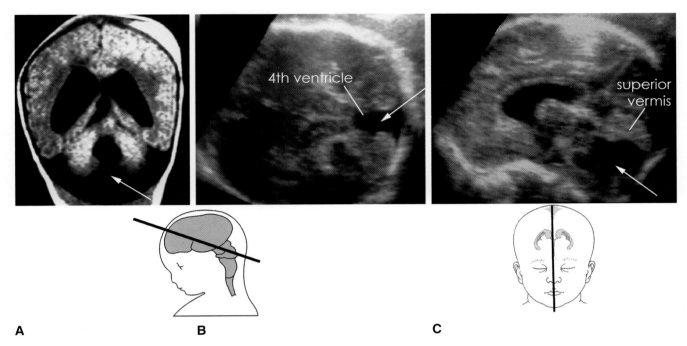

Figure 5–12. Classic Dandy–Walker malformation demonstrated by postnatal MRI and prenatal ultrasound. **A.** The postnatal MRI. **B.** A large defect of the cerebellar vermis *(arrow)* connects the fourth ventricle with a large cerebello-medullar cistern (cisterna magna). **C.** The median view confirms the connection between the cistern and the area of the fourth ventricle. Only the superior portion of the cerebellar vermis can be demonstrated.

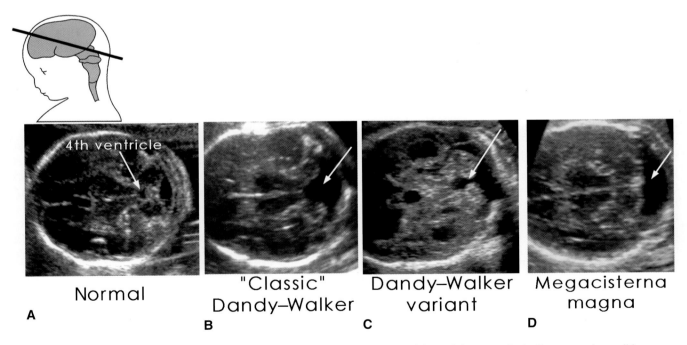

Figure 5–13. The spectrum of Dandy–Walker complex demonstrated by axial scans. **A.** In the normal condition, the cavity of the fourth ventricle *(arrow)* is separated by the cerebello-medullar cistern (cisterna magna) from the inferior cerebellar vermis. **B.** In the classic type of Dandy–Walker malformation, the vermis is largely absent, the cerebellar hemispheres are splayed apart *(arrow),* and the cistern greatly enlarged. **C.** With the Dandy–Walker variant, a thin communication *(arrow)* is found between the cavity of the fourth ventricle and the cistern. **D.** Megacisterna magna is featured by an enlarged cistern *(arrow)* with a seemingly intact cerebellum.

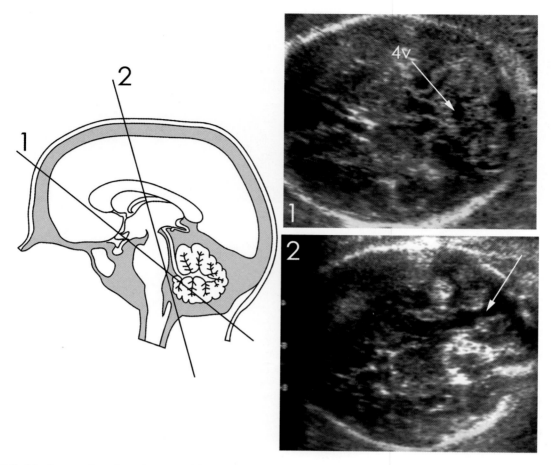

Figure 5–14. A scanning plane to steep (almost coronal) into the fetal head may lead to the erroneous impression that the fourth ventricle (4v) communicates posteriorly with the cisterna cerebello-medullaris (magna). 1. Slightly slanted axial plane. 2. The steep, almost coronal plane.

fluid normally present between the cerebellar tonsils and the brain stem (Fig. 5–14). Visualization of the posterior fossa in the median plane may be helpful in these cases in that it allows demonstration of the vermis in the sagittal plane. It is unlikely however that even this approach will solve the problem of a subtle dysgenesis of the cerebellum. We have recently seen several fetuses on antenatal ultrasound that had either an isolated enlargement of the cerebello-medullar cistern or an image suggestive of a small vermian defect that were not confirmed by postnatal follow-up (Figs. 5–15 and 5–16). On the other hand, despite meticulous multiplanar imaging, we have been unable to demonstrate any cerebellar defect in a fetus with a slightly enlarged cistern that was found at birth to have Dandy–Walker variant and overt ventriculomegaly requiring neurosurgery.[85]

These results are well correlated both with a recent clinical series describing a normal outcome in 7 of 13 infants with an antenatal diagnosis of Dandy–Walker variant,[86] and with an autopsy series, attesting that antenatal ultrasound in generally works poorly both in recognizing as well as excluding the Dandy–Walker complex, with about 50% false positives.[87]

In conclusion, the experience thus far indicates that it may be impossible to solve antenatally the doubt of either a large cerebello-medullar cistern or a defect of the cerebellar vermis. A targeted scan to exclude associated anomalies is certainly indicated, and even fetal karyotyping has been suggested. How to counsel the patients in which the abnormal findings in the fetal posterior fossa are isolated remains however uncertain. Indeed, these findings may represent an artifact, and the fetal brain may prove to be entirely normal. On the other hand, the clinical significance of the minor varieties of the Dandy–Walker complex is scarcely known. An association with neurologic compromise

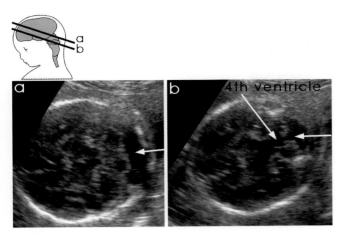

Figure 5–15. a. at 22 postmenstrual weeks, ultrasound reveals borderline ventriculomegaly and a slightly enlarged cerebello-medullar cistern (cisterna magna) (depth 11 mm). b. A low axial plane reveals an image suggesting a communication between the area of the fourth ventricle and the cisterna magna. The patient requested pregnancy termination and pathology revealed a small, hypoplastic cerebellum with a very small defect of the lower vermis.

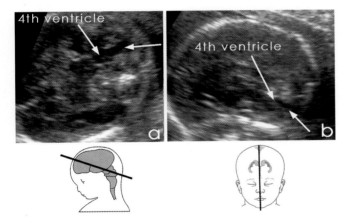

Figure 5–16. a. At 22 postmenstrual weeks, ultrasound reveals an image suggestive of a communication between the fourth ventricle and the cisterna magna, which has, however, a normal size. b. a median plane section seems to confirm the finding, although it is unclear whether the impression is due to increased rotation of the cerebellum, a normal anatomic variant. Following termination of pregnancy, pathology revealed a small and possibly hypoplastic cerebellum, but failed to demonstrate a defect in the vermis.

TABLE 5–3. ABNORMALITIES ASSOCIATED WITH DANDY–WALKER COMPLEX AFTER MURRAY[74]

Mendelian
  Warburg (AR)
  Aase–Smith (AD)
  Ruvalcaba syndrome (AD/X-linked)
  Coffin–Siris (AR)
  Oro-facio-digital syndrome type II (AR)
  Meckel–Gruber syndrome (AR)
  Aicardi syndrome (X-linked dominant)
  Ellis Van Creveld (AR)
  Fraser cryptophthalmus (AR)
Chromosomal
  45,X
  6p−
  9q+
  Dup 5p
  Dup 8p
  Dup 8q
  Trisomy 9
  Triploidy
  Dup 17q
Environmental
  Rubella
  Coumadin
  Alcohol use
  CMV
  Diabetes
  Isotretinoin
Multifactorial
  Congenital heart disease
  Neural tube defects
  Cleft lip/palate
Sporadic
  Holoprosencephaly
  Cornelia de Lange syndrome
  Goldenhar syndrome
  Kidney abnormalities
  Facial hemangiomas
  Klippel–Feil syndrome
  Polysyndactyly

AR, autosomal recessive; AD, autosomal dominant.

certainly exists, but no clear-cut prognostic data are available. Sonologists should be well aware of all these limitations. Whether or not intrauterine magnetic resonence can be of value in these cases remains to be demonstrated. Dandy–Walker malformation has been diagnosed in utero with magnetic resonance.[88] However, the relatively limited spatial resolution and the difficulty of obtaining exact sagittal planes with current magnetic resonance technology makes one wonder whether this technique will prove any better than ultrasound in recognizing or excluding defects of the cerebellar vermis, particularly at midgestation.

REFERENCES

1. De Myer W. Classification of cerebral malformations. *Birth Defects.* 1971; 7:78–93.
2. Fitz CR. Midline anomalies of the brain and spine. *Radiol Clin North Am.* 1982;20:95–104.
3. Leech RW, Shuman RM. Holoprosencephaly and related midline cerebral anomalies. *J Child Neurol.* 1986;1:3–18.
4. DeMyer W. Zeman W. Alobar holoprosencephaly (arhinencephaly) with median cleft lip and palate: Clinical electroencephalographic and nosologic considerations. *Confin Neurol.* 1963;23:1–36.
5. DeMyer W. Holoprosencephaly. In: Vinken PJ, Bruyn GW, eds. *Handbook of Clinical Neurology.* Amsterdam: Elsevier, 1977:431–478.
6. Matsunaga E, Shiota Y. Holoprosencephaly in human embryos: Epidemiological studies of 150 cases. *Teratology.* 1977;16:261–72.
7. Cohen MM. An update on the holoprosencephalic disorders. *J Pediatr* 1982;101:865–9.
8. Triulzi F, Parazzini C, Bianchini E. La oloprosencefalia lobare tipo B. Valutazione RM di una disgenesia della linea mediana. In: Scotti G, ed. *Neuradiologia.* Udine: Centauro; 1992:103–108.
9. Pilu G, Ambrosetto P, Sandri F et al. Intraventricular fused fornices: A specific sign of fetal lobar holoprosencephaly. *Ultrasound Obstet Gynecol.* 1994;4:65-7.
10. DeMyer W, Zeman W, Palmer CG. The face predicts the brain. Diagnostic significance of median facial anomalies for holoprosencephaly (arhinencephaly). *Pediatrics.* 1964;34:259–62.
11. Rizzo N, Pittalis MC, Pilu G, et al. Prenatal karyotyping in malformed fetuses. *Prenat Diagn.* 1990;10:17–23.
12. Hill LM, Breckle R, Bonebrake CR. Ultrasonic findings with holoprosencephaly. *J Reprod Med.* 1982; 27:172–5.
13. Blackwell DE, Spinnato JA, Horsch G, et al. Prenatal diagnosis of cyclopia. *Am J Obstet Gynecol.* 1982;143:848–52.
14. Chervenak FA, Isaacson G, Mahoney MJ, et al. The obstetric significance of holoprosencephaly. *Obstet Gynecol.* 1984;63:115–21.
15. Benacerraf BR, Frigoletto FD, Bieber FR. The fetal face. Ultrasound examination. *Radiology.* 1984;153:495–7.
16. Filly RA, Chinn DH, Callen PW. Alobar holoprosencephaly. Ultrasonographic prenatal diagnosis. *Radiology.* 1984;151:455–9.
17. Pilu G, Romero R, Rizzo N, et al. Criteria for the antenatal diagnosis of holoprosencephaly. *Am J Perinatol.* 1987;4:41–9.
18. Pilu G, Reece EA, Romero R et al. Prenatal diagnosis of cranio-facial malformations by sonography. *Am J Obstet Gynecol.* 1986;155:45–50.
19. Blaas HG, Eik-Nes SH, Kiserud T, et al. Early development of the forebrain and midbrain: A longitudinal study from 7 to 12 weeks of gestation. *Ultrasound Obstet Gynecol.* 1994;3:183–92.
20. Bronshtein M, Weiner Z. Early sonographic diagnosis of alobar holoprosencephaly. *Prenat Diagn.* 1991;11:459–62.
21. Cayea PD, Balcar I, Alberti O, et al. Prenatal diagnosis of semilobar holoprosencephaly. *Am J Roentgenol.* 1984;142:401–2.
22. Fitz CR. Holoprosencephaly and related entities. *Neuroradiology.* 1983;25:225–38.
23. Altman NR, Altman DH, Sheldon JJ, et al: Holoprosencephaly classified by computed tomography. *Am J Neuroradiol.* 1984;5:433–7.
24. Hoffman-Tretin JC, Horoupian DS, Koenigsberg M, et al. Lobar holoprosencephaly with hydrocephalus: Antenatal demonstration and differential diagnosis. *J Ultrasound Med.* 1986;5:691–7.
25. Pilu G, Sandri F, Perolo A, et al. Prenatal diagnosis of lobar holoprosencephaly. *Ultrasound Obstet Gynecol.* 1992;2:88–94.
26. Osaka K, Matsumoto S. Holoprosencephaly in neurosurgical practice. *J Neurosurg.* 1978;48:787–91.
27. de Morsier G. Etudes sur le dysraphies cranioencephaliques. III. Agenesie du septum pellucidum avec malformations du traits optique: la dysplasie septo-optique. *Schweiz Arch Neurochir Psychiatry.* 1956;77:267–75.
28. Menelfe C, Rocchioli P. CT of septo-optique dysplasia. *AJR.* 1979;133:1157–61.
29. Williams JL, Faerber EN. Septo-optic dysplasia (de Morsier syndrome). *J Ultrasound Med.* 1985;4:265–69.
30. Pilu G, Sandri F, Cerisoli M, Alvisi C, Salvioli GP, Bovicelli L. Sonographic findings in septo-optic dysplasia in the fetus and newborn infant. *Am J Perinatol.* 1990;7:337–9.
31. Grogono JL. Children with agenesis of the corpus callosum. *Dev Med Child Neurol.* 1968;10:613–6.
32. Han J, Benson JE, Kaufman B, et al. MR imaging of pediatric cerebral abnormalities. *J Comput Assist Tomogr.* 1985;9:103–114.
33. Jeret JS, Serur D, Wisniewski K, et al. Frequency of agenesis of the corpus callosum in the developmentally disabled population as determined by computerized tomography. *Pediatr Neurosci.* 1986;12:101–3.
34. Young ID, Trounce JQ, Levene MI, et al. Agenesis of the corpus callosum and macrocephaly in siblings. *Clin Genet.* 1985;28:225–8.
35. Kaplan P. X-linked recessive inheritance of agenesis of the corpus callosum. *J Med Genet.* 1983;20:122–4.
36. Dobyns WB, Pagon RA, Armstrong D, et al: Diagnostic criteria for Walker–Warburg syndrome. *Am J Med Genet.* 1989;32:195–210.
37. Andermann F, Andermann E, Joubert M, et al. Familial agenesis of the corpus callosum with anterior horn cell disease. A syndrome of mental retardation and paresis. *Trans Am Neurol Assoc.* 1972;97:242–7.
38. Schinzel A, Schnid W. Hallux duplication, postaxial polydactily, absence of corpus callosum, severe mental retardation and additional anomalies in two unrelated patients. A new syndrome. *Am J Med Genet.* 1980;6:241–6.

39. Opitz JM, Richieri da Costa A, Aase JM et al. FG syndrome update 1988. Note of 5 new patients and bibliography. *Am J Med Genet.* 1988;30:309–28.

40. Ayme S, Julian C, Gambarelli D et al. Fryns syndrome. Report on 8 new cases. *Clin Genet.* 1989;35:191–201.

41. Salinas CF, Pai GS, Vera CL, et al. Variability of expression of the orofaciodigital syndrome type I in black females. Six cases. *Am J Med Genet.* 1991;38:574–79.

42. Donnenfeld AE, Packer RJ, Zackai EH, et al: Clinical, cytogenetic and pedigree findings in 18 cases of Aicardi syndrome. *Am J Med Genet.* 1989;32:461–7.

43. Cohen MM, Sedano HO, Gorlin RJ. Frontonasal dysplasia (median cleft face syndrome). Comments on etiology and pathogenesis. *Birth Defects.* 1971;7:117–9.

44. Bamforth F, Bamforth S, Poskitt K, et al. Abnormalities of the corpus callosum in patients with inherited metabolic diseases. *Lancet.* 1988;2:451.

45. Barkovich AJ, Norman D. Anomalies of the corpus callosum. Correlation with further anomalies of the brain. *Am J Roentgenol.* 1988;151:171–9.

46. Holman CB, MacCarthy CA. Cerebral angiography in agenesis of the corpus callosum. *Radiology.* 1959;72:317.

47. Baarsma R, Martijn A, Okken A. The missing pericallosal artery on sonography. A sign of agenesis of the corpus callosum in the neonatal brain? *Neuroradiology.* 1987;29:47–52.

48. Parrish M, Roessman U, Levinsohn M. Agenesis of the corpus callosum: A study of the frequency of associated malformations. *Ann Neurol.* 1979;6:349–54.

49. Pilu G, Sandri F, Perolo A, et al. Sonography of fetal agenesis of the corpus callosum: A survey of 35 cases. *Ultrasound Obstet Gynecol.* 1993;3:318–29.

50. Mulligan G, Meier P. Lipoma and agenesis of the corpus callosum with associated choroid plexus lipomas. In utero diagnosis. *J Ultrasound Med.* 1989;8:583–8.

51. Serur D, Jeret JS, Wisniewski K. Agenesis of the corpus callosum. Clinical, neuroradiological and cytogenetic studies. *Neuropediatrics.* 1986;19:87–91.

52. Pilu G, De Palma L, Romero R et al. The fetal subarachnoid cisterns. An ultrasound study with report of a case of congenital communicating hydrocephalus. *J Ultrasound Med.* 1986;5:365–72.

53. Monteagudo A, Reuss ML, Timor-Tritsch IE. Imaging the fetal brain in the second and third trimester using transvaginal sonography. *Obstet Gynecol.* 1991;77:27–32.

54. Gebarski SS, Gebarski KS, Bowerman RA, et al. Agenesis of the corpus callosum. Sonographic features. *Radiology.* 1984;151:443–8.

55. Babcock DS. The normal, absent and abnormal corpus callosum. Sonographic findings. *Radiology.* 1984;151:449–52.

56. Sandri F, Pilu G, Cerisoli M, et al. Sonographic diagnosis of agenesis of the corpus callosum in the fetus and newborn infant. *Am J Perinatol.* 1988;5:226–31.

57. Comstock CH, Culp D, Gonzalez J: Agenesis of the corpus callosum in the fetus. Its evolution and significance. *J Ultrasound Med.* 1985;4:613–6.

58. Vergani P, Ghidini A, Mariani S, et al. Antenatal sonographic findings of agenesis of the corpus callosum. *Am J Perinatol.* 1988;5:105–8.

59. Bertino RE, Nyberg DA, Cyr DR, et al. Prenatal diagnosis of agenesis of the corpus callosum. *J Ultrasound Med.* 1988;7:251–60.

60. Lockwood CJ, Ghidini A, Aggarwal R, et al. Antenatal diagnosis of partial agenesis of the corpus callosum. A benign cause of ventriculomegaly. *Am J Obstet Gynecol.* 1988;159:184–6.

61. Hilpert PL, Kurtz AB. Prenatal diagnosis of agenesis of the corpus callosum using endovaginal ultrasound. *J Ultrasound Med.* 1990;9:363–5.

62. Filly RA, Cardoza JD, Goldstein RB, et al. Detection of fetal central nervous system anomalies. A practical level of effort for a routine sonogram. *Radiology.* 1988;172:403–8.

63. Goldstein RB, La Pidus AS, Filly RA, et al. Mild lateral cerebral ventriculomegaly: clinical significance and prognosis. *Radiol.* 1990;176:237–92.

64. Ettlinger G. Agenesis of the corpus callosum. In: Vinken P, Bruyn G, eds. *Handbook of Clinical Neurology.* Vol. XXX. New York: American Elsevier; 1974:285–312.

65. Gupta JK, Lilford RJ. Assessment and management of fetal agenesis of the corpus callosum. *Prenat Diagn.* (in press)

66. Vergani P, Ghidini A, Strobelt N, et al. Prognostic indicators in the prenatal diagnosis of agenesis of the corpus callosum. *Am J Obstet Gynecol.* 1994;170:753–7.

67. Fischer M, Ryan SB, Dobyns WB. Mechanisms of interhemispheric transfer and patterns of cognitive functions in acallosal patients of normal intelligence. *Arch Neurol.* 1992;49:271–7.

68. Karnath HO, Schumacher M, Wallesch CW. Limitations of interhemispheric extracallosal transfer of visual information in callosal agenesis. *Cortex.* 1992;27:345–52.

69. Jeeves MA. Stereoperception in callosal agenesis and partial callosotomy. *Neuropsychologia.* 1991;29:19-34.

70. Temple CM, Jeeves MA, Villaroya OO. Reading in callosal agenesis. *Brain Lang.* 1990;39:235–53.

71. Temple CM, Jeeves MA, Villaroya OO. Ten pen men: Rhyming skills in two children with callosal agenesis. *Brain Lang.* 1989;37:548-64.

72. Swayze VM, Andreasen NC, Ehrardt JC, et al. Developmental abnormalities of the corpus callosum in schizophrenia. *Arch Neurol.* 1990;47:805–11.

73. Osenbach RK, Menezes AH. Diagnosis and management of the Dandy–Walker malformation: 30 years of experience. *Pediatr Neurosurg.* 1991;18:179–83.

74. Murray JC, Johnson JA, Bird TD. Dandy–Walker malformation: Etiologic heterogeneity and empiric recurrence risk. *Clin Genet.* 1985;28:272–81.

75. Dandy WE. The diagnosis and treatment of hydrocephalus due to occlusion of the foramina of Magendie and Luschka. *Surg Gynecol Obstet.* 1921;32:112–128.

76. Taggart JK, Walker AE. Congenital atresias of the foramens of Luschka and Magendie. *Arch Neurol Psychiatr.* 1942;48:583–495.

77. Barkovich AJ, Kjos BO, Normal D, et al. Revised classification of the posterior fossa cysts and cystlike malformations based on the results of multiplanar MR imaging. *AJNR.* 1990;10:977–82.

78. Pilu G, Romero R, DePalma L, et al. Antenatal diagnosis and obstetric management of Dandy–Walker syndrome. *J Reprod Med.* 1986;31:1017–1022.

79. Pilu G, Goldstein I, Reece EA, et al. Sonography of fetal Dandy–Walker malformation: A reappraisal. *Ultrasound Obstet Gynecol.* 1992;2:151–157.

80. Achiron R, Achiron A. Transvaginal ultrasonic assessment of the early fetal brain. *Ultrasound Obstet Gyn.* 1991;1:336–342.

81. Nyberg DA, Mahony BS, Hegge FN, et al. Enlarged cisterna magna and the Dandy–Walker malformation: Factors associated with chromosome abnormalities. *Obstet Gynecol.* 1991;77:436–42.

82. Estroff JA, Scott MR, Benacerraf BR. Dandy–Walker variant: Prenatal sonographic diagnosis and clinical outcome. *Radiology.* 1992;185:755–8.

83. Bromley B, Nadel AS, Pauker S, Estroff JA, Benacerraf BR. Closure of the cerebellar vermis: Evaluation with second trimester US. *Radiology.* 1994;193:761–763.

84. Babcock CJ, Chong BW, Salamat MS, Ellis WG, Goldstein RB. Sonographic anatomy of the developing cerebellum: Normal embryology can resemble pathology. *AJR.* 1996;166:427–433.

85. Pilu G, Falco P, Gabrielli S, Perolo A, Sandri F, Bovicelli L. The clinical significance of fetal isolated cerebral borderline ventriculomegaly: Report of 31 cases and review of the literature. *Ultrasound Obstet Gynecol.* 1999;14:320–326.

86. Ecker JL, Shipp TD, Bromley B, Benacerraf B. The sonographic diagnosis of Dandy–Walker and Dandy–Walker variant: associated Findings and outcomes. *Prenat Diagn.* 2000;20:328–332.

87. Carroll SGM, Porter H, Abdel-Fattah S, Kyle PM, Soothil PW. Correlation of prenatal ultrasound diagnosis and pathologic findings in fetal brain abnormalities. *Ultrasound Obstet Gynecol.* (in press)

88. Levine D, Barnes PD, Madsen JR, Abbot J, Tejas Mehta T, Edelman R. Central nervous system abnormalities assessed with prenatal magnetic resonance. *Obstet Gynecol.* 1999;94:1011–1019.

CHAPTER SIX

Ultrasonography of the Fetal Face

Israel Meizner

Ultrasonography has greatly improved our understanding of normal and abnormal embryonic development of the face and the neck. Imaging of the fetal face is feasible quite early in gestation, using the transvaginal approach. With this modality, studies of the fetal face may begin as early as the 11th to 12th weeks of pregnancy for the bony elements. Soft tissue parts may be observed at 14 weeks. Thus, the fetal face, an area of considerable information, may be included in every scan dedicated for the early detection of fetal abnormalities.

Grossly, facial abnormalities may be classified into two major categories: (1) isolated malformations limited to the facial region and (2) abnormalities representing syndromes of multisystem anomalies, some of which are associated with an abnormal karyotype. Indeed, the early detection of a facial defect should initiate a thorough survey for other structural malformations in the fetus, as well as a cytogenetic analysis. The survey of the fetal face should therefore be incorporated into all scans dedicated for the early detection of fetal malformations. This chapter provides an overview of normal and abnormal findings in ultrasonographic imaging of the fetal face. It also supplies the reader with a systematic approach to the diagnosis and recognition of the numerous possible malformations of this complex region. The reader should consider Chapters 2, 3, 4, 5, and 9 for a better understanding of the diverse aspects of facial pathology.

EMBRYOLOGY OF THE FACE

The development of the fetal face occurs chiefly between the fourth and eighth conceptual weeks.[1,2] In describing the method of face construction, it is practical to say that several "processes" meet and merge.

These components are mere elevations, or ridges of central mesenchymal proliferations, covered by a sheet of continuous epithelium. Early in development, the face of the embryo appears as an area bounded cranially by the neural plate (unpaired frontonasal elevation or process), laterally by the paired maxillary processes of the first branchial arch, and caudally by the paired mandibular processes. In the center of this area exists a depression in the ectoderm, known as the stomodeum (Fig. 6–1A).

The further development of the face is dependent on the approach and merging of a number of important processes: the frontonasal, maxillary, and mandibular processes. By the end of the fourth postconceptual week, bilateral oval thickenings of the surface ectoderm, called nasal placodes, appear on each side of the lower part of the frontonasal process. Mesenchyme proliferates at the margins of these placodes, producing convex medial and lateral nasal elevations. These elevations are situated in depressions called olfactory, or nasal, pits (Fig. 6–1B). The maxillary processes grow rapidly and approach each other in the medial nasal elevation. A definite separation between each nasal elevation and the maxillary processes exists and is called the nasolacrimal groove. By the end of the fifth postconceptual week, the eyes are slightly forward on the face and the external ears have begun to appear.

Meanwhile, the maxillary process grows out from the upper edge of each first arch and passes medially, forming the inferior border of the developing orbit. During the sixth and seventh postconceptual weeks, the medial nasal elevations fuse with the maxillary processes. As these elevations merge, they form an intermaxillary segment of the upper jaw, which will later give rise to (1) the middle portion of the upper lip (philtrum), (2) the middle por-

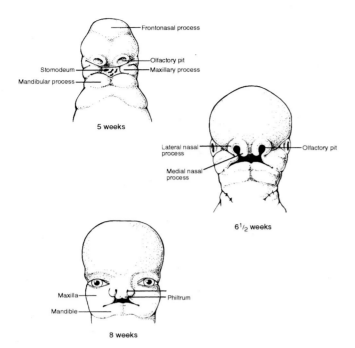

Figure 6–1. The different stages of the developing fetal facial structures by weeks from conception. **A.** Five weeks. **B.** Six and one half weeks. **C.** Eight weeks.

TABLE 6–1. FATES OF STRUCTURES CONTRIBUTING TO FACIAL FORMATION

Elevation	Derivatives
Frontonasal process	Forehead, nasal bridge, lateral and medial nasal prominences
Lateral nasal elevation	Side and wing of the nose
Medial nasal elevation	Philtrum of the upper lip, fleshy nasal septum, median part of the upper lip and the gum, frenulum
Maxillary process	Upper cheek regions, most of the upper lip and the gum
Mandibular process	Lower cheek regions, lower lip, gum, and chin

tion of the upper jaw and its associated gingiva, and (3) the primary palate. The lateral parts of the upper lip, the upper jaw, and the secondary palate form from the maxillary processes. These processes merge laterally with the mandibular processes and reduce the size of the mouth. The primitive lips and cheeks are invaded by mesenchyme, derived from the second branchial arch, which creates the facial muscles. The frontonasal process forms the forehead and the dorsum and apex of the nose. The sides of the alae of the nose are derived from the lateral nasal elevations (Fig. 6–1C). The mandibular processes merge in the fourth week, and the groove between them disappears by the end of the fifth postconceptual week. The mandibular processes give rise to the lower jaw, the lower lip, and the lower part of the face.

When it is first formed, at 5 postconceptual weeks, the nose is broad and flat, with the nostrils set far apart and directed forward. In later fetal months the bridge of the nose is elevated and prolonged into the apex and the nostrils point downward. Accompanying this relative narrowing of the nose, the head broadens behind the eyes and causes them to be directed forward. The eyelids arise as simple folds of the skin. The lips begin to split away from the gum regions of the jaws in the seventh week. The chin is a median projection grown forward

from the fused mandibular processes. The external ear is developed around the first branchial groove by the appearance of small tubercles that merge as the auricle. The tissue of the auricle is furnished by both the first (mandibular) and second (hyoid) branchial arches. Table 6–1 describes the fates of the facial components according to embryonic parts.

The final development of the face occurs slowly and results mainly from changes in the relative proportion and position of the facial components. One should bear in mind that the smallness of the fetal face at birth results from (1) the rudimentary upper and lower jaws, (2) the unruptured teeth, and (3) the small size of the nasal cavities and the maxillary air sinuses.

Most congenital malformations of the facial region originate during the transformation of the branchial apparatus into adult structures. The most sensitive period for the induction of congenital malformations extends from the initiation of first branchial arch morphogenesis (fourth postconceptual week) through the 12th postconceptual week of fetal development.

FACIAL MALFORMATIONS: GENERAL CONSIDERATIONS

Birth Prevalence of Different Facial Anomalies

It is difficult to estimate correctly the birth prevalence of all facial malformations due to the fact that some of them are extremely rare, or represent part of a rare syndrome. Furthermore, in some of the syndromes, not all affected fetuses have the specific facial expression. The data currently available concerning the birth prevalence of facial malformations are summarized in Table 6–2. It should be stressed that the true prevalence of many specific malformations is either unknown or extremely rare.

TABLE 6–2. BIRTH PREVALENCE OF SPECIFIC FACIAL MALFORMATIONS

Facial Malformation	Birth Prevalence
Isolated malformations	
Facial clefts	1:700–1:1000
Arhinia	Extremely rare
Cyclopia	1:40,000
Cebocephaly	1:16,000
Pierre Robin syndrome	1:30,000
Otocephaly	Extremely rare
Congenital cataract	<0.5% of live births
Goldenhar's syndrome	1:3000–1:5000
Treacher Collins syndrome	>250 cases reported
Nager syndrome	>22 cases reported
Beckwith–Wiedemann syndrome	>200 cases reported
Seckel syndrome	Rare
Part of a syndrome	
Trisomy 21	1:660
Trisomy 13	1:5000
Trisomy 18	0.3:1000
Hypotelorism	Very rare
Hypertelorism	Rare

Classification

A uniform classification of facial malformation does not exist. From the clinical point of view, it is easy to classify these anomalies based on their location: forehead, nose, lips, chin, etc. However, this does not apply in all cases. A more reasonable classification is suggested here, dividing all facial malformations into four categories: (1) isolated facial malformations (e.g., facial hemangioma or cebocephaly), which may be subdivided according to the anatomic site of appearance; (2) part of a syndrome (e.g., Nager syndrome or Beckwith–Wiedemann syndrome); (3) malformations associated with chromosomal aberrations (e.g., all trisomies); and (4) malformations resulting from cranial deformities (e.g., craniosynostosis or encephalocele).

Terminology

The description of facial anatomy and associated malformation is based on the recognition of specific terms applied to these structures. These terms may be derived from embryonic nomenclature or may represent Greek terms. Useful terms associated with facial malformations or with their diagnosis appear in Table 6–3.

SCANNING TECHNIQUES AND APPROACH TO THE DIAGNOSIS OF FACIAL ANOMALIES

Ultrasound is quite accurate in detecting facial malformations in utero. Several studies have indicated that a systematic examination of facial anatomy may reveal most facial abnormalities.[3–5] Most fetal facial anomalies are present in the setting of other obvious fetal organ malformations, presence of polyhydramnios, presence of chromosomal abnormalities, or, rarely, history of a previous facial anomaly or maternal teratogen exposure.

Although the fetal face can be studied quite early in pregnancy using the transvaginal approach, the examination may sometimes be difficult and time consuming. Features of the fetal facial anatomy may be observed as early as 10 postmenstrual weeks. By 14 postmenstrual weeks, soft tissues as well as bony structures may be easily recognized. The normal facial anatomy should be studied systematically in three planes: sagittal, axial, and coronal (Fig. 6–2).[6] Paramedian as well as multiple axial planes may sometimes be helpful in detecting specific anatomic landmarks. (See Chapter 2 for detailed explanations on the sonographic planes useful in scanning studies.)

The *median* plane is useful for observing the fetal profile: forehead, nasal bridge, upper and lower lips, and jaw. Mouth-opening movements as well as protrusion of the tongue are easily observed in this plane (Figs. 6–3 through 6–5).

The *paramedian sagittal* planes may provide information regarding orbital dimensions, presence, and transparency of the lenses (Fig. 6–6), and an extremely lateral sagittal image is the best plane for visualization of the ears since it is tangential to the skull. A detailed auricular anatomy can sometimes be observed, including the helix, antihelix, tragus, antitragus, scaphoid fossa, triangular fossa, concha, and lobule. However, visualization of all ear structures is rarely achieved (Fig. 6–7).

The *coronal* planes are the most useful in identifying the integrity of the facial anatomy, especially the lips, nose, and orbital structures. This view includes soft tissues of the nose (tip, alae nasi, and nostrils), soft tissues of the lips (including the philtrum), and bony structures of the maxilla and the orbits (Figs. 6–8 through 6–10). The lens of the eye is observed as a small echogenic circle within the bony orbit; and the eyelids and, at times, the eyelashes can be examined (Figs. 6–11 and 6–12). Movements of both eyeballs may be detected. Opening of the mouth, "chewing" and "sucking" movements ("mouthing"), and tongue protrusion are seen. The movements of the eyeballs, mouth, and tongue become important as fetal behavioral status is considered (Chapter 15).

The *axial* planes are best used to evaluate the orbital region (see also Chapter 7). Orbital abnormalities such as hypotelorism and hypertelorism are best detected in this plane, since this is the plane

TABLE 6–3. TERMINOLOGY AND NOMENCLATURE OF USEFUL TERMS FREQUENTLY ASSOCIATED WITH FACIAL MALFORMATIONS

Acrania	Complete or partial absence of the skull
Anencephaly	Congenital defective development of the brain, with absence of the bones of the cranial vault, the cerebral and cerebellar hemispheres, a rudimentary brain stem, and traces of basal ganglia
Anodontia	Absence of the teeth
Anophthalmia	Congenital absence of all tissues of the eyes
Arhinia	Absence of the nose
Cataract	Loss of transparency of the lens of the eye or its capsule
Cebocephaly	A malformation with a tendency toward cyclopia, with defective or absent nose and close-set eyes
Craniosynostosis	Premature ossification of the skull and obliteration of the sutures
Cryptophthalmos	Congenital absence of the eyelids, with the skin passing continuously from the forehead onto the cheek over a rudimentary eye
Cyclopia	A congenital defect in which the two orbits merge to form a single cavity containing one eye
Encephalocele	A congenital gap in the skull with herniation of brain substance
Epignathus	A teratoma arising from the oral cavity or the pharynx
Ethmocephaly	A malformation with a tendency toward cyclopia, with extreme hypotelorism, arhinia, and presence of a proboscis
Holoprosencephaly	Failure of the forebrain to divide into hemispheres or lobes
Hypertelorism	Extreme width between the eyes due to an enlarged sphenoid bone
Hypotelorism	Abnormal closeness of the eyes
Macroglossia	Enlargement of the tongue
Macrognathia	Enlargement or elongation of the jaw
Macrostomia	Abnormal wideness of the mouth
Microcephaly	Abnormal smallness of the head
Micrognathia	Abnormal smallness of the jaws, especially of the mandible
Microstomia	Smallness of the mouth
Otocephaly	An anomaly characterized by absence or hypoplasia of the mandible, proximity of the temporal bones, and abnormal horizontal position of the ears
Philtrum	Depression on the upper lip
Proboscis	A cylindrical protuberance of the face which, in cyclopia or ethmocephaly, represents the nose
Prognathism	Abnormal forward projection of one or both jaws beyond the established normal relationship with the cranial base

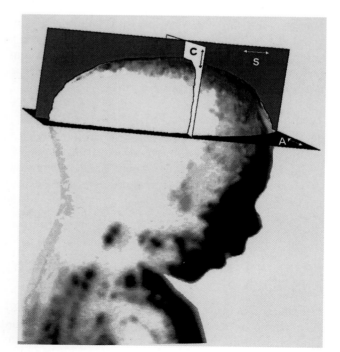

Figure 6–2. Illustration of the three scanning planes used for identifying fetal facial structures. A, axial; C, coronal; S, sagittal.

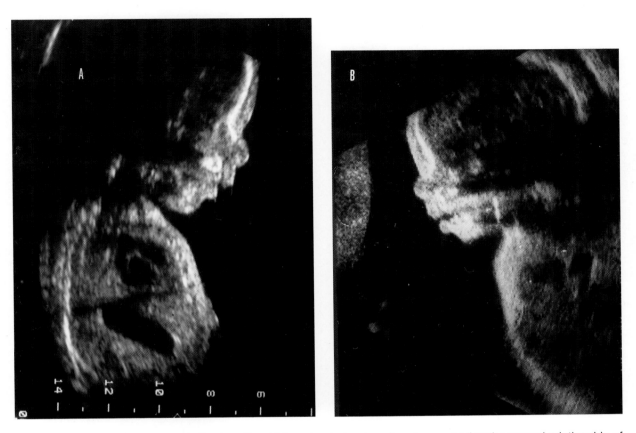

Figure 6–3. **A.** Median view of the fetal profile at 20 postmenstrual weeks, demonstrating the normal relationship of the forehead, nasal bridge, lips, and mandible. **B.** Median view at 24 weeks of gestation.

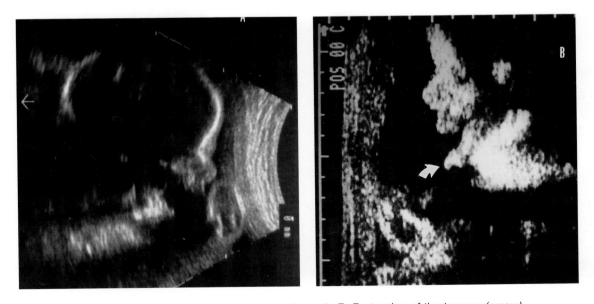

Figure 6–4. **A.** Sagittal view of an opened mouth. **B.** Protrusion of the tongue (arrow).

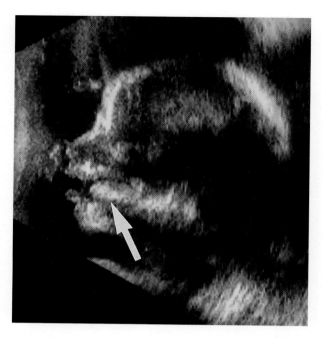

Figure 6–5. Median sonogram of the fetal face at 28 post-menstrual weeks, demonstrating a normally positioned tongue *(arrow)*.

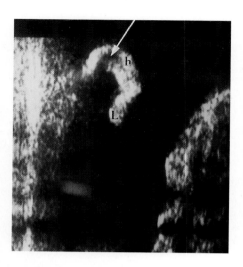

Figure 6–7. Extremely lateral sagittal scan at 24 postmenstrual weeks, showing the fetal ear. h, Helix; L, lobule; *thin arrow,* scaphoid fossa.

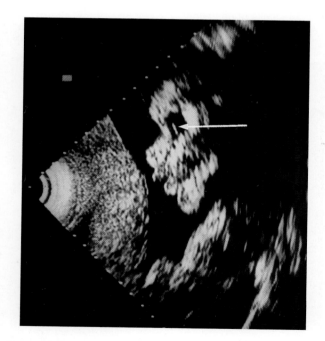

Figure 6–6. Paramedian image of the fetal face at 20 post-menstrual weeks, showing a normal orbit. Note the lens *(arrow)*.

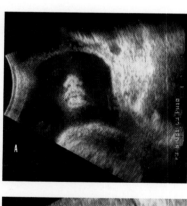

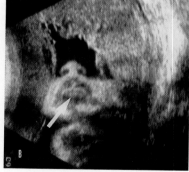

Figure 6–8. A. Coronal view of the fetal face, showing the nose, nostrils, and upper and lower lips. **B.** A slightly more posterior coronal view. Note the midline position of the tongue *(arrow)*.

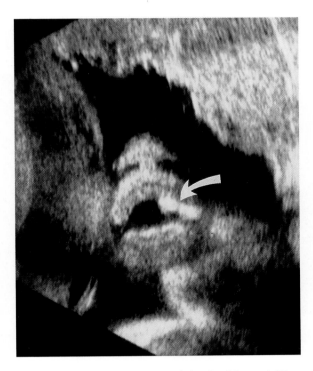

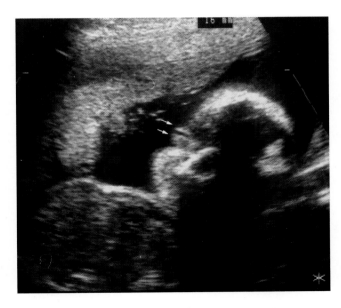

Figure 6–11. Coronal sonogram obtained at 20 postmenstrual weeks, showing the eyelids *(small arrows)*.

Figure 6–9. Coronal sonogram of the fetal face at 21 postmenstrual weeks, showing a finger *(arrow)* inside an opened mouth. Note the integrity of both lips.

used for measurement of interorbital distance (see also Chapter 3). Several nomograms for binocular distance are currently available (Figs. 6–13 and 6–14).[7,8] Other axial planes may reveal the anatomy of the maxilla and the mandible and, by slight angulation, allow identification of the tongue within the oral cavity and the oropharynx (Figs. 6–15 and 6–16). The axial plane also allows visualization of the tooth buds (Fig. 6–17). In the last few years three-dimensional ultrasound technology became advanced enough to be used in clinical practice. Still, the as-

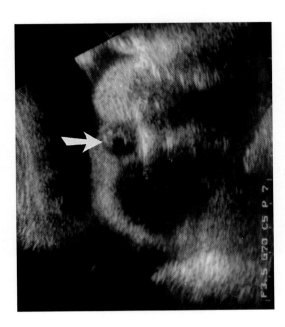

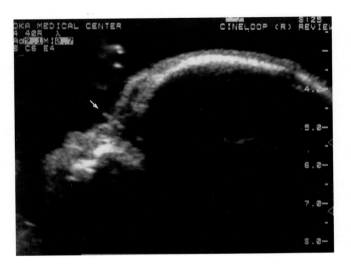

Figure 6–10. Coronal sonogram demonstrating a normal lens *(arrow)* within the orbit.

Figure 6–12. Paramedian view at 30 postmenstrual weeks, demonstrating eyelashes *(arrow)*.

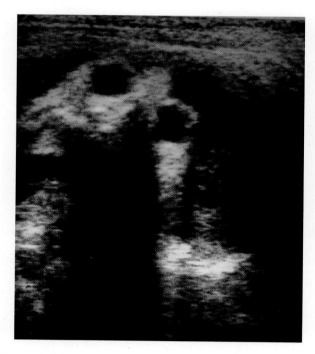

Figure 6–13. Axial sonogram through the fetal orbits.

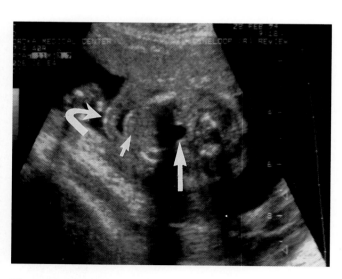

Figure 6–15. Axial scan of the fetal face at the level of the base of the skull (21 postmenstrual weeks). Note the oropharynx *(straight arrow)* and the tongue *(small arrow)*. The *curved arrow* indicates the upper lip.

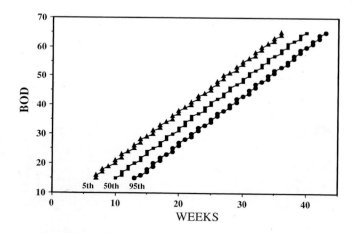

Figure 6–14. Growth of the biorbital diameter across gestational age.

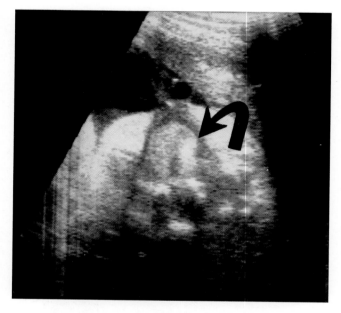

Figure 6–16. Axial sonogram demonstrating the tongue *(black arrow).*

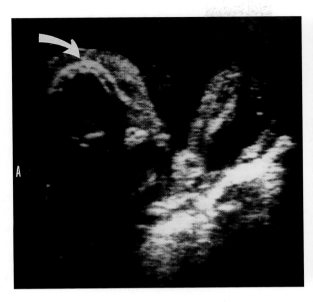
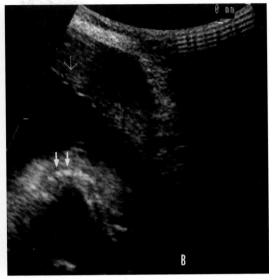

Figure 6–17. Axial sonogram through the fetal mandible. **A.** Tooth sockets *(curved arrow).* **B.** The tooth buds are imaged *(small arrows).*

sessment of this new technology and determination of its realistic advantage in the clinical management of selected cases require many years of well-planned and carefully conducted research. The fetal face is among the organs that can be particularly well analyzed by three-dimensional ultrasonography (Fig. 6–18). It is possible to verify a correct profile with the simultaneous image display. In the surface mode, it is possible to detect facial abnormalities, even small ones like facial clefts. The ability to rotate every region of interest into an adequate position allows the examiner to investigate the fetal head from a side view as well. More detailed data employing three-dimensional ultrasound in the evaluation of the fetal face is found in Chapter 9.

The diagnostic approach for the detection of facial abnormalities should be based on the following.

1. Adherence to strict evaluation of the facial anatomy by all three anatomic planes.
2. Visualization of all anatomic structures by site.
3. Observation of functional capacities of the facial organs (e.g., mouth-opening or eye movements).
4. Meticulous scanning of the skull anatomy (e.g., bony skull andbrain anatomy, including the spine).
5. Consideration of the associated extrafacial malformations (e.g., holoprosencephaly or encephalocele).

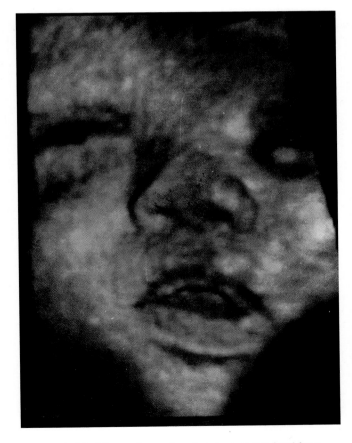

Figure 6–18. Three-dimensional picture of the fetal face.

6. Consideration of sonographic markers associated with facial anomalies (e.g., polyhydramnios, which is associated with facial clefts and micrognathia).

It is best to start viewing the fetal profile by obtaining the median plane. This provides initial information regarding the mandible and the integrity of the lips. If no pathology is encountered, one should proceed to a coronal plane through the lips and the nose. If the lips and the nostrils are detected and found to be normal, the orbital region should be sought and the eyelids and lenses should be located. Axial planes are reserved to the end, for the evaluation of the palate.

In all scans one should try to answer the following questions.

1. Is the median plane in this fetus intact? Were the forehead, nasal bridge, lips, and chin observed?
2. Has the chin been detected in a coronal plane? (Its absence will hint toward micrognathia.)
3. Has the upper lip been viewed on an axial plane as well as longitudinally? Have both nostrils been located?
4. Are the binocular distances normal? Are the orbits of normal size?
5. Has the anatomy of the ears been observed, and are they normally positioned?
6. Is the tongue enlarged or protuberant?
7. Is there a widely opened mouth?
8. Have "mouthing" movements occurred?
9. Have any abnormal structures (e.g., proboscis or hemangiomas) been observed throughout the scan?
10. Has the skull been thoroughly examined? Is it adequately ossified? Is the brain anatomy normal?

DETECTION OF SPECIFIC MALFORMATIONS BY SITE OF APPEARANCE

Malformations Involving the Orbital Region

Imaging the anatomy of the orbital region anatomy is not a time-consuming task. Indeed, if one uses coronal and axial views, information regarding the normalcy of the orbits and the eyes is easily obtained. A helpful diagnostic tool is the measurement of the binocular distance (Fig. 6–13). Identification of the eyelids and the lenses is feasible in most cases by using the coronal planes. Chapter 7 deals further with the sonographic evaluation of the fetal eye.

Hypertelorism

Hypertelorism is a rare deformity that may appear sporadically as a primary defect or may be secondary to specific malformations involving the skull or the face. It is defined as an increased width between the orbits and is bilateral in the majority of reported cases. There are numerous conditions associated with hypertelorism, including facial clefting, brain defects (e.g., encephalocele, hydrocephaly, and agenesis of corpus callosum), skeletal deformities and dysplasias (e.g., arthrogryposis multiplex congenita, multiple pterygium syndrome, and achondroplasia), chromosomal aberrations, and other miscellaneous conditions.[9] By far, the most frequent conditions associated with hypertelorism are syndromes of craniosynostosis, such as Apert syndrome, Crouzon's disease, cleft lip and cleft palate, frontal encephaloceles and arthrogryposis multiplex congenita (Pena–Shokeir type) (Figs. 6–19 through 6–21).

The sonographic diagnosis of hypertelorism may rely on measuring the interorbital distance[7] in a coronal or axial view. If a frontal encephalocele is suspected, the sagittal view may be helpful. The prenatal diagnosis of hypertelorism has been reported in several isolated case reports; however, information from large series of cases is not yet available.[10,11]

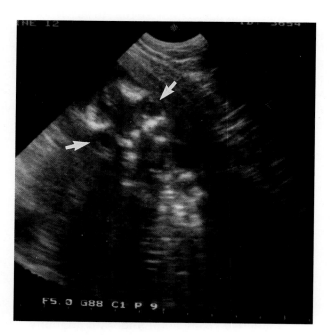

Figure 6–19. Multiple pterygium syndrome. Transvaginal coronal sonogram of a fetus with multiple pterygium syndrome at 15 postmenstrual weeks. Hypertelorism is evident (the *arrows* mark the orbits).

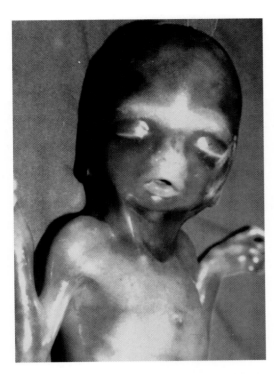

Figure 6–20. Photograph of the abortus with multiple ptery-gium syndrome, showing the hypertelorism. Micrognathia is also present. (See Figs. 9–17 and 9–20.)

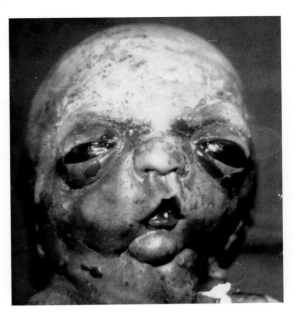

Figure 6–21. Postmortem photograph at 28 postmenstrual weeks of another fetus with multiple pterygium syndrome, showing obvious hypertelorism.

Hypotelorism

Hypotelorism is a result of a severe brain anomaly in most reported cases. In the vast majority of cases, the underlying cause is the wide spectrum of the holoprosencephaly sequence.[12] Other conditions associated with hypotelorism may include chromosomal abnormalities (trisomy 13), 18p–syndrome, microcephaly, Meckel–Gruber syndrome, myotonic dystrophy, and trigonocephaly (Fig. 6–22).

Holoprosencephaly is the term applied to a variety of anomalies resulting from incomplete cleavage of the primitive prosencephalon, or forebrain, during organogenesis. Various midline facial anomalies have been described with this entity. The incidence has been reported to vary between 0.6 and 1.9 per 10,000 births.[13] The condition may be divided into alobar, semilobar, and lobar categories, depending on the degree of separation of the cerebral hemispheres.[14] Alobar holoprosencephaly is the most severe form, characterized by no evidence of division of the cerebral cortex and absence of the falx cerebri and the interhemispheric fissure, thus producing a single common ventricle. Furthermore, the corpus callosum is deficient in most cases. This variety is associated with a wide spectrum of midline facial malformations, including cyclopia, ethmocephaly, cebocephaly, hypotelorism, and midline facial clefts.

In cyclopia a single median bony orbit exists with a fleshy proboscis above it (Figs. 6–23 and 6–24).[15] In ethmocephaly the nose is absent and a proboscis is found between two narrowly placed orbits. In cebocephaly hypotelorism is present, accompanied by a normally placed nose and a single nostril (Figs. 6–25 and 6–26). It should be stressed that not all patients with alobar holoprosencephaly may have facial deformities, and the condition may be associated with only milder forms of midline facial dysplasia or normal facies (Fig. 6–27).[16] The prognosis of alobar holoprosencephaly is poor, and most infants die shortly after birth. In utero diagnosis of holoprosencephaly has been reported on several occasions.[17–19] It is also of importance that the proboscis can be seen as early as 9 postmenstrual weeks (Fig. 6–23B). The sonographic markers leading to correct diagnosis of this condition may include the presence of hypotelorism, facial midline clefts, the presence of a proboscis, and an abnormal brain anatomy. Chromosomal analysis is mandatory in all of these cases. When holoprosencephaly is suspected, the diagnosis requires visualization of the facial and intracranial anatomy in all planes, especially sagittal and axial views (see Chapter 4). Other extrafacial anomalies are also present in the holoprosencephaly sequence and include cardiac, skeletal, renal, and gastrointestinal malformations.

Trigonocephaly, a form of craniosynostosis, is a congenital cranial anomaly characterized by a small,

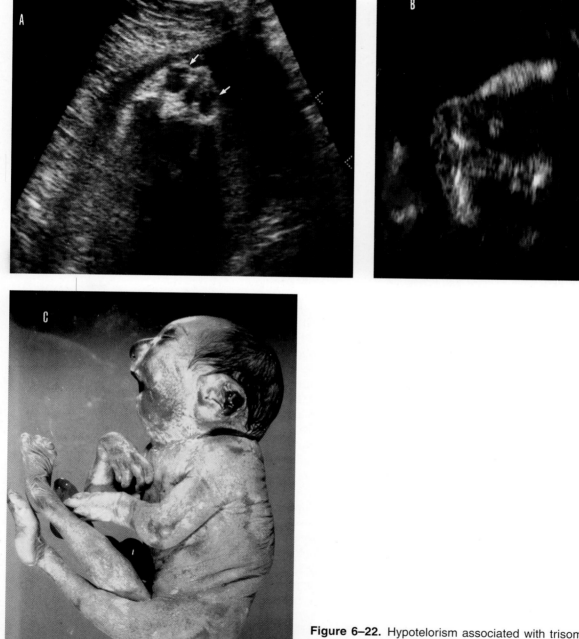

Figure 6–22. Hypotelorism associated with trisomy 13 syndrome at 17 postmenstrual weeks. **A.** Note the extreme proximity of the orbits *(arrows)* in an axial plane and **(B),** the flattened forehead in a mid-sagittal plane. **C.** Photograph of the aborted fetus. Note the presence of other structural anomalies typical of this trisomy.

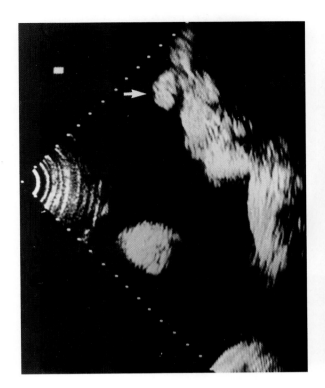
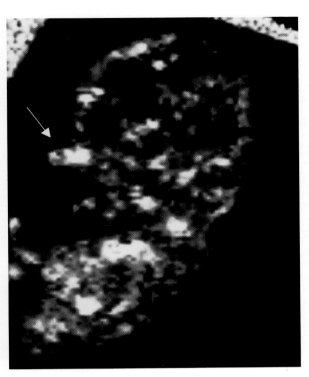

Figure 6–23. A. Cyclopia. Median ultrasound scan demonstrating a proboscis *(arrow)* protruding from the fetal fore-head. *(From Meizner and Bar-Ziv, 1993,*[15] *with permission.)* **B.** Detection of the proboscis in a case of holoprosen-cephaly at 10 postmenstrual weeks *(arrow). (Courtesy of Dr Harm-Gerd Blaas, Troudheim, Norway.)*

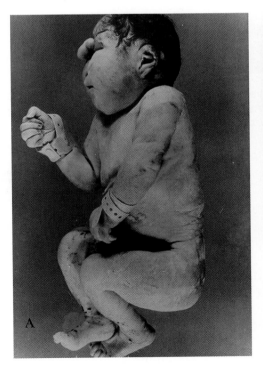
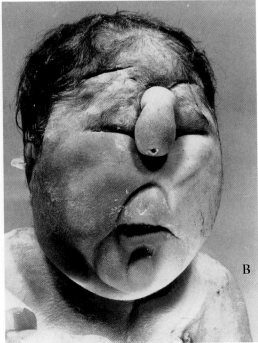

Figure 6–24. Cyclopia. Postmortem pictures of the newborn (see Fig. 6–22), showing the proboscis. **A.** Lateral view. **B.** Frontal view. Microcephaly was also present. *(From Meizner and Bar-Ziv, 1993,*[15] *with permission.)*

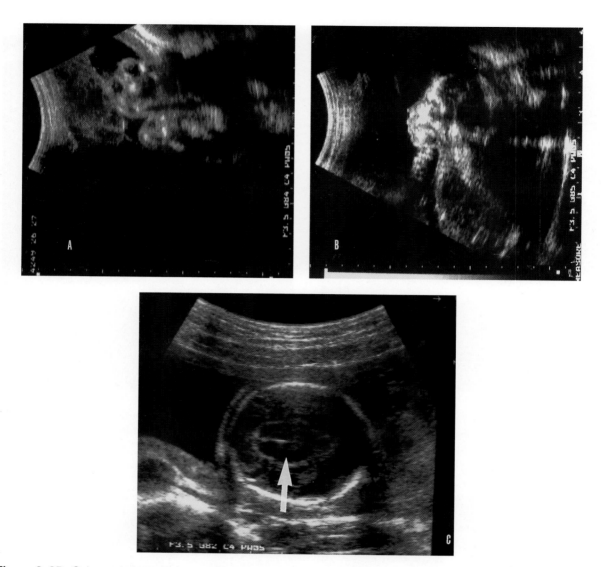

Figure 6–25. Cebocephaly associated with trisomy 13. Ultrasound scan of the fetal face in the **(A)** coronal and **(B)** median planes. Note the hypotelorism and the flat face. **C.** Axial sonogram of the fetal brain, showing enlarged thalami *(arrow)*. A single ventricle was also present. *(From Meizner and Bar-Ziv, 1993,[15] with permission.)*

pointed forehead and attributed to premature ossification and closure of the metopic sutures. The resulting decreased transverse dimension of the frontal bone gives a triangular configuration to the cranium.

Diprosopus

Diprosopus is an extremely uncommon malformation occurring in craniopagus conjoined twins. In this form of severe craniopagus, there is craniofacial duplication but only one neck and body.[20] There are variable forms of appearance, ranging from two midline globes that may be fused or separate within a central orbit up to completely separate orbits. An-

tepartum demonstration of this pathology using ultrasonography has been described previously.[21,22] To establish a correct diagnosis, coronal and sagittal views should be consecutively taken. Associated malformations include central nervous system anomalies and spina bifida. Polyhydramnios may accompany the disorder.

Otocephaly (Synotia)

Otocephaly (synotia) is a rare anomaly characterized by hypoplasia or absence of the mandible, proximity of the temporal bones, and approximation or fusion of auricles beneath the maxilla. Cyclopia and en-

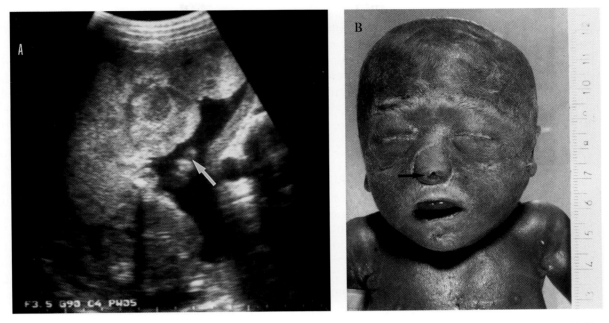

Figure 6–26. Cebocephaly associated with trisomy 13. **A.** Prenatal coronal sonogram of the fetal nose. **B.** Postmortem picture of the abortus. Note the single nostril *(arrow). (From Meizner and Bar-Ziv, 1993,*[15] *with permission.)*

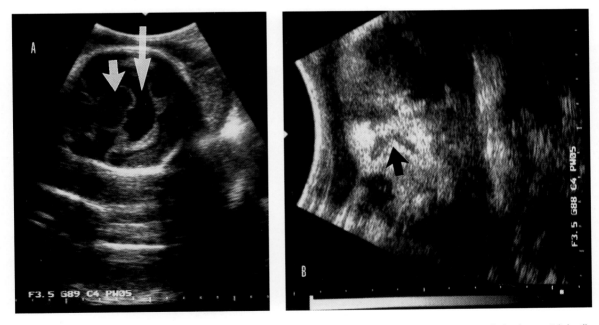

Figure 6–27. Holoprosencephaly. **A.** Axial ultrasound scan of the fetal brain, showing a dilated single ventricle *(long arrow)* and the fused thalami *(short arrow).* **B.** Coronal sonogram of the fetal face, showing a large midline defect *(arrow). (From Meizner and Bar-Ziv, 1993,*[15] *with permission.)*

cephalocele may be associated with otocephaly. The etiology is unknown, and associated malformations include holoprosencephaly, presence of a proboscis, neural tube defects, cardiac anomalies, adrenal anomalies, and tracheoesophageal fistula. Otocephaly is incompatible with life. Prenatal sonograms may rely on a previously reported case,[23] in which the fetal cranium was poorly defined, the orbits were absent, an anterior cephalocele was obvious, and two soft tissue structures resembling ears were observed in the midfacial region.

Microphthalmos and Anophthalmia Syndromes

Microphthalmos refers to smallness of the eyeballs, and *anophthalmia* means "absence of the eyes." Microphthalmos is found in many specific syndromes and can be unilateral or bilateral. This entity should not be confused with cryptophthalmos, a condition characterized by fusion of the eyelids, often associated with microphthalmos (see also Chapter 7). Anophthalmia is less frequent than microphthalmos and results from lack of formation of the optic vesicle. Several conditions may be associated with anophthalmia, including trisomy 13, Goldenhar–Grolin syndrome, and Lenz's syndrome. The prognosis relies on the underlying etiology. Sonographic diagnosis may rely on measurements of the orbital diameters.[24,25]

Congenital Cataract

A cataract is any opacity of the crystalline lens sufficient to cause visual impairment. Congenital lens opacities occur in less than 0.5% of live births and account for about 10% of blindness in preschool children.[26,27] Approximately one third of the cases are idiopathic, and many of these are familial. Congenital cataract may be associated with infections (rubella, toxoplasmosis, cytomegalovirus, herpes simplex, and or varicella), chromosomal anomalies (trisomies 13, 18, 20, and 21), and systemic isolated disorders.[28] The sonographic appearance of congenital cataract is characterized by an opaque echogenic fetal lens (Fig. 6–28).[29]

It is sometimes possible to observe the hyaloid artery, which originates from the ophthalmic artery, runs through the center of the eye, and terminates at the posterior surface of the lens. This vessel normally regresses at the beginning of the third trimester. The hyaloid artery was clearly observed in fetuses of 16 to 29 postmenstrual weeks.[30] The importance of these observations needs further clarification (see also Chapter 7).

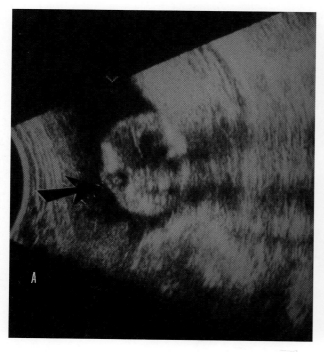
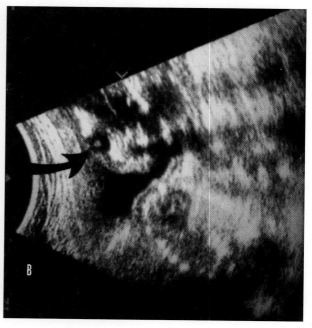

Figure 6–28. Congenital cataract in two siblings with multiple pterygium syndrome. An opaque echogenic lens is demonstrated by the *arrows* in coronal sonograms **(A, B).**

Periorbital Protrusions

Two major types of congenital masses may be encountered in the fetal periorbital region: lacrimal duct cysts (dacryocystoceles) and hemangiomas. The nasolacrimal duct develops as a linear thickening of ectoderm on the developing face and extends from the medial canthus of the developing eye to the region of the developing nose. This thickening forms, in its upper end, the lacrimal sac. Further cellular proliferation results in the formation of the lacrimal ducts, which enter each eyelid. The nasolacrimal duct usually becomes patent by 18 postmenstrual weeks, although almost 30% of newborns will have an obstructed duct.[31] Atresia of the nasolacrimal duct is a common anomaly and is caused by failure in canalization of the developing duct. The usual location of a lacrimal duct cyst is inferior and medial to the orbit. The differential diagnosis may include a dermoid tumor (typically superolateral to the eyeball), an encephalocele, and hemangioma (Fig. 6–29). Doppler signals may help in distinguishing the hemangioma from a simple dacryocystocele.

Aside from different sites of appearance, congenital hemangiomas tend to be larger and echogenic than nasolacrimal cysts (a few centimeters versus 1 cm in diameter, respectively).[32] Whenever a solid facial tumor suspicious of hemangioma is detected by ultrasonography, one should look for areas of calcifications. The calcifications can be gross and therefore can suggest the possibility of a teratoma. However, calcifications can be very small and widely scattered, giving rise to homogeneous echogenicities. This homogeneous echogenicity also could be attributed to the multiple interfaces between the walls of the cavernous sinuses and the blood within them, as described in cases of hemangioma of the liver.[33]

Malformations Involving the Nose, Lips, Mouth, and Tongue

Facial Clefts

Cleft lip and cleft palate are common congenital defects, resulting from errors in the complex modeling process of the facial region. The incidence is estimated to be 1 in 800 to 1 in 1000 births.[34] Cleft lip most commonly involves the upper lip. Cleft lip and cleft palate result from failure of the facial prominence to coalesce during the embryonic period.

Normally, the lip is formed between the fourth and seventh weeks of gestation by a series of complex morphogenetic movements and consequent coalescence of the maxillary and nasal prominences. The development of the secondary palate begins during the seventh postmenstrual week and is completed by the 12th postmenstrual week, when the two palatal processes fuse at the midline. There are two groups of clefts, which apparently differ in their etiology: (1) the group with cleft lip with or without

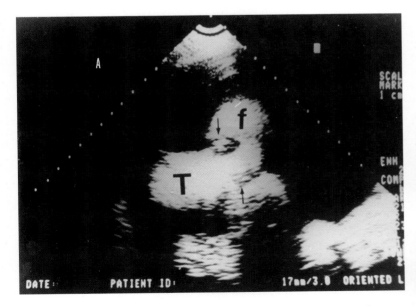
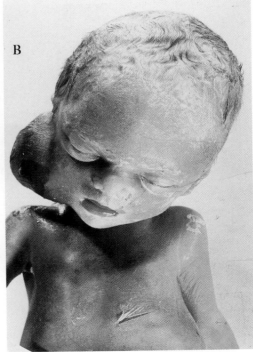

Figure 6–29. Facial hemangioma. **A.** Coronal ultrasound scan demonstrating an echogenic mass protruding from the right fetal infraorbital region. The *upper arrow* indicates the eyelids, and the *lower arrow* marks the mouth. T, Tumor; f, forehead. **B.** Postmortem photograph of the newborn. *(From Meizner and colleagues, 1985,[32] with permission.)*

a consequent cleft palate and (2) the group with a cleft of the secondary palate alone. Several forms of facial clefts have been described.

Unilateral cleft upper lip (cheiloschisis), also inappropriately called harelip, which is usually unilateral and more often on the left side. This cleft may vary from a slight notch (Figs. 6–30 and 6–31) to a complete separation extending into the nostril. The defect is usually limited to the fleshy lip alone, but it may involve the bony upper jaw as well. The cause lies in a faulty spread of mesenchyme into the normally merging maxillary and median nasal processes at one side, with the other side remaining intact. Virtual absence of mesenchyme at the line of junction can lead to actual separation of these parts.

Ultrasonographic recognition of this cleft may best be achieved using all three: axial, median and coronal planes. Although for first impression it is best to scan the face in the median plane, thus exploring the disruption in the integrity of the lips, it is probably better to view the lips in the axial as well as in the coronal planes for the detection of this type of cleft (Fig. 6–32). In most cases these planes demonstrate the unilateral cleft lip as early as the beginning of second trimester of pregnancy.

Bilateral cleft lip is caused by failure of both maxillary processes to fuse with the medial nasal process, which then remains as a central flap of tis-

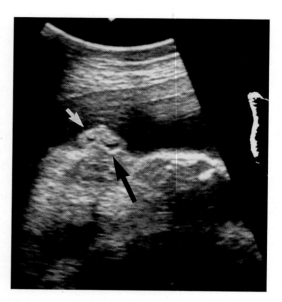

Figure 6–31. Cleft lip. Coronal ultrasound scan showing an incomplete cleft lip *(black arrow)* causing minor deformity of the left nostril. The *white arrow* marks the nose.

sue. This type of cleft is the easiest to diagnose, because disruption of the facial integrity is remarkable. Recognition of this defect is made due to the large gap appearing in the upper lip, coupled by the protrusion of a central fleshy flap of tissue. A flattened, widened appearance of the nose may also be visualized.[35,36]

Median cleft lip is very rare and is caused by the failure of fusion of the globular processes of the median nasal process. Identification of this type of cleft is accomplished using both coronal and median views (Figs. 6–33 and 6–34).

Oblique facial cleft is a rare condition in which the cleft lip on one side extends to the medial margin of the orbit. This is caused by failure of the maxillary process to fuse with the lateral and median nasal processes. A slanting furrow that extends from the mouth up the cheek to the eye is evident.

Cleft lower lip is extremely rare. It is exactly central and is caused by failure or incomplete fusion of the mandibular processes.

Isolated cleft palate represents a diagnostic challenge. This is because, in many cases, only the soft palate is affected, in these cases the cleft is not detected prenatally. However, clefts of the bony palate may be diagnosed in utero using modified axial views.

In most cases cleft lip and cleft palate diagnosed in utero represent a manifestation of a syndrome or are associated with congenital abnormalities.[4,37,38] Congenital anomalies have been described in 50% of the fetuses with isolated cleft lip and in 9% of those

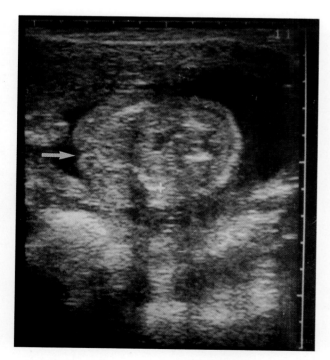

Figure 6–30. Cleft lip. Axial sonogram demonstrating a small incomplete cleft upper lip *(arrow).*

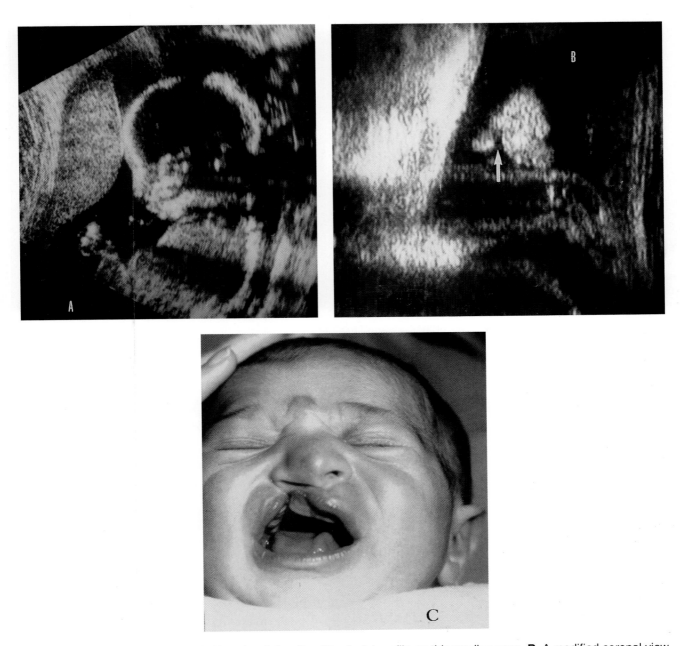

Figure 6–32. Unilateral cleft lip. **A.** Note the deformity of the facial profile on this median scan. **B.** A modified coronal view demonstrates the cleft *(arrow)*. **C.** Photograph of the newborn.

with combined cleft lip and palate.[39] Facial clefts are common in specific chromosomal abnormalities, especially trisomies 13 and 18.[40] There are now over 150 recognized syndromes that include cleft lip, cleft palate, or both. Over 50% are manifestations of mutant genes; about half of these are autosomal dominant, half are autosomal recessive, and a few are X-linked. The remainder do not seem to be familial.

The prenatal detection of a facial cleft warrants a complete survey of the fetus for other structural malformations. Lately 3D evaluation of the lips is suggested as an adjunct in establishing the correct diagnosis and to aid in counseling. Fetal karyotyping analysis should be performed to exclude chromosomal aberrations. In the absence of other fetal malformations and with a normal karyotype, parents can be adequately counseled regarding surgical correction of the defect. However, a thorough explanation concerning the possibility of respiratory and feeding difficulties is mandatory.

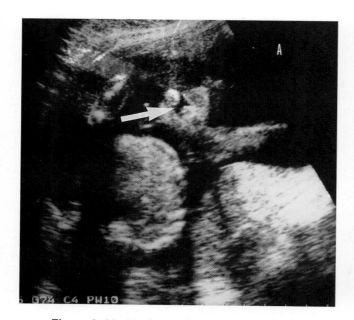
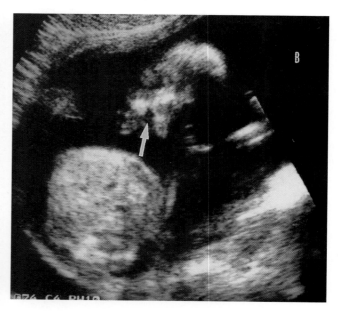

Figure 6–33. Median cleft lip. **(A, B)** Coronal sonograms demonstrating a large median cleft lip *(arrow)* in two cases.

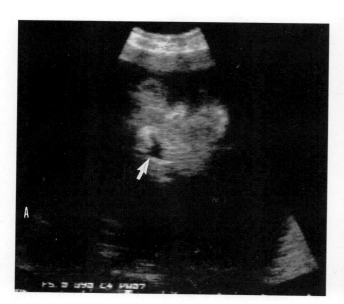
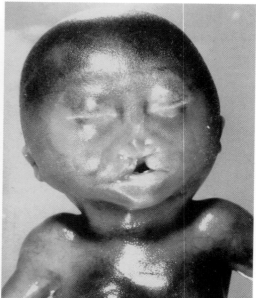

Figure 6–34. Median cleft lip associated with trisomy 18. **A.** Coronal transvaginal ultrasound image demonstrating the median cleft *(arrow)*. **B.** Photograph of the abortus. *(From Meizner and Bar-Ziv, 1993,[15] with permission.)*

Fetal "Mustache"

This is a small skin tag appearing on the upper lip of the fetus early in pregnancy, and is not associated with cleft lip or any other malformation of the lips (Fig. 6–35). This skin tag appears at around 14 to 16 weeks of gestation, and is not found on repeated sonograms performed at around week 22.[41] The etiology of this finding is unknown. The formation of the upper lip is a multistep process leading to a fusion of the epithelial sheets of the two maxillary processes. This is followed by degeneration of the fused sheet and invasion by connective tissue of the

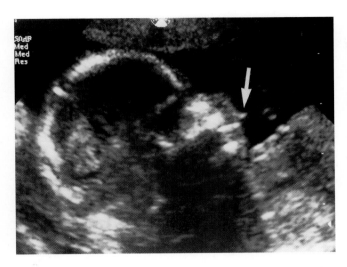

Figure 6–35. A fetal "mustache." Note the skin tag coming from the upper lip *(arrow)* in a transverse oblique view of a 15-week-old fetus.

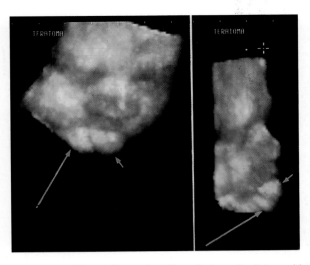

Figure 6–36. Three-dimensional rendering of a fetus with a teratoma *(long arrow)* protruding at the side of the tongue *(short arrow)*. *(Courtesy of Ilan E. Timor-Tritsch.)*

lip growing through it.[42] It is speculated that the fetal "mustache" represents a delay in the normal embryonic process of degeneration of the epithelial remnants, which are formed during the process of lip fusion. The early detection of a fetal "mustache" on the upper, otherwise normal, fetal lip is therefore not a pathology. It probably represents a variant of the development of the upper lip.

Epignathus

Epignathus is a pharyngeal teratoma arising from the oral cavity or the pharynx. This tumor mass protrudes through the mouth and may vary in size and composition. It may arise from the sphenoid bone, palate, pharynx, tongue, or jaw. The tumor is mostly benign in nature and comprises the three germinal layers. About 6% of these tumors may have associated anomalies, especially facial clefts, congenital heart defects, and umbilical hernia.[43] Management may involve cesarean section to avoid dystocia in labor and immediate resuscitation of the newborn to establish an open airway. Surgical excision of the tumor is associated with a 30% to 40% rate of survival.[44]

The composition of adipose tissue, bone, cartilage, and nerve tissue may be reflected on ultrasonography as a mixture of echogenic and sonolucent echoes coming from the protruding mass. Thus, the diagnosis depends on the demonstration of a solid tumor originating from the fetal oral cavity, with both cystic and solid components visualized (Fig. 6–36).[45]

Granular Cell Myoblastoma

Congenital tumors arising from the oropharyngeal region are extremely rare. Granular cell tumor of infancy (congenital epulis, granular cell myoblastoma) refers to a rare intrabucal tumor of unknown origin, presenting either in utero or during early infancy. This tumor probably relates to a large group of granular cell tumors seen in all age groups in multiple anatomic sites. The tumor is usually situated in the alveolar ridge, predominantly in the maxilla.[46] The size may vary from several millimeters to several centimeters in diameter. Although the etiology is enigmatic, there is an 8:1 ratio of female predominance.[47] No sex predilection, however, exists in tumors appearing in older children or adults (Fig. 6–37 A–D).

The differential diagnosis of congenital tumors of the oropharyngeal region includes teratoma, hemangioma, lymphangioma, neurofibroma, and granular cell tumor. A large oropharyngeal tumor may cause partial or complete obstruction of the fetal mouth, thus causing polyhydramnios in late pregnancy. After birth, acute airway obstruction and feeding problems may be encountered. Therefore, early surgical removal of the tumor is required. After surgical removal, no recurrence or malignant changes have been reported.[48]

Since these tumors represent one of those conditions where the prenatal diagnosis can make the difference between life and death of a neonate, correct counseling of the parents is mandatory to assure a safe treatment regime. Delivery should occur in a

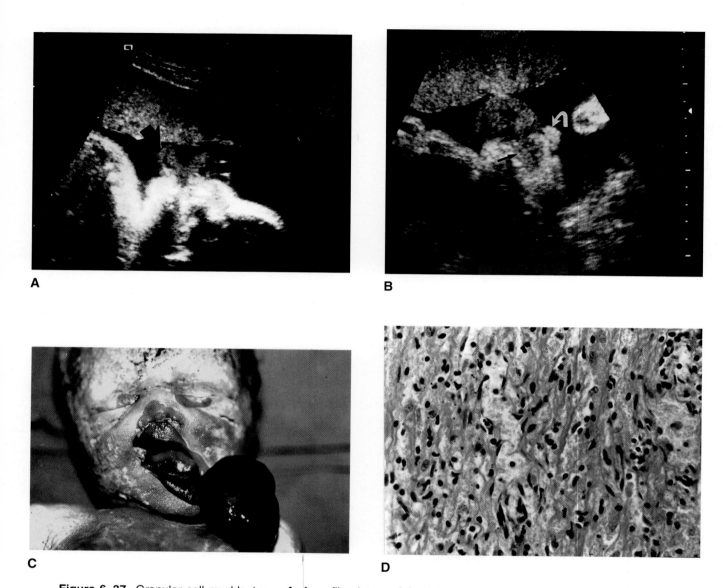

Figure 6–37. Granular cell myoblastoma. **A.** A profile picture of the fetal face showing the proximity of the tumor mass *(arrow)* to the face. **B.** Coronal sonogram of the fetal face. Notice the normal appearance of the lips *(arrows),* nose *(curved arrow),* and nostrils. The tumor mass is located to the right of the mouth (m). **C.** Postmortem picture of the newborn shown in the two previous pictures. **D.** High power microscopic picture small revealing large cells with abundant granular cytoplasm and hyperchromatic nucleus (hematoxylin and eosin, × 250). *(By permission. From Meizner et al* J Ultrasound Med. *2000;19:337.)*

tertiary center, capable of handling such cases that require complicated procedures.

Macroglossia

Ultrasonography can detect macroglossia quite easily using both median and coronal views. The midsagittal view is far better, since it enables the examiner to clearly delineate the tongue from its origin to its tip. Macroglossia is a feature of Beckwith–Wiedemann syndrome, characterized by visceromegaly, macroglossia, omphalocele, and renal hyperplasia and dysplasia (Fig. 6–38).[49] The most striking sonographic findings include macroglossia and omphalocele.[50] Several cases have been described in the English literature; however, macroglossia was observed in only one.[51] Protrusion of the tongue is not sufficient for making the diagnosis of macroglossia. The tongue should remain outside the mouth, regardless of swallowing movements of the lips. The differential diagnosis of macroglossia should include trisomy 21 (Fig. 6–39), tumors of the tongue, and hypothyroidism.

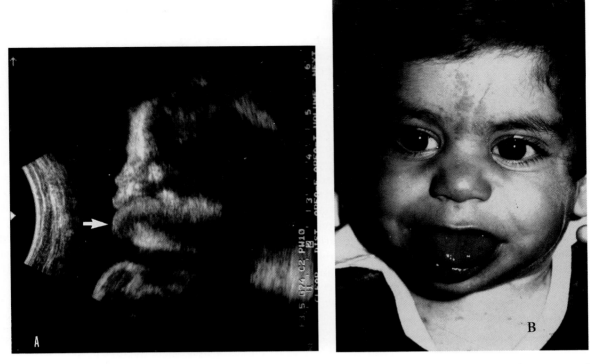

Figure 6–38. Beckwith–Wiedemann syndrome. **A.** Median sonogram of the fetal face, demonstrating a protruding enlarged tongue *(arrow).* **B.** Photograph of the infant's face. Note the large protruding tongue and the capillary nevus flammeus on the central forehead, typical of this syndrome.

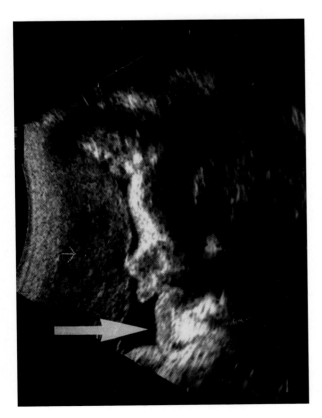

Figure 6–39. Macroglossia *(arrow)* in a case of trisomy 21 syndrome.

Malformations Involving the Mandible

Malformations affecting the mandible represent mainly those associated with first branchial arch syndrome. This syndrome consists of several malformations resulting from the disappearance of or abnormal development of various components of the first pharyngeal arch. It is postulated that the origin of the malformations is probably due to a deficiency of neural crest cells as a result of insufficient migration, cell necrosis, or decreased cell proliferation. Factors responsible for these changes may be genetic or environmental. Furthermore, because neural crest cells contribute to septation of the aortic and pulmonary arteries, first arch syndrome is often associated with cardiac anomalies such as transposition of the great vessels and interrupted aortic arch. The main syndromes encountered in first arch syndrome include Treacher Collins syndrome (mandibulofacial dysostosis), Nager syndrome, and Pierre Robin syndrome. The term *first arch syndrome* was coined by McKenzie in 1966.[52]

Treacher Collins Syndrome

Treacher Collins syndrome is an autosomal dominant disorder affecting structures derived from the first branchial arch. It is characterized by malformations of the eyes, ears, and mandible. Manifestations include antimongoloid slant of the palpebral fissures, hypoplasia of the malar bones and the man-

dible, abnormalities of the auricle, high arched or cleft palate, external ear canal defects, and abnormal hair growth on the cheeks.[53] Prenatal diagnosis of Treacher Collins syndrome has been documented.[54,55]

The differential diagnosis includes Goldenhar's syndrome (oculoauriculovertebral dysplasia), which is familial, is almost always unilateral, and involves notching of the upper rather than the lower lid. Hemifacial microsomia may be a variant of this. In Nager's acrofacial dysostosis mandibulofacial dysostosis occurs with preaxial reduction defects of the hands.[56] Inheritance is autosomal recessive. The sonographic approach to the diagnosis of all first arch syndrome malformations should rely on the midsagittal view of the face. The profile view demonstrates pathologies of the mandible—the most striking feature of the syndrome (Figs. 6–40 through 6–42).

Pierre Robin Syndrome

Pierre Robin syndrome is another first arch syndrome characterized by micrognathia (mandibular hypoplasia), cleft palate, and glossoptosis.[57] Defects of the ears and the eyes may also appear. Most cases are sporadic. Most of the reported familial cases appear to represent cases of Strickler syndrome

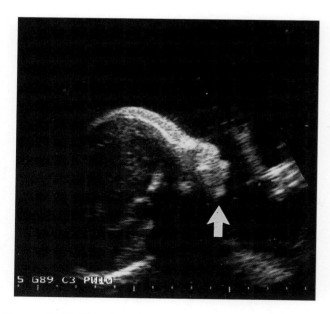

Figure 6–40. Treacher Collins syndrome. Median scan of the fetal profile. Note the micrognathia *(arrow). (From Meizner and colleagues, 1991,*[50] *with permission.)*

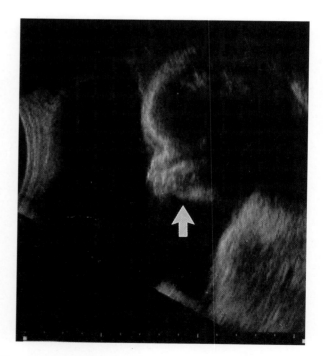

Figure 6–41. Treacher Collins syndrome. Sagittal scan of the fetal face and thorax. The *arrow* indicates the extremely hypoplastic mandible. Polyhydramnios is evident. *(From Meizner and colleagues, 1991,*[50] *with permission.)*

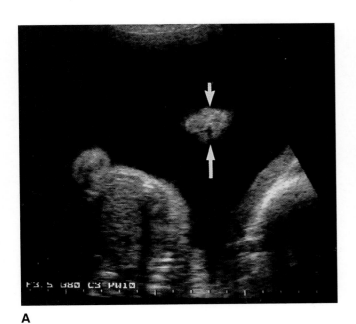

A

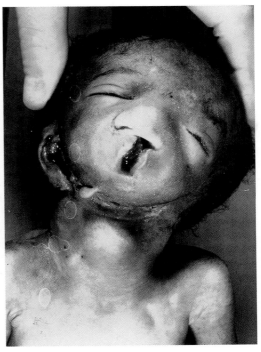

B

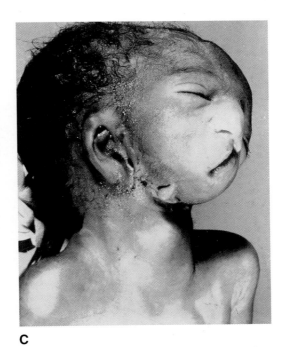

C

Figure 6–42. Treacher Collins syndrome. **A.** Coronal scan through the fetal nose at 31 postmenstrual weeks *(arrowhead).* Note the cleft lip *(arrow).* **B.** Photograph of the newborn. Note the hypoplastic mandible and the facial cleft. **C.** Lateral view of the newborn face, showing the malformed ear. *(From Meizner and colleagues, 1991,[50] with permission.)*

(associated with eye problems) or Weissenbacher–Zweymüller syndrome (rhizomelic dwarfism).[58]

The diagnosis, again, is based on a midsagittal view of the face marking the severe micrognathia (Figs. 6–43 and 6–44). Because glossoptosis is a main feature in this syndrome, associated polyhydramnios due to lack of swallowing is a common finding.

Micrognathia of Various Etiologies

Fetal micrognathia may appear in many syndromes. The most frequent ones include Seckel syndrome, lethal multiple pterygium syndrome, trisomy 13, trisomy 18, and skeletal dysplasias (e.g., camptomelic dwarfism or achondrogenesis).[11] As in Pierre Robin anomalad, in all of these cases polyhydramnios may appear. The sonographic detection of micrognathia, with or without accompanying polyhydramnios, presents a diagnostic challenge to the examiner. This finding is associated with many syndromes, therefore, a careful anatomic survey of the fetus coupled with fetal karyotyping is warranted.

Miscellaneous Facial Deformities

Numerous facial deformities associated with specific syndromes, which cannot be adequately classified into groups, may be encountered in this category. One may include in this category the following anomalies.

Facial Malformations Associated with Skeletal Dysplasias

Two major facial defects may appear in this unique group of anomalies: frontal bossing and depressed nasal bridge (saddle nose). Frontal bossing is found in cases of achondroplasia, dyssegmental dysplasia, short rib–polydactyly syndrome types I through III, and many more (Figs. 6–45 and 6–46).[59,60] In some dysplasias a cloverleaf skull may be present, which may cause deformation of the face (Fig. 6–47). In short rib–polydactyly syndrome severe edema of the face may be found, which can be detected by ultrasonography (Fig. 6–48).

In cases of osteogenesis imperfecta, demineralization of the calvarium may cause deformation of the face, with prominence of the eyes. A case of association between osteogenesis type II and micrognathia has also been reported.[61] Micrognathia may accompany several skeletal disorders, e.g., Weissenbacher–Zweymüller syndrome.

Three-dimensional ultrasound rendering of the face in cases of skeletal dysplasia may be a significant aid to the diagnostic algorythm (Fig. 6–49).

Facial Malformations Associated with Neural Tube Defects

Facial malformations of various forms may accompany neural tube defects involving the cranial vault. Cranial anomalies affecting facial morphol-

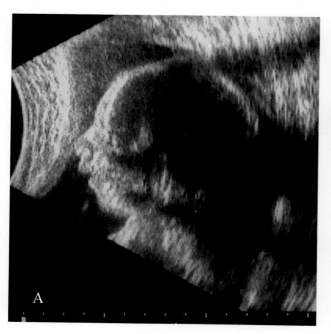
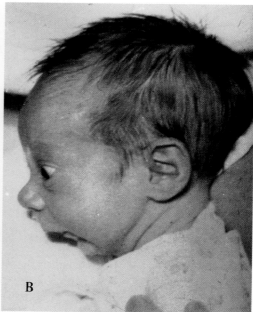

Figure 6–43. Pierre Robin anomalad. **A.** Median view of the fetal face, showing the recessed jaw. **B.** Photograph of the newborn, showing severe micrognathia.

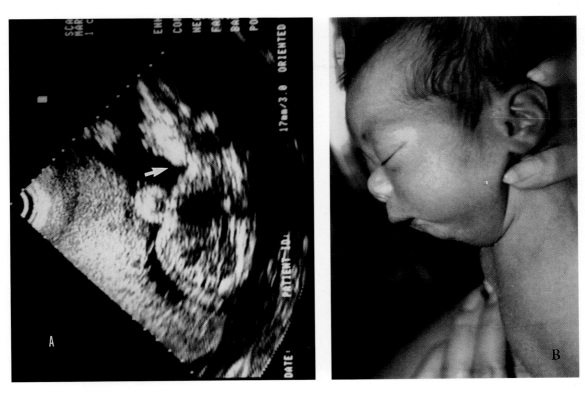

Figure 6–44. Weissenbacher–Zweymüller syndrome. **A.** Longitudinal scan of the fetus at 18 weeks of gestation. Micrognathia is evident *(arrow).* **B.** Photograph of the newborn, showing micrognathia. Cleft palate was also present. *(From Meizner and Bar-Ziv, 1993,[15] with permission.)*

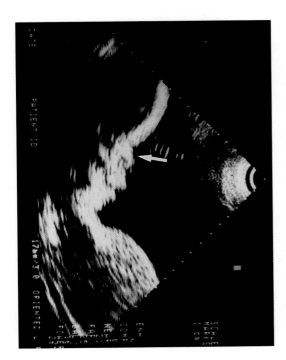

Figure 6–45. Achondroplasia. Profile sonogram of the fetus, showing frontal bossing and depression of the nasal bridge *(arrow).*

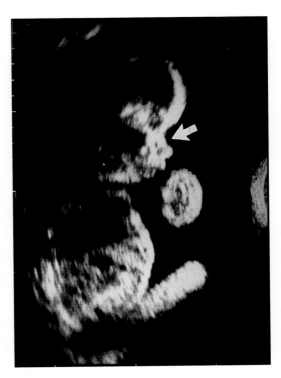

Figure 6–46. Dyssegmental dysplasia. Fetal profile at 22 weeks of gestation, showing a depressed nasal bridge *(arrow).*

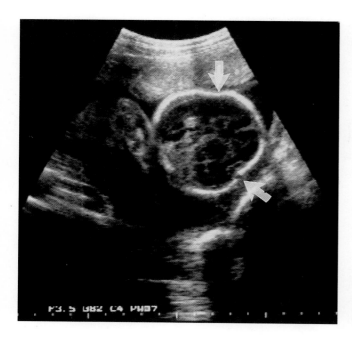

Figure 6–47. Thanatophoric dysplasia diagnosed at 19 postmenstrual weeks. The sonogram demonstrates a typical cloverleaf skull. The *arrows* mark the closure of the coronal sutures. *(From Meizner and Bar-Ziv, 1993,[15] with permission.)*

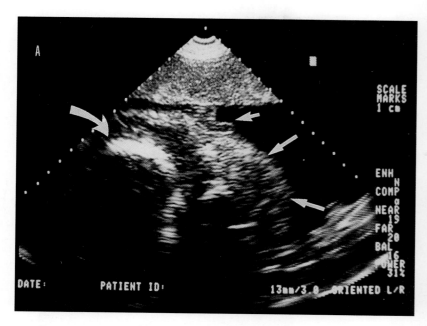

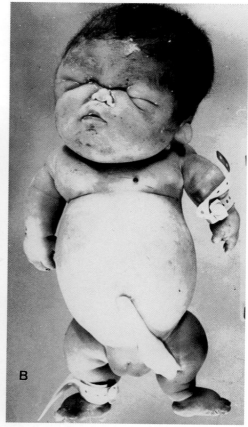

Figure 6–48. Short rib–polydactyly syndrome type III. **A.** Semicoronal scan of the fetal face, showing extreme edema of the cheek. The *long arrows* indicate the edema, and the *short arrow* marks the ear. The *curved arrow* points to the skull. **B.** Postmortem photograph of the newborn, showing the facial edema. *(From Meizner and Bar-Ziv, 1993,[15] with permission.)*

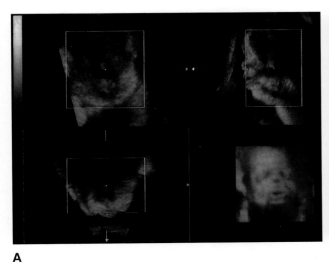
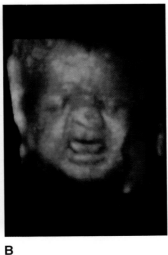
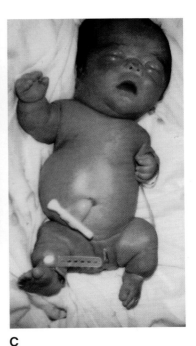

A

B

Figure 6–49. Three-dimensional rendering of the face in a case of skeletal dysplasia (achrondroplasia). **A.** The three-dimensional rendering process of the face. **B.** The final image of the face. **C.** The expired neonate. *(Courtesy of Ilan E. Timor-Tritsch.)*

C

ogy include anencephaly, encephalocele, and iniencephaly.

Anencephaly is a lethal congenital malformation characterized by absence of the cerebral hemispheres and the cranial vault. On ultrasonography absence of the cranial vault and the brain cephalad to the orbits is diagnostic of this pathology.[62] Both orbits are large and prominent, simulating the appearance of a frog. Polyhydramnios is a common finding (Figs. 6–50 through 6–52). Facial clefts are also common (see also Chapter 4).

The term *encephalocele* describes herniation of the brain or the meninges through a cranial defect.[63] With the presence of a large mass of brain protruding through the skull defect, secondary facial changes may appear. These include hypotelorism with downslanting of the palpebral fissures and flattening of the forehead as a result of secondary microcephaly (Fig. 6–53).

Iniencephaly designates anomaly in the brain and the neck (inion). The head is retroflexed and there is exaggerated cervicothoracic lordosis. The head is large in relation to the shortened body, the face looks upward, and the neck is absent. Occipital encephalocele, rachischisis, anencephaly, and, at times, omphalocele are part of the anomaly.[64] Targeted coronal ultrasonography of the fetal face demonstrates both the orbits and the nose resembling those of an owl (Fig. 6–54). This specific view is obtained due to the severe lordosis of the cervical spine, causing extreme retroflexion of the head (see also Chapter 4). (See also Fig. 4-15, 16)

Fetal Hydrops

In cases of immune and nonimmune fetal hydrops, severe edema of the body is present. This generalized edema does not skip the facial region and presents a grotesque sonographic appearance of the fetal face (Fig. 6–55). Edema of the soft tissue distorts the normal facial profile.

Fetal Goiter

A fetal goiter may occur as a consequence of either hypothyroidism (most common) or hyperthyroidism, both of which may be associated with persistent neurological and developmental sequela in the newborn. Goiters associated with hypothyroidism are due to iodine deficiency, iodine intoxication, maternal antithyroid medications, or inborn errors in thyroid hormone synthesis. Goiters associated with hyperthyroidism are the result of transplacental transfer of maternal LATS (long active thyroid stimulating) antibodies whether or not the mother has active Graves' disease. Ultrasonography has allowed the early detection of fetal goiter and fetal blood sampling now facilitates direct evaluation of fetal thyroid hormone status. Knowledge of the cause and severity of abnormal fetal thyroid function permits rational treatment of the affected fetus. Evidence of thyroid dysfunction in the presence of fetal goiter should be aggressively managed, either by treatment of the maternal cause or direct fetal therapy.

Ultrasound diagnosis relies on the appearance of an enlarged thyroid represented by a symmetrical

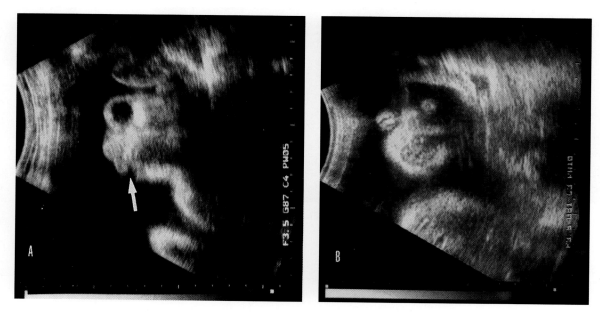

Figure 6–50. Anencephaly. **(A)** Median and **(B)** coronal sonograms of a fetus with anencephaly at 21 postmenstrual weeks. Note the absence of the calvarium, the bulging eyes, and the cleft lip *(arrow)*. *(From Meizner and Bar-Ziv, 1993,[15] with permission.)*

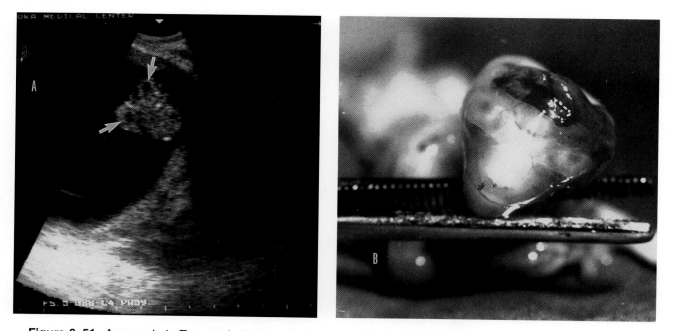

Figure 6–51. Anencephaly. Transvaginal scan of a fetus with anencephaly (10 postmenstrual weeks). **A.** Coronal view of the fetal face. Note the bulging orbits *(arrows)* and the absence of the calvarium. **B.** Photograph of the face of the abortus. *(From Meizner and Bar-Ziv, 1993,[15] with permission.)*

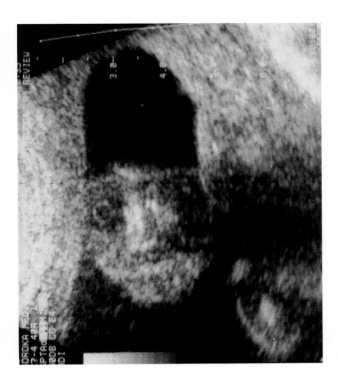

Figure 6–52. Anencephaly. Coronal view of the fetal face, demonstrating the lens of the right eye. Note the absence of the skull (20 postmenstrual weeks).

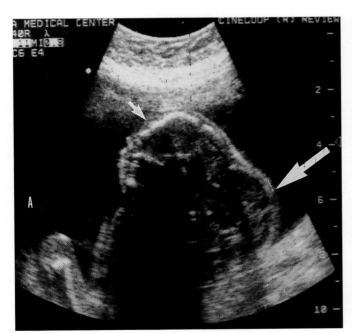

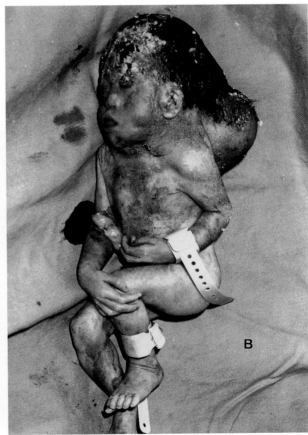

Figure 6–53. Encephalocele. **A.** Large occipital encephalocele *(arrow)*. Note the flattening of the forehead due to the microcephaly caused by protrusion of most of the brain through the skull defect. The *small arrow* indicates the flattened forehead. **B.** Postnatal photograph of the stillborn. *(From Meizner and Bar-Ziv, 1993,*[15] *with permission.)*

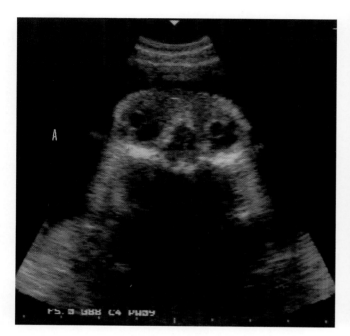
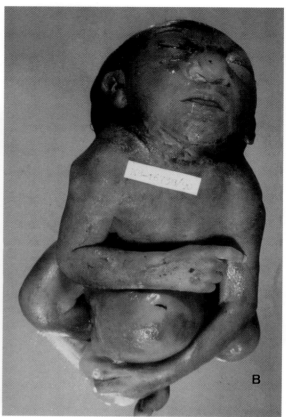

Figure 6–54. Iniencephaly detected at 18 postmenstrual weeks. **A.** Image of the fetal face, showing both eye lenses. This image was obtained separately from the rest of the body because of the marked retroflexion of the head (transvaginal approach). **B.** Photograph of the face of the abortus. *(From Meizner, 1993,[15] with permission.)*

echogenic mass in the neck. Polyhydramnios may appear due to esophageal compression (Fig. 6–56 A and B). Antenatal treatment, although controversial, is possible by intra-amniotic, intravascular and intramuscular injection of thyroxin.[65] The intra-amniotic route is preferred because of the relative ease of the technique and the longer intervals between administration. Two hundred to 500 mg at 7 to 10 day intervals seems to be a reasonable regimen based on the limited information available.[66]

Teratoma of the Neck and the Face

Teratomas are neoplasms derived from pluripotent cells and composed of a wide diversity of tissues foreign to the anatomic site in which they arise.[67] These tissues are derived from precursors in three different germinal layers. Most cervical teratomas are benign and tend to appear as an isolated anomaly. Teratomas of the neck may present as a mixture of solid and cystic components. Calcified foci may be present in almost 50% of the cases in neonates,[68] but

these have not been reported on prenatal sonograms.[69,70] The differential diagnosis may include cystic hygroma, goiter, and branchial cleft cyst.

Antenatal detection is feasible, relying on the demonstration of a complex mass in the cervical region compressing and distorting the fetal face (Fig. 6–57). Polyhydramnios is a frequent associated finding.[71] The early detection of this pathology allows the physician to establish a strategy as to mode and time of delivery. Cesarean section is indicated once lung maturity is achieved, especially in cases with large teratomas, which may cause dystocia. Immediate resuscitation and intubation may be necessary.

Congenital Ichthyosis (Harlequin Fetus)

The term *harlequin fetus* refers to a severe and dramatic form of congenital ichthyosis. Whereas mild and moderately severe forms of ichthyosis are relatively common disorders, harlequin fetus represents a rare condition with fewer than 100 cases described in the world literature.[72] Because of the rarity of

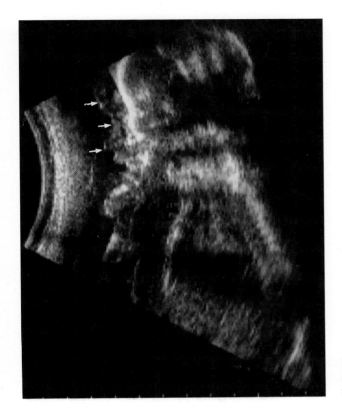

Figure 6–55. Fetal hydrops. Median sonogram showing severe edema of the fetal face. The *small arrows* indicate the severity of the facial edema.

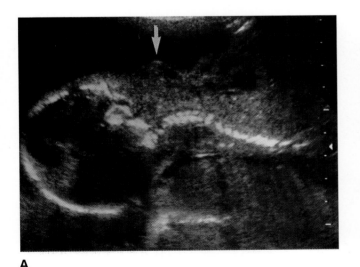

A

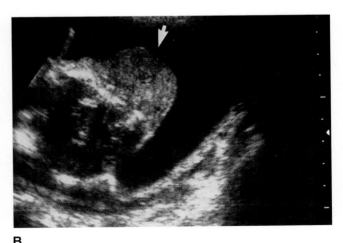

B

Figure 6–56. Fetal goiter. **A.** Longitudinal scan of the fetus. Notice the bulging tumor mass at the cervical region *(arrow)*. **B.** Coronal scan of the fetal neck. The large goiter is evident *(arrow)*.

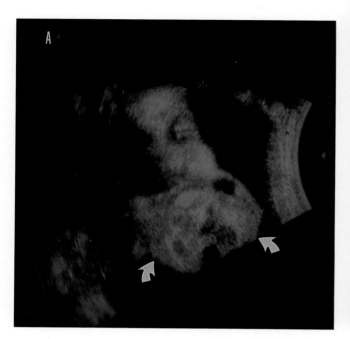
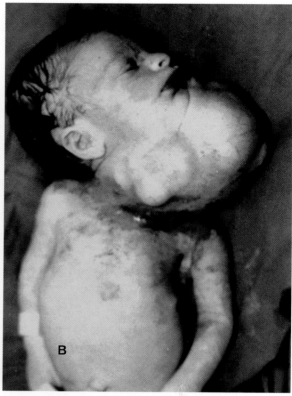

Figure 6–57. Cervical teratoma. **A.** Coronal sonogram demonstrating a large, semisolid mass coming from the left side of the neck and the face. The *arrows* mark the mass. **B.** Photograph of the newborn after failed resuscitation.

this condition and the short life span of affected individuals (6 weeks or less), the place of this disorder in the spectrum of ichthyosis remains controversial. The skin of the fetus is hard, brown, cracked, and rigid. Rigidity of the skin about the eyes results in marked ectropion, everted O-shaped lips with a gaping fish-mouth deformity, and a distorted, flattened, and undeveloped appearance of the nose and the ears, all of which add to the grotesque, clownlike appearance of the infant (Fig. 6–58).

The sonographic signs leading to prenatal diagnosis of this disorder may include (1) a widely opened mouth, (2) an absent nose with evident apertures corresponding to the nostrils, (3) large, "bulging" eyes, (4) a lack of fetal and breathing movements, and (5) "edematous-like" limbs.[73]

SUMMARY

The impressive advances in sonographic imaging of the fetus over the last decade have made possible the detailed evaluation of the fetal face in the majority of cases. A logical sonographic approach to the diagnosis of fetal facial malformations must be based

on recognition of the normal sonographic anatomy of the face as well as understanding of facial pathology and the abnormalities associated with specific pathological entities.

Lately, three-dimensional ultrasound rendering of the fetal face proved to be of real clinical value. Centers with the required three-dimensional ultrasound equipment should add this important imaging modality to the armamentarium of imaging the fetal face in case of suspected anomalies. Showing the rendered image to the plastic surgeon enables a better understanding of the lesion and appropriate counseling of the patient.

Incorporation of facial imaging into the basic examination of the fetus is highly recommended, because facial abnormalities may reflect intracranial pathologies and may assist in the process of decision making regarding the performance of invasive procedures for fetal karyotyping. Examination of the face after delivery in a neonate in whom congenital malformation was diagnosed or suspected is of the utmost importance in order to best counsel the parents with regard to management and future childbearing. It is equally important to obtain a

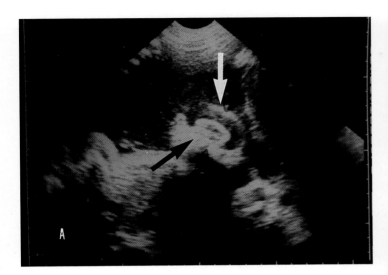

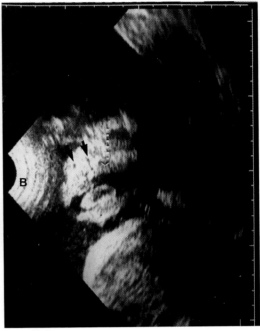

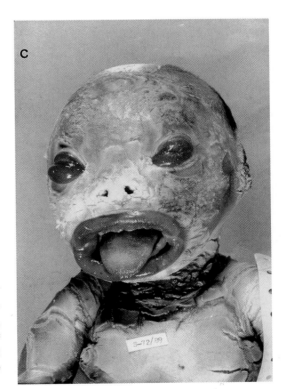

Figure 6–58. Congenital ichthyosis. **A.** Coronal ultrasound scan of the fetal face. The *arrows* indicate the widely opened mouth. Note the tongue in the center of the mouth. **B.** Oblique coronal scan of the fetal face. The *arrows* mark the apertures where the nose would have been. **C.** Picture of the grotesque, clownlike appearance of the infant. *(From Meizner, 1992,[66] with permission.)*

pathological specimen if a midtrimester abortion was performed or intrauterine fetal death occurred. The postmortem examination and an accurate description of the facial dysmorphology should be documented, together with photographs taken from various angles.

REFERENCES

1. Shell RS. *Clinical Embryology for Medical Students.* Boston: Little, Brown; 1975:111–118.
2. Arey LB. *Developmental Anatomy.* Philadelphia: WB Saunders; 1974:199–207.
3. Hegge FN, Prescott GH, Watson PT. Fetal facial abnormalities identified during obstetric sonography. *J Ultrasound Med.* 1986;5:679–684.
4. Meizner I, Katz M, Bar-Ziv J, et al. Prenatal sonographic detection of fetal facial malformations. *Isr J Med Sci.* 1987;23:881–885.
5. Pilu G, Reece A, Romero R, et al. Prenatal diagnosis of craniofacial malformations with ultrasonography. *Am J Obstet Gynecol.* 1986;155:45–50.
6. Benacerraf B. Ultrasound evaluation of the fetal face. In: Callen PW, ed. *Ultrasound in Obstetrics and Gynecology.* Philadelphia: WB Saunders; 1994:235–253.
7. Jeanty P, Cantraine F, Cousaert E. The binocular distance: A new way to estimate fetal age. *J Ultrasound Med.* 1984;3:241–243.
8. Mayden KL, Tortora M, Berkovitz RI. Orbital diameters: A new parameter for prenatal diagnosis and dating. *Am J Obstet Gynecol.* 1982;144:289–297.
9. Smith DW. *Recognizable Patterns of Human Malformations.* 4th ed. Philadelphia: WB Saunders; 1988: 714–715.
10. Chervenak FA, Tortora M, Mayden K. Antenatal diagnosis of median cleft face syndrome: Sonographic demonstration of cleft lip and hypertelorism. *Am J Obstet Gynecol.* 1984;149:94–97.
11. Meizner I, Hershkovitz R, Carmi R, et al. Prenatal ultrasound diagnosis of a rare occurrence of lethal multiple pterygium syndrome in two siblings. *Ultrasound Obstet Gynecol.* 1993;3:1–5.
12. Fitz CR. Holoprosencephaly and related entities. *Neuroradiology.* 1983;25:225–238.
13. Saunders ES, Shortland D, Dunn PM. What is the incidence of holoprosencephaly? *J Med Genet.* 1984;21: 21–24.
14. DeMyer W. Classification of cerebral malformations. *Birth Defects Orig Artic Ser.* 1971;7:78–93.
15. Meizner I, Bar–Ziv J. *In Utero Diagnosis of Skeletal Disorders.* Boca Raton, Fla: CRC Press; 1993.
16. DeMyer W, Zeman W. Alobar holoprosencephaly (arhinencephaly) with median cleft lip and palate. *Confin Neurol.* 1963;23:1–6.
17. Greene MF, Benacerraf BR, Frigoletto FD. Reliable criteria for the prenatal sonographic diagnosis of alobar holoprosencephaly. *Am J Obstet Gynecol.* 1987; 156:687–689.
18. Nyberg DA, Mack LA, Bronstein A. Holoprosencephaly: Prenatal sonographic diagnosis. *AJR.* 1987; 149:1051–1058.
19. Pilu G, Romero R, Rizzo N. Criteria for the prenatal diagnosis of holoprosencephaly. *Am J Perinatol.* 1987; 4:41–49.
20. Chervenak FA, Pinto MM, Heller CI. Obstetric significance of fetal craniofacial duplication: A case report. *J Reprod Med.* 1985;30:74–76.
21. Okazaki JR, Wilson JL, Holmes SM. Diprosopus: Diagnosis in utero. *AJR.* 1987;149:147–148.
22. Strauss S, Tamarkin M, Engelberg S. Prenatal sonographic appearance of diprosopus. *J Ultrasound Med.* 1987;6:93–95.
23. Cayea PD, Bieber FR, Ross MJ. Sonographic findings in otocephaly (synotia). *J Ultrasound Med.* 1985;4: 377–379.
24. Feldman E, Shalev E, Weiner E. Microphthalmia: Prenatal ultrasound diagnosis. *Prenat Diagn.* 1985;5: 205–207.
25. Tamas DE, Mahony BS, Bowie JD. Prenatal sonographic diagnosis of hemifacial microsomia (Goldenhar–Grolin syndrome). *J Ultrasound Med.* 1986;5: 461–463.
26. Kohn BA. The differential diagnosis of cataracts in infancy and childhood. *Am J Dis Child.* 1976;130: 184–192.
27. Nelson LB. Diagnosis and management of cataracts in infancy and childhood. *Ophthalmic Surg.* 1984;15: 688–697.
28. Zimmer EZ, Bronshtein M, Ophir E, et al. Sonographic diagnosis of fetal congenital cataracts. *Prenat Diagn.* 1993;13:503–511.
29. Bronshtein M, Zimmer EZ, Gershoni-Baruch R, et al. First and second trimester diagnosis of fetal ocular defects and associated anomalies: Report of eight cases. *Obstet Gynecol.* 1991;7:443–449.
30. Birnholz JC, Farrell EE. Fetal hyaloid artery: Timing of regression with ultrasound. *Radiology.* 1988;166: 781–783.
31. Davis WK, Mahony BS, Carroll BA. Antenatal sonographic detection of benign dacryocystoceles (lacrimal duct cysts). *J Ultrasound Med.* 1987;6:461–465.
32. Meizner I, Bar-Ziv J, Holcberg G. In utero prenatal diagnosis of fetal facial tumor–hemangioma. *J Clin Ultrasound.* 1985;13:435–437.
33. McArdle CR. Ultrasonic appearance of the hepatic hemangioma. *J Clin Ultrasound.* 1978;5:122–124.
34. Gorlin RJ, Cervenka J, Pruzansky S. Facial clefting and its syndromes. *Birth Defects Orig Artic Ser.* 1971; 7:3–9.
35. Saltzman DH, Benacerraf BR, Frigoletto FD. Diagnosis and management of fetal facial clefts. *Am J Obstet Gynecol.* 1986;155:377–382.
36. Seeds JW, Cefalo RC. Technique of early sonographic diagnosis of bilateral cleft lip and palate. *Obstet Gynecol.* 1983;62:2S.
37. Kraus BS, Kitamura H, Ooe T. Malformations associated with cleft lip and palate in human embryos and fetuses. *Am J Obstet Gynecol.* 1963;86:321–326.

38. Benacerraf BR, Miller WA, Frigoletto FD. Sonographic detection of fetuses with trisomies 13 and 18. Accuracy and limitations. *Am J Obstet Gynecol.* 1988; 158:404–409.
39. Ingalls TH, Taube IE, Klingberg MA. Cleft lip and cleft palate: Epidemiologic considerations. *Plast Reconstruct Surg.* 1964;34:1–8.
40. Benacerraf BR, Frigoletto FD, Greene MF. Abnormal facial features and extremities in human trisomy syndromes: Prenatal ultrasound appearance. *Radiology.* 1986;159:243–248.
41. Bronstein M, Zimmer EZ, Offir H, et al. Fetal mustache in early pregnancy. *Ultrasound Obstet Gynecol.* 1998;12:252.
42. Avery JA. Prenatal fetal growth. In Enlaw DH, ed. *Handbook of Facial Growth.* 3rd ed. Philadelphia: WB Saunders; 1990:18.
43. Carney JA, Thompson DP, Johnson CL. Teratomas in children: Clinical and pathologic aspects. *J Pediatr Surg.* 1972;7:271–275.
44. Holmgern G, Rydnert J. Male fetus with epignathus originating from the ethmoidal sinus. *Eur J Obstet Gynecol Reprod Biol.* 1987;24:69–72.
45. Chervenak FA, Tortora M, Moya FR. Antenatal sonographic diagnosis of epignathus. *J Ultrasound Med.* 1984;3:235–237.
46. Pellicano M, Zulo F, Castizone, et al. Prenatal diagnosis of congenital granular cell epulis. *Ultrasound Obstet Gynecol.* 1998;11:144.
47. Rainey JB, Smith J. Congenital epulis of the newborn. *J Pediatr Surg.* 1984;9:305.
48. Jenkins HR, Hill CM: Spontaneous regression of congenital epulis of the newborn. *Arch Dis Child.* 1989;64:145.
49. Beckwith JB. Macroglossia, omphalocele, adrenal cytomegaly, gigantism and hyperplastic visceromegaly. *Birth Defects Orig Artic Ser.* 1969;5:188–193.
50. Meizner I, Katz M, Carmi R, et al. In utero prenatal diagnosis of Beckwith–Wiedemann syndrome. *Eur J Obstet Gynecol Reprod Biol.* 1989;32:259–264.
51. Cobellis G, Iannoto P, Stabile M. Prenatal ultrasound diagnosis of macroglossia in the Weidemann–Beck with syndrome. *Prenat Diagn.* 1988;8:79–81.
52. McKenzie J. The first arch syndrome. *Dev Med Child Neurol.* 1966;8:55–62.
53. Poswillo D. The pathogenesis of Treacher Collins syndrome (mandibulofacial dysostosis). *Br J Oral Surg.* 1975;13:1–7.
54. Crane JP, Beaver HA. Midtrimester sonographic diagnosis of mandibulofacial dysostosis. *Am J Med Genet.* 1986;25:251–255.
55. Meizner I, Carmi R, Katz M. Prenatal ultrasonic diagnosis of mandibulofacial dysostosis (Treacher–Collins syndrome). *J Clin Ultrasound.* 1991;19:124–129.
56. Benson CB, Pober BR, Hirsh MP, et al. Sonography of Nager acrofacial dysostosis syndrome in utero. *J Ultrasound Med.* 1988;7:163–167.
57. Pilu G, Romero R, Reece EA, et al. The prenatal diagnosis of Robin anomalad. *Am J Obstet Gynecol.* 1986; 154:630–632.
58. Chemke J, Carmi R, Galil A, et al. Weissenbacher–Zweymüller syndrome. A distinct autosomal recessive skeletal dysplasia. *Am J Med Genet.* 1992;43:989–993.
59. Filly RA, Golbus MS, Carey JC. Short-limbed dwarfism: Ultrasonographic diagnosis by measurement of fetal femoral length. *Radiology.* 1981;138: 653–656.
60. Meizner I, Bar-Ziv J. Prenatal ultrasonic diagnosis of short rib polydactyly syndrome, type I. A case report. *J Reprod Med.* 1989;34:668–670.
61. Meizner I, Levy A, Yosef S, et al. Prenatal ultrasonic diagnosis of type II osteogenesis imperfecta in the second trimester. *Isr J Med Sci.* 1991;2:26–28.
62. Cunningham ME, Walls WJ. Ultrasound in the evaluation of anencephaly. *Radiology.* 1976;118:165–167.
63. Meizner I, Bar-Ziv J, Katz M. Prenatal ultrasonic diagnosis of occipital encephalocele. *Harefuah.* 1984;56: 263–264.
64. Meizner I, Bar-Ziv J. Prenatal ultrasonic diagnosis of iniencephaly apertus. *J Clin Ultrasound.* 1987;15: 200–203.
65. Thorpe-Beeston G. Goitre. In Fisk NM, Moise Jr KJ, eds. *Fetal Therapy.* Cambridge: Cambridge University Press; 1977:252.
66. Abuhamad AZ, Fisher DA, Warsof SL, et al. Antenatal diagnosis and treatment of fetal goiterous hypothyroidism: Case report and review of the literature. *Ultrasound Obstet Gynecol.* 1995;6:368.
67. Gonzalez-Crussi F, Winkler RF, Merkin BL. Sacrococcygeal teratomas in infants and children. *Arch Pathol Lab Med.* 1978;102:420–425.
68. Gadwood KA, Reynes CJ. Prenatal sonography of metastatic neuroblastoma of neck. *J Clin Ultrasound.* 1983;11:512–514.
69. Goodwin BD, Gay BB. The roentgen diagnosis of teratoma of the thyroid region. *AJR.* 1965;95:25–31.
70. Gundry SR, Westey JR, Klein MD. Cervical teratomas in the newborn. *J Pediatr Surg.* 1983;18:382.
71. Rosenfeld CR, Coln CD, Duenhoelter JH. Fetal cervical teratomas as a cause of polyhydramnios. *Pediatrics.* 1979;64:176–178.
72. Buxhan M, Goodkin PE, Fahrenbach WH. Harlequin ichthyosis with epidermal lipid abnormality. *Arch Dermatol.* 1979;115:189–191.
73. Meizner I. Prenatal ultrasonic features in a rare case of congenital ichthyosis (harlequin fetus). *J Clin Ultrasound.* 1992;20:132–134.

week. At the end of the fifth week, the optic capsule is completely surrounded by a loose mesenchyme. This tissue differentiates into an inner layer comparable to the pia mater of the brain and an outer layer comparable to the dura mater. At 6 to 7 weeks, the choroid originates from the inner layer and the outer layer develops into the sclera. The anterior chamber of the eye comes from the mesenchyme that overlies the lens. At 8 weeks, the cornea forms from the outer layer of the anterior chamber. The eyelids are mesodermal folds lined with ectoderm that meet in front of the cornea by the eighth week.

The hyaloid artery originates from the ophthalmic artery. It runs through the center of the eye and terminates at the posterior surface of the lens (Fig. 7–2).[9–11] The primary function is to nourish the developing lens. There is a normal process of regression of the vessel toward the end of pregnancy.[9–12] A delay in the process of regression is associated with fetal abnormalities mainly of the central nervous system.[12] The flow in the hyaloid artery can be seen using color Doppler sonography. Figure 7–2B depicts arterial flow at 16 weeks.

Ocular growth during fetal life was studied in products of spontaneous and induced abortions.[13,14] The development of the diameter and circumference of the eyeball showed an almost linear increase during gestation. The horizontal diameter of the eyeball was longer than the sagittal, and the vertical diameter was the shortest one. The average diameters of the eye in male fetuses were longer than in female fetuses.[13] At birth, the various dimensions of the eyeball were one third of the adult size.

When eyeball measurements were compared to gestational age weight, height, head circumference, and abdominal circumference, it was found that the fetal head circumference correlated best with ocular growth.[14]

ULTRASONOGRAPHIC EVALUATION OF THE FETAL EYE

Technique

A detailed ultrasonic examination of the fetal eye was first reported by Birnholz[15] and de Elejalde and Elejalde.[16] The eyes were analyzed in both transverse and coronal plane. In the transverse plane, the transducer was moved from the top of the skull across the fetal face. In the coronal plane, the transducer was moved from the tip of the nose to the posterior aspect of the eye. In both these studies, the eyelids, lens, cornea, sclera, irides, hyaloid artery, retina, and optic nerve were observed. However, such a detailed examination is difficult and sonologists are advised to refer to these studies in order to better understand the ultrasonic features of these different parts of the eye. For practical purposes, most sonologists examine the size and location of the orbits, the eyelids, hyaloid artery, and the lens (Figs. 7–2 through 7–7).

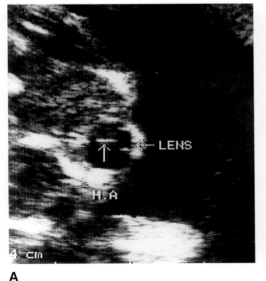

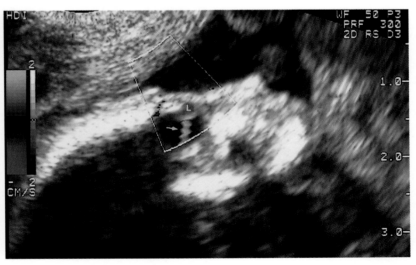

A   **B**

Figure 7–2. A. The fetal eye. The borders of the lens are imaged as two parallel echogenic lines. The hyaloid artery (HA) appears as a smooth reflective structure traversing the vitreous. **B.** Color-flow imaging reveals the active arterial flow in the hyoloid artery *(arrow)* toward the lens (L).

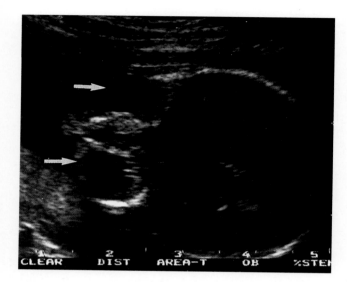

Figure 7–3. Axial section of the fetal head at postmenstrual 15 weeks demonstrates two normal sized orbits *(arrows)*.

Biometric Measurements

The eyes are best visualized by scanning the fetal face in coronal, axial, and corono-axial planes. The eyes appear as two symmetrical structures on both sides of the nose. Nomograms have been constructed for the following measurements.[17–19]

1. Ocular or orbital diameter
2. Inner orbital distance
3. Outer orbital or biocular diameter
4. Diameter of the lens

These nomograms are of importance in the detection of many fetal eye and face malformations (Tables 7–1 and 7–2). See also Chapter 2.

The Lens

The normal lens appears on the coronal ultrasonic facial view as a smooth hyperechogenic circular line with a hypoechogenic circular line with hypoechogenic content (Figs. 7–4 and 7–5). In the axial view of the fetal head and orbits, the lens is depicted in the form of a pair of small dotted echoes originating from the near and far margins of the lens (Fig. 7–2).

Pathology of the Lens
Cataracts

Cataract is any opacity of the lens that causes visual impairment. It can be unilateral or bilateral. It was estimated that this anomaly accounts for about 10% of blindness in preschool children.[20,21] Approximately one third of cataract cases are idiopathic and many of these are familial. Both autosomal dominant and autosomal recessive inheritance have been reported.[22,23]

In most cases of cataract, a possible associated etiologic factor has been suggested, mainly intrauterine infections, chromosomal disorders, or sys-

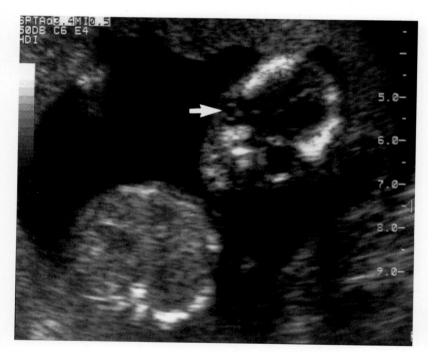

Figure 7–4. Coronal section of the fetal face. The round ring of the lens is imaged inside the eye *(arrow)*

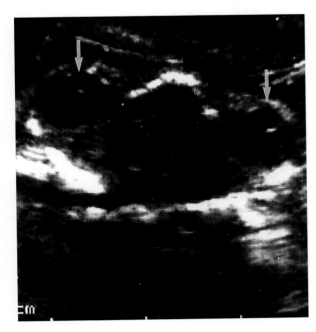

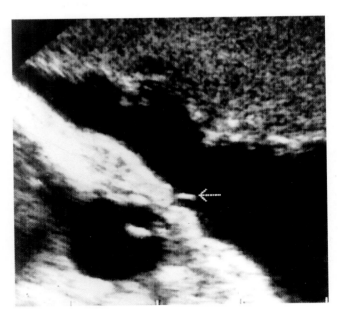

Figure 7–7. Eyelashes *(arrow)* observed in front of the fetal eye.

Figure 7–5. Cross section of the fetal face at postmenstrual 15 weeks. The lenses can be seen inside the orbits *(arrows)*.

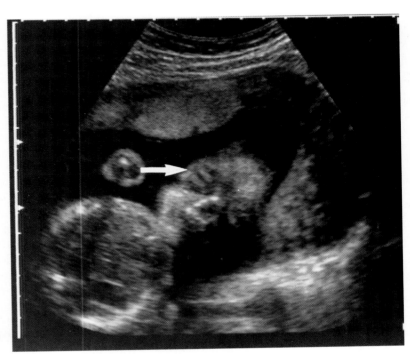

Figure 7–6. The eyelids are visualized in a cross section of the fetal face *(arrow)*.

TABLE 7–1. GROWTH OF THE OCULAR PARAMETERS

Age (postmenstrual weeks)	Binocular Distance (mm)			Interocular Distance (mm)			Ocular Diameter (mm)		
	5th	*50th*	*95th*	*5th*	*50th*	*95th*	*5th*	*50th*	*95th*
11	5	13	20	—	—	—	—	—	—
12	8	15	23	4	9	13	1	3	6
13	10	18	25	5	9	14	2	4	7
14	13	20	28	5	10	14	3	5	8
15	15	22	30	6	10	14	4	6	9
16	17	25	32	6	10	15	5	7	9
17	19	27	34	6	11	15	5	8	10
18	22	29	37	7	11	16	6	9	11
19	24	31	39	7	12	16	7	9	12
20	26	33	41	8	12	17	8	10	13
21	28	35	43	8	13	17	8	11	13
22	30	37	44	9	13	18	9	12	14
23	31	39	46	9	14	18	10	12	15
24	33	41	48	10	14	19	10	13	15
25	35	42	50	10	15	19	11	13	16
26	36	44	51	11	15	20	12	14	16
27	38	45	53	11	16	20	12	14	17
28	39	47	54	12	16	21	13	15	17
29	41	48	56	12	17	21	13	15	18
30	42	50	57	13	17	22	14	16	18
31	43	51	58	13	18	22	14	16	19
32	45	52	60	14	18	23	14	17	19
33	46	53	61	14	19	23	15	17	19
34	47	54	62	15	19	24	15	17	20
35	48	55	63	15	20	24	15	18	20
36	49	56	64	16	20	25	16	18	20
37	50	57	65	16	21	25	16	18	21
38	50	58	65	17	21	26	16	18	21
39	51	59	66	17	22	26	16	19	21
40	52	59	67	18	22	26	16	19	21

From Romero and colleagues, 1988,[42] with permission.

temic syndromes.[23,24] The mechanism of cataract formation is denaturation of lens protein and formation of an opaque insoluble precipitate that causes loss of lens translucency.[20]

In cases of cataract, the image of the lens is affected to various degrees. Thick, irregular or crenated hyperechogenic borders, clusters of hypoechogenic material, or homogeneous opacity may be observed (Figs. 7–8 through 7–11).[25–31] In some cases of cataract, the authors failed to demonstrate the hyaloid artery. It is possible that the opacity of the lens interfered with the visualization of this vessel. It can also be speculated that there is an association between congenital cataract and pathology of the hyaloid artery.

It should be noted that demonstration of clear lenses on ultrasound does not exclude the presence of cataract. The authors failed to diagnose some cases of mild cataract.[24] It can, therefore, be summarized that at present the threshold for the ultrasonic identification of cataract is still uncertain and mild to moderate or even severe cases might not be sufficiently abnormal for recognition.[26,27]

Pathology of the Eyelids

Because the normal eyelid and its opening and closure can be detected, it is expected that a thorough, targeted examination of the eyelids can potentially detect abnormality. Figure 7–11 depicts a fetus with

TABLE 7–2. THE DIAMETER OF THE FETAL LENS (MM)

GA (postmenstrual weeks)	Mean	95% CI	Centiles				
			10	25	50	75	90
14	2.5	2.3–2.7	2.1	2.4	2.5	2.7	2.9
15	2.9	2.9–3.0	2.7	2.8	2.9	3.1	3.2
16	2.9	2.8–3.0	2.7	2.8	2.9	3.1	3.2
17–18	3.3	3.0–3.6	2.8	2.9	3	3.3	5
19–20	4.1	4.0–4.3	3.6	4	4	4.3	5
21	4.4	4.1–4.6	3.7	3.9	4	5	5
22	4.4	4.2–4.7	3.9	4	4.3	5	5
23	4.6	4.3–4.8	3.8	4	5	5	5
24	4.6	4.4–4.8	4	4.3	4.6	5	5
25	4.8	4.6–5.0	4.2	4.6	5	5.1	5.2
26	5	4.8–5.2	4.4	4.8	5.1	5.2	5.5
27	5	4.8–5.2	4.4	4.8	5.1	5.2	5.5
28	5.1	5.0–5.2	4.5	5	5.2	5.2	5.5
29	5.3	5.1–5.5	4.6	5.2	5.2	5.5	5.9
30–31	5.3	5.2–5.5	4.8	5.1	5.5	5.5	5.7
32–33	5.6	5.4–5.8	4.8	5.2	5.5	5.9	6.2
34–36	5.8	5.6–6.0	5.4	5.5	5.7	6	6.5

GA, gestational age; CI, confidence interval.
From Goldstein and colleagues, 1998,[19] *with permission.*

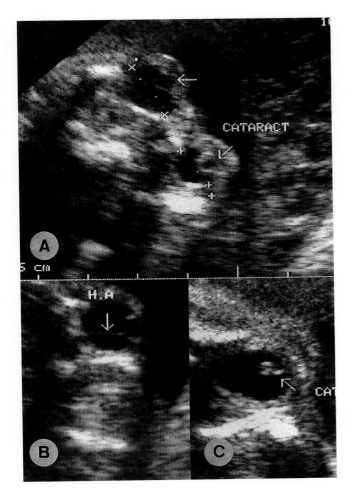

Figure 7–8. A. The right eye is smaller than the left eye and contains a hyperechogenic lens. **B.** Medial (nasal) insertion of the hyaloid artery (HA). **C.** In a plane slightly caudal to the one shown in **(A)** debris of hyperechogenic material was detected. *(From Zimmer and colleagues, 1993,*[26] *with permission.)*

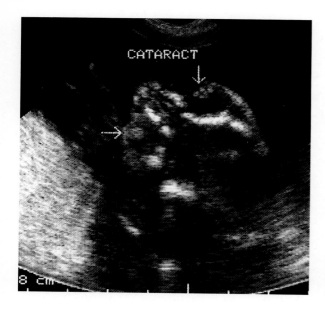

Figure 7–9. Homogeneous hyperechogenicity of the right lens and clusters of hyperechogenic material in the left eye (cataract). *(From Zimmer and colleagues, 1993,[26] with permission.)*

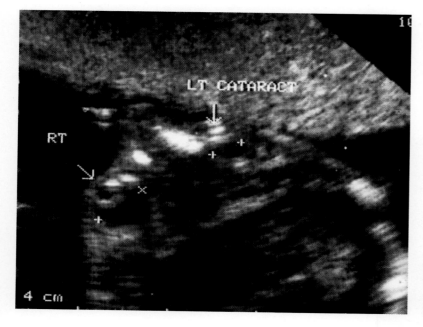

Figure 7–10. Microphthalmia with cataract. A normal orbit and lens are imaged on the right side (RT). On the left side, the orbit is small and the lens contains hypoechogenic material.

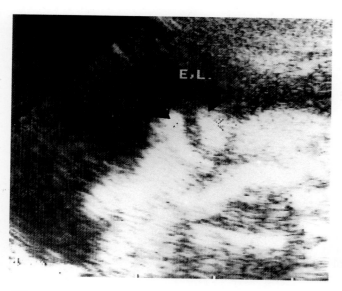

Figure 7–11. Eyelids (EL). The upper and lower eyelids were small *(arrows)* and open throughout the ultrasound examination. Partial atrophy was therefore suggested.

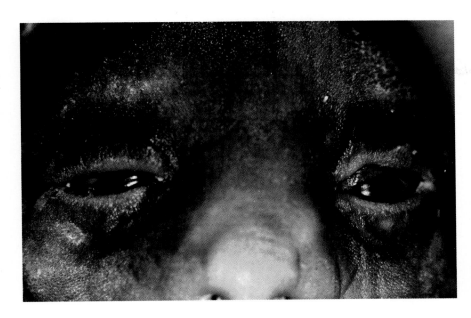

Figure 7–12. The aborted fetus with Neu–Laxova syndrome. There is partial atrophy of the eyelids as well as cataract.

fixed, partially open eyelids detected during ultrasonography. Examination of the stillborn fetus confirmed this finding. The syndrome detected was the Neu–Laxova syndrome (Fig. 7–12), suggested also by the report of Shapiro and associates.[25]

PATHOLOGY OF THE EYEBALL

Microphthalmia and Anophthalmia

Congenital microphthalmia can be sporadic or hereditary.[32–34] Some sporadic cases are secondary to exogenous factors such as infections (e.g., rubella, syphilis). Sutcliffe and colleagues[35] reported two cases of bilateral severe microphthalmia and one case of anophthalmia associated with treatment of carbamazepine during pregnancy.

Microphthalmia may present as an isolated anomaly or may be a component of multiple malformation syndrome. All patterns of mendelian inheritance have been reported.[32–34] Right and left eyes alone or together are about equally affected.[32] These eyes are blind or have poor vision due to disorganization of the globe as a whole or of one or more of its constituent parts. Common associated anomalies are cataract, corneal scarring or vascularity colobomas of iris or choroid, Fraser syndrome, and Walker–Warburg syndrome.[32–34]

Anophthalmia or complete absence of ocular primordia is considered as the most extreme form of microphthalmia. Clinical distinction between severe microphthalmia and anophthalmia might be difficult and the accurate diagnosis can be done only after a pathological examination.[32,33]

The sonographic diagnosis of microphthalmia should be suggested in cases of a small orbital diameter that does not fit the accepted nomograms of orbital growth (Figs. 7–10, 7–13, and 7–14). The prenatal diagnosis of microphthalmia was reported by several investigators.[35–40] Both isolated cases as well as microphthalmia in multiple malformation syndromes have been identified. The earliest gestational age of detection was reported by Porges and collaborators,[38] who found the anomaly in a fetus of 11 weeks of gestation.

Sonographic diagnosis of anophthalmia has also reported.[40–43] However, sonographers should be cautious because fetal head position, especially a cephalic prone position with the head dipping into the pelvis, might preclude visualization of the eyes. In such cases, vaginal sonography might be of value

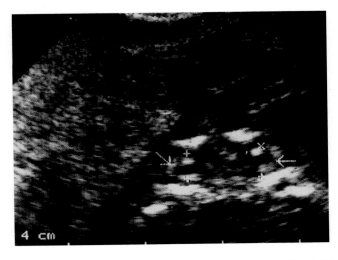

Figure 7–13. Bilateral microphthalmia at postmenstrual 15 weeks. The orbits are marked by an *arrow* and *crosses*.

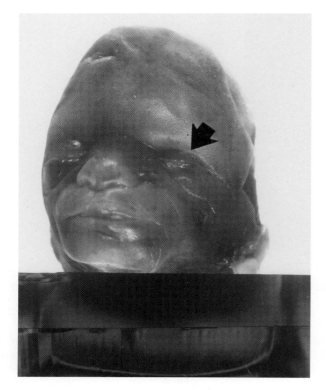

Figure 7–14. An aborted fetus with anophthalmia.

even in advanced pregnancy. The sonographic diagnosis of anophthalmia should, therefore, be suggested in cases in which a complete view of the fetal face failed to demonstrate one or both orbits. However, we are aware of two cases in which a normal orbit was observed in early pregnancy but at delivery, anophthalmia was found. The reason for this unexpected sequence of events is still unclear.

Exophthalmos

Prominent eye or exophthalmos are a result of shallow orbits or large eye balls. The ultrasonographic diagnosis is done by imaging the protrusion of the eye on axial section, which is used for interorbital and biocular biometry (Fig. 7–15). Exophthalmos may appear with various fetal abnormalities. Prenatal sonographic diagnosis was reported in cases of holoprosencephaly,[37] Saethre–Chotzen syndrome,[44] Crouzon syndrome,[45] Roberts syndrome,[46] and akinesia hypokinesia sequence.[47]

PATHOLOGY OF THE INTERORBITAL DISTANCES

Hypotelorism

Hypotelorism is a decreased interorbital distance (Fig. 7–16). It is usually associated with other fetal

abnormalities, mainly holoprosencephaly (arhinencephaly).[48,49] Cyclopia is the most severe form of malformation marked by midline deficiencies in facial development and incomplete morphogenesis of the forebrain. There is a single eye or partially divided eye in a single orbit and arhinia with proboscis. In most cases, extracephalic malformations are present as well.[48–54] Of the various karyotypes associated with cyclopia, trisomy D has been described with the greatest frequency.[55–57]

Environmental factors like viremia or salicylates have also been suggested as a possible cause of this abnormality.[58] In ethmocephaly, there is extreme hypotelorism, but separate orbits, and arhinia with proboscis. In cebocephaly, hypotelorism is associated with a proboscis-like nose or a single nostril nose, but there is no median or cleft lip.[44,48,59,60] An accurate sonographic diagnosis of these three different types of orbital anomalies is not easy. It might be difficult to differentiate between a single orbital cavity and very close or fused orbits. Furthermore, in some cases the observers failed to identify the orbits and the diagnosis relied on the demonstration of a proboscis in a fetus with a brain anomaly.[51,53]

Hypertelorism

Hypertelorism is a craniofacial defect that consists of abnormally spaced orbits. The sonographic diagnosis, therefore, relies on the interorbital distance. This abnormality may be an isolated finding or a secondary feature of many malformation syndromes. Romero and colleagues[49] summarized nearly 150 fetal abnormalities in which hypertelorism was reported. Most common associations are with cran-

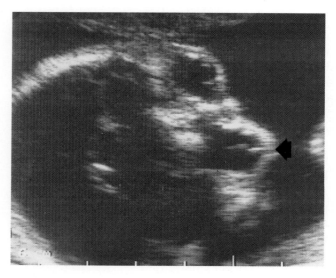

Figure 7–15. Exophthalmos of the right eye in a 19-week-old fetus.

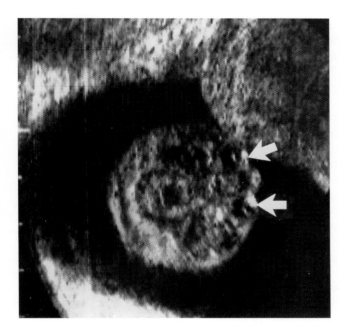

Figure 7–16. Hypotelorism. The orbits *(arrows)* of this 15-week-postmenstrual fetus are very close to each other.

iosynostosis syndromes and the median facial cleft syndrome. Prenatal sonographic diagnosis was reported by several investigators in various fetal abnormalities.[35,41,49,53,54,61–64]

Retina

Prenatal sonographic diagnosis of retinal detachment and dysplasia was reported in a few cases.[65–67] There are reports on fetuses with the Walker–Warburg syndrome. The characteristics of this syndrome are diffuse neurodysplasia with brain and eye anomalies and muscular dystrophy. Ultrasound of the fetal eye revealed a conical structure within the globe with its conical base toward the lens and its apex pointing posteriorly toward the optic nerve. In one case,[65] this ultrasonic image was obtained in one eye only. However, at the time of autopsy, the anomaly was identified in both eyes.

In another case,[66] a similar conical structure was seen on ultrasound of the fetal orbits. Ultrasonographic examination of the newborn showed disorganized fibrous structures within the vitreous cavity. On physical examination, absence of the irides and pupils was noted.

Bilateral retinal detachment was also imaged by ultrasound in a fetus with Norrie disease.[67] The principal feature of this disease is retinal dysplasia with resultant retinal detachment.

Maat-Kievit and colleagues[68] reported on the detection of a large retinoblastoma in a fetus at 21 postmenstrual weeks of gestation. The oval shaped tumor protruded from the right side of the fetal face. The right orbit as well as the fetal nose and mouth could not be imaged and a deformity of the normal anatomy of the facial bones was noted.

CONGENITAL NASOLACRIMAL DUCT CYST

Congenital nasolacrimal obstruction occurs in 1.75% to 6% of newborns.[69,70] The abnormality may be unilateral or bilateral. Epiphora is the only clinical sign in most cases and spontaneous resolution occurs during infancy. However, in some cases cysts are formed because of mucus accumulation. Complete obstruction may lead to an increased respiratory effort or even respiratory distress. In such cases, probing of the duct or silicone intubation is indicated.[71] Prenatal sonographic diagnosis should be suggested if a cystic mass is visualized adjacent to the orbit and the base of the nose (Figure 7–17).[72–75] The differential diagnosis includes other anomalies in this region such as encephalocele or hemangioma.

TRAUMA OF THE EYE DURING AMNIOCENTESIS

The possible association between amniocentesis and fetal damage is well known. However, there are only a few cases reports on ophthalmic complications.[76–81] Cystic lesions, perforations, and scars were noted in the different parts of the eye. In some cases, the damage could be corrected by surgery. In other cases, the damage was severe, leading to hemianopia, gaze palsy,[80] microphthalmia, and total blindness.[77]

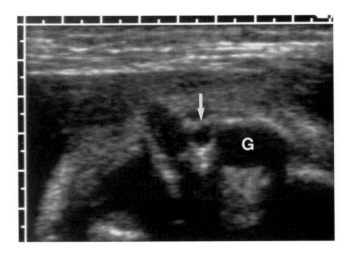

Figure 7–17. At 33 postmenstrual weeks, a 13 × 7 mm hypoechoic mass *(arrow)* was detected inferior and medial to the right globe. Synchronous fetal eye motion was demonstrated. Polyhydramnios was the only other abnormality. *(From Davis and colleagues, 1987,[72] with permission.)*

Ultrasound guided amniocentesis has now become the standard of care. It is expected that this technique will decrease the incidence of fetal trauma during the procedure.

PHYSIOLOGICAL ASPECTS OF THE FETAL EYE

Fetal Eye Movements

Fetal eye movements are best evaluated by ultrasonographic observation of positional changes of the lens. The pattern of fetal eye movements was studied and correlated with the emergence of fetal behavior states.

Birnholz[82] recognized four types of eye movements.

1. Type I: single transient linear deviation, usually from mid-position to a lower, outer orbital margin, followed by a slightly slower return to the initial position.
2. Type II: prolonged, but single deviation to a medial or lateral position.
3. Type III: complex sequence of deviations including rotatory components without apparent spatial or temporal periodicity (these movements are typically brisk and jerky).
4. Type IV: repetitive or nystagmoid deviations.

Birnholz regarded type I and II movements as slow eye movements, and type III and IV as rapid eye movements. Arduini and coworkers[83] considered as rapid eye movements, rapid nystagmus-like movements with a frequency greater than six every minute. Eye movements with a frequency of less than six every minute were regarded as slow eye movements.

Horimoto and associates[84] noted two types of eye movements. Those with a duration of 0.07 up to 0.6 to 0.8 second were regarded as rapid eye movements. The others, with a duration of 0.6 to 0.8 up to 4 to 5 seconds were considered as slow eye movements. Differences in gestational age distribution of the various types of eye movements have been observed. Birnholz[82] reported that type I movements were apparent between 16 and 26 weeks of gestation, whereas type IV movements were recognized only after 32 postmenstrual weeks.

The patterns of eye movements as well as the periodicity of absent eye movements are important in the definition of fetal behavioral states. Nijhuis and collaborators[85] defined four types of fetal behav-

ior at 36 to 40 postmenstrual weeks. According to their classification, there is absence of fetal eye movements in state 1F. In the other three states, 2F, 3F, and 4F, both slow and rapid eye movements are continually present. (See Chapter 15)

Arduini's group[83] reported that during quiet phases of fetal behavior, slow eye movements as well as absence of eye movement were recorded. Rapid eye movements were never observed at this phase of fetal activity. On the other hand, during the active phases of fetal activity, both slow and rapid eye movements, as well as the absence of eye movement could be noted. However, after 36 postmenstrual weeks, a significant prevalence of rapid eye movements during the active phases and absence of eye movement during the quiet phases was observed.

A change in fetal eye movements (blinking response) may be induced by vibroacoustic stimulation. This response is part of the startle response and change in state obtained in healthy fetuses following stimulation.[86]

Horimoto and colleagues[87] evaluated changes in pupillary diameters in relation to fetal eye movements. Pupillary diameters were found to be differentiated with statistical significance into two groups: 9.7% for the dilated pupil (range 2.1 to 3.4 mm) and 90.3% for the constricted pupil (range 1.4 to 1.9 mm). The percentage of dilated pupils during eye movement period (14.3%) was significantly greater than that during no eye movement period (2.3%). This relation between pupillary diameter and eye movement is in agreement with data from adults.

SUMMARY

The eye can be abnormal in several diseases as a single malformation or in association with a variety of abnormalities involving other organ systems. Any alteration in the size of the orbits or in the appearance of the eye should be carefully evaluated as a possible sign of fetal abnormality. At present, ultrasonography is a well-established technique for biometric measurements of the orbits. However, there are still only limited data on the ultrasonographic features of the different abnormalities of the fetal eye. Further experience is required to improve the ability to prenatally diagnose malformations of the eye.

REFERENCES

1. Robinson GC, Jan JE, Kinnis C. Congenital ocular blindness in children, 1945 to 1984. *Am J Dis Child.* 1987;141:1321–1324.

2. Goggin M, O'Keefe M. Childhood blindness in the Republic of Ireland: A national survey. *Br J Ophthalmol.* 1991;75:425–429.

3. Foster A, Gilbert C. Epidemiology of childhood blindness. *Eye.* 1992;6:173–176.

4. Stoll C, Alembik Y, Dott B, Roth MP. Epidemiology of congenial eye malformations in 131,760 consecutive births. *Ophthalmic Pediatr Genet.* 1992;13:179–186.

5. Jay B. Causes of blindness in school children. *Br Med J.* 1987;294:1183–1184.

6. Phillips CI, Levy AM, Newton M, Stokoe NL. Blindness in school children: Importance of heredity, congenial cataract and prematurity. *Br J Ophthalmol.* 1987;71:578–584.

7. Nicolaides KH, Salversen DR, Sijders RJM, Gosdes CM. Fetal facial defects: Associated malformations and chromosomal abnormalities. *Fetal Diagn Ther.* 1993;8:1–9.

8. Wilkie AOM, Amberger JS, McKusick VA. The gene map of congenital malformations. *J Med Genet.* 1994;31:507–517.

9. Sadler TW, ed. Eye. In: *Langman's Medical Embryology.* 6th ed. Williams & Wilkins; 1990:338–346.

10. Larsen WJ (ed). Development of the eyes. In: *Human Embryology.* Churchill Livingstone; 1993:341–351.

11. Ko M-K, Chi JG, Chang B-L. Hyaloid vascular pattern in the human fetus. *J Pediatr Ophthalmol Strabismus.* 1985;22:188–193.

12. Birnholz JC, Farrell EE. Fetal hyaloid artery: Timing of regression with US. *Radiology.* 1988;166:781–783.

13. Harayama K, Amemiya T, Nishimura H. Development of the eyeball during fetal life. *J Pediatr Ophthalmol Strabismus.* 1981;18:37–40.

14. Denis D, Righini M, Scheiner C, et al. Ocular growth in the fetus. I. Comparative study of axial length and biometric parameters in the fetus. *Ophthalmologica.* 1993;207:117–124.

15. Birnholz JC. Ultrasonic fetal ophthalmology. *Early Hum Dev.* 1985;12:199–209.

16. de Elejalde MM, Elejalde BR. Ultrasonographic visualization of the fetal eye. *J Craniofac Genet Dev Biol.* 1985;5:319–326.

17. Jeanty P, Dramaix-Wilmet M, Van Gansbeke D, Van Regemorter N, Rodesch F. Fetal ocular biometry by ultrasound. *Radiology.* 1982;143:513–516.

18. Mayden KL, Tortora M, Berkowitz RL, Bracken M, Hobbins JC. Orbital diameters: A new parameter for prenatal diagnosis and dating. *Am J Obstet Gynecol.* 1982;144:289–297.

19. Goldstein I, Tamir A, Zimmer EZ, Itskovitz-Eldor J. Growth of the fetal orbit and lens in normal pregnancies. *Ultrasound Obstet Gynecol.* 1998;12:175–-179.

20. Kohn BA. The differential diagnosis of cataracts in infancy and childhood. *Am J Dis Child.* 1976;130:184–192.

21. Nelson LB. Diagnosis and management of cataracts in infancy and childhood. *Ophthalmic Surg.* 1984;15:688–697.

22. Merin S, Crawford JS. The etiology of congenital cataracts: a survey of 386 cases. *Can J Ophthalmol.* 1971;6:178–182.

23. Taylor D. Congenital cataract: the history, the nature and the practice. *Eye.* 1998;12:9–36.

24. Walton DS. Eye evaluation in the newborn. In: Oski FA, DeAngelis CD, Feigin RD, Warshaw JB, eds. *Principles and Practice of Pediatrics.* Philadelphia 1990:468–470.

25. Shapiro I, Borochowitz Z, Degni S, Dar H, Ibschitz I, Sharf M. Neu-Laxova syndrome: Prenatal ultrasonographic diagnosis, clinical and pathological studies and new manifestations. *Am J Med Genet.* 1992; 43: 602–605.

26. Zimmer EZ, Bronshtein M, Ophir E, et al. Sonographic diagnosis of fetal congenital cataracts. *Prenat Diagn.* 1993;13:503–511.

27. Gaary EA, Rawnsley E, Marin-Padilla JM, Morse CL, Crow HC. In utero detection of fetal cataracts. *J Ultrasound Med.* 1993;12:234–236.

28. Monteagudo A, Timor-Tritsch IE, Friedman AH, Santos R. Autosomal dominant cataracts of the fetus: Early detection by transvaginal ultrasound. *Ultrasound Obstet Gynecol.* 1996;8:104–108.

29. Drysdale K, Kyle PM, Sepulveda W. Prenatal detection of congenital inherited cataracts. *Ultrasound Obstet Gynecol.* 1997;9:62–63.

30. Romain M, Awoust J, Dugauquier C, van Maldergem L. Prenatal ultrasound detection of congenital cataract in trisomy 21. *Prenat Diagn.* 1999;19: 780–782.

31. Pedreira DAL, Diniz EMA, Schultz R, Faro LB, Zugaib M. Fetal cataract in congenital toxoplasmosis. *Ultrasound Obstet Gynecol.* 1999;13:266–267.

32. Zeiter HJ. Congenital microphthalmus. *Am J Ophthalmol.* 1963;55:910–922.

33. Duke-Elder S, Cooke C. Microphthalmos. Congenital deformities. In: Duke-Elder S, ed. *System of Ophthalmology.* Vol 3. CV Mosby 1964:488–495.

34. Warburg M. Genetics of microphthalmos. *Int Ophthalmol.* 1981;4:45–65.

35. Sutcliffe AG, Jones RB, Woodruff G. Eye malformations associated with treatment with carbamazepine during pregnancy. *Ophthalmic Genet.* 1998;19:59–62.

36. Schauer GM, Dunn LK, Godmilow L, Eagle RC, Knisely AS. Prenatal diagnosis of Fraser syndrome at 18.5 weeks gestation, with autopsy finding at 19 weeks. *Am J Med Genet.* 1990;37:583–591.

37. Bronshtein M, Zimmer EZ, Gershoni-Baruch R, Yoffe N, Meyer H, Blumenfeld Z. First and second trimester diagnosis of fetal ocular defects and associated anomalies: Report of eight cases. *Obstet Gynecol.* 1991;77:443–449.

38. Porges Y, Gershoni-Baruch R, Leibu R, et al. Hereditary microphthalmia with colobomatous cyst. *Am J Ophthalmol.* 1992;114:30–34.

39. Shulman LP, Gordon PL, Emerson DS, Wilroy RS, Elias S. Prenatal diagnosis of isolated bilateral microphthalmia with confirmation by evaluation of products of conception obtained by dilation and evacuation. *Prenat Diagn.* 1993;13:403–409.

40. Cayea PD, Beiber FR, Ross MJ, Davidoff A, Osathanondh R, Jones TB. Sonographic findings in otocephaly (synotia). *J Ultrasound Med.* 1985;4:377–379.

41. Pilu G, Reece EA, Romero R, Bovicelli L, Hobbins JC. Prenatal diagnosis of craniofacial malformations with ultrasonography. *Am J Obstet Gynecol.* 1986;155:45–50.

42. Tomas DE, Mahoney BS, Bowie JD, Woodruff WW, Kay HH. Prenatal sonographic diagnosis of hemifacial microsomia (Goldenhar-Gorlin syndrome). *J Ultrasound Med.* 1986;5:461–463.

43. Lee A, Deutinger J, Bernaschek G. Three dimensional ultrasound: Abnormalities of the fetal face in surface and volume rendering mode. *Br J Obstet Gynecol.* 1995;102:302–306.

44. Turner GM, Twining P. The facial profile in the diagnosis of fetal abnormalities. *Clin Radiol.* 1993;47:389–395.

45. Menashe Y, Ben Baruch G, Rabinovitch O, Shalev Y, Katznelson MBM, Shalev E. Exophthalmus—Prenatal ultrasonic features for diagnosis of Crouzon syndrome. *Prenat Diagn.* 1989;9:805–808.

46. Gershoni-Baruch R, Drugan A, Bronshtein M, Zimmer EZ. Roberts syndrome or "X linked amelia"? *Am J Med Genet.* 1990;37:569–572.

47. Bocino CA, Platt LD, Garber A, et al. Fetal akinesia hypokinesia sequence: Prenatal diagnosis and intrafamilial variability. *Prenat Diagn.* 1993;13:1011–1019.

48. DeMyer W, Zeman W, Palmer CG. The face predicts the brain: Diagnostic significance of median facial anomalies for holoprosencephaly (arhinencephaly). *Pediatrics.* 1964;34:256–263.

49. Romero R, Pilu G, Jeanty P, Chidini A, Hobbins JC, eds. The face. In: *Prenatal Diagnosis of Congenital Anomalies.* Appleton & Lange 1988:81–113.

50. Khudr G, Olding L. Cyclopia. *Am J Dis Child.* 1973;125:120–122.

51. Elejalde BR, de Elejalde MM, Hamilton PR, Christenson R, Broekhuizen F. Prenatal diagnosis of cyclopia. *Am J Med Genet.* 1983;14:15–19.

52. Toth Z, Csecsei K, Szeifert G, Papp Z. Early prenatal diagnosis of cyclopia associated with holoprosencephaly. *J Clin Ultrasound.* 1986;14:550–553.

53. Meizner I, Drawall D, Mazor M, Katz M. Sonographic findings in a rare case of fetal cyclopia. *Isr J Med Sci.* 1987;23:910–912.

54. Van Allen MI, Ritchie S, Toi A, Fong K, Winsor E. Trisomy 4 in a fetus with cyclopia and other anomalies. *Am J Med Genet.* 1993;46:193–197.

55. Arakaki DT, Waxman SH. Trisomy D in a cyclops. *J Pediatr.* 1969;74:620–622.

56. Jaschevatzky OE, Goldman B, Georghiou P, Grunstein S, Pevzner S. Trisomy D in a cyclops with cardiovascular defects. *Acta Obstet Gynecol Scand.* 1976;55:73–76.

57. Taysi K, Tinaztepe K. Trisomy D and the cyclops malformation. *Am J Dis Child.* 1972;124:710–713.

58. Mollica F, Pavone L, Nuciforo G, Gorge G. A case of cyclopia. Role of environmental factors. *Clin Genet.* 1979;16:69–71.

59. Bundy AL, Lidov H, Soliman M, Doubilet PM. Antenatal sonographic diagnosis of cebocephaly. *J Ultrasound Med.* 1988;7:395–398.

60. Rolland M, Sarramon MF, Bloom MC. Astomia–agnathia–holoprosencephaly association. Prenatal diagnosis of a new case. *Prenat Diagn.* 1991;11:199–203.

61. Chervenak FA, Tortora M, Mayden K, et al. Antenatal diagnosis of median cleft face syndrome: Sonographic demonstration of cleft lip and hypertelorism. *Am J Obstet Gynecol.* 1984;149:94–97.

62. Shever DM, Shah YG, Wang N, Metlay LA, Wood JR Jr. Prenatal diagnosis and subsequent management of a fetus with a 46 XYr (4) (p15-q35) karyotype. *Am J Perinatol.* 1991;8:53–55.

63. Trout T, Budorick NE, Pretorius DH, McGahan JP. Significance of orbital measurements in the fetus. *J Ultrasound Med.* 1994;13:937–943.

64. Bernstein PS, Gross SJ, Cohen DJ, et al. Prenatal diagnosis of type 2 Pfeiffer syndrome. *Ultrasound Obstet Gynecol.* 1996;8:425–428.

65. Farrel SA, Leadman TML, Davidson RG, Caco C. Prenatal diagnosis of retinal detachment in Walker—Warburg syndrome. *Am J Med Genet.* 1987;28:619–624.

66. Vohra N, Ghidini A, Alvarez M, Lockwood C. Walker–Warburg syndrome: Prenatal ultrasound findings. *Prenat Diagn.* 1993;13:575–579.

67. Redmond RM, Vaughan JI, Jay M, Jay B. In utero diagnosis of Norrie disease by ultrasonography. *Ophthalmol Pediatr Genet.* 1993;14:1–3.

68. Maat-Kievit JA, Oepkes D, Hartwig NG, Vermeij-Keers C, Van Kamp IL, Van De Kamp JJP. A large retinoblastoma detected in a fetus at 21 weeks of gestation. *Prenat Diagn.* 1993;13:377–384.

69. Kushner BJ. Congenital nasolacrimal system obstruction. *Arch Ophthalmol.* 1982;100:597–600.

70. Harris GJ, DiClementi D. Congenital dacryocystocele. *Arch Ophthalmol.* 1982;100:1763–1765.

71. Paul TO, Shepard R. Congenital nasolacrimal duct obstruction: Natural history and the timing of the optimal intervention. *J Pediatr Opthalmol Strabismus.* 1994;31:362–367.

72. Davis WK, Mahoney BS, Carroll BA, Bowie JD. Antenatal sonographic detection of benign dacrocystoceles (lacrimal duct cysts). *J Ultrasound Med.* 1987;6:461–465.

73. Alper CM, Chan KH, Hill LM, Chenevey P. Antenatal diagnosis of congenital nasolacrimal duct cyst by ultrasonography: a case report. *Prenat Diagn.* 1994;14:623–626.

74. Walsh G, Dubbins PA. Antenatal sonographic diagnosis of dacryocystocele. *J Ultrasound Med.* 1994;22:457–460.

75. Sharony R, Raz J, Aviram R, Cohen I, Beyth Y, Tepper R. Prenatal diagnosis of dacryocystocele: A possible marker for syndromes. *Ultrasound Obstet Gynecol.* 1999;14:71–3.

76. Cross HE, Maumenee AE. Ocular trauma during amniocentesis. *Arch Ophthalmol.* 1973;90:303–304.

77. Merin S, Beyth Y. Uniocular congenital blindness as a

complication of midtrimester amniocentesis. *Am J Ophthalmol.* 1980;89:299–301.

78. Isenberg SJ, Heckenlively JR. Traumatized eye with retinal damage from amniocentesis. *J Pediatr Ophthalmol Strabismus.* 1985;22:65–67.

79. Admoni MM, Ben Ezra D. Ocular trauma following amniocentesis as a cause of leukocoria. *J Pediatr Ophthalmol Strabismus.* 1988;25:196–197.

80. Naylor G, Roper JG, Willshaw HE. Ophthalmic complications of amniocentesis. *Eye.* 1990;4:845–849.

81. Rummelt V, Rummelt C, Naumann GOH. Congenital nonpigmented epithelial iris cyst after amniocentesis. Clinicopathologic report on two children. *Ophthalmology.* 1993;100:776–781.

82. Birnholz JC. The development of human fetal eye movement patterns. *Science.* 1981;213:679–681.

83. Arduini D, Rizzo G, Giorlandino C, Valensise H, Dellacqua S, Romanini C. The development of fetal behavioral states: A longitudinal study. *Prenat Diagn.* 1986;6:117–124.

84. Horimoto N, Koyanagi T, Satoh S, Yoshizato T, Nakano H. Fetal eye movement assessed with real time ultrasonography: Are these rapid and slow eye movements? *Am J Obstet Gynecol.* 1990;163:1480–1484.

85. Nijhuis JG, Prechtl HFR, Martin BR Jr, Bates RSGM. Are there behavioral states in the human fetus? *Early Hum Develop.* 1982;6:177–195.

86. Birnholz JC, Benacerraf BR. The development of human fetal hearing. *Science.* 1983;222:516–518.

87. Horimoto N, Koyanagi T, Takashima T, Akazawa K, Nakano H. Changes in pupillary diameter in relation to eye movement and no eye movement periods in the human fetus at term. *Am J Obstet Gynecol.* 1992;167:1465–1469.

CHAPTER EIGHT

Magnetic Resonance Imaging of the Fetal Brain

Maurizio Resta
Vincenzo D'Addario
Pantaleo Greco
Gilda Caruso
Nicola Medicamento
Nicola Burdi

In the last 3 years, no significant changes in domain of prenatal diagnosis occurred. Nevertheless, the technical advances in the magnetic resonance imaging (MRI) were notable and some concepts have been reviewed.[1] This chapter will discuss important changes in MRI technique and new knowledge in fetal brain anatomy.

Ultrasonography (US) remains the method of choice to image the fetus. High-resolution real-time scanners and transvaginal probes[2,3] allow accurate and detailed evaluation of the fetal anatomy. However, there are some circumstances, such as maternal obesity, severe oligohydramnios, and rare and complex malformations, in which even expert sonologists may need alternative imaging procedures.

The goal in fetal imaging is to obtain detailed pictures by using harmless techniques. Computed tomography (CT) has never been considered an acceptable imaging modality in fetal imaging because it uses ionizing radiations. MRI, however, has not been reported to cause harm to the fetus. The only known biologic effect, induced by the static magnetic field and the radiofrequency radiation, is a mild increase in body temperature and heart rate.[4–7] Recent reports refer that MRI at high field strengths with powerful gradients does not change fetal car-

diotocographic parameters.[8] Although we do not propose that MRI will replace US in pregnancy, we believe that it can play a role in prenatal imaging as an ancillary tool when US fails for technical reasons. Now, ultrafast MRI sequences corroborate and refine more and more US diagnoses.

HISTORY

Many articles during the last 10 years have confirmed the potential application of this technique in pregnancy. The use of MRI for the study of fetal anomalies was first reported in the literature in the early 1980s.[9,10] Nevertheless, its use for diagnostic imaging during pregnancy was not regulated and generally it was not recommended in Protection Board suggested guidelines for the use of MRI during the second and third trimesters of pregnancy.[11] However, MRI investigation during pregnancy was limited to patients at high risk for obstetric disease or fetal abnormality, following approval by ethics committees.

In 1985, McCarthy and colleagues[12,13] reported their first experience with MRI evaluation of the maternal and fetal anatomy. They emphasized the difficulty of obtaining detailed magnetic resonance images of the fetal brain because of the lack of differentiation between gray and white matter. These authors used medium-field strength equipment, and fetal motion did not seem to impair image quality. Other authors complained about image degradation due to fetal activity and suggested the use of fetal neuromuscular blockage.

Transient fetal paralysis was achieved by injecting a neuromuscular blocking agent into the umbilical vein or into the fetal musculature.[14–20] This obtained a period of transient fetal paralysis ranging from 40 to 90 minutes. In this condition, several authors found that both spin-echo (SE) pulse sequences with a long repetition time (TR) and a short or long echo time (TE), and SE sequences with a short TR produced good anatomic details.[12,21–24] In contrast, other authors suggested the use of only T1-weighted images. Wrongly, the T2-weighted images were supposed to be useless in the fetal brain because of the incomplete differentiation between gray and white matter.[22,24,25] Also, the inversion recovery (IR) sequences[21,26] and gradient echo (GRE) sequences were used.

Afterward, very short GRE breath-hold sequences and fast imaging with steady-state procession, with acquisition time ranging from 20 to 40 seconds, obtaining T1-weighted sections were introduced. Furthermore, it became mandatory to attempt fetal MRI without any maternal[27,28] or fetal medication.[29–32]

Because fetal activity increases 30 minutes to 1 hour after intravenous or oral glucose administration and fetal movements are more numerous in the evening than in the morning, a simple but partial solution is to examine the fetus during the morning hours, following overnight fasting.[33] Some authors propose special maternal positions, such as the left lateral position, to minimize fetal movements.[34]

At least, in the last few years ultrafast MR sequences were improved and progressively applied. Half-Fourier acquisition single-shot turbo spin-echo (HASTE) or half-Fourier single-shot rapid acquisition with relaxation enhancement (RARE) techniques revealed the ability to generate T2-weighted images in less than 1 second, reducing fetal movements artifacts.[35]

EXAMINATION AND IMAGING TECHNIQUE

The experience of the authors is based on about 200 fetal MRI examinations. Three different types of MRI equipment have been used: a 1.5 Tesla (T) superconducting system (Magnetom 63 SP Siemens, Erlangen, Germany); a 1 T superconducting system (Impact Siemens, Erlangen, Germany), and more re-

cently, a 2 T superconducting system (Prestige Elscint, Israel).

The examination usually begins with the acquisition of three scout images on the axial, coronal, and sagittal planes using conventional SE or GRE sequences. Once the fetal position is identified, different pulse sequences and different techniques in the oblique, axial, sagittal, and coronal planes can be performed.

In the past on "paralyzed" fetuses, SE pulse sequences with a short TR and a short TE were used with satisfactory results. We experienced and applied very short GRE "breath-hold" FLASH-2D sequences or fast imaging with steady-state procession (FISSP), with acquisition times ranging from 20 to 40 seconds, obtaining eight T1-weighted sections. A body receiver–transmitter coil is routinely used or, when possible, a couple of surface coils, sandwiched and placed on the pregnant abdomen, may be used with good results.[36]

On the 2 T equipment, we optimized the ultrafast sequences based on the half-Fourier single-shot fast spin-echo technique. Two main pulse sequences were preferred: single-shot fast spin-echo (SSFSE) and rapid fast spin-echo (SSE).

SSFSE is a conventional HASTE that involves 7.2 msec of echo space, 65 msec echo time, echo train length of 80, 2 acquisitions, 6-mm section thickness, 40 × 40 cm field of view, and 144 × 256 acquisition matrix. The imaging time for 12 images acquired with a single sequence is 22 seconds using TR of 11,000 msec.

SSE is a high-speed sequence that produces a heavy T2 contrast. It involves 11 msec of echo space, 406 msec of echo time, echo train length of 115, 2 acquisitions, 5-mm section thickness, 40 × 40 cm field of view, and 160 × 256 acquisition matrix. The scan time is of 400 msec per slice.

BRAIN ANATOMY

The aim of this section is to describe the fetal brain anatomy pertaining to the specific requirements of MRI. In the last 3 years, the advent of ultrafast MRI sequences has completely changed the imaging of the fetal brain and has improved the sensitivity and the accuracy of the technique.

The fetal brain is grossly developed at about 20 weeks. The aspect and the morphology of the brain at this gestational age, however, is different from that at the third trimester and at the term of pregnancy. The different features are due to the formation, maturation of brain neocortex and white matter, as well as developmental morphology of the subarachnoidal space.[37–39]

The gyration of the cerebral neocortex depends on the migration of the neurons from the germinal matrix surrounding the lateral ventricle. The germinal zone presents its maximal volume at 26 weeks of pregnancy and the gyration is complete only at the end of the pregnancy.[24,37,40]

At about 20 weeks of pregnancy, indeed, the surface of the fetal brain is absolutely flat (Fig. 8–1). Proceeding with the gestational age, at the beginning of the third trimester (about 26–28 weeks of pregnancy), the cortical ribbon starts to inflect and the sulci and gyri appear starting from parietal lobes (Fig. 8–2). Approaching term, gyration proceeds to the remaining lobes with the frontal having the least number of gyri (Fig. 8–3). In the past, the MRI visualization of the germinal matrix was an occasional finding seen as a periventricular hyperintense signal in T1-weighted images (Fig. 8–4).[40] With the new ultrafast T2-weighted images, the germinal zone and the cortical ribbon are always evident, presenting a hypointense signal.

The basal ganglia and thalami originate from cells of neural epithelium around the diencephalon and the third ventricle. They are usually not able to be visualized on MRI, but sometimes they can express a high signal in T1-weighted images that is similar to what can be observed in the newborn.[41] Thanks to HASTE–RARE new sequences, the hippocampus and the choroidal fissure can be recognized. (Fig. 8–2)

Myelination is mostly a postnatal process, however, it starts toward the beginning of the third trimester[38,42] and occurs in a caudal to rostral gradient. The structures already myelinated at birth are the perirolandic areas, the posterior limb of the internal capsule, the corona radiata, and, in the posterior fossa, the brain stem and the superior and inferior cerebellar peduncles.

Similar to the newborn, any differentiation between gray and white matter can be appreciated because of their similar relaxation times. Using heavily T2-weighted images of the ultrafast turbo spin-echo sequences, it is now possible to visualize the white matter where it is very dense. For this reason, the corpus callosum is occasionally recognizable as a hypointense structure above the third ventricle (Fig. 8–3).

The cavum septi pellucidi and the cavum vergae are normal structures in fetal period and are easily identified (Figs. 8–1, 8–2, and 8–3). The orbital cavities, the eyeballs, and the cristallyne lens are always well depicted (Figs. 8–2 and 8–3). The posterior fossa structures[43–45] are evident early in the second trimester (Fig. 8–1).

The cerebral ventricles, hypointense in T1-weighted images, are now imaged as hyperintense signal in fast turbo-SE sequences. The third and the fourth ventricle[41,43] are recognizable at the 20th postmenstrual week, and their morphology remains unchanged until term (Figs. 8–1, 8–2, and 8–3). Sometimes in the early gestational age, axial views fail to visualize the fourth ventricle, which is easily depicted on sagittal and coronal sections (Figs. 8–1, 8–2, and 8–3).

On the contrary, the lateral ventricles[41,45,47] undergo wide variations in morphology and size, which justify their varying appearance at different gestational ages. During the second trimester they are typically prominent compared to those of the fetus at term, and contain large choroid plexuses at the level of the ventricular bodies and atria. Approaching term, the lateral ventricles become similar to those of the newborn (Figs. 8–1, 8–2, and 8–3).

The subarachnoid spaces[39,41,43] undergo wide variations in size and appear hypointense in T1-weighted images and hyperintense in T2-weighted images. This is due to the long relaxation times of cerebrospinal fluid. The sylvian fissure, the interhemispheric fissure, and the perivermian cistern are the first subarachnoid spaces to be imaged. The sylvian fissure is large and vertically oriented. Its width tends to shrink toward the end of the pregnancy, as happens for the other fetal cisterms, such as central sulcus (Rolando), cisterna ambiens, posterior fossa cisterns, and the cisterna magna (Figs. 8–1, 8–2, and 8–3).

BRAIN ANOMALIES

Neural Tube Defects

The earliest abnormality of the fetal central nervous system organogenesis is represented by the severe forms of neural tube defects such as anencephaly, iniencephaly, and cephalocele.[17,19,20,24,48–54] These malformations are easily detected with US; prenatal MRI is rarely needed. However, MRI can be useful when the morphology of a cephalocele is doubtful, when the relationship between the malformed encephalic plate and the placenta is unclear—such as in cases of amniotic band syndrome (Fig. 8–5)—or when the lesion is so small that is requires more detailed anatomical topography (for example, parietal or occipital atretic meningoceles (Fig. 8–6).

Holoprosencephaly

Holoprosencephaly, another early alteration of brain organogenesis, results from cleavage failure of the primitive prosencephalon. The degree of the severity of this anomaly are classically reported: *alobar* holo-

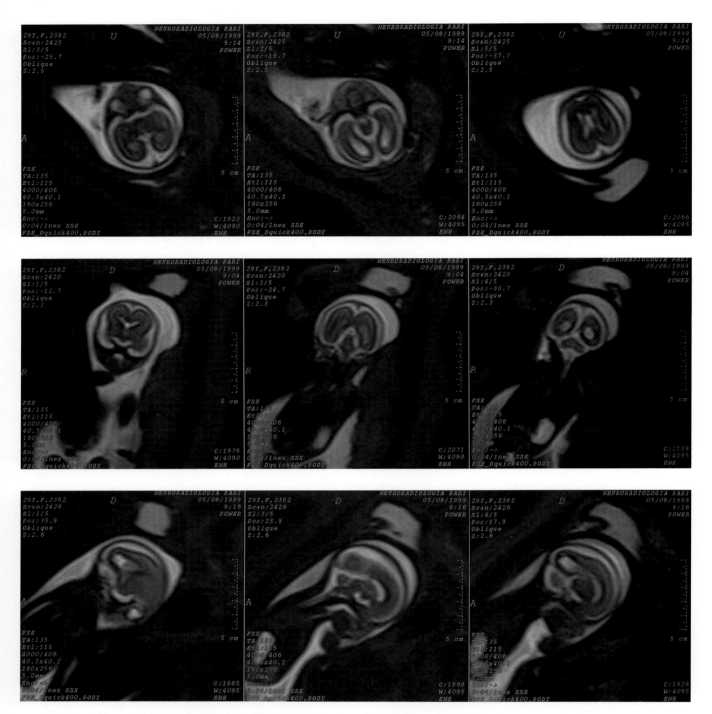

Figure 8–1. Normal anatomy by magnetic resonance image of the fetal brain at 21 postmenstrual weeks. **A.** SSE (TR 4000, TE 406, ETL 115) Axial views. At this early gestational age, the cerebral surface presents a pachygyric aspect due to the incomplete neuronal migration. The atria and the posterior horns are physiologically enlarged (A2) and the choroid plexuses are very large (A1). The lateral ventricles at level of cella media are normally wide (A3). The cavum of septi pellucidi is recognizable. The cisterns are diffusely enlarged particularly at level of the perimesencephalic region in this case. **B.** SSE (TR 4000, TE 406, ETL 115) Coronal views. The same findings shown in axial views are confirmed. Note that the falx and the cerebellar tentorium are already formed. The posterior fossa with the cerebellum is better represented than in the axial scans, at this gestational age (B3). **C.** SSE (TR 4000, TE 406, ETL 115) Sagittal views. On the sagittal sections, the absence of gyri is well depicted in all the brain lobes. The isolated dilatation of the atria and the posterior horns are also appreciated (C1). The fourth ventricle and the cerebellar vermis, already completely formed, are perfectly depicted (C2). Note the enlarged perivermian cisterns.

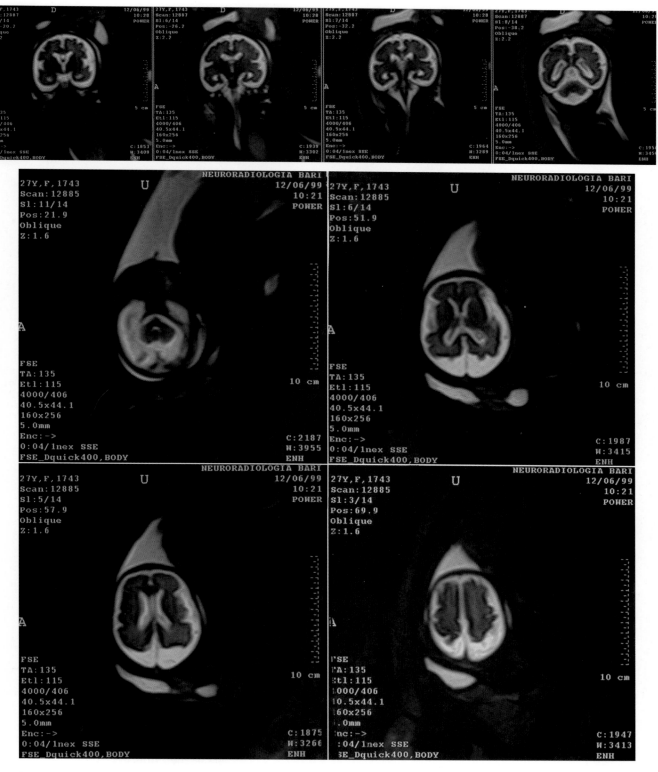

Figure 8–2. Normal anatomy by magnetic resonance image of the fetal brain at 28 postmenstrual weeks. **A.** SSE (TR 4000–TE 406–ETL 115) Coronal views. The sylvian fissures are still open. The early gyri are evident in the parietal region. The hippocampus and choroidal fissures are already structured. The corpus callosum is well evident just below the inter-hemispheric fissure and cynguli. The cavum septi pellucidi presents as a normal structure. The fourth ventricle, the cerebellar hemispheres, and the brain stem are well evident under the cerebellar tentorium. The atria are slightly enlarged but the proportionally wide choroid plexuses indicate a normal anatomy at this gestational age. The cisterna magna is wide as usual. **B.** SSE (TR 4000–TE 406–ETL 115) Axial views. The normal cerebellum, the fourth ventricle, and the middle cerebellar peduncuII are evident. The cerebral cisterns are wide as usual at this gestational age. The choroid plexuses are large in the wide atria. The septum pellucidum appears like an enlarged fissure. The sulci are evident in the insuloparietal region (perirolandic).

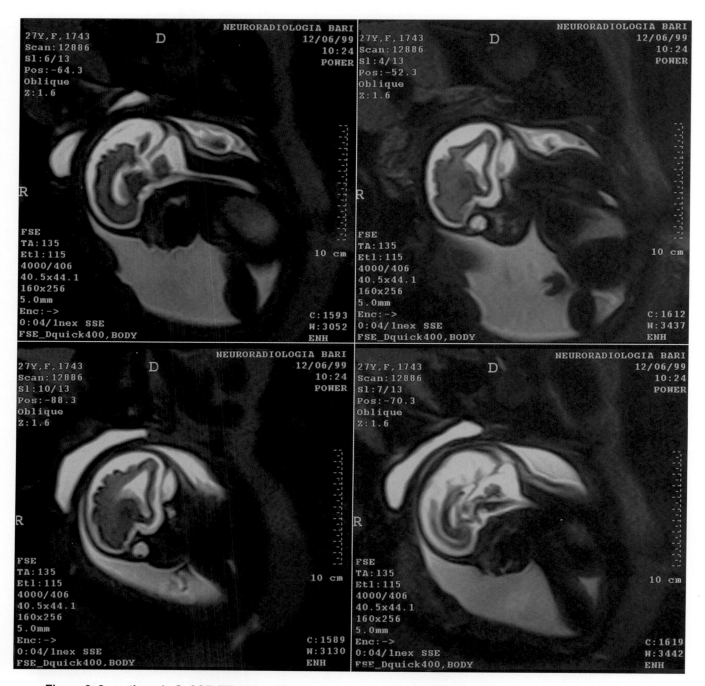

Figure 8–2 continued. C. SSE (TR 4000–TE 406–ETL 115) Sagittal sections. The eyeballs and lenses are well depicted. The frontal and temporal cortex presents pachygyric aspect while the sulci and gyri are already evident in parietal regions. The corpus callosum is normal and evident as a hypointense signal line from the rostrum to the splenium. The brainstem, fourth ventricle, and cerebellar vermis are successfully imaged. Note the wide vermian cistern and mega-cisterna magna.

Figure 8–3. Normal anatomy by magnetic resonance image of the fetal brain at 35 postmenstrual weeks. **A.** SSE (TR 16000, TE 406, ETL 115) Axial views. The fourth ventricle and the middle cerebellar peduncle are similar to those of the newborn. The subarachnoid space around the temporal lobe is still large (A1). The atria and the posterior horns are smaller and similar to those of the newborn. The cerebral peduncles and the base of the frontal lobes are evident. The cisterna ambiens remains wide (A2). On the convexity, the *gyration* is well depicted on the parietal lobes (A3).

(Continued)

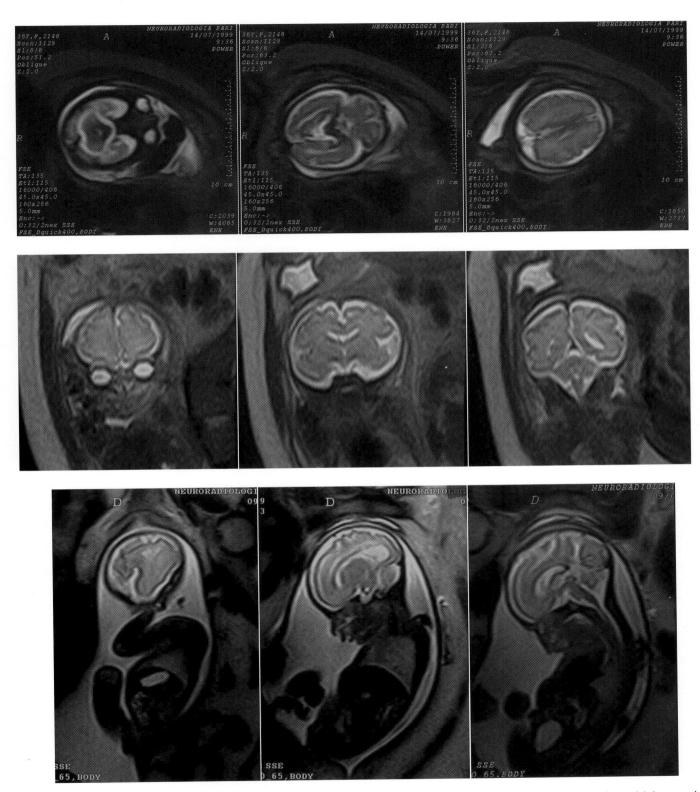

Figure 8–3 continued. B. SSFSE (TR 5000, TE 65, ETL 80) Coronal views. The gyri are evident on the frontal lobes and equally represented in the parietal regions (B1). The opercula are proceeding toward closure. The corpus callosum is formed and evident above the anterior horns and the cingulate gyri are normally oriented. The cavum of septi pellucidi is still present. Note the cortical ribbon hipointensity (B2). The falx and the cerebellar tentorium are normally formed; the ventricular atria show normal size and minimal dimensional asymmetry, which is not a pathological finding (B3). **C.** SSFSE (TR 11000, TE 65, ETL 80) Sagittal views. On a lateral section, the opercula and the cortical ribbon are evident. Note also the diaphragma, the fetal lung, and the gastric bubble (C1). On a paramedian section, in this case, the gyri are more pronounced in the parietal region than in the previous ones (C2). In the midline the corpus callosum, the brainstem, and the upper cervical spinal cord are visualized (C3).

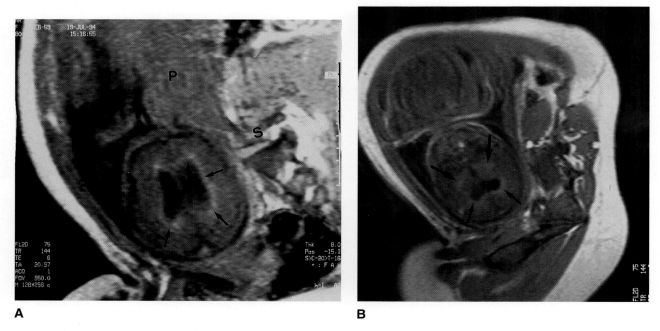

A   **B**

Figure 8–4. Germinal matrix of the fetal brain. **A.** Parasagittal maternal FL2D T1-weighted image (breath hold) at 35 postmenstrual weeks. The fetal head is in axial view. P, Placenta; S, maternal spine. **B.** Axial oblique maternal FL2D T1-weighted image of the same case shown in **A.** The fetal head is in a coronal view. Moderate ventriculomegaly is evident. The hyperintense signal of the germinal matrix is clearly depicted close to the lateral ventricles *(arrows)*. Note the hyperintensity of the basal ganglia *(large arrows)* in **B.**

prosencephaly is characterized by a normal posterior fossa, fused thalami, absent falx cerebri, and a large holoventricular cavity (Fig. 8–7); in the *semilobar* form, the cerebral hemispheres are partially separated, even though a single holoventricle is still present (Fig. 8–8); in the case of *lobar* holoprosencephaly, only a mild ventriculomegaly can be present, mainly at the level of the anterior horns, due to the absent septum pellucidum. At least, in the alobar and semilobar holoprosencephaly, the fetal MRI has an anecdotic value and is substantially useless because the US is very sensitive and conclusive. A certain role the fetal MRI maintains in less severe lobar form when the distinction from other similar features—such as septo-optic dysplasia—is required.[55–62]

Neuronal Migration Anomalies

Potentially, neuronal migration anomalies can be diagnosed with MRI, but only when they cause a severe distortion of the brain morphology, such as hemimegalencephaly, hemilissencephaly (Fig. 8–9)[63] or schizencephalic porencephaly. Milder neuronal migration anomalies cannot be diagnosed prenatally with MRI. Coronal heterotopias can be identified due to the absence of the myelinization, which causes the contrast between gray and white matter.

Similarly, macrogyria and polymicrogyria resulting from a gyration abnormality can be recognized only on postnatal MRI.[37,41]

In rare circumstances, the germinal matix can be completely *absent,* leading to a severe, true microcephaly called microcephalia vera.[37] The prenatal MRI helps to differentiate this rare anomaly from other microcephalies that are part of different complexes.

Dysgenesis of the Corpus Callosum

Dysgenesis of the corpus callosum is a frequent brain malformation easily diagnosed by US (Fig. 8–10); however, the prenatal MRI can offer more detailed anatomic information. Corpus callosum dysgenesis consists of the complete or partial absence of this major brain commissural structure. The absence of the corpus callosum produces three morphological changes in the brain: anteriorly, fibers that fail to cross on the controlateral hemisphere bend posteriorly (Probst's bundles), producing a typical crescent-like impression on the medial surface of the frontal horn (Fig. 8–10); posteriorly, the absent crossing of the callosal fibers produces an alteration of the periventricular white matter, with consequent abnormal dilatation of the atria and the

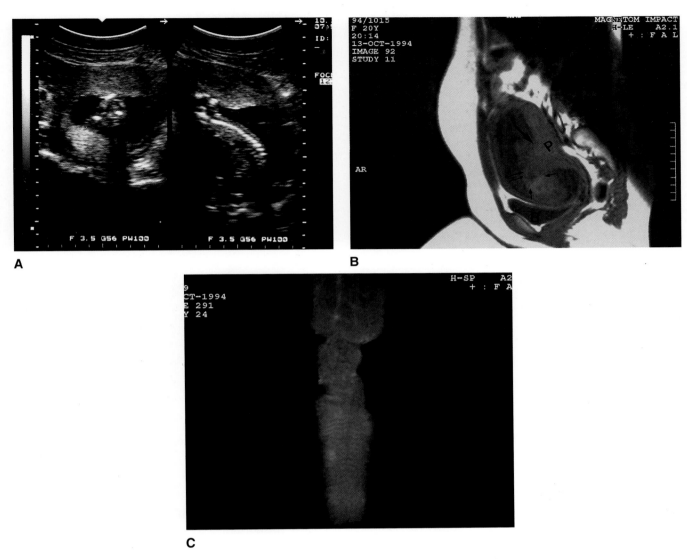

Figure 8–5. Anencephaly due to an amniotic band at 17 postmenstrual weeks. **A.** Transabdominal sonography in the axial and parasagittal plane. The anencephaly can be easily diagnosed, but the relationship with the placenta is unclear. *(Courtesy of Dr. R. Mastronardi, Taranto, Italy.)* **B.** Sagittal oblique maternal spin echo T1-weighted image. Due to early pregnancy, the fetal image is difficult to interpret. However, the expert magnetic resonance imager cannot fail to recognize the fetus in coronal section and in the breech presentation. The *small arrows* point to the fetal diaphragm between the hyperintense fetal liver and the hypointense fetal lung *(double arrow)*. The cephalic plate is clearly fused with the placenta (P) *(large arrow),* allowing the diagnosis of amniotic band syndrome. B, Maternal bladder. **C.** Magnetic resonance image of the aborted fetus in coronal view. The placenta shows fusion with the anencephalic fetal head.

posterior horns (colpocephaly) (Fig. 8–10); and the third ventricle is dorsally displaced, and in the most severe forms, may communicate with the interhemispheric fissure or with an interhemispheric cystic malformation (Fig. 8–10).[38,41,42,64–66]

Posterior Fossa Abnormalities

Abnormalities of the posterior fossa are mainly cystic in nature and include a variety of syndromes defined as Dandy–Walker complex. In its most severe form, the classic Dandy–Walker malformation is characterized by the cystic dilatation of the fourth ventricle due to the atresia of the median aperture (foramen Magendie). Hydrocephaly is almost always associated with this severe form of the malformation (Fig. 8–11). Similar to other severe conditions, US is generally sufficient. Prenatal MRI in major forms of Dandy–Walker also may be useful to understand the actual pathogenetic mechanism and the evolution (Fig. 8–12).

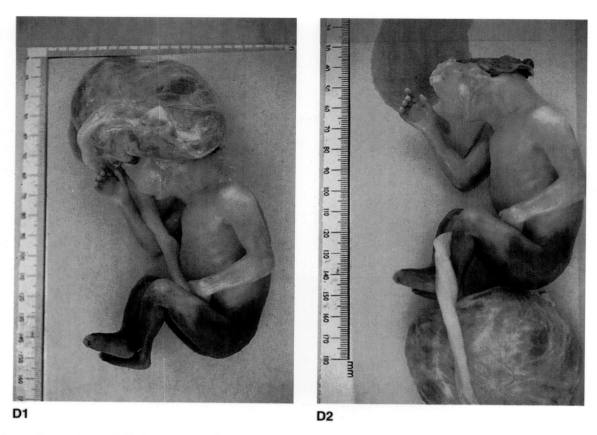

D1   **D2**

Figure 8–5 continued. D. Appearance of the aborted fetus before (1) and after (2) anatomic dissection of the placenta from the cephalic plate. *(Courtesy of Dr. V. Suma, Taranto, Italy.)*

The minor forms of Dandy–Walker complex include the Dandy–Walker variant anomaly (hypoplasia or dysplasia of the inferior cerebellar vermis with the caudal part of the fourth ventricle communicating with the medullocerebellar cistern) (Fig. 8–11 and Fig. 8–13) and the enlarged cisterna magna, where the only anatomic feature is a prominent medullocerebellar cistern (Fig. 8–14).[45,67–70]

Chiari Malformation

Another posterior fossa abnormality is the Chiari malformation.[44,71] Two more frequent forms have been recognized: type I and type II. The evidence of a small posterior fossa with herniation of the cerebellar tonsils and of the brain stem is characteristic of the Chiari type II malformation. The association with a spinal defect is uniformly present, however, on the basis of our preliminary prenatal MRI results, it seems not to be absolutely mandatory.[19,20] Ventriculomegaly, on the contrary, is almost always present (Fig. 8–15). In the Chiari type I malformation, the characteristic structural finding is the caudal ectopia of the cerebellar tonsils (amygdala), not always associated with syringomyelia, and bone anomalies of the craniocervical joint.

Hydrocephaly

Hydrocephaly is easily recognized with US beginning in the second trimester.[46] As is the case with US, the diagnosis of hydrocephaly with MRI is based on

Figure 8–6. Parietal atretic meningocele. Comparison between prenatal (29 postmenstrual weeks) and neonatal MRI. **A.** Axial sections passing through the vertex and the superior parietal regions. The small lesion presents inhomogeneous isohyperintense signal and a transosseous path may be supposed (A1, A3) whereas is well evident in the neonatal MRI (A2, A4). **B.** Sagittal paramedian sections (upside-down image). In prenatal a MRI (B1), the small lesion is confused with the amniotic hyperintensity and it was recognized only after neonatal MRI (B2).

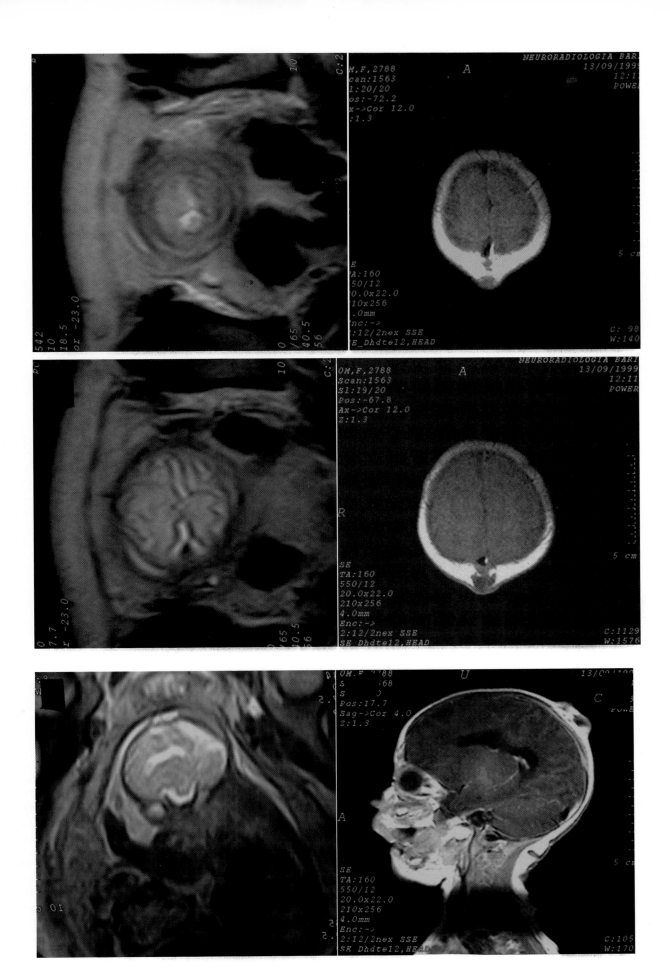

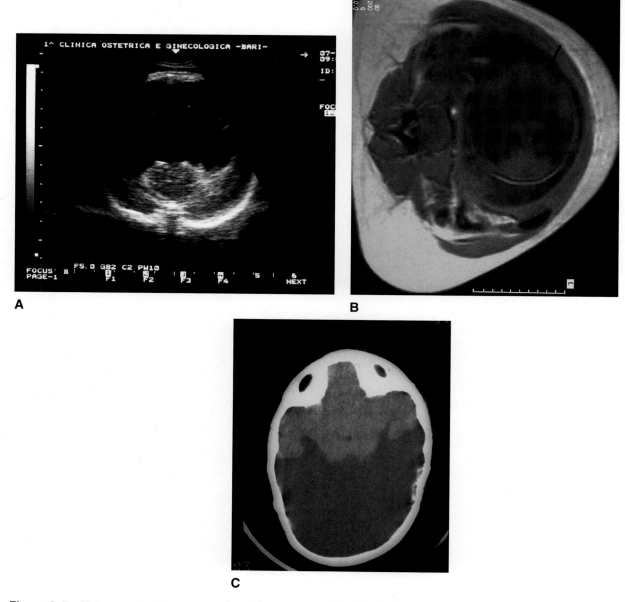

Figure 8–7. Alobar holoprosencephaly at 28 postmenstrual weeks. **A.** Transvaginal sonography of the fetal head in axial view. A wide ventricular cavity and the fused thalami can be visualized. **B.** Axial maternal FL2D T1-weighted image of the fetal head in axial view. The posterior fossa structures are normal *(arrow),* the thalami are partially fused *(double arrow),* and the malformed frontal lobes are evident anteriorly *(large arrows).* **C.** Postnatal computed tomogram. The diagnosis of alobar holoprosencephaly was confirmed.

Figure 8–8. Semilobar holoprosencephaly at 23 (case I) and 27 (case II) postmenstrual weeks. Case I: **A.** Coronal maternal spin echo T1-weighted image with two sandwiched surface coils (rotated) at 23 postmenstrual weeks. The fetal head is in sagittal view. The frontal lobe appears wide and contains a rudimentary ventricular cavity *(arrow).* A large holoventricular cavity is evident posteriorly *(double arrow).* Note the prominent eyeball *(small arrow).* **B.** Axial oblique maternal FL2D T1-weighted image. The fetal head is seen in axial view. The frontal lobes are fused *(arrows),* and the malformed ventricular cavities are evident *(arrowheads).* The *open arrow* indicates the posterior holoventricular cavity. **C.** Appearance of the fetal brain corresponding to the axial prenatal magnetic resonance image. Case II: **D.** Sagittal oblique maternal spin echo T1-weighted image at 27 postmenstrual weeks. The fetus is in the parasagittal plane. The picture is similar to the previous case, with a malformed rostral parenchymal remnant and a posterior holoventricular cavity, however anteriorly, at the level of the fetal face, a pathological soft tissue mass is evident, which can be interpreted as a cephalocele *(arrow).* Note also the fetal heart with the interventricular septum *(double arrow).* **E.** Appearance of the newborn with the anterior cephalocele.

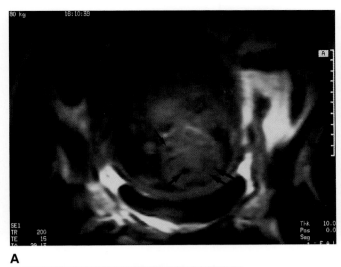

A

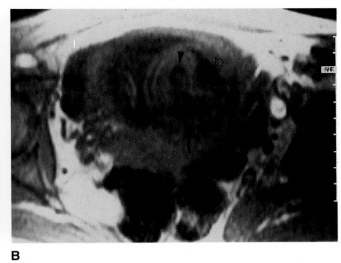

B

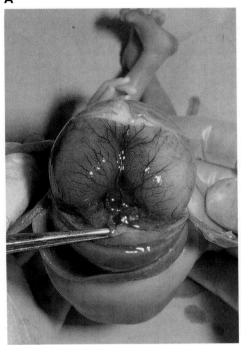

C

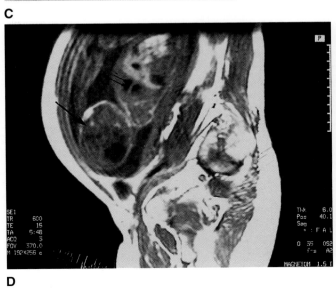

D

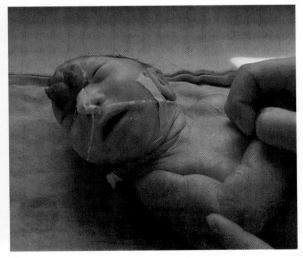

E

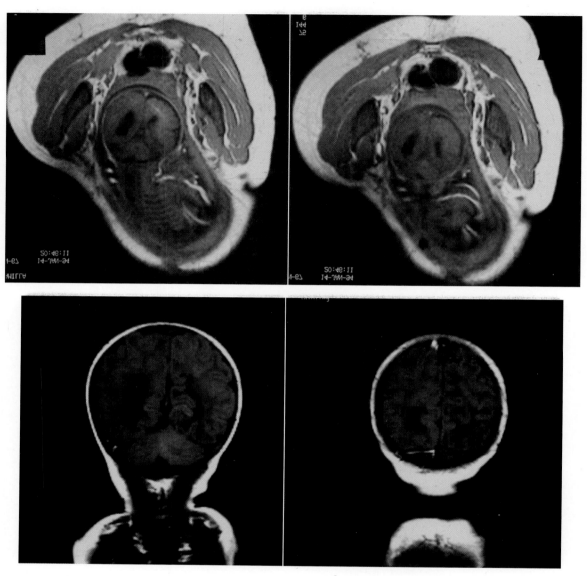

Figure 8–9. Emilissencephaly comparison between prenatal (36 postmenstrual weeks) and neonatal MRI. *(Ultras Obstet Gynecol 12:276–279;1998.)* **A.** Prenatal MRI coronal sections through ventricular atria and posterior fossa (upside-down images). The right hemisphere with the lateral ventricle is clearly enlarged and the cortical brain surface appears smooth. On the other hemisphere, sulci and gyri are recognizable. **B.** Post-natal MRI coronal section through the same planes before. The severe form of neuronal migration disturbance is easily diagnosed. Note the absolute absence of gray and white matter differentiation.

Figure 8–10. Dysgenesis of the corpus callosum at 30 (case I) and 32 (case II) postmenstrual weeks. Case I: **A.** Transvaginal ultrasonography at 30 postmenstrual weeks. A sagittal view of the fetal brain shows the absence of the corpus callosum and the typical radial array of the gyri and fulci on the medial aspect of the hemispheres. **B.** Oblique sagittal maternal spin echo T1-weighted image. The third ventricle is dorsally displaced *(double arrows).* Note the crescentlike appearance of the anterior horn due to Probst's bundles *(arrow).* **C.** Axial maternal oblique scan. The fetal head is in axial view. The severe dilatation of the atria and the posterior horns (colpocephaly) is well imaged. Case II: **D.** Coronal maternal spin echo T1-weighted image at 32 postmenstrual weeks. The fetus is in coronal view. Because of the complete absence of the corpus callosum, the third ventricle directly communicates with an interhemispheric fissue *(arrow).* **E.** Axial maternal scan. The fetal head is seen in the axial plane. Note the interhemispheric cyst and the colpocephaly. **F.** Pathological specimen of the stillborn, confirming the complete communication between the interhemispheric fissure and the third ventricle.

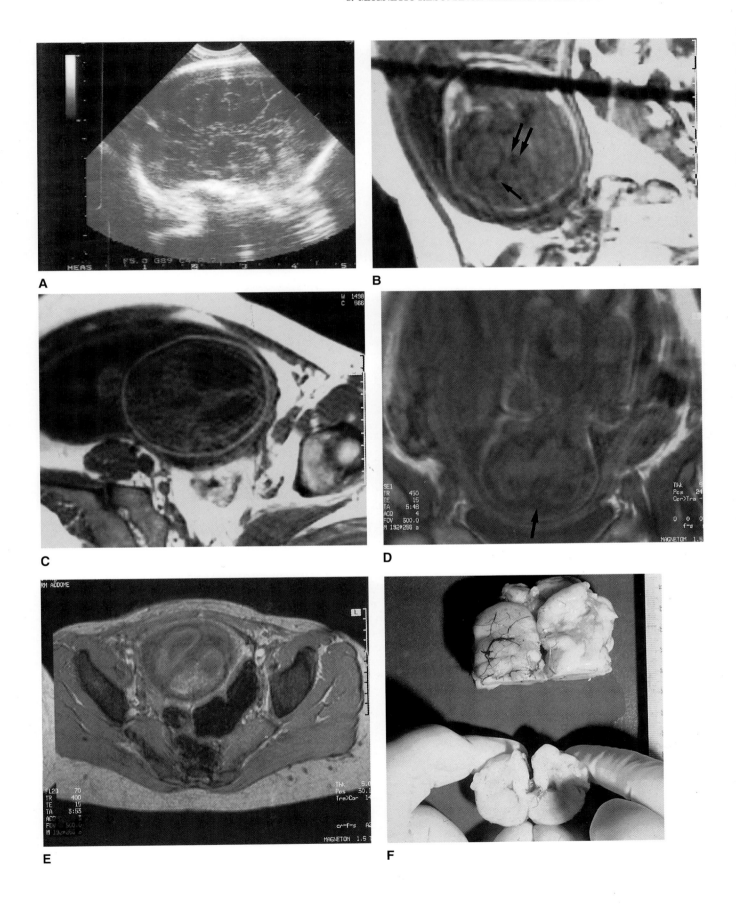

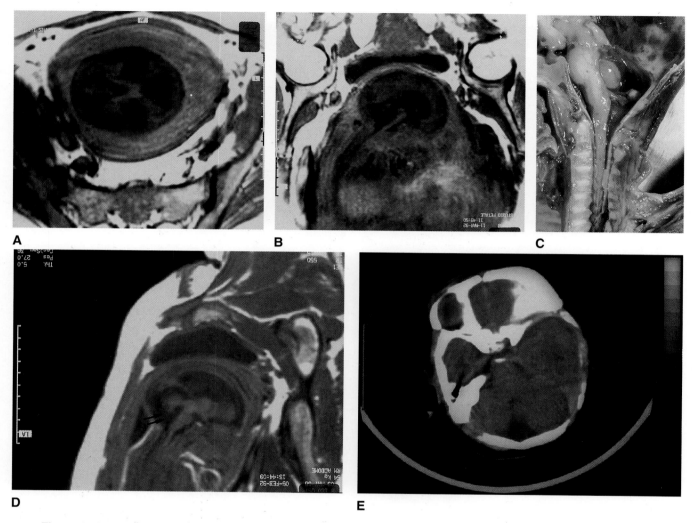

Figure 8–11. Dandy–Walker complex at 24 (case I) and 32 (case II) postmenstrual weeks. Case I: **A.** Axial maternal spin echo T1-weighted image at 24 postmenstrual weeks. The fetal head is seen in the axial view. Cystic dilatation of the fourth ventricle and hydrocephaly are accurately imaged. **B.** Coronal maternal spin echo T1-weighted image. The fetus is seen in the sagittal view. The fourth ventricle is severely enlarged, but its morphology is still recognizable. **C.** Pathological specimen of the aborted fetus. Case II: **D.** Coronal oblique maternal spin echo T1-weighted image at 32 postmenstrual weeks. The fetus, in sagittal view, shows agenesis of the corpus callosum associated with a Dandy–Walker variant malformation. The cerebello-medullar cistern is enlarged and communicates with the inferior surface of the fourth ventricle *(double arrow)*. Note the dysplasia of the inferior cerebellar vermis *(arrow)*. **E.** Postnatal computed tomogram confirming the Dandy–Walker variant anomaly. Reil's vallecula is almost absent due to dysplasia of the inferior cerebellar vermis; the cerebello medullar cistern is prominent.

the recognition of enlarge ventricles with loss of the typical external concavity of the lateral walls of the lateral ventricles and shrunken choroid plexuses inside the ventricular cavities (Fig. 8–16). In the severe forms of hydrocephaly, MRI can be useful only in recognizing or better defining associated brain malformations.[72] Thanks to new ultrafast MRI sequences, the better visualization of cerebrospinal fluid cavities has improved the capability in the comprehension of pathogenesis and evolution of fetal hydrocephaly.

Porencephaly

Porencephaly is a rare, destructive condition of the brain tissue secondary to vascular or infective insults in the fetal period. Given the various possible etiologies for the defect, almost any location in the brain is possible, and the defects may be single or multiple (Fig. 8–17). Sometimes, the brain tissue loss is subventricular and may produce a rapid monoventricular enlargement (Fig. 8–18).

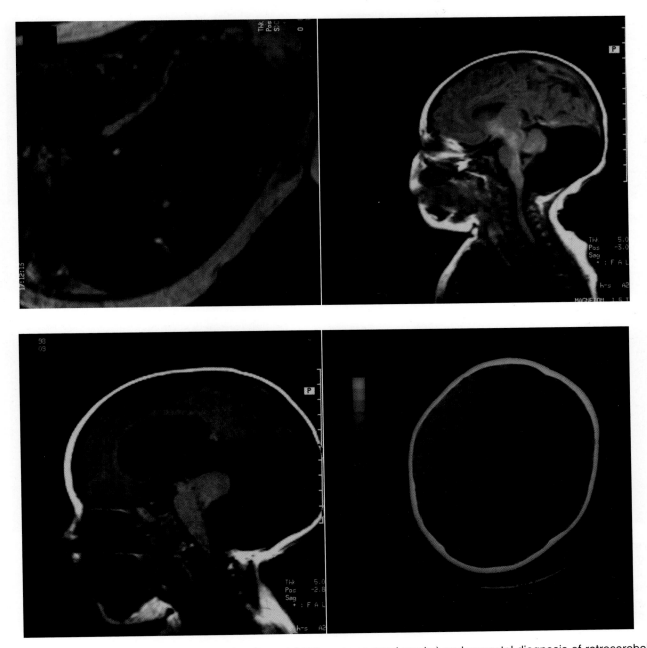

Figure 8–12. Dandy–Walker complex. Prenatal (30 postmenstrual weeks) and neonatal diagnosis of retrocerebellar cyst. The same case, major Dandy–Walker malformation diagnosis, at 6 months after birth. *(Rivista di Neuroradiologia 12:13–20;1999.)* **A.** Comparison between prenatal (A1) and neonatal (at birth) (A2) MRI sagittal midline sections. The fourth ventricle seems to be normal; a retrocerebellar cyst is well evident and apparently does not communicate with fourth ventricle. No hydrocephaly is evident. **B.** MRI sagittal section (B1) and axial CT scan (B2) 6 months after birth. The fourth ventricle is no more recognizable. The retrocerebellar cyst is under pressure and severe hydrocephaly formed. The picture is now typical of Dandy–Walker malformation despite the prenatal and neonatal appearance.

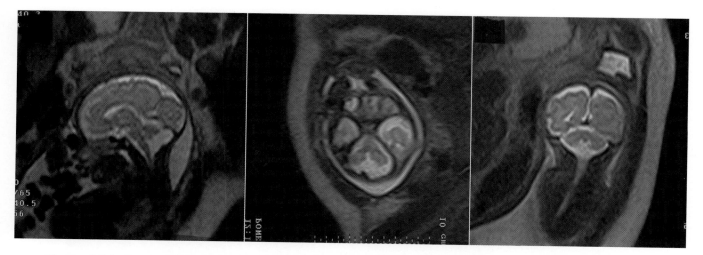

Figure 8–13. Dandy–Walker variant malformation. Prenatal (31 postmenstrual weeks.) MRI sagittal, axial, and coronal views. The fourth ventricle is not enlarged and communicates with the prominent cerebello medullar cistern. In the axial view the absence of Reil's vallecula is well evident.

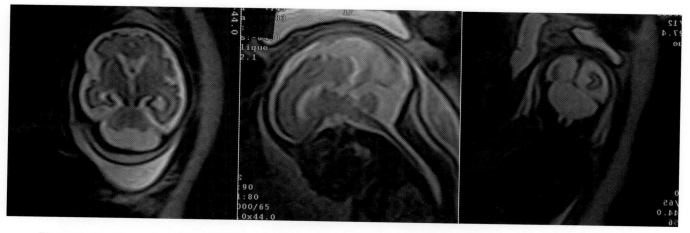

Figure 8–14. Mega-cisterna magna. Prenatal MRI (28 postmenstrual weeks). **A.** Axial section passing through third ventricle and posterior fossa. The mega-cisterna magna is evident. The lateral ventricles and the third ventricle are not enlarged. **B.** Median section. Fourth ventricle, brainstem and cerebellar vermis are regular. The superior vermian cistern is wide as usual at this age of pregnancy. The cerebello–medullar cistern is severely enlarged (mega-cisterna magna). **C.** Coronal section. The scan through the cyst shows the cerebellar tentorium, the falx, and the occipital lobes.

Tumors

Tumors of the fetal brain are very rare prenatal conditions. Prenatal ultrasonographic diagnosis of the choroid plexus papilloma has been reported.[73] Two cases in our series have shown that prenatal MRI can be as accurate as US in diagnosing neoplastic pathology (Fig. 8–19). Prenatal MRI may help to better characterize the tumor on the basis of the signal evaluation of the pathological tissues or of the hemorrhagic foci (Fig. 8–20).

SUMMARY AND CONCLUSIONS

US is and will continue to be the primary diagnostic tool for evaluating fetal brain. Fetal MRI can be helpful in those rare cases when US diagnosis is doubtful such as maternal obesity, and severe oligohydramnios, where the transvaginal approach is not possible.

Thanks to the new ultrafast MRI sequences, in the last 3 years, many advances have been obtained and the fetal brain anatomy as seen by MRI has been rewritten. However, the routine use of fetal

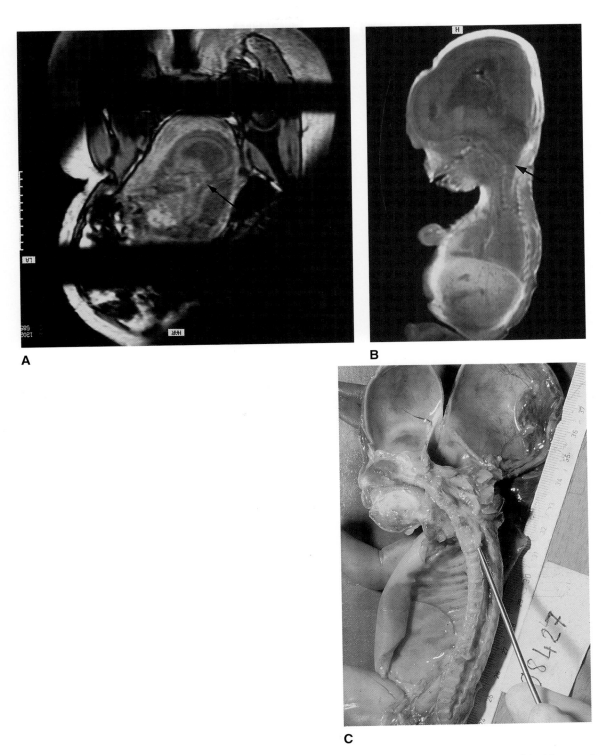

Figure 8–15. Chiari malformation with severe hydrocephaly. **A.** Coronal oblique maternal fast low-angle shot two-dimensional T1-weighted image at 21 postmenstrual weeks. The fetus is in sagittal view. The posterior fossa is very small, and the herniation of both the cerebellar tonsils and the brain stem in the upper cervical canal can be suspected *(arrow)*. Note also the severe hydrocephaly. No spinal defect was detected with either ultrasonography or magnetic resonance imaging. The use of four presaturation bands was necessary. **B.** This magnetic resonance image of the aborted fetus seems to confirm the prenatal diagnosis *(arrow)*. **C.** Pathological specimen of the aborted fetus. After removal of the fetal brain, the hypoplasia of the posterior fossa is well evident and the herniation of the brain stem and the cerebellum is confirmed. No spinal defect was present.

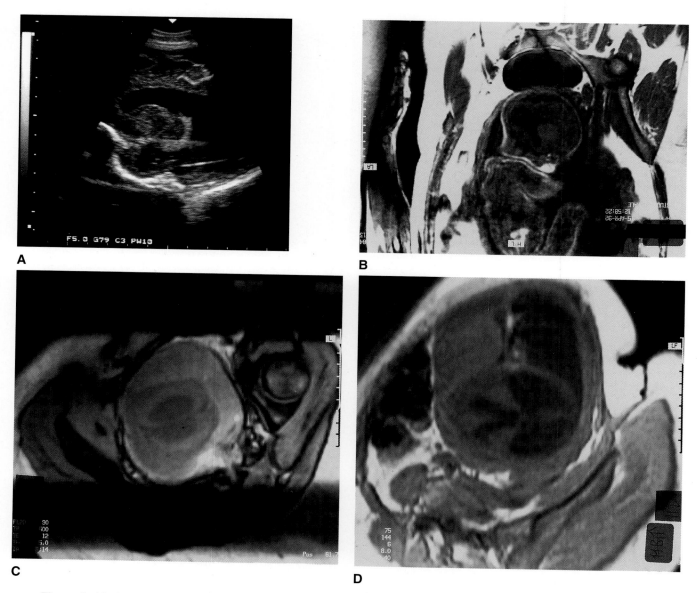

Figure 8–16. Hydrocephaly at different ages of pregnancy and different degrees of severity. **A.** Case I: Transvaginal sonography in a moderate hydrocephaly at 22 postmenstrual weeks. Paramedian view shows that the lateral ventricle is enlarged and the choroid plexus is shrunken. **B.** Coronal oblique maternal spin echo T1-weighted image. The fetal head is in paramedian view. The lateral ventricle is enlarged and the choroid plexus is not well evident, perhaps due to its close location to the thalami. **C.** Axial oblique maternal fast FL2D T1-weighted image. The fetus is in axial view. Note the loss of the typical concavity of the lateral wall of the ventricular cavities. **D.** Case II: Axial oblique maternal FL2D T1-weighted image at 30 postmenstrual weeks. The fetus is in axial view. The severe hydrocephaly is easily recognizable.

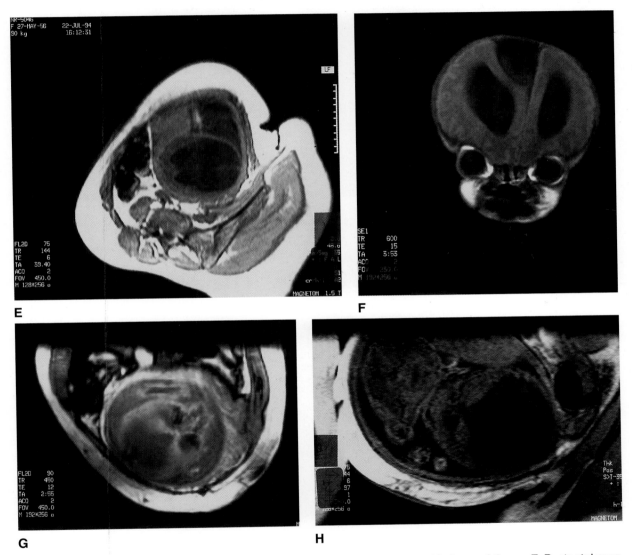

Figure 8–16 continued. E. In a more cranial section the brain appears as a thin layer of tissue. **F.** Postnatal magnetic resonance image shows hydrocephaly associated with an interhemispheric (probably aradinoid) cyst. **G.** Case III: Axial oblique maternal FL2D T1-weighted image at 27 postmenstrual weeks. The fetal head is in coronal view. Severe hydrocephaly is evident, but the morphology of the anterior horns is still preserved. **H.** Magnetic resonance imaging (MRI) control at 31 postmenstrual weeks. Axial oblique maternal FL2D T1-weighted image (rotated). The hydrocephaly is clearly in progress, and the lateral ventricle morphology cannot be recognized. The correct diagnosis of evolutive hydrocephaly was possible only because of the previous MRI examination, avoiding the incorrect diagnosis of hydranencephaly.

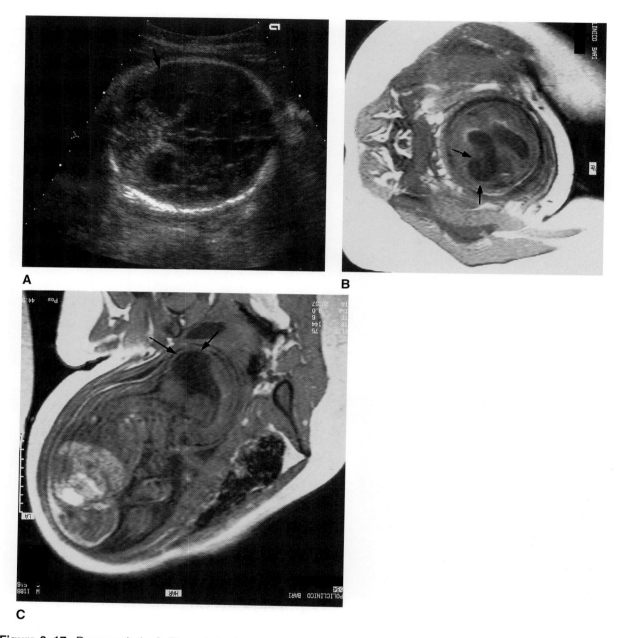

Figure 8–17. Porencephaly. **A.** Transabdominal ultrasonography at 35 postmenstrual weeks. The diagnosis of hydrocephaly is easy, and an asymmetrical dilatation of the right posterior horn was described *(arrows)*. **B, C.** Axial maternal FL2D T1-weighted image and coronal oblique maternal FL2D T1-weighted image of the fetus in axial and parasagittal views, respectively. The prenatal magnetic resonance images offer a more detailed anatomic evaluation, allowing the sure diagnosis of a porencephalic cavity communicating with the lateral ventricle *(arrows)*.

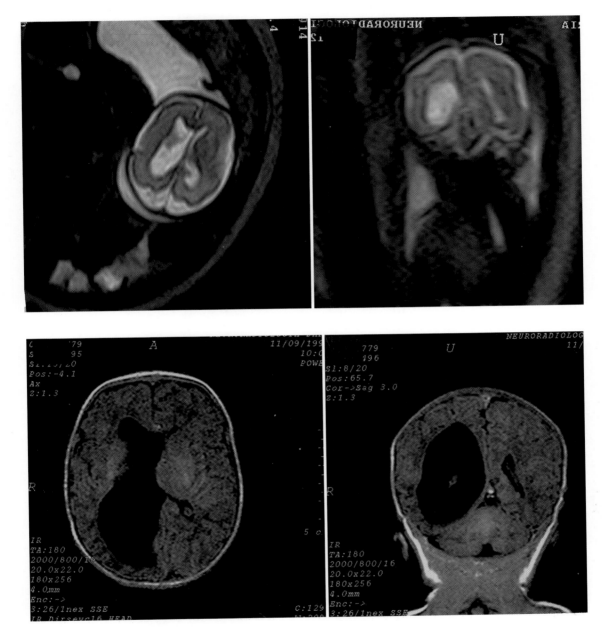

Figure 8–18. Monoventricular hydrocephaly secondary to subventricular destructive lesions. **A.** Prenatal MRI at 28 postmenstrual weeks in axial and coronal views. The destructive lesion is present and monoventricular dilatation is well evident. **B.** Postnatal MRI through the same planes as before. The scans confirm that the monoventricular dilatation is not under pressure validating the destructive pathogenesis.

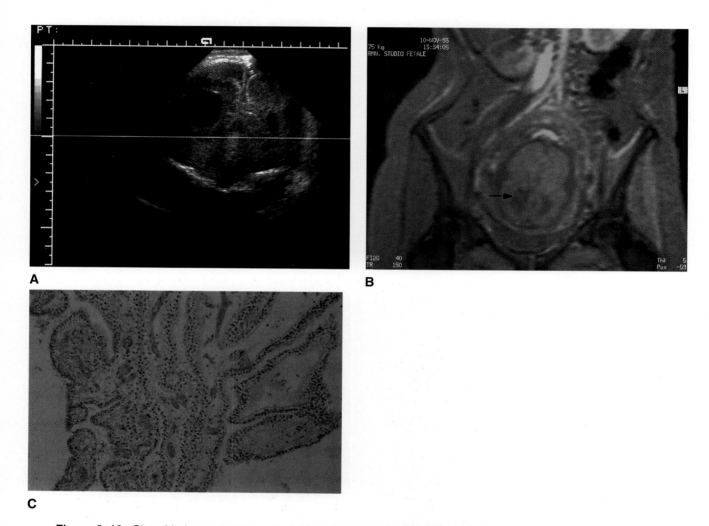

Figure 8–19. Choroid plexus papilloma. **A.** Transvaginal ultrasonography at 36 postmenstrual weeks. Only a diagnosis of monoventricular hydrocephaly is possible. **B.** Coronal oblique maternal FL2D T1-weighted image. In the enlarged right atrium a hypertrophic choroid plexus can be clearly visualized *(arrow),* suggesting the diagnosis of papilloma. **C.** Histology confirmed the prenatal diagnosis.

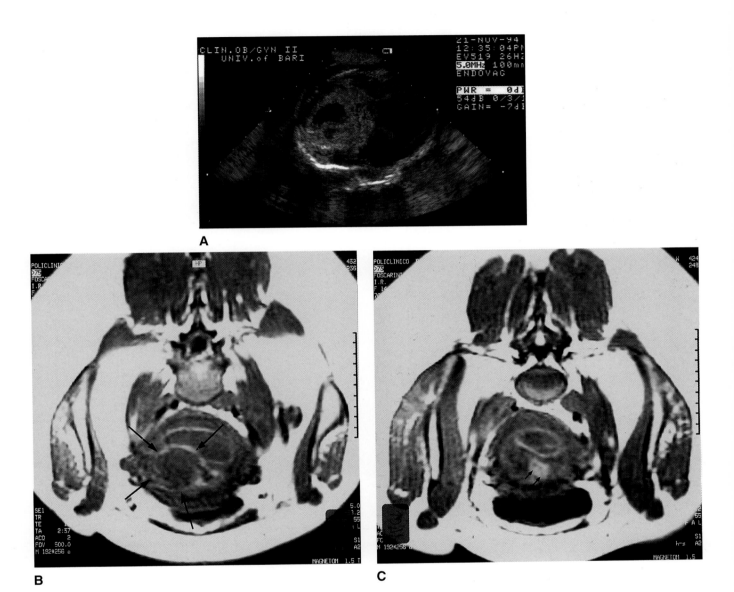

Figure 8–20. Intra-axial large hemorrhagic tumor. **A.** Transvaginal ultrasonography at 23 postmenstrual weeks. The fetus was stillborn, and in the right frontal region a large, round echogenic mass with anechoic foci was diagnosed. **B, C.** The patient voluntarily underwent magnetic resonance imaging even though the fetus was dead. Axial oblique maternal spin echo T1-weighted images. The large intra-axial frontal mass was confirmed *(arrows),* and in the more cranial section **(C)** a hyperintensive signal *(double arrow)* made possible the hypothesis of intraneoplastic hemorrhage.

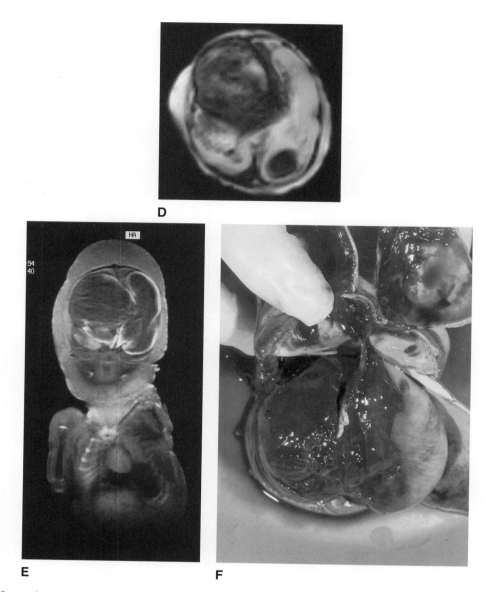

Figure 8–20 continued. D, E. Magnetic resonance image of the aborted fetus. The mass is clearly depicted, and the gradient echo sequence **(E)** confirmed the intraneoplastic hemorrhagic signal. **F.** Pathology confirmed the hemorrhagic aspect of the tumor, and histology allowed the diagnosis of a primitive neuroectodermic hemorrhagic tumor.

MRI is very far from being widely implemented. On the contrary, very interesting is the speculative evaluation of the MRI data in the interpretation of different nosological entities and physiological cerebral activities. Functional MRI of the fetus is already proposed,[74] representing a fascinating field of research.

REFERENCES

1. Levine D, Barnes PD, Edelman RR. Obstetric MR imaging. *Radiology.* 1999;211:609–617.

2. Benaceraff BR, Estroff JA. Transvaginal sonographic imaging of the low fetal head in the second trimester. *J Ultrasound Med.* 1989;8:325.

3. Monteagudo A, Reuss ML, Timor-Tritsch IE. Imaging of the fetal brain in the second and third trimester using transvaginal sonography. *Obstet Gynecol.* 1991;77:27–32.

4. Kido DK, Morris TW, Erickson JL, Plewes DB, Simon JH. Physiologic changes during high field strength MR imaging. *AJNR.* 1987;8:263–266.

5. Wolff S, James TL, Young GB, Margulis AR, Bodycote J, Afzal V. Magnetic resonance imaging: Absence of in vitro cytogenetic damage. *Radiology.* 1985;155:163–165.

6. Wolff S, Crooks LE, Brown P, et al. Tests for DNA and chromosomal damage induced by nuclear magnetic resonance imaging. *Radiology.* 1980;136:707–710.

7. Shellock FG, Crues JV. Temperature changes caused by MR imaging of the brain with a head coil. *AJNR.* 1988;9:287–291.

8. Poutamo J, Partanen K, Vanninen R, Vainio P, Kirkinen P. MRI does not change fetal cardiotocographic parameters. *Prenat Diagn.* 1998;18:1149–1154.

9. Johnson II, Symonds E, Kean A, et al. Imaging the pregnant human uterus with nuclear magnetic resonance. *Am J Obstetr Gynecol.* 1984;148:1136–1139.

10. Weinreb JC, Lowe TW, Santos-Ramos R, Cunningham FG, Parkey R. Magnetic resonance imaging in obstetric diagnosis. *Radiology.* 1985;154:157–161.

11. Smith FW, Adam AM, Phillips WDP. NMR imaging in pregnancy. *Lancet.* 1983;1:61–62.

12. McCarthy SM, Filly RA, Stark DD, Callen PW, Golbus MS, Hricak H. Magnetic resonance imaging of the fetal anomalies in utero: Early experience. *AJR.* 1985;14:677–682.

13. McCarthy SM, Stark DD, Filly RA, Callen PW, Hricak H, Higgins CB. Obstetrical magnetic resonance imaging: maternal anatomy. *Radiology.* 1985;154:421–425.

14. Daffos F, Forestier F, McAleese J, et al. Fetal curarization for prenatal magnetic resonance imaging. *Prenatal Diagn.* 1988;8:311–314.

15. Moise KJ, Carpenter RJ, Deter RL, Kirshon B, Diaz SF. The use of fetal neuromuscular blockade during intrauterine procedures. *Am J Obstet Gynecol.* 1987;157:874–879.

16. Seeds JW, Corke BC, Spielman FJ. Prevention of fetal movements during invasive procedures with pancuronium bromide. *Am J Obstet Gynecol.* 1986;155:818–819.

17. Wenstrom KD, Williamson RA, Weiner CP, Sipes SL, Yuh WTC. Magnetic resonance imaging of fetuses with intracranial defects. *Obstet Gynecol.* 1991;77:529–532.

18. Toma P, Lucigrai G, Bodero P, et al. Prenatal detection of an abdominal mass by MR imaging performed while the fetus is immobilized with pancuronium bromide. *AJR.* 1990;154:1049–1050.

19. Resta M, Greco P, D'Addario V, et al. MRI in pregnancy. Study of cerebral fetal malformations. *Ultrasound Obstet Gynecol.* 1994;4:7–20.

20. Resta M, Spagnolo P, DiCuonzo F, et al. La RM. Parte II: quadri patologici. *Rivista di Neuroradiologia.* 1994;7:557–571.

21. Smith FW, Kent C, Abramovich DR, Sutherland HW. Nuclear magnetic resonance imaging: A new look at the fetus. *Br J Obstet Gynaecol.* 1985;92:1024–1033.

22. McCarthy SM, Filly RA, Stark DD, et al. Obstetrical magnetic resonance imaging: Fetal anatomy. *Radiology.* 1985;154:427–432.

23. Powell MC, Worthington BS. MRI: A new milestone in modern OB care. *Diagn Imaging.* 1986;April:86–91.

24. Weinreb JC, Lowe T, Coen JN, Kutler M. Human fetal anatomy: MR imaging. *Radiology.* 1985;157:715–720.

25. Williamson RA, Weiner CP, Yuh WTC, Abu-Yousef MM. Magnetic resonance imaging of anomalous fetuses. *Obstet Gynecol.* 1989;73:952–956.

26. Smith FW, Sutherland HW. Short T1 inversion recovery (STIR) imaging in human pregnancy. *Magn Reson Imaging.* 1986;4:137.

27. Birger M, Homburg R, Insler V. Clinical evaluation of fetal movements. *Int J Gynaecol Obstet.* 1980;18:337–382.

28. Resta M, Spagnolo P, DiCuonzo F, et al. La RM del feto. Parte I: storia, tecnica d' esame ed anatomia cerebrale normale. *Rivista di* Neuroradiologia. 1994;7:53–65.

29. Greco P, Vimercati A, Resta M, Loizzi V, Selvaggi L. Magnetic resonance imaging in prenatal diagnosis. In: Monduzzi ed. Women's health in the 2000. From reproduction to menopause" *Int Proceed Div* 1999;157–162.

30. Resta M, Medicamento N, Dicuonzo F, Burdi N. La RM fetale: Esperienza di 5 anni. *Rivista di Neuroradiologia* 1999;12:13–20.

31. Resta M, Burdi N, Medicamento N. Magnetic resonance imaging of normal and pathological fetal brain. *Child Nerv Syst.* 1998;14:151–154.

32. Vimercati A, Greco P, Resta M, Loizzi V, Selvaggi L. The diagnostic role "in utero" of magnetic resonance imaging. *J Perinat Med.* 1999; 27: 303–308.

33. Gelmann SR. Fetal movements and ultrasound effects of intravenous glucose administration. *Am J Obstet Gynecol.* 1980;137:459–461.

34. Minors DS, Waterhose JM. The effects of maternal posture, meals, and time of day on fetal movements. *Br J Obstet Gynecol.* 1979;86:717–723.

35. Levine D, Barnes PD, Sher S, et al. Fetal fast MR imaging: Reproducibility, technical quality, and conspicuity of anatomy. *Radiology.* 1998;206:549–554.

36. Revel MP, Pons JC, Lelairder C, et al. MRI of the fetus: A study of 20 cases performed without curarization. *Prenat Diagn.* 1993;13:775–799.

37. Barkovich AJ, Gressens P, Evrard P. Formation, maturation, and disorders of brain neocortex. *AJNR.* 1992;13:423–446.

38. Barkovich AJ, Lyon G, Evrard P. Formation, maturation, and disorders of white matter. *AJNR.* 1992;13:447–461.

39. McLone DG, Naidich TP. Developmental morphology of the subaracnoid space, brain vasculature, and contiguous structures, and the cause of the Chiari II malformation. *AJNR.* 1992;13:463–482.

40. Trefelner E, McCarthy S, Kier L. Developmental fetal anatomy with MRI. *Magn Reson Imag.* 1989;7:170.

41. Barkovich AJ. *Pediatric Neuroimaging.* New York: Raven Press; 1990:5–13.

42. Evrard P, de Saint Georges P, Kadhim H, et al. Pathology of prenatal encephalopathies. In: French J, ed. *Child Neurology and Developmental Disabilities.* Baltimore: Paul H. Brookes; 1989:153–176.

43. Normann MG. In: Dimmick JE., Kalousek DK, eds. *Developmental Pathology of the Embryo and Fetus.* Philadelphia: JB Lippincott; 1992:341–348.

44. Barkovich AJ, Norman D. Anomalies of the corpus callosum: Correlation with further anomalies of the brain. *AJNR.* 1985;9:493–501.

45. Raybaud C. Cystic malformations of the posterior fossa: Abnormalities associated with development of the roof of the fourth ventricle and adjoint meningeal structures. *J Neuroradiol.* 1982;9:103–133.

46. Chinn DH, Calle PW, Filly RA. The lateral ventricle in early second trimester. *Radiology.* 1983;148:529–531.

47. Hadlock FP, Deter RL, Park SK. Real-time sonography: Ventricular and vascular anatomy of the fetal brain in utero. *AJR.* 1981;136:133–137.

48. Aleksic S, Budzilovi CG, Greco MA, et al. Iniencephaly: Neuropathologic study. *Clin Neuropathol.* 1983;2:55–61.

49. Foderaro AE, Abu Yousef MM, Benda JA, et al. Antenatal ultrasound diagnosis of iniencephaly. *J Clin Ultrasound* 1987;15:550.

50. Friedle RL. Anencephaly, rachischisis and encephaloceles. In: *Developmental Neuropathology.* Part 2. New York: Springer-Verlag; 1975:230–240.

51. Lemire RJ, Beckwith JB, Warkany J. *Anencephaly.* New York: Raven Press; 1978.

52. Naidich TP. Cranial CT signs of the Chiari II malformation. *J Neuroradiol.* 1986;8:233–239.

53. Rakestraw MR, Massod S, Ballinger WE. Brain heterotopia and anencephaly. *Arch Pathol Lab Med.* 1987;111:858.

54. Scherrer CC, Hammer F, Schinzel A, et al. Brain stem and cervical spine cord dysraphic lesions in iniencephaly. *Pediatr Pathol.* 1992;12:469–476.

55. Cohen MM, Jirasek JE, Guzman RT, et al. Holoprosencephaly and facial dysmorphia: Nosology, etiology and pathogenesis. *Birth Defects.* 1971;7:125–135.

56. Nyberg DA, Mack LA, Bronstein A, et al. Holoprosencephaly: Prenatal sonographic diagnosis. *AJNR.* 1987;8:871–878.

57. Müller F, O'Rahilly R. Mediobasal prosencephalic defects, including holoprosencephaly and cyclopia, in relation to the development of the human forebrain. *Am J Anat.* 1989;40:409.

58. Jellinger K., Gross H, Kaltenback E, et al. Holoprosencephaly and agenesis of the corpus callosum: Frequency of associated malformations. *Acta Neuropathol.* 1981;55:1.

59. Leech RW, Shuman RM. Holoprosencephaly and related cerebral midline anomalies: A review. *J Child Neurol.* 1986;1:3–18.

60. Fitz CR. Holoprosencephaly and related entities. *Neuroradiology.* 1983;25:225–238.

61. De Myer W. Holoprosencephaly. In: Vinicken PJ, Bruyn GW, eds. *Handbook of Clinical Neurology.* Amsterdam: North Holland Publishing; 1977:30.

62. Filly RA, Chinn DH, Callen PW. Alobar holoprosencephaly: Ultrasonic prenatal diagnosis. *Radiology.* 1984;151:455–459.

63. Greco P, Resta M, Vimercati A, et al. Antenatal diagnosis of isolated lissencephaly by ultrasound and magnetic resonance imaging. *Ultrasound Obstet Gynecol.* 1998;12:276–279.

64. Barkovich AJ. Apparent atypical callosal dysgenesis: Analysis of MR findings in six cases and their relationship to holoprosencephaly. *AJNR.* 1990;11:333–340.

65. Ettlinger G. Agenesis of the corpus callosum. In: Vinicken PJ, Bruyn GW, eds. *Handbook of Clinical Neurology.* Amsterdam: North Holland Publishing; 1997;30:431–478.

66. Kendall BE. Dysgenesis of the corpus callosum. *Neuroradiology.* 1983;25:239–256.

67. Barkovick AJ, Kjos BO, Norman D, Edwards MS. Revised classification of posterior fossa cysts and cystlike malformations based upon the results of multiplanar MR imaging. *AJNR.* 1989;10:977–988.

68. Barkovich AJ, Kjos BO, Normann D, et al. New concepts of posterior fossa cysts in children (abstract). *AJNR.* 1988;9:1007.

69. Barkovich AJ, Wippold FJ, Shermann JL, et al. Significance of cerebellar tonsillar ectopia on MR. *AJNR.* 1986;7:795–799.

70. Hirsch JF, Pierre Kahn A, Renier D, et al. The Dandy–Walker malformation. *J Neurosurg.* 1984;61:515–522.

71. Naidich TP, Altman NR, Braffman BH, McLone DG, Zimmerman RA. Cephaloceles and related malformations. *AJNR.* 1992;13:655–690.

72. Fiske CE, Filly RA, Callen PW. Sonographic measurement of lateral ventricle width in early ventricular dilatation. *J Clin Ultrasound.* 1981;9:303–307.

73. Cappe IP, Lam AH. Ultrasound in the diagnosis of choroid plexus papilloma. *J Clin Ultrasound.* 1985;13:122.

74. Hykin J, Moore R, Duncan K, et al. Functional brain activity demonstrated by functional magnetic resonance imaging. *Lancet.* 1999;354:645–646.

CHAPTER NINE

Three-Dimensional Sonographic Evaluation of the Fetal Brain

Ana Monteagudo
Ilan E. Timor-Tritsch
Patricia Mayberry

Until recently, physicians could translate a standard, two-dimensional (2D) ultrasonographic image of a fetus into a three-dimensional (3D) model only in their mind. This mental "exercise" was based on years of experience and on their concept of the structure or the malformation in question. Now, however, modern ultrasonographic machines equipped with new hardware and powerful software can create a 3D image of structures such as the fetal face, hand, or spine, surrounded by the amniotic fluid or other internal organs. This 3D picture is not only useful to the physician evaluating the fetus, but it may be much more meaningful to the neonatologist, pediatric neurologist, or surgeon, as well as the parents.

As the experience with this technology grows and better ultrasound machines with better resolution are now available, distinct advantages are emerging for both fetal and gynecologic evaluation. Initially, the main thrust of the manufacturers and the research teams was to produce surface renderings of the fetal body. This required a well defined interface (e.g., tissue to fluid) to create a 3D picture. At present, some 3D ultrasound equipment still focuses on surface rendering only.

With improving two-dimensional gray scale technology, excellent sectional images of the fetal body with its internal organs are generated. Because the 3D data represented in the volume is obtained by a multitude of successive 2D sectional images, it became possible to recreate any desired image by "slicing" the volume in any direction using any imaginable plane (sometimes called "anyplane"). Planes can be created that are virtually impossible to obtain by 2D scanning. Most of the time, it is possible to obtain any two of the three classical planes (coronal, sagittal, or axial) of a fetal head or the brain; however, it is virtually impossible to obtain all three planes unless the fetus does not change its position significantly during the scan.

Using the volume acquisition of the 3D equipment, it became feasible to obtain simultaneously displayed images of a volume scan, among others, in the three classical planes (coronal, sagittal, and axial planes) of the body. Not only can the three simultaneously displayed images, that are perpendicular to each other, be seen, but these planes can be followed as they can be moved back and forth, up and down, and from side-to-side. This enables free movement (scrolling or navigating) in the volume. This special form of imaging in the three simultaneously displayed planes is called *multiplanar imaging*. If we acquire a volume we can obtain the above mentioned three planes. The display of the three planes at right angles to each other is called the *orthogonal display*. This feature is currently available on some, but not all, 3D ultrasound machines.

The objective of 3D imaging is to obtain a set of data points that are stored as a volume—usually in a Cartesian system—for later reformatting in a multiplanar fashion. The system in this case is a three-dimensional Cartesian coordinate system in which the coordinate of a point in the volume are its distances from each of three perpendicular lines that intersect at an origin. In such a system, all points in any plane are described by Cartesian coordinates. This data can both elucidate spatial relationships between the scanned structures and provide more accurate linear and, in most cases, volumetric measurements. The end result is that in certain display modes an image will appear simultaneously in the three orthogonal planes, will appear as an x-ray picture (transparency mode), or it will be shown as a 3D photograph of an organ.

While performing 3D imaging of the fetal brain, we employ the multiplanar orthogonal display modality and scroll or navigate freely in all three planes to scrutinize the brain.

EQUIPMENT

For a detailed description and functioning of a 3D ultrasound system including the explanation of the physics behind the different display modalities, we refer the reader to several well-written texts.[1,2]

The "front end" of every system, regardless of the differences in the display software used, are the transducers. Two kinds of transducers are available: the transabdominal transducers and the transvaginal transducers. In most transducers, a motor moves the crystal array, thus the scanning plane to section the volume at precise time intervals. This enables measurements to be made in the volume itself. This is not possible using hand-held transducers, which rely on the movement of the operator through the volume at the time of the acquisition. Therefore, in the latter external position, sensors are necessary to ascertain the correct incremental spatial storage of the data.

The main system requirements for 3D ultrasonography are the position sensors within or outside the transducer, for the ability to form volume sets in the storage area, 3D surface and/or volume-rendering capability, and the algorithms for determining measurements within the volume. A basic diagram of the 3D ultrasound system is shown in Figure 9–1. Some systems may differ in their algorithms.

The end result of the processing module is displayed on the monitor. The displayed picture can be modified using the master control panel of the unit.

The main avenues in displaying the scan are: the three *orthogonal planes,* the *surface rendering,* and the *x-ray* or *transparency modes.*

The most frequently used display modes are the orthogonal and surface rendering modes. In addition, the images can also be displayed in the transparency (x-ray) mode, in which only the strong echoes are retained. This is also called the **maximum mode.** As bones usually provide the strongest echoes, the image looks like an x-ray because the weaker tissue echoes are surpressed. This mode is particularly helpful for enhancing the fetal skeleton in examining the spine for neural tube defects.

The reconstruction and examination of organs or organ systems take a relatively long time after the acquisition has taken place. Should the operator want to study the acquired volume, he or she would "tie up" the machine, which precludes the scanning of a subsequent patient. There are two concepts of examining the stored volume; one combines the acquisition and the postprocessing in the same unit (e.g., Medison, GE, ATL 1500). The other utilizes a separate workstation to scrutinize the volume acquired data while the acquiring ultrasound unit continues to scan patients without interruption (e.g., ATL 5000). The two concepts are different only from the standpoint of enabling or precluding the continuous work of the ultrasound machine. A relatively fast desktop computer can theoretically be used as an off-line workstation for any ultrasound machine. The time invested for the actual examination by the operator remains the same regardless of the way the postacquisition work is done.

Sophisticated software incorporated in a small dedicated but powerful computer box attachable to any computer and any transducer has been designed. The heart of the equipment is a sensitive motion detector (gyroscope). At the time of this writing, clinically useful surface segmentation and rendering was possible with this device based on ingenious surface tracking software. It is probably a question of time until such devices will be able to produce multiplanar imaging.

It is worth mentioning here that the Medison 3D system enables the use of one or several desktop workstations (or laptop computers) using a software package called "3D view." This software enables the user to utilize the following: (1) multiplanar image display and analysis of 3D data sets; (2) measuring in the data set; (3) interactive 3D rendering (surface, x-ray, grayscale, and angio modes); (4) use of the electronic scalpel and electronic eraser; and (5) producing BMP files for teaching and printouts. Furthermore, the following DICOM functions are also enabled: (1) receiving 3D datasets from the Voluson 530D system; (2) sending images to the picture archiving system of the hospital and; (3) sending images to DICOM printers.

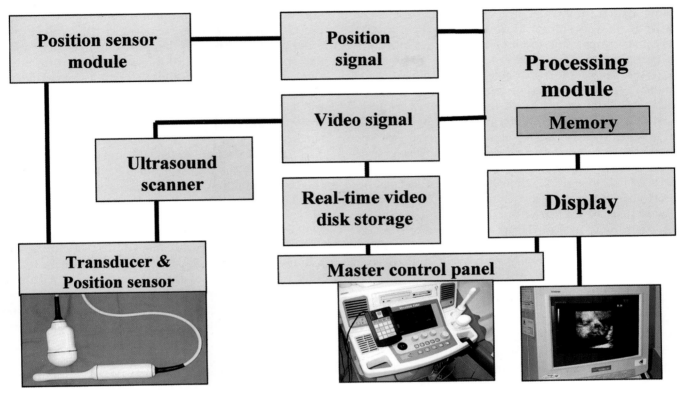

Figure 9–1. The basic block diagram of the three-dimensional machine.

ADVANTAGES AND DISADVANTAGES OF THREE-DIMENSIONAL FETAL ULTRASOUND

The advantages and disadvantages of 3D ultrasound in general, and the 3D neuroscan in particular, have to be considered. Concerning the general use of 3D ultrasound, one advantage over conventional 2D imaging is that it allows the physician to view the structure or organ of interest simultaneously in the coronal, sagittal, and axial planes. If surface rendering is used, images can be rotated and viewed from a variety of angles. This enhances the assessment of malformations by allowing images to be resliced and viewed from angles that are not available with 2D ultrasonography.

Also, both the volume and the images can be stored for future reevaluation. This stored volume can be sent over networks or via the Internet to specialists anywhere in the world for evaluation and consultation. Recipients can then further manipulate the volume to obtain the desired sections and planes.

Another advantage is that the surface-rendering mode produces an image similar to a photograph, which is especially useful in patient education and counseling. A patient viewing a small fetal omphalocele, encephalocele, or a facial abnormality may be better informed as she notes the appearance and size of the anomaly. Finally, 3D imaging may reduce scanning time, allowing for more efficient use of staff and equipment.

In discussing the advantages of 3D ultrasound in performing a fetal neuroscan, we must mention that only the multiplanar orthogonal display mode is used to scroll or "navigate" in the volume most of the time. By doing this, views can be obtained that are impossible (or extremely hard) to obtain by traditional transabdominal sonography (TAS) or the more advanced transvaginal transfontanelle scanning route.

The most important attribute of the 3D fetal neuroscan using the Medison Voluson-530 digital ultrasound equipment is the use of the **marker dot.** This dot is generated by the intersection of the three planes. It is freely movable by the user and marks the same spot (or technically the same voxel) within the volume. In our hands the liberal use of this **marker dot** constituted the most valuable feature of the software in the machine, without which it would be extremely hard to pinpoint the exact same structure on the three orthogonal simultaneously displayed planes. More importantly, it would be almost impossible to pinpoint the exact locations of pathological structures.

Another useful feature of 3D ultrasound equipment in fetal brain scanning is the power angio or the color Doppler mode. In selected cases, volume scans can be obtained using the power angio feature to image various main vessels in the brain. We are mainly interested in the course of the anterior cerebral artery and one of its branches: the pericallosal artery. On a median 2D image, these arteries can be seen only if one stays within the strictly median plane. If, however, the artery deviates to one side or another due to pressure from a structure (such as a cyst), the course of the displaced artery can be followed using 2D scans only with great difficulty or not at all. Using the 3D volume to trace the artery with the power angio mode, one can relatively easily follow the deviant course of any artery by maneuvering the **marker dot.**

In general, the limitations of 3D ultrasound are few. It has a relatively long learning curve.[3] A drawback of surface rendering is that, as with 2D ultrasound, it is difficult to obtain a good image in pregnant patients who are obese or with oligohydramnios. Other factors that can compromise image quality include fetal position, a fetal hand over the fetal face, or a fetal face too close to the anterior placenta. Some of these limitations can be overcome by using the **electronic scalpel** or the **electronic eraser** to eliminate structures that are not desired or that block the target structure. The special software program enables surface tracking within the volume thus creating a "clean" 3D image. Fetal motion may preclude the acquisition of a good 3D volume making it necessary to obtain additional volumes. This may not be a problem once acquisition time approaches real time.

The 'sine qua non' for a good 3D image is to generate good quality 2D pictures on good ultrasound machines. Finally, 3D ultrasonography is more expensive than 2D imaging; at least for now its use is limited by its availability and by financial aspects. However, respectable ultrasound laboratories and hospital centers probably will include a 3D study in the overall cost of a malformation work-up.

The limitations of using 3D during a fetal neuroscan are few. A high-frequency transvaginal ultrasound probe produces better images with higher resolution. The fetus must be in vertex presentation to perform a transvaginal transfontanelle neuroscan. A breech presentation will generally preclude acquisition of a good set of volume data. A

transabdominal volume acquisition should always be tried; however, in our experience, this will rarely yield good quality and diagnostic images. At times external version of the fetus into vertex presentation is warranted, especially in fetuses with strong suspicion of a brain anomaly. Another limiting factor is the rare case of craniosynostosis. The early fusion of the sutures limits easy scanning access to the brain.

As gestation advances, the best way to obtain 3D images of the fetal vertebral column is by using the transabdominal ultrasound probes.

The biggest obstacles to the widespread use of 3D are: lack of equipment and operator inexperience and/or the lack of knowledge regarding the procedure. These can be overcome by first becoming familiar with the developmental fetal neuroanatomy, then with the fetal neuroscan, and finally, with the 3D scanning technique and its literature. We are confident that in the near future, most top-of-the-line ultrasound machines will feature the 3D scanning option.

TECHNIQUE OF THE THREE-DIMENSIONAL FETAL NEUROSCAN

All patients should first undergo fetal neurosonography using the transabdominal and/or the transvaginal 2D scanning approach. The technique is extensively described in Chapter 2 as well as in several articles in the literature.[4-7] After identification of the anterior fontanelle or the superior sagittal sinus, an adequate 2D transvaginal picture of the fetal brain is obtained. The 3D volume acquisition is then started. The fetal head should be gently manipulated and controlled by the examiner's free hand. Once the ultrasound beam has been aligned with the longitudinal axis of the fetal brain through the anterior fontanelle or the sagittal suture and a clear and diagnostically good 2D image of the fetal brain is seen, a volume scan of the brain can be obtained by adjusting the size of the region of interest in the x and the y planes (Fig. 9–2) to generate and by using the sweep mode of the ultrasound machine. A second volume with the fetal head in the short axis should also be obtained by rotating the probe 90 degrees from the median section of the fetal brain. Care should be given to the orientation of the images. A description of this process is given in Chapter 14. The process is similar using the transvaginal probe; however, by transvaginal scanning (TVS) it is hard to "see" the orientation of the fontanelle and one has to rely on finding which way the face is oriented. This is to ensure the acquisition of a techni-

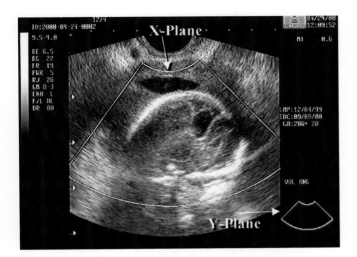

Figure 9–2. During the three-dimensional volume acquisition the first step is to select the region of interest. The task is to fit the fetal head into the box within which the data points will be used for reformatting and reslicing. The *x* and *y* planes can be made larger and smaller and moved in any desired position on this Medison 530 Voluscan machine's monitor.

cally good volume. The volume should then be processed as follows.

- The three boxes containing the orthogonal displays are called box 'A' (upper left), box 'B' (upper right), box 'C' (lower left), and box 'D' (lower right). This arrangement refers to the display of the Medison Voluson 530 machine (Figs. 9–3 through 9–5).
- Box 'B' should display the fetal head in the sagittal plane when the fetus "looks" to the left of the screen. This way, in box 'A' the right and left sides will be displayed as in traditional imaging. In box 'C,' the forehead will be on the bottom (Figs. 9–3 through 9–5).
- Coronal sections of the brain should be restored and displayed in the **active box** or box 'A,' which is the upper left side of the monitor (recognizable by its rectangular frame), in which the successive coronal sections are seen scrolled from anterior to posterior. At the same time on the sagittal image in the upper right box (box 'B') of the quartered field of the monitor screen, the moving vertical line displays the level at which the picture in box 'A'; is seen (Fig. 9–3).
- By transferring the **active box** to the sagittal image (box 'B') of the upper right

side of the monitor, it is possible to view all sagittal sections from side-to-side (temporal-to-temporal) following the planes of the sections in the upper left coronal image (Fig. 9–4 box 'A').
- Finally, moving the **active box** to the lower left image (box 'C'), we obtain successive horizontal (axial) views of the brain from the base of the skull to the "top-of-the-head" by following the changing planes, which are simultaneously moving in boxes 'A' and 'B' (Fig. 9–5).
- In box 'D,' the orientation of the volume and the scanning planes are represented.

THE THREE-HORN VIEW

One of the tasks of the fetal neuroscan is to study the lateral ventricles. The traditional lateral ventricular measurement is performed by measuring the atrium (or body) of the lateral ventricle in the horizontal plane.[4,5] Other kinds of measurements of the ventricular system using transabdominal (TAS)[6–8] and transvaginal scanning techniques have been previously published.[14]

The posterior horn is the first to change in size and shape during progressive developing ventriculomegaly. The anterior horn is the last to dilate.[9,10] Normally, the anterior horn is large before 14 weeks and narrows progressively at or after 20 to 22 weeks. The inferior horn is either barely visible or not visible earlier in pregnancy.

Our observations lead us to believe that the "classical" measurement of the lateral ventricular body in the horizontal plane cannot represent the dynamic and progressive change in shape and size occurring in all three horns. We, therefore, looked for a single scanning plane to see and measure all three horns of both lateral ventricles on one image. This scanning plane was termed the three-horn view (3HV).

The three-horn view is easy to obtain using both the traditional 2D as well as the 3D transvaginal transfontanelle approach. It takes somewhat longer to obtain both the left and the right views by 2D than by the 3D method. After obtaining a technically good 3D volume of the fetal brain, it takes only several minutes to perform the necessary measurements on the reconstructed 3HV.

Based on the anatomy of the brain, it is important to remember that the lateral ventricles are not oriented in perfect sagittal or coronal planes but are oriented obliquely. On the horizontal sections, the

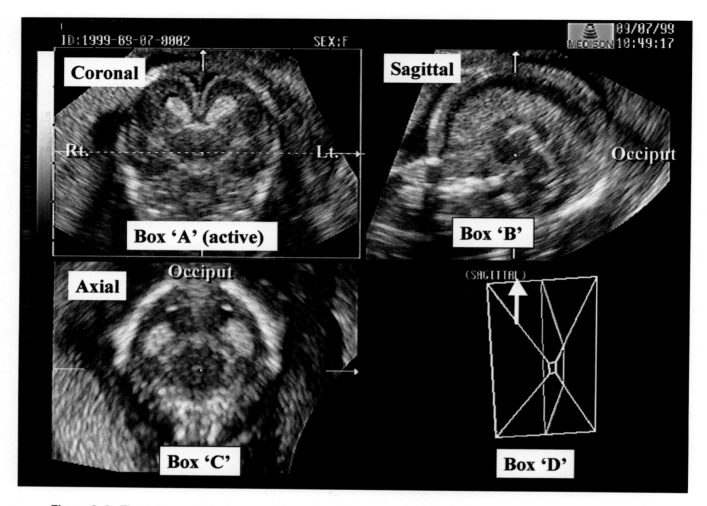

Figure 9–3. The orthogonal display. Once the volume is acquired and stored in a Cartesian system, it is displayed on the monitor. Using the agreed upon positioning controls, the following is the basic orientation of the cranium and the brain. *Box 'A'* contains all coronal views. In this picture box 'A' is the **active box** and it is bordered by a square around it. Fetal right is on the left of the picture. *Box 'B'* contains the sagittal planes, in this case the median plane is seen. The coronal view in the active box 'A' is generated using the plane across the white arrow under box 'B.' The fetus faces the left. *Box 'C'* contains the axial (horizontal) views. This view is generated using the plane across the horizontal dotted line in box 'A.' The occiput is marked. *Box 'D'* may contain the orientation of the plane seen in 'B.' It also may display the rendered picture once the rendering mode is activated.

distance between the anterior horns is smaller than the distance between the posterior horns. The distance between the inferior horns is even larger. The coronal sections are the same. This is evident on the line drawing in Figure 2–45, Chapter 2. The three-horn plane is divergent from anterior to posterior, and in the sagittal and the coronal planes, is not part of the classical, conventional, and scanning planes. It is easy to create such a "hybrid" plane (through the three horns) by manipulating the 3D volume scan.

A simultaneous three-horn view can be accomplished by the following.

1. Placing the coronal plane (as before) in the upper left (box 'A'), the sagittal (median) plane in the upper right (box 'B') and the axial (horizontal) plane in the lower left (box 'C') (Fig. 9–6A).
2. Placing the **active box** on box 'A' and rotating in the Y axis to image the right lateral ventricle. During this rotation, the cross section of the sagittal sinus should move to the right (Figure 9–6B).
3. Activating box 'B' and using the main **section control knob.** Using this control, the sagittal plane in box 'A' is moved

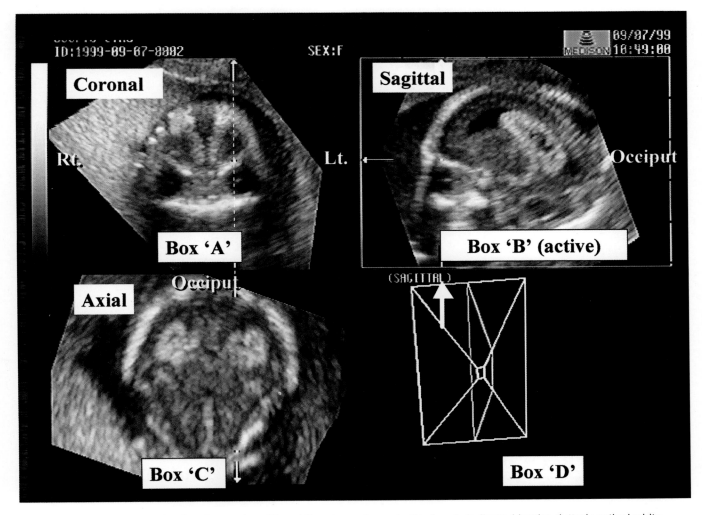

Figure 9–4. The active box is now box 'B' and the plane shown in this box is indicated by the dotted vertical white line box 'A.'

toward the right of the screen and placed on the left lateral ventricle. The left lateral ventricle is kept in the vertical position in box 'C.' The three-horn view appears in box 'B' (Fig. 9–6B). The same steps must be followed in the opposite direction to see the right three-horn view (Fig. 9–6C and D).

The three horns should be considered abnormal if on the three-horn view:

a. *The anterior horn height* is in excess of 8.7 mm at 14 weeks and 6.9 mm at 40 weeks, which represents the 95th percentile for these measurements (Chap. 3, Table 3–32);

b. *The posterior horn height* is larger than 11 mm at 14 weeks and 14 mm at 39 weeks, which represents the 95th percentile for these measurements (Chap. 3, Table 3–34);

c. The posterior horn measurement from the *posterior tip of the thalamus to the posterior tip of the horn* is in excess of 2.6 mm at 14 weeks to 3.4 mm at 40 weeks, which represents the 95th percentile for this measurement (Chap. 3, Table 3–35); and/or

d. *The inferior horn* is obvious to any degree.

It is redundant to obtain the 3HV of the fetal brain where there is major pathology and the diagnosis or the prognosis is obvious. However, in cases where borderline ventriculomegaly (a frequently used term with a variety of definitions and prognoses) or an incipient and mild ventriculomegaly is

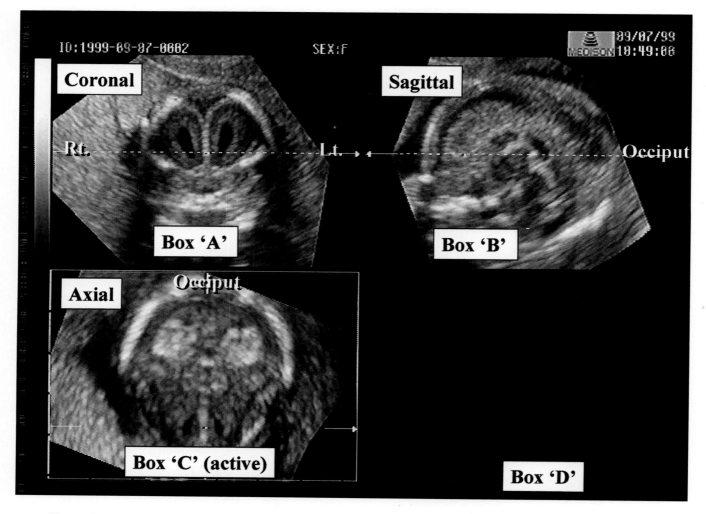

Figure 9–5. The active box is transferred to box 'C' and the picture seen in this box is generated along the level of the horizontal dotted white line in boxes 'A' and 'B.'

seen, the 3HV may present an objective measure of the severity. If serial observations are necessary to follow ventricle size, using the 3HV is an objective way to evaluate the size as a function of time.

Even the smallest dilatation of the inferior horn is considered by us the most reliable sign of lateral ventriculomegaly. In a normal fetal brain scan after 14 to 16 weeks one should not see an open inferior horn on the 2D Oblique–1 plane or the 3D three-horn view!

Using the 3HV makes it possible to compare objectively the appearance and the size of the ventricular horns over time or as a single observation. Another use of the 3HV may lie in the recognition of colpocephaly. Colpocephaly, a pathological and persistent dilatation of the posterior horn, has frequent associations with agenesis of the corpus callosum and other syndromes affecting the midbrain, such as obstruction of the aqueduct.[11] Some believe that not all cases of colpocephaly are a result of pressure related anomalies but may be a result of an error in morphogenesis.[12]

Using computed tomography (CT), Heinz and coworkers[13] were able to distinguish between obstructive and atrophic dilatation of the lateral ventricles in 92 infants and children using CT imaging. Obstructive dilatations showed a much larger measurement of the inferior and anterior horns than the posterior horn. However, in cases of atrophic dilatation, colpocephaly was more prominent. It seems logical to employ the 3HV to determine the relative dilatation of the anterior, posterior, and inferior horns and their deviation from normal in order to separate the above mentioned obstructive and atrophic entities.

The 3HV can be used to compare the size and shape of the left lateral ventricle to the right lateral ventricles in the same fetus as seen in Figure 9–9c.

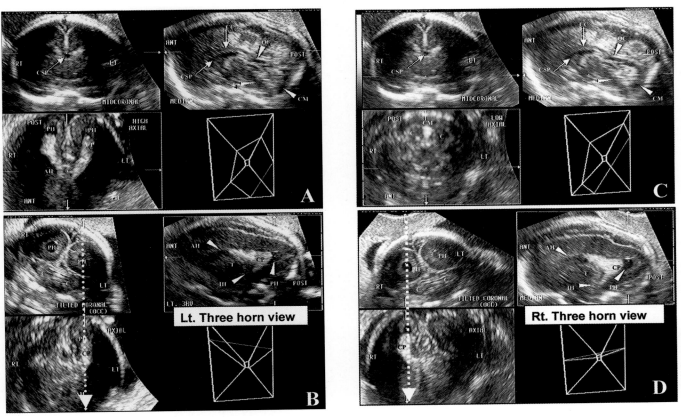

Figure 9–6. The three-horn views. **A.** To generate the left three-horn view first the desired coronal and axial planes are selected. Box 'B' contains the median plane. **B.** The coronal plane in box 'A' is titled clockwise. The active box is transferred to box 'B.' The line of the section (*dotted vertical line with arrow* through box 'A' and 'C') has to be placed to traverse the left lateral ventricle. The left three-horn view is seen in box 'B.' CSP, Cavum septi pellucidi; CC, corpus callosum; QC, corpora quadrigemina; U, fourth ventricle; AH, anterior horn; PH, posterior horn; IH, inferior horn; CP, choroid plexus; C, cerebellum. **C.** To obtain the right three horn view, the first step is identical to that of obtaining the left three-horn view. **D.** The coronal planes in box 'A' is now tilted counter-clockwise. The active box is transferred to box 'B.' The line of the section (*dotted vertical line*) has to transect the right lateral ventricle. The right three-horn view is seen in box 'B.'

Although minimal asymmetry between the lateral ventricles may exist,[14–16] precise measurements of the size of the left and right lateral ventricles in cases of lateral ventricular asymmetry contributed to the identification of pathological unilateral dilatation.[17] Objective measuring of the lateral ventricles utilizing the left and the right 3HV will probably add to our understanding of this apparently normal variant.

DIFFERENCES BETWEEN THE TWO-DIMENSIONAL AND THREE-DIMENSIONAL FETAL BRAIN STUDIES

Before addressing the differences between the two techniques associated with the fetal neuroscan, it is important to review the development of fetal brain ultrasound scanning. First, the fetal brain was imaged by conventional transabdominal scanning.

Later, the transvaginal transfontanelle approach was developed, which emulates the neonatal neuroscan and applies it to fetal brain imaging.[18–20]

The planes and sections of the transvaginal fetal neuroscan yield sequential coronal and sagittal "slices" of the fetal brain.[7] It is possible to mentally recreate the three-dimensional anatomy of the fetal brain by using these consecutive "slices." This is what the imaging specialists do: mentally recreate three-dimensional structures based upon sequential two-dimensional images. However, using 3D technology, volume acquisition and reslicing the volume in any desired plane present clear differences and advantages.

The main differences between 2D and 3D studies are the following.

1. During a transvaginal study, transfontanelle examination of the axial section

can be reconstructed only by using the 3D technique. This is a distinct advantage because the axial section is rarely seen with 2D transvaginal scanning. However, the images of the axial sections seem to be somewhat less sharp than those of the coronal and sagittal sections, especially as the gestational age increases. This is because, in recreating the axial plane, the computer uses a larger number of artificially inserted average points between the divergent planes.

2. The sections recreated from the 3D volume are *parallel* to each other and not *radiating* from a common point (the fontanelle) as is the case of conventional 2D transvaginal transfontanelle neurosonography. This makes the 3D scanning of the fetal brain similar to conventional imaging using CT and MRI. However, 3D ultrasound images will definitely differ somewhat from the neonatal 2D ultrasound images obtained by the transfontanelle scanning method. It would be advantageous to standardize the prenatal and neonatal neuroscans by using the 3D ultrasound imaging methods both in the prenatal and neonatal period (see Chap. 14).

3. When 3D volumes are examined the posterior fossa is probably seen better in the coronal and the sagittal sections. In addition, by scanning through the *posterior fontanelle,* or the *posterior section of the sagittal suture,* the image of the posterior fossa is much clearer (Fig. 9–7).

4. When 2D studies are compared to 3D studies, the main advantage of navigating within-the-volumes is the ability to follow the **marker dot.** The **marker dot** indicates the same anatomical spot on all three orthogonal planes. By placing this dot on various normal (or abnormal) structures, it is possible to know their exact location.

5. Another difference between 2D and 3D fetal brain imaging is the use of the preselected planes and sections.[5] Using the 2D transfontanelle approach, we arbitrarily decided on "coronal" and "sagittal" sections that we felt were representative of the 2D brain scan. These predetermined sections were felt to be important because "snapshots" of the fe-

tal brain in the "coronal" and in the "sagittal" plane had to be taken on hard copies for subsequent "reconstruction" of the anatomy or the location of the pathology. Using the 3D volume scan, these sections could easily be placed at the level of predetermined anatomic structures, as we did when using the 2D transvaginal fetal neuroscan. However, because it is so easy to navigate within the volume and to scroll at will through the sections in all three planes, there maybe little need to have predetermined standard 3D sections. This seems to be a distinct advantage of multiplanar imaging.

6. Another advantage of 3D multiplanar imaging using the orthogonal display is the ease with which any existing pathology can be conveyed to the surgeon, pediatric neurologist, or neurosurgeon. Having experienced the customary approach of the neurologist's and neurosurgeon's in the past it was astounding to see the change in approach to discussing the case with the parents after they were presented with a volume scan and the physicians demonstrated the multiplanar navigation within the volume. The parents' understanding of the pathology was better and faster. The physicians were able to provide more focused and precise postnatal management and counseling based on the objective evaluation of the pathology.

NORMAL FETAL NEURO-ANATOMY BY THREE-DIMENSIONAL ULTRASOUND

The first attempts to obtain a 3D ultrasound image of the embryonic brain or primitive brain cavities were made by Blaas and colleagues in Trondheim, Norway.[21–24] Some of the anatomic pictures were presented and discussed in Chapter 2. Their study was preformed using a special Tomtec 3D transvaginal annular array mechanical ultrasound probe with a main frequency of 7 MHz and a narrow focus rendered by the annular crystal array to obtain high-resolution pictures. Analyzing the sequential sections, this group was the first to publish neuromorphometic data on live embryos.[9]

In France, Dr. Benoit (unpublished communication) recorded exceptional 3D images of embryos and late first trimester fetal brain using the Medison transvaginal ultrasound probe.

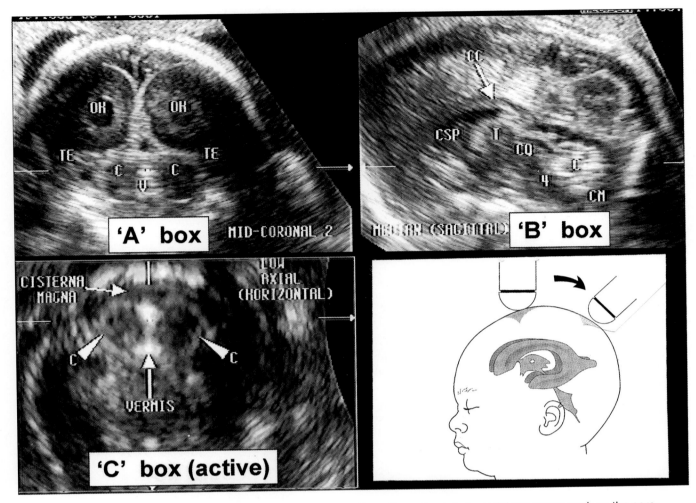

Figure 9–7. Viewing the structures in the posterior fossa. Sometimes, the infratentorial structures such as the cerebellum (C), the vermis (V), the fourth ventricle (4), and the cisterna magna (CM) are blurred. If so, the following should be attempted using the abdominally placed hand. Maneuvering the head, the transvaginal probe should be slid posteriorly along the sagittal suture as close as possible to the smaller posterior fontanelle *(line drawing).* Being closer to the posterior fossa may improve picture quality.

Our impression is that at this point in early gestation (i.e., up to about 12 postmenstrual weeks), the brain can probably be scanned better using a high-resolution transvaginal probe and top-of-the-line ultrasound machines than with the existing 3D equipment.[25]

Currently available 3D ultrasound transvaginal probes produce diagnostic quality volume scans at or after 14 to 15 postmenstrual weeks.

Figure 9–8 demonstrates the ability of transvaginal transfontanelle 3D imaging at 16 postmenstrual weeks and 2 days.

Before starting to scroll up and down, back and forth, and from side-to-side in the acquired volume, one has to remember that the number of possibilities is virtually endless. However using five to seven

(maximum eight) continuous coronal, three sagittal, and three axial sections, it is possible to get an excellent impression about the anatomy of the brain. This can be done in less than five minutes after the perfect orientation of the volume was achieved. What is left to do is examine the anatomy in the active boxes. Figure 9–8 A, B, and C, demonstrates the subsequent *coronal planes* from anterior to posterior depicting only the active boxes (boxes 'A') pasted side to side for easier comprehension.

The right and left parasagittal planes are shown on Figure 9–8D as they appear in the active box (box 'B'). The anterior and the posterior horns, the choroid plexus, and the median plane are also demonstrated. Note that on the median plane the corpus callosum is not seen since only a small

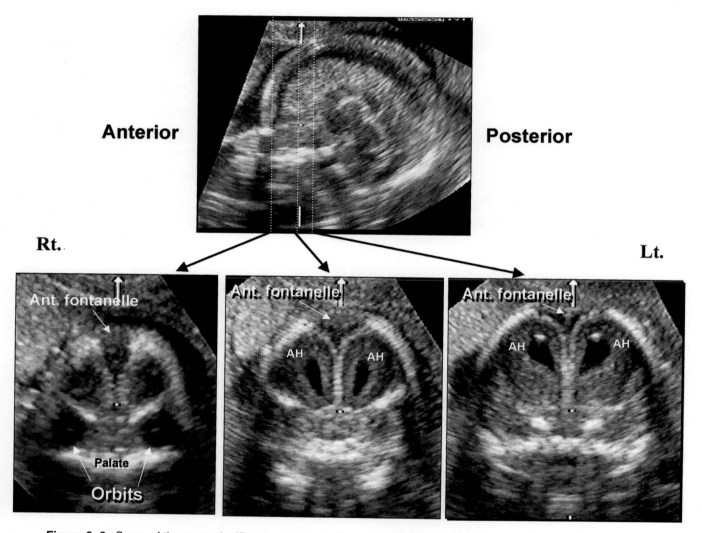

Figure 9–8. Some of the more significant coronal, sagittal, and axial planes in a 16 postmenstrual weeks fetus obtained through the anterior fontanelle using a transvaginal ultrasound probe are shown. **A.** Three anterior coronal planes across the vertical white lines in the upper sagittal image are shown. AH, Anterior horns.

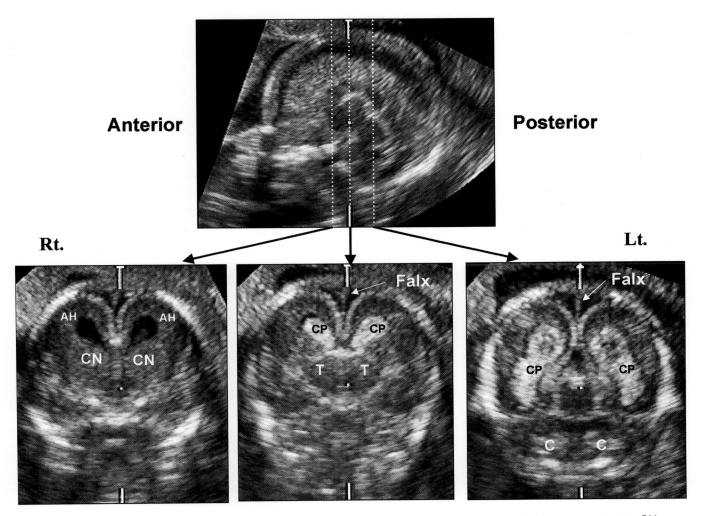

Figure 9–8. B. Three midcoronal planes across the vertical white lines in the upper, sagittal image are shown. CN, Caudate nucleus; T, thalamus; CP, choroid plexus, C, cerebellum.

Anterior   **Posterior**

Rt.   **Lt.**

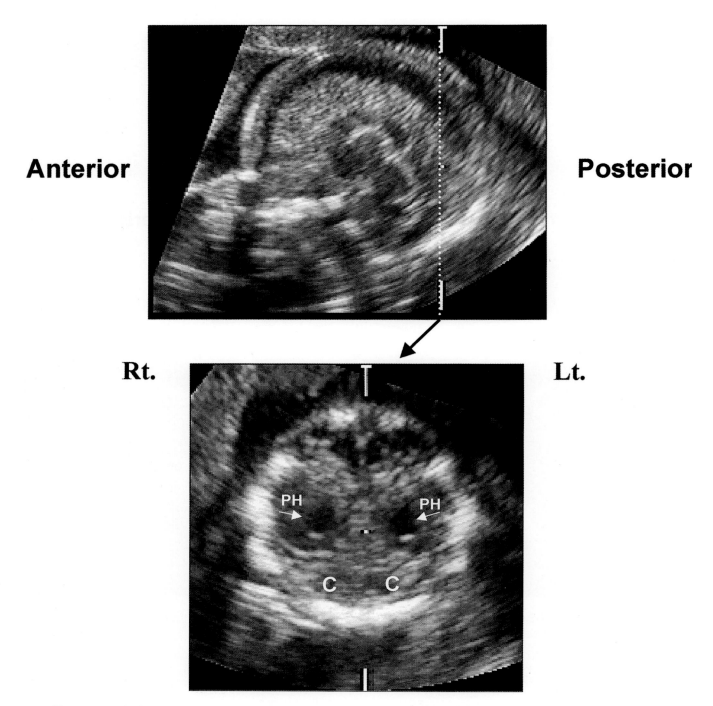

Figure 9–8. C. One posterior coronal plane across the white line in the upper, sagittal image is shown. PH, Posterior horn; C, cerebellum.

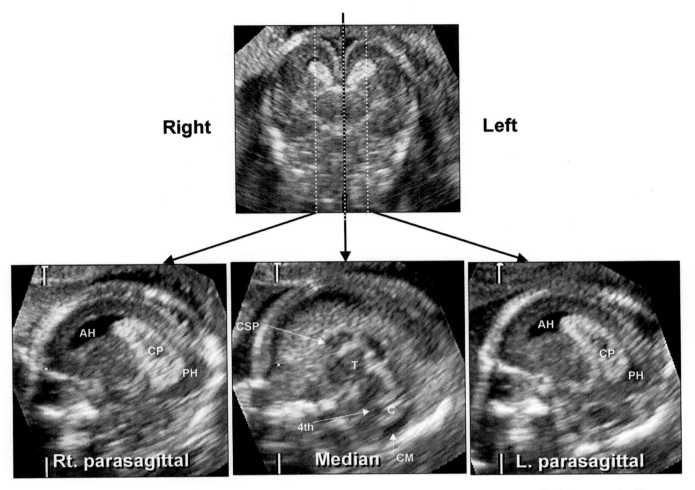

Figure 9–8. D. Three sagittal images, across a right parasagittal, a median, and a left parasagittal plane marked by the vertical white lines in the upper, coronal image are shown. AH, Anterior horn; CP, choroid plexus; PH, posterior horn; T, thalamus; C, the vermis of the cerebellum, 4th, fourth ventricle; CM, cisterna cerebello-medullaris (magna).

portion of the genu corporis callosi is formed at 16 weeks. On the two parasagittal planes that cross the choroid plexus only the anterior and the posterior horns are seen. The inferior horns, found more laterally in the temporal direction, are not included in this plane. The three axial planes in Figure 9–8E created empirically at the levels shown demonstrate the normal anatomy. On this plane, it is important to observe the lateral ventricles.

All those who are interested in learning and understanding fetal neuroanatomy must realize that the anatomy and the structural interrelationships change continuously during the pregnancy. It is mandatory that the sonologist, sonographer, and the perinatologist understand three-dimensional normal neuroanatomy. This can be achieved by reading basic brain anatomy books. Only if the normal brain

anatomy and the normal variants are understood can we get one step closer diagnosing brain pathology.

Once the brain volume is scrutinized in the three orthogonal planes, other artificially generated sections and planes can be generated at will. One set of such artificial planes is the 3HV mentioned earlier and demonstrated in Figure 9–6.

Another example of a normal 3D transvaginal neuroscan is shown in Figure 9–10. This depicts the brain of a fetus at 22 postmenstrual weeks. It is important to recognize normal brain anatomy at this age as most structural fetal evaluations are performed at 20 to 22 postmenstrual weeks. Also, the midbrain and corpus callosum are well developed and can be easily seen at this age. Performing a 3D volume scan of the fetus at this gestational age, particularly if an anomaly is suspected or has to be

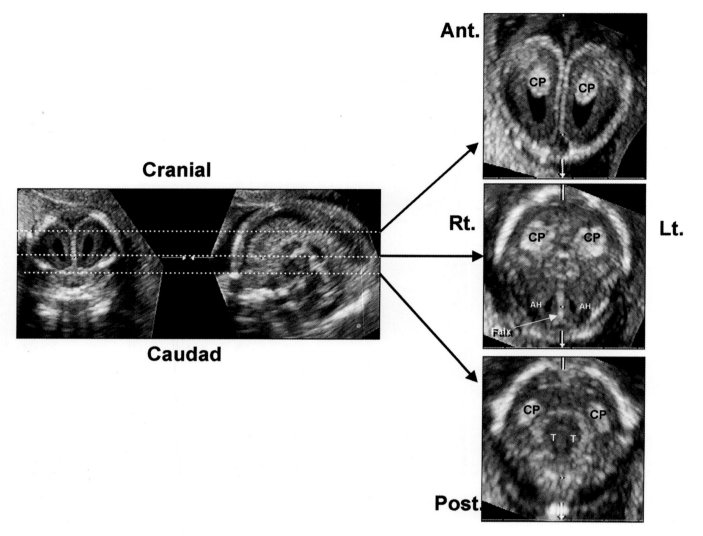

Figure 9–8. E. Three axial (horizontal) images across the three horizontal white lines in the two left pictures are shown. CP, Choroid plexus; AH, anterior horn; T, thalamus.

ruled out, is highly indicated if the equipment is available.

ABNORMAL FETAL NEUROPATHOLOGY BY THREE-DIMENSIONAL ULTRASOUND

It would be counterproductive to duplicate every single malformation of the fetal brain using the 3D technique. However, we will present several typical and more frequent anomalies or variants of normal to illustrate the power of this imaging modality.

Agenesis of the Corpus Callosum (ACC)

Since many fetal brain pathologies are present with symmetric ventriculomegaly, it is of utmost importance to scrupulously study every such case to de-

tect the underlying cause, one of which may be pathology of the corpus callosum. Partial or total agenesis may ultimately lead to dilatation of the lateral ventricles. Figure 9–9 illustrates a partial agenesis of the corpus callosum. In such cases, a small anterior portion of the genu corporis callosi as well as a small cavum septi pellucidi may be seen. Use of color or power Doppler is helpful to detect the anterior portion (but not the entire) pericallosal artery branching off the anterior cerebral artery (Fig. 9–9B inset). Inspecting the anatomic site of the corpus callosum, the pericallosal artery, and the cavum septi pellucidi on the median plane and detecting their absence is probably the only direct site-specific finding to enable the diagnosis of ACC. All the other sonographic signs of ACC described as follows are

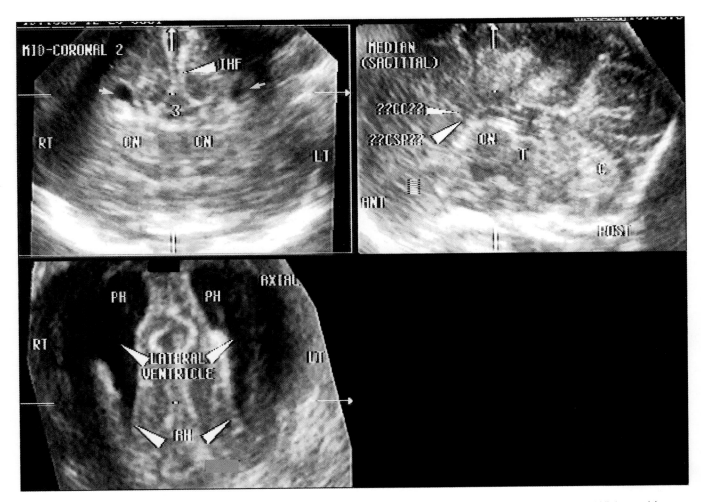

Figure 9–9. Agenesis of the corpus callosum at 22 postmenstrual weeks. **A.** The upper left box (box 'A') is a mid-coronal section showing the laterally displaced anterior horns *(small arrows),* the upward displaced third ventricle (3). Box 'B,' the upper left box, demonstrates that the cavum septi pellucidi and the corpus callosum are missing. The lower left box (box 'C') obtained at the level of the lateral ventricles clearly demonstrates the dilatation of the posterior horn (PH) and the tear drop shaped ventricles. IHF, Interhemispheric fissure; AH, anterior horn; CN, caudate nucleus; CC, corpus callosum; CSP, cavum septi pellucidi; T, thalamus; C, cerebellum).

indirect signs resulting from the missing corpus callosum.

The typical "sunburst" pattern of the gyri and sulci are seen on the median plane while the mid-coronal sections demonstrate the widely displaced and upward pointing anterior horns of the lateral ventricles. On the same plane, the upward displaced third ventricle may also become visible. On the simultaneously displayed axial planes, it is possible to scroll up and down to reveal bilateral colpocephaly, a characteristic of this pathological entity. The pathognomonic teardrop shaped lateral ventricles with dilated posterior horns are also seen in this plane. On the 3HV (Fig. 9–9C), the entire dilated lateral ventricular system is evident with the overly dilated posterior horn (colpocephaly).

Another case, in which the initial diagnosis of only ventriculomegaly/hydrocephaly was made, is seen in Figure 9–10. Although the hydrocephaly and the colpocephaly are clearly seen on the coronal and the axial images respectively, only the median plane reveals the true diagnosis. On this plane the short, small, and undeveloped corpus callosum is seen above an equally small and underdeveloped cavum septi pellucidi. On the 3HV (Fig. 9–10C), all three horns of the lateral ventricle appear extremely dilated. The colpocephaly is better seen on the axial planes.

Figure 9–9B shows the typical use of 3D color Doppler. After the power Doppler was turned on, a 3D volume was acquired concentrating only on the area of the corpus callosum. Clearly, only the first

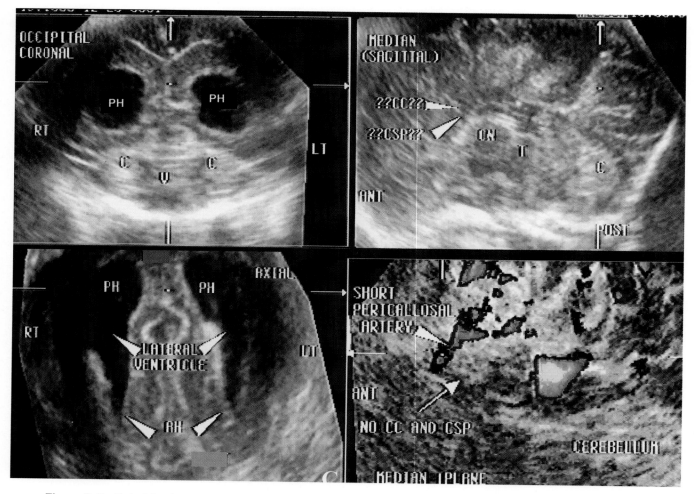

Figure 9–9. B. In this picture, box 'A' represents a posterior coronal plane showing the dilated posterior horns (PH). Box 'B' and 'C' are identical to those on panel **A.** Box 'D' (lower right) is an insert: trial to detect the pericallosal artery was made. Only the incipient 1.5 cm of this artery is seen, confirming the fact that the corpus callosum is missing. V, Vermis; C, cerebellum.

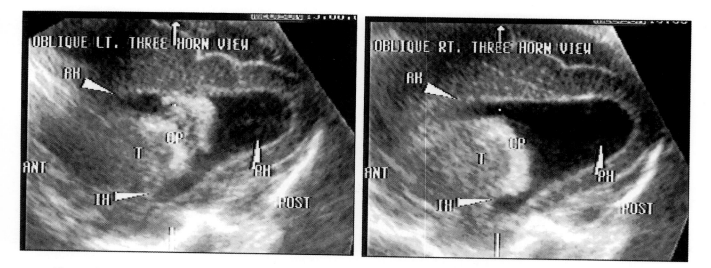

Figure 9–9. C. The left and the right three horn views are shown. Note that in both the posterior horns (PH) are dilated. In addition, the inferior horns (IH) are open or, in other words, dilated. AH, Anterior horn; T, thalamus; CP, choroid plexus.

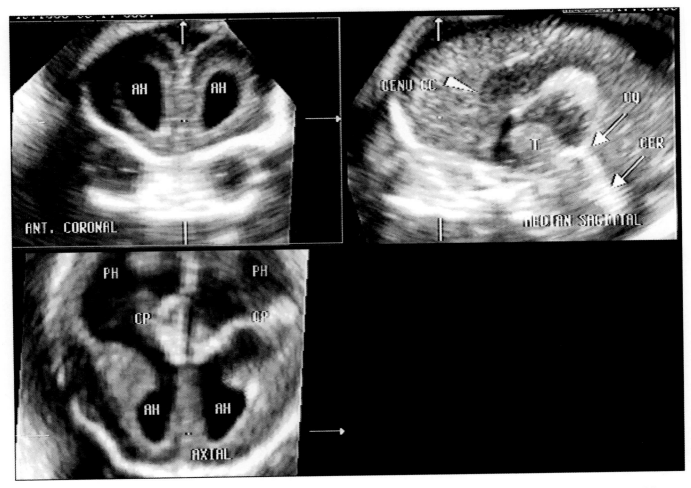

Figure 9–10. Partial agenesis of the corpus callosum with significant ventriculomegaly and colpocephaly at 23 postmenstrual weeks. **A.** In box 'A' an anterior coronal plane is depicted. Box 'B' is the median plane showing only the knee of the corpus callosum (CC). Box 'C' is a horizontal plane demonstrating the severe dilatation of the posterior horns termed colpocephaly (PH). CP, Choroid plexus; AH, anterior horn; T, thalamus; CQ, corpora quadrigemina; CER, cerebellum.

segment of the pericallosal artery was seen at 20 postmenstrual weeks, confirming the diagnosis of (partial) agenesis of the corpus callosum.

Because cephalocele is a relatively frequent occurrence, exact localization and the extent of the bulging brain tissue is easily performed by the 3D scanning method (Fig. 9–11).

Arachnoid Cysts

Arachnoid cysts can be located in various parts of the brain; at its surface, between the lobes, and even in the depth of the brain originating at various sites (see Chap. 4). Utilization of three-dimensional ultrasound was important in a case of quadrigeminal plate arachnoid cyst (Fig. 9–12 A and B). The 3D gray scale localized the cyst slightly off the median plane (Fig. 9–15A). Color 3D enabled the tracking of

the pericallosal artery confirming the present but laterally displaced corpus callosum (Fig. 9–12 C and D). The finding of the corpus callosum pushed to one side by the arachnoid cyst changed the prognosis of a poor fetal outcome to a more favorable one. If needed, a 3D rendering can also be performed (Fig. 9–12E) showing the spatial arrangement of these vessels. The 3D images and the possibility of slicing within the volume gave important clinical information to the pediatric neurosurgeon and played a practical role in patient counseling.

Three-Dimensional Imaging of the Fetal Vertebral Column

Sonographic evaluation of the fetal vertebral column is an essential part of a malformation workup. Because the spinal cord is part of the CNS and it is

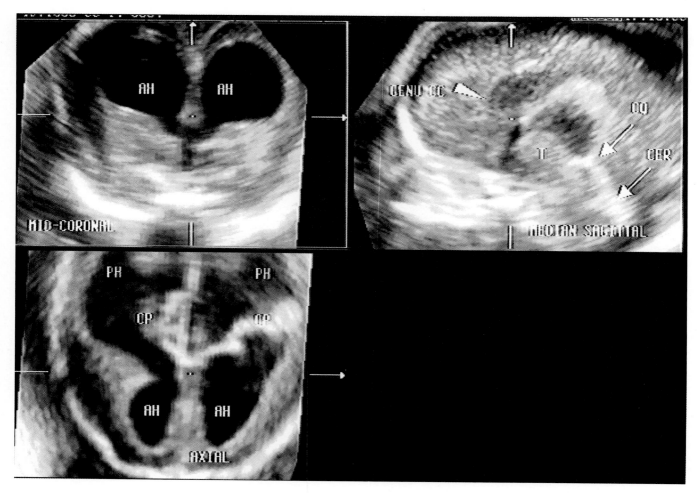

Figure 9–10. B. The only change from panel **A** is in box 'A' where a mid-coronal plane is shown. AH, Anterior horn; T, thalamus; CP, choroid plexus; PH, posterior horn.

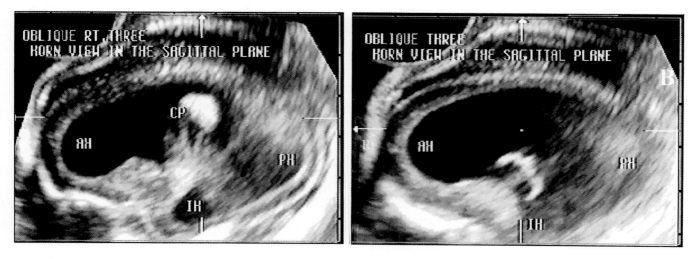

Figure 9–10. C. The left and the right three horn views are shown. All three horns, the anterior (AH), posterior (PH), and inferior horns (IH), are severely dilated. CP, Choroid plexus.

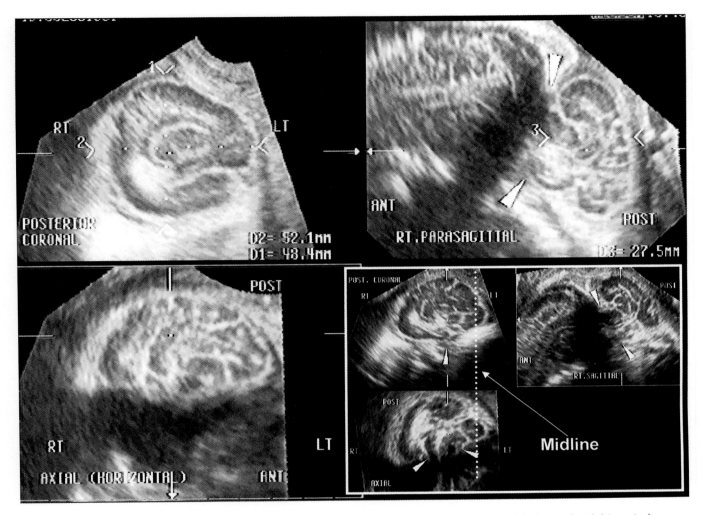

Figure 9–11. Posterior coronal (box 'A'), right parasagittal (box 'B'), and an axial (box 'C') views of a right posterior parietal encephalocele is imaged. The inset (lower right) contains the same three planes, however, the median plane (*white line*) is shown. This makes the localization of the lesion easier. The two *arrowheads* point to the gap in the calvarium through which the brain tissue protrudes.

found within the vertebral canal, it is imperative to examine the bony casing of the spinal cord. During the ultrasound scan, we use two longitudinal median and left and right paramedian sections and the horizontal sections. If feasible, a coronal section should also be generated.

On the median and the paramedian planes the vertebrae generate the appearance of two interrupted parallel lines often referred to as railroad tracks. On the horizontal (also called transverse or axial/view), the vertebrae appear as three echogenic structures (ossification centers) arranged in a triangular shape. One of them (usually the largest) is the vertebral body, the other two are the transverse processes.[26] Clinical diagnoses rely on identifying the ossification centers and assessing their appear-

ance, distances from each other, the symmetry of the transverse processes and so forth.[27]

Two-dimensional gray scale ultrasound was and continues to be used widely in the structural evaluation of fetuses from 10 to 11 postmenstrual weeks onward with excellent results.

It is not our intention to review the existing literature and textbooks on the use of 2D gray scale transvaginal and transabdominal sonography in the evaluation of the fetal vertebral column. But to concentrate the use of 3D scanning to image the fetal spine.

The basic concepts of general 3D ultrasound and 3D in obstetrics and gynecology has been covered in other textbooks.[28–30]

With the slowly spreading use of 3D ultrasound machines and the possibility of pre- and post-pro-

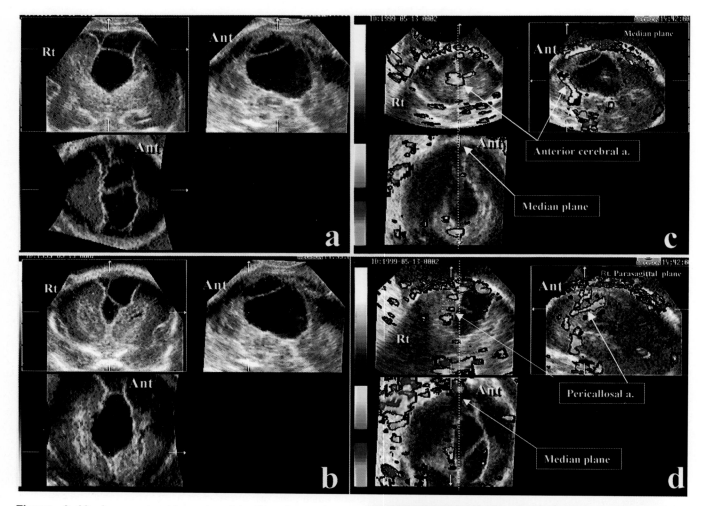

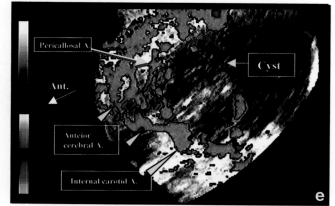

Figure 9–12. An arachnoid cyst originating from the quadrigeminal plate at 23 postmenstral weeks. **A.** The septated cyst displacing the falx to the right is shown by the coronal (box 'A'), sagittal (box 'B'), and axial (box 'C') planes. **B.** Another set of orthogonal planes were selected to study the extent of the lesion. **C.** Color Doppler study. The picture in the active box (box 'B') highlighted by the frame is generated in the median plane (*vertical dotted white line* through boxes 'A' and 'C') only the anterior cerebral artery, but no pericallosal artery is seen (the latter should be evident in this plane). **D.** The plane is moved to the right. Now the active box (box 'B') is generated in the right parasagittal plane. In this plane the pericallosal artery is clearly detected. This proves that the corpus callosum is not destroyed by the cyst. The *dotted vertical white line* was kept to mark the median plane. **E.** A three-dimensional color flow rendering of the anterior cerebral and the pericallosal arteries. The approximate place of the arachnoid cyst is marked.

cessing to emphasize bony structures, articles describing 3D volume scanning started to appear in the early 1990s.[31–34]

Toward the mid-1990s, articles devoted predominantly to scanning the fetal skeleton by 3D "x-ray" (transparency or maximum mode) appeared and made their way into the literature.[35–40] All of these included or dealt specifically with the fetal spine.

Nelson and Pretorius, pioneers of 3D ultrasound in the United States, stated that fetal vertebral bodies and ribs were identifiable on 3D sonograms that clearly showed the structural continuity of these structures as well as details of the vertebrae.[35] The same group studied the fetal spine at a mean age of 21 postmenstrual weeks in 20 normal and five pathological cases using transabdominal 3D scans. They could see the vertebral column, clavicles, scapula, and the iliac bones in the rendered images. In their opinion, it improved comprehension of complex anatomy by providing a simultaneous display of all orthogonal sectional planes.[36] A later work by Johnson and coworkers[37] completed a three-dimensional study of the fetal spine looking at 28 fetuses (16 normal and 12 abnormal). Fifteen of the 16 normal fetal spines were visualized completely. In the cases of neural tube defects, 3D was able to better identify the level of the lesion in three out of the five cases. Scoliosis was easily recognized on the rendered image. Their conclusion, among others, was that the ability to review volume data using 3D techniques not available in 2D ultrasound may enable the observers to evaluate the extent of neural tube defects with more accuracy.

In Germany, Schild and colleagues[38] used 3D ultrasound to calculate the volume of the thoracolumbar spine between 16 and 25 postmenstrual weeks. The Austrian group of the University Hospital of Vienna, who did much of the work in developing some of the first 3D ultrasound equipment, evaluated the fetal spine length between 14 and 24 postmenstrual weeks.[39]

A three-dimensional study was performed by Wallery and colleagues[40] to determine the size of the lumbar spinal canal. No clinical use was suggested.

An important additional value of 3D compared to traditional 2D evaluation of the fetal skeleton and fetal spine was echoed in studies by Garjian and coworkers[41] and by Yanagihara and Hata.[42] Both articles emphasize the ability of 3D ultrasound to review the anatomic orientation and evaluate skeletal dysplasias in conjunction with the 2D grayscale imaging.

The Technique

Transabdominal and transvaginal transducers can be used to obtain the volume. The choice of transducers depends upon the orientation of the spine and its size (e.g., age of the fetus). The volume is obtained in the usual manner and saved in the machine's computer. The next step is to rotate the spine to obtain perfect sagittal and coronal planes (Fig. 9–13 a and c). The rendered 3D image appears in box 'D.' The necessary post-processing to obtain the x-ray or transparency display is performed as a final step (Fig. 9–13 b and d).

As far as the CNS is concerned, the main effort is usually directed toward evaluating the integrity of the vertebral arches and to rule out spina bifidia aperta or occulta as well as hemivertebrae.

Spina Bifida Aperta

Once again, it is not our intention to present all pathological cases involving the vertebral column. Those having a direct or indirect bearing on the fetal CNS are adequately covered in Chapter 13.

One of the examples we show here in the case of an open spina bifidia at 22 weeks (Fig. 9–14). The volume was acquired and then displayed in the three orthogonal planes. Using the steps described previously to create a 3D rendering of the face, the vertebral column is rendered. By adjusting the level of transparency, the desired image of the lesion is obtained (Fig. 9–14b).

Hemivertebrae

Figure 9–15 illustrates the ability of the x-ray or transparency mode to study the vertebral bodies. In this case, the missing side of the vertebra is clearly visible. The same is shown in Figure 9–16, where a hemivertebra was suspected at 16 postmenstrual weeks. At this point in gestation, despite the hemivertebra, no scoliosis was seen as in the case shown in Figure 9–15. The use of the marker dot is clearly demonstrated in Figure 9–16, where it was placed on the site of the missing vertebral structure.

In summary, 3D rendering of the vertebral column using the transparency feature of the 3D machine valuable information can be added to that obtained by the 2D method.

THREE-DIMENSIONAL IMAGING OF THE FETAL FACE AND CALVARIA

A large number of anomalies of the CNS also involve the face. Table 9–1 summarizes most of these associations. It can be said with a fair amount of confidence that the shape of the head and the face are a mirror of the CNS pathology.

Sonographic imaging of the fetal face by two-dimensional gray scale is an integral part of fetal structural evaluation and is considered to be the "gold standard" in clinical use.

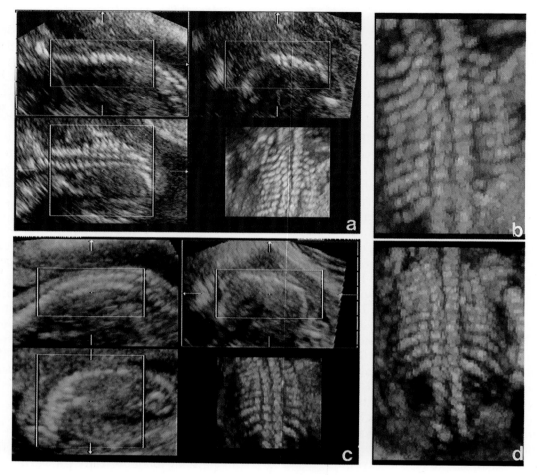

Figure 9–13. Transparency (x-ray) views of a normal fetal spine at 32 postmenstrual weeks. **A.** The volume is displayed in the orthogonal planes and a sagittal as well as an axial plane (boxes "A" and "B" are brought close to the upper horizontal line of the rendering boxes). **B.** The rendered image of the thoracic spine with the ribs. **C.** The same process is repeated for the lumbar vertebrae. **D.** The thoracic and lumbar vertebrae are seen.

A detailed discussion of ultrasonography of the fetal face is included in Chapter 6. This discussion of the 3D imaging was included to describe the technique and the potential usefulness of this emerging imaging technology. It was not intended to present all or even part of the pathologies of the face. The examples were those at hand at the writing of the chapter.

One of the first attempts to use 3D imaging of the head was done by Pretorius and Nelson,[43] who used it to depict fetal cranial sutures and fontanelles. In 1995, a string of articles appeared in the literature heralding the clinical use of 3D imaging of the fetal face.[44–51] These were the "opening arguments" presented to the readers in which the authors compared 2D and 3D imaging to produce clinically useful clear images. At that time, volume data acquisition (about 10 seconds), reconstruction of the image (about 5 sec-

onds), and surface rendering of the fetal face (2 to 10 minutes) required a relatively long time.[51] Currently, this entire process may take a fraction of the time (about 10 seconds or even less). If certain circumstances (adequate amount of amniotic fluid around the face) are present, an almost real-time surface rendering and continuous "updating" of the data points of the face is possible every 1 to 2 seconds using several commercially available machines.

One should not forget that the post-processing of the volume and the rendered surface image may require much longer time depending on each and every case and the operator's experience.

Following the first set of "basic" articles, several authors published additional articles attesting to the clinical usefulness of imaging of the fetal face by 3D ultrasound.[57,58] The diagnoses of syndromes and facial abnormalities are reported.[44–46,47,49,51–57]

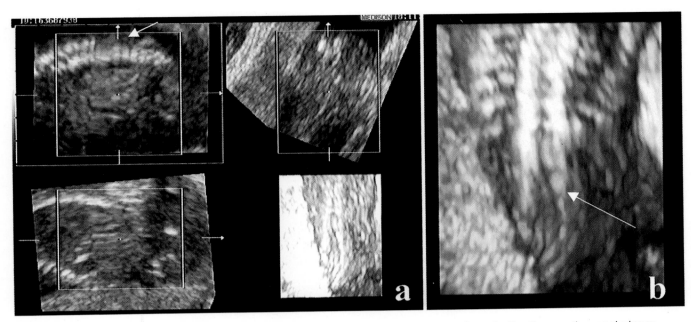

Figure 9–14. Spina bifidia at the level of L 3–4 *(arrows)*. **A.** Displaying the volume in the three orthogonal planes and rendering the area of interest. The *arrow* points to the defect. **B.** Using the transparency (x-ray) mode the defect is shown *(arrow)*.

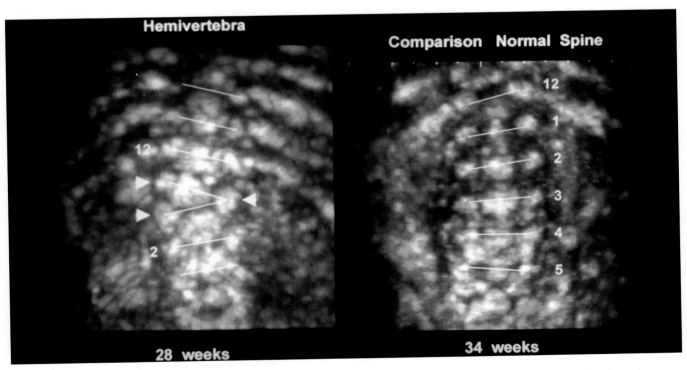

Figure 9–15. To demonstrate the ability of the 3D transparency (x-ray) display mode for imaging the fetal spine a fetus at 28 postmenstrual weeks with a hemivertebra of the L2 level is shown. The 12th rib is marked. For comparison, a normal spine at 34 postmenstrual weeks is shown. *(Courtesy of Drs. Gary Thieme and John Hobbins, Denver, Colorado.)*

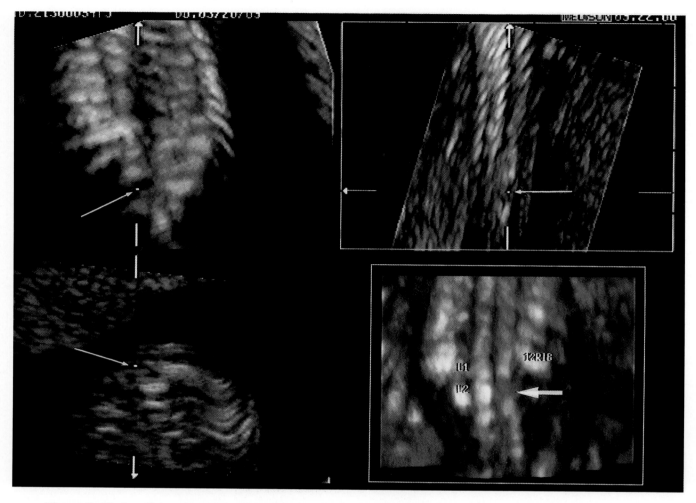

Figure 9–16. Localizing the place of a missing vertebral structure using 3D transparency mode and the **marker dot.** An isolated hemivertebra (L2) was diagnosed in this fetus *(large arrow)* at 17 postmenstrual weeks. Note that the marker dot is placed on the sonolucent spots *(arrows),* at the site of the missing vertebral structure. Box "D" is the x-ray rendering of the vertebrae.

An interesting, simple, inexpensive technique to image the fetal face has to be mentioned here. Kossoff and colleagues[57,58] suggested using a certain technique with 2D gray scale technique and an inexpensive defocusing lens attached to the transabdominal transducer. With this it is possible to obtain a 2D image of the face with a 3D effect. To obtain this, the angle of insonation between the beam and the surface to be scanned has to be equal or larger than the critical angle for a total reflection of the ultrasound beam. This 3D effect can be enhanced by rotating the probe around structures of interest.[58] The authors suggested that this simple technique can be used as a complementary method to study the surface of different fetal structures such as the face. It is clear that in the future, with

the spread of true 3D imaging, this quasi-3D technology will be mentioned as a "poor-man's" 3D, as the author once referred to it.

The Technique

The most useful fetal face display is obtained by three-dimensional surface rendering. The method is described as follows.

1. A reasonably good quality fetal profile should be obtained. If this is not possible, then a 2 to 3 cm fluid pocket in front of the face should be looked for. If the face or part of it is touching the uterine wall, a limb, or the placenta, it will be extremely hard to eliminate these

TABLE 9–1. ABNORMALITIES COMMON TO THE CENTRAL NERVOUS SYSTEM (CNS) AND THE FACE

Syndrome	CNS Abnormalities	Facial Abnormalities
Gorlin	Macrocephaly; ventriculomegaly; calcification of the falx; agenesis of the corpus callosum*	Prognathism; cleft lip and palate; frontal bossing; hypertelorism
Hydrolethalus	Ventriculomegaly; neural tube defect	Micrognathia; cleft lip and palate; low-set ears
Joubert	Dandy–Walker variant	Micrognathia
Meckel–Gruber	Ventriculomegaly; microcephaly; posterior encephalocele; cerebellar hypoplasia; agenesis of the corpus callosum; Dandy–Walker abnormalities; Arnold–Chiari malformation	Micrognathia; cleft palate; microphthalmia
Neu-Laxova	Microcephaly; lissencephaly; absent corpus callosum; hypoplastic cerebellum and cerebrum; Dandy–Walker malformation*; ventriculomegaly*	Micrognathia; hypertelorism with protruding eyes and absent lids; cataracts; microphthalmia; facial clefting*
Walker–Warburg	Microcephaly; agyria; lissencephaly; ventriculomegaly; occipital encephalocele; Dandy–Walker malformation; agenesis of the corpus callosum	Microphthalmia; cataracts; cleft lip*
Ectrodactyly ectodermal dysplasia clefting (EEC)	Semilobar holoprosencephaly*	Cleft lip with or without cleft palate; facial cleft; choanal atresia*; micrognathia*; malformed ears*
Multiple pterygium (lethal type)	Microcephaly*; ventriculomegaly*	Micrognathia; cleft palate; hypertelorism
Roberts	Microcephaly; ventriculomegaly*; craniosynstosis*; encephalocele*	Micrognathia; cleft lip; hypertelorism; microphthalmia*; cataracts
Thrombocytopenia absent radius (TAR)	Vermian hypoplasia*	Micrognathia*
Achondroplasia (heterozygous)	Megalocephaly; mild ventriculomegaly*	Frontal bossing; depressed nasal bridge
Camptomelic dysplasia	Ventriculomegaly	Cleft palate; hypertelorism; depressed nasal bridge*; micrognathia*
Chondrodysplasia punctata, rhizomelic type	Ventriculomegaly	Hypertelorism; cataracts
Majewski (Short rib polydactyly, type II)	Small cerebellar vermis*	Facial cleft
Apert (Acrocephalosyndactyly, type I)	Agenesis of the corpus callosum; mild ventriculomegaly	High forehead; flat face; hypertelorism
Crouzon (Craniofacial dysostosis, type I)	Ventriculomegaly*; agenesis of the corpus callosum	Beaked nose; micrognathia; hypertelorism or hypotelorism; cleft lip and palate*
Pfeiffer (Acrofacial dysostosis)	Ventriculomegaly*	Depressed nasal bridge; hypertelorism; choanal atresia*
Fryns	Ventriculomegaly; Dandy–Walker malformation; agenesis of the corpus callosum	Micrognathia; cleft lip and palate; broad nasal bridge; abnormal ear shape; microphthalmia*
Amniotic band sequence	Encephalocele; asymmetric anencephaly	Micrognathia; facial cleft
Arthrogryposis	Ventriculomegaly*; lissencephaly*; agenesis of the corpus callosum*; vermian agenesis*; microcephaly*	Facial defects*; cataracts*
Caudal regression	Neural tube defect*	Facial cleft*
Charge association	Mild ventriculomegaly*; Dandy–Walker variant*	Hypoplastic nose; malformed ears; micrognathia*; cleft lip and palate*; hypertelorism*; microphthalmia*

Continued.

TABLE 9–1. ABNORMALITIES COMMON TO THE CENTRAL NERVOUS SYSTEM (CNS) AND THE FACE—Cont'd

Syndrome	CNS Abnormalities	Facial Abnormalities
Holoprosencephaly sequence (alobar)	Absent inner hemispheric fissure of third ventricle and olfactory bulb; single central ventricle; fused thalami; microcephaly or macrocephaly*; dorsal cyst*	Cyclopia; hypotelorism; cebocephaly; maxillary hypoplasia or absent premaxilla with hypotelorism; cleft lip and palate
Pentalogy of cantrell	Neural tube defect*	Facial defects*
Alcohol	Microcephaly	Ear deformities; low forehead; depressed nasal bridge; micrognathia; cleft lip and palate; ophthalmic abnormalities
Aminopterin	Incomplete skull ossification; ventriculomegaly; microcephaly; neural tube defect	Micrognathia; low-set ears
Carbamazepine (Tegretol)	Meningomyelocele	Nasal hypoplasia; cleft lip; hypertelorism
Codeine	Ventriculomegaly	Facial cleft
Cortisone (hormone)	Ventriculomegaly	Cleft lip and palate
Coumadin (anticoagulant)	Encephalocele; anencephaly; spina bifida	Choanal atersia; nasal hypoplasia; depressed nasal bridge; cataracts
Ethosuximide (anticonvulsant)	Ventriculomegaly	Facial cleft
Hydantoin (anticonvulsant)	Microcephaly*; holoprosencephaly*	Hypertelorism; depressed nasal bridge
Hyperthermia	Microcephaly; neural tube defect	Facial defects
Imipramine (tranquilizer, antidepressant)	Exencephaly	Cleft palate
Quinine (antibiotic)	Ventriculomegaly	Facial defects
Radiation (large dosage)	Microcephaly; spina bifida	Facial defects
Trimethadione (anticonvulsant)	Microcephaly	Broad nasal bridge; low-set ears
Valproic acid (anticonvulsant)	Microcephaly; meningomyelocele	Low-set ears; facial cleft; depressed nasal bridge; micrognathia
Rubella	Microcephaly	Cataracts; microphthalmia
Toxoplasmosis	Ventriculomegaly; microcephaly; intracranial calcifications	Cataracts
Deletion 4P (Wolf–Hirschhorn)	Microcephaly; agenesis of the corpus callosum	Micrognathia; hypertelorism; cleft lip and palate
Deletion 11Q (Jacobsen)	Microcephaly; ventriculomegaly*; holoprosencephaly*	Hypertelorism; depressed nasal bridge; micrognathia; ear malformations
Tetrasomy 12P (Pallister–Killian)	Cerebellar hypplasia	Facial dysmorphism; hyertelorism; low-set ears
Triploidy	Ventriculomegaly; agenesis of the corpus callosum; Dandy–Walker malformation; holoprosencephaly meningomyelocele	Hypertelorism; microphthalmia; micrognathia
Trisomy 9	Microcephaly; cerebellar anomalies; ventriculomegaly; neural tube defect	Cleft lip and palate; micrognathia; microphthalmia
Trisomy 13 (Patau)	Holoprosencephaly; ventriculomegaly; enlarged cisterna magna; microcephaly; agenesis of the corpus callosum; neural tube defect	Cleft lip and palate; midface hypoplasia; cyclopia; hypotelorism; microphthalmia
Trisomy 18 (Edwards)	Agenesis of corpus callosum; choroid plexus cysts; posterior fossa abnormalities; meningomyelocele*; ventriculomegaly*	Micrognathia; low-set ears; microphthalmia; hypertelorism; lip and palate*
Trisomy 21 (Down)	Ventriculomegaly	Flat facies; small ears

*Occasionally occurring features.
From Benacerraf BR. Ultrasound of Fetal Syndromes *New York: Saunders, 1999.* pp. 358–405

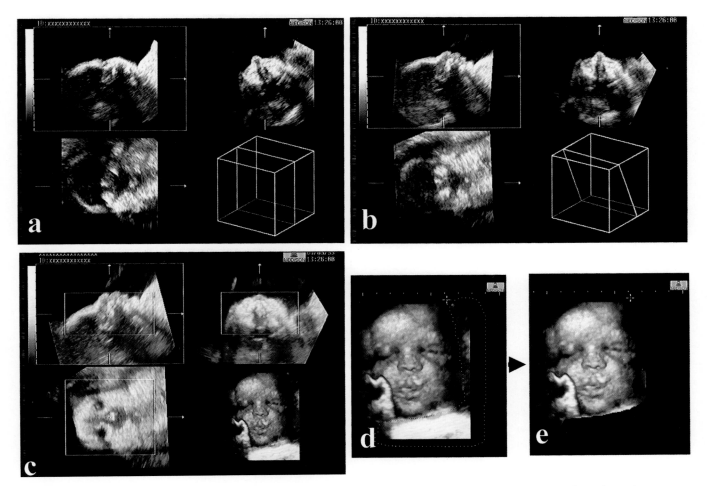

Figure 9–17. The major steps in imaging rendering and post processing a normal fetal face. **A.** The volume is acquired and displayed in the three orthogonal planes. **B.** In boxes 'A' and 'B,' the fetal profile and symmetrically oriented axial section is obtained. **C.** The rendering process begins with bringing the sagittal and the axial contours in boxes 'A' and 'B' close to the *horizontal upper* (green) *line* of the rendering boxes. In box 'D,' the face is rendered. **D.** The use of the **electronic scalpel** is demonstrated. Unwanted areas are encircled by the dotted line and the function is activated to remove these areas (the **electronic eraser** is operated the same way). **E.** The result after removing the area shown in **D.**

and produce a reasonable, clinically useful rendering. The volume acquisition is then activated, which results in a orthogonal 3D display on the monitor (Fig. 9–17A).

2. The fetal face is then rotated, tilted, and moved, into its most favorable position to be able to start the rendering process. This procedure displays the profile in 'box A' (sagittal plane), the horizontal section in 'box B' (axial plane), and a coronal plane (when important at this point) in 'box C.' The 'D box' displays the shape of the volume (Fig. 9–17B).

3. The next step is to save the region (volume) of interest in the memory of the computer in a Cartesian system. Figure 9–17C demonstrates that the region to be rendered (in this case the face) has to be positioned as close as possible to the upper horizontal (green) lines of the volume rectangles seen in boxes 'A' and 'B.' As the appropriate control key is touched, box 'D' will display the rendered face.

4. Several post-processing features are available including:

   a. An almost endless string of gray scale levels, colors, and levels of transparency.

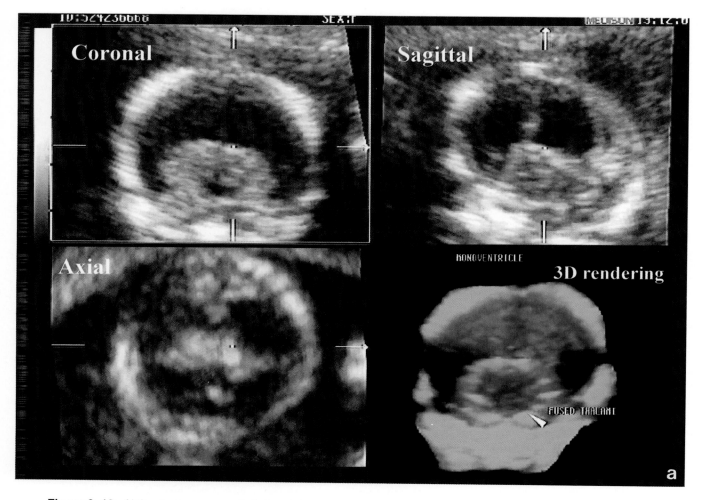

Figure 9–18. Alobar holoprosencephaly in a 17 postmenstrual week fetus. **A.** The multiplanar views with a 3D rendering demonstrating the lack of the falx and the fused thalami.

b. The **electronic scalpel** (Fig. 9–17D), which enables eliminating, or cutting off desired areas of the volume to get rid of structures (e.g., placenta, cord, a hand, etc.) that obliterate the view to the face (Fig. 9–17E).
c. The **eraser** will let the user rub off minor structures to fine tune the rendering.
5. During the process of post-processing of the rendered face, it is possible to rotate the face in any desired position.

Although the above process was described using the Medison 530 digital 3D equipment, we are confident that the volume acquisition and its processing to obtain the 3D orthogonal planes (Fig. 9–18A) strengthened the diagnosis made by 2D scans. In

addition, the desired display will be similar using other commercial equipment.

In a case of holoprosencephaly detected at 17 postmenstrual weeks, we were able to obtain a 3D rendering of the face, which clearly indicated the proboscis and the one orbit (cyclops) making the diagnosis easier (Fig. 9–18B and C). More importantly, it conveyed the notion and the severity of the anomaly to the parents, making their decision to terminate the pregnancy easier.

In another case, a tumor arising from the oral cavity was studied by 3D rendering of the face (Fig. 9–19). In this case, the tumor protruding through the mouth and displaced the tongue up and to the left. The differential diagnosis was anterior (ethmoidal) cephalocele and teratoma of the pharyngeal region. The brain scan was normal and the diagnosis of teratoma was confirmed at birth.

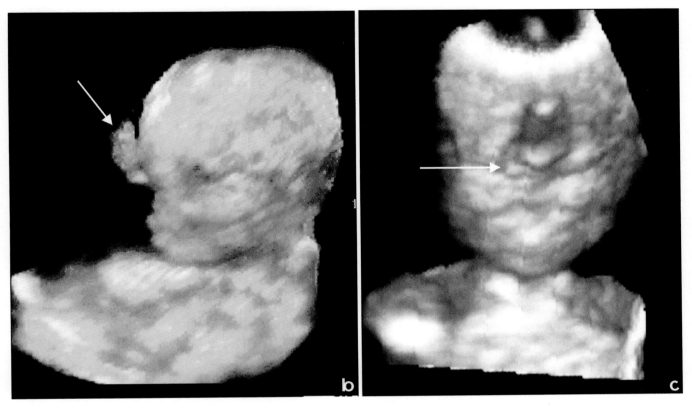

Figure 9–18. **B** and **C.** The profile and the face of the fetus with the proboscis (*arrow* in B) and the single orbit (*arrow* in C).

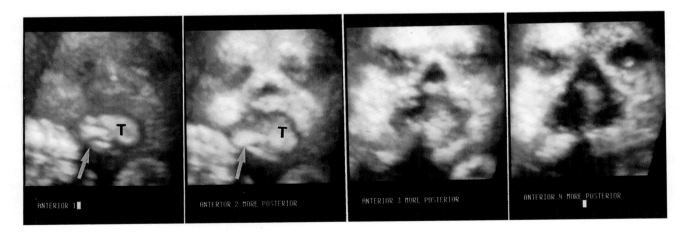

Figure 9–19. Workup of a tumor originating in the oral cavity of a fetus at 32 postmenstrual weeks. These are consecutive coronal sections. The first two on the left are showing the tongue (T) on the left and the tumor on the right *(arrows)* protruding from the mouth. The last two were directed toward depicting the palate. A defect in the palate was diagnosed. This was a benign teratoma.

SUMMARY

In summary, the present 3D imaging technology available on several commercially available ultrasound machines is acceptable and produces clinically useful rendered images. If available, this scanning modality should be employed in clinical cases where information obtained by surface rendering, multiplanar-orthogonal-imaging, and transparency mode facilitates the diagnostic process.

Additional value of using this technology in scanning the fetal brain, vertebral column, and the face are the following.

- Short acquisition time allows high patient through-put.
- The volume can be analyzed and scrutinized time and again without the need to rescan the patient.
- Several display modes are available.
- An infinite number of different planes can be generated using the multiplanar modality.
- Electronic transmittal is available.
- An unsurpassed patient counseling tool.
- An excellent teaching modality.
- Provides valuable information to consulting pediatric surgeons, plastic surgeons, neonatologists, neurologists, and neurosurgeons.

As computers become faster and smaller, miniature devices will become easier to incorporate in a larger number of machines. In the not-so-far future, 3D technology will be available on almost every ultrasound machine to serve larger and larger patient populations. Three-dimensional fetal CNS scanning should be considered the ultimate imaging modality to obtain an insight into the normal and abnormal fetal brain, vertebral column, and the face.

REFERENCES

1. Baba K, Jurkovic D. *Three-Dimensional Ultrasound in Obstetrics and Gynecology.* New York: The Parthenon Publishing Group; London and NY, 1997.
2. Nelson TR, Downey DB, Pretorius DH, Fauster A. *Three-Dimensional Ultrasound.* Philadelphia: Lippincott Williams & Wilkins 1999.
3. Platt LD, Santulli T Jr, Carlson DE, et al. Three-dimensional ultrasonography in obstetrics and gynecology: Preliminary experience. *Am J Obstet Gynecol.* 1998;178:1199–1206.
4. Denkhaus H, Winsberg F. Ultrasonic meaasurement of the fetal ventricular system. *Radiology.* 1979;131: 781–787.
5. Cardoza JD, Goldstein RB, Filly RA. Exclusion of fetal ventriculomegaly with a single measurement: The width of the lateral ventricular atrium. *Radiology.* 1988;169:711–714.
6. Goldstein I, Reece EA, Pilu G, et al. Sonographic evaluation of the normal developmental anatomy of the fetal cerebral ventricles. I: The frontal horn. *Obstet Gynecol.* 1988;72:588–592.
7. Goldstein I, Reece EA, Pilu G, et al. Sonographic evaluation of the normal developmental anatomy of the fetal cerebral ventricles. IV: The posterior horn. *Am J Perinatol.* 1990;7:79–83.
8. Monteagudo A, Timor-Tritsch IE, Moomjy M. Nomograms of the fetal lateral ventricles using transvaginal sonography. *J Ultrasound Med.* 1993;5:265–269.
9. Naidich TP, Schott LH, Baron RL. Computed tomography in evaluation of hydrocephalus. *Radiol Clin North Am.* 1982;20:143–167.
10. Epstein F, Naidich T, Kricheff I, et al. Role of computerized axial tomography in diagnosis, treatment and follow-up of hydrocephalus. *Child's Brain.* 1977;3: 91–100.
11. Noorani PA, Bodensteiner JB, Barnes PD. Colpocephaly: Frequency and associated findings. *J Child Neurol.* 1988;2:100–104.
12. Garg BP. Colpocephaly. An error of morphogenesis? *Arch Neurol.* 1982;4:243–246.
13. Heinz ER, Ward A, Drayer BP, Dubois PJ. Distinction between obstructive and atrophic dilatation of ventricles in children. *J Comput Assist Tomogr* 1980;3: 320–325.
14. Shapiro R, Galloway SJ, Shapiro MD. Minimal asymmetry of the brain: A normal variant. *AJR Am J Roentgenol.* 1986;147:753–756.
15. Horbar JD, Heahy KA, Lucey JF. Ultrasound identification of lateral ventricular asymmetry in the human neonate. *J Clin Ultrasound.* 1983;11:67–69.
16. Achiron R, Yagel S, Rotstein Z, Inbar O, Mashiach S, Lipitz S. Cerebral lateral ventricular asymmetry: Is this a normal ultrasonographic finding in the fetal brain? *Obstet Gynecol.* 1997;89:233–237.
17. Reeder JD, Kaude JV, Setzer ES. The occipital horn of the lateral ventricles in premature infants. An ultrasonographic study. *Eur J Radiol.* 1983;3:148–150.
18. Monteagudo A, Timor-Tritsch IE, Moomjy M. Nomograms of the fetal lateral ventricles using transvaginal sonography. *J Ultrasound Med.* 1993;12:265–269.
19. Monteagudo A, Timor-Tritsch IE, Moomjy M. In utero detection of ventriculomegaly during the second and third trimesters by transvaginal sonography. *Ultrasound Obstet Gynecol.* 1994;4:193–198.
20. Timor-Tritsch IE, Monteagudo A. Transvaginal fetal neurosonography: Standardization of the planes and sections used by anatomic landmarks. *Ultrasound Obstet Gynecol.* 1996;8:42–47.

21. Blass HG, Eik-Nes SH, Kiserud T, et al. Three-dimensional imaging of the brain cavities in human embryos. *Ultrasound Obstet Gynecol.* 1995;5:228–232.

22. Blass HG, Eik-Nes SH, Kiserud T, et al. Early development of the forebrain and midbrain: A longitudinal ultrasound study from 7 to 12 weeks gestation. *Ultrasound Obstet Gynecol.* 1994;4:183–192.

23. Blass HG, Eik-Nes SH, Kiserud T, et al. Early development of the hindbrain: A longitudinal ultrasound study from 7 to 12 weeks of gestation. *Ultrasound Obstet Gynecol.* 1995;5:151–160.

24. Blass HG, Eik-Nes SH, Berg S, Torp H. In-vivo three-dimensional ultrasound reconstruction of embryos and early fetuses. *Lancet.* 1998;352:1182–1186.

25. Monteagudo A, Timor-Tritsch I, Reuss M, et al. Transvaginal sonography of the second and third trimester fetal brain. In: Timor-Tritsch I, Rottem S, eds. *Transvaginal Sonography.* New York: Chapman & Hall; 1991; 393–426.

26. Noback CR, Robertson GG. Sequences of appearance of ossification centers in the human skeleton during the first five prenatal months. *Am J Anat.* 1951;89: 1–28.

27. Filly RA, Golbus MS. Ultrasonography of the normal and pathologic fetal skeleton. *Radiol Clin North Am.* 1982;20:311–323.

28. Baba K, Jurkovic D. Three dimensional ultrasound in obstetrics and gynecology. New York: The Parthenon Publishing Group; 1997.

29. Nelson TR, Downey DB, Pretorius DH, Fenster A. Three-dimensional ultrasound. Philadelphia: Lippincott Williams & Wilkins; 1999.

30. Merz E. 3D ultrasound in obstetrics and gynecology. Philadelphia–New York–Baltimore; Lippincott Williams & Wilkins, 1998.

31. Merz E, Bahlmann F, Weber G, Macchiella D. Three-dimensional ultrasonography in prenatal diagnosis. *J Perinat Med.* 1995;23:213–222.

32. Steiner H, Spitzer D, Weiss-Wichert PH, Graf AH, Standach A. Three-dimensional ultrasound in prenatal diagnosis of skeletal dysplasia. *Prenat Diagn.* 1995;15:373–377.

33. Mueller GM, Weiner CP, Yankowitz J. Three-dimensional ultrasound in the evaluation of fetal head and spinal anomalies. *Obstet Gynecol.* 1996;88:372–378.

34. Platt LD, Santuli T Jr., Carlson DE, Greene N, Walla CA. Three-dimensional ultrasonography in obstetrics and gynecology: Preliminary experience. *Am J Obstet Gynecol.* 1998;178:1199–1206.

35. Nelson TR, Pretorius DH. Visualization of the fetal thoracic skeleton with three-dimensional sonography: A preliminary report. *Am J Roentgenol.* 1995;164: 1485–1488.

36. Riccabona M, Johnson D, Pretorios DH, Nelson TR, Three dimensional ultrasound: display modalities in the fetal spine and thorax. *Eur J Radiol.* 1996;22: 141–145.

37. Johnson DD, Pretorius DH, Riccabona M, Budorick NE, Nelson TR. Three-dimensional ultrasound of the fetal spine. *Obstet Gynecol.* 1997;89:434–438.

38. Schild RL, Wallny T, Fimmers R, Hansmann M. Fetal lumbar spine volumetry by three-dimensional ultrasound. *Ultrasound Obstet Gynecol.* 1999;13:335–339.

39. Ulm MR, Kratochwil A, Oberhuemer U, Ulm B, Blaicher W, Bernaschek G. Ultrasound evaluation of fetal spine length between 14 and 24 weeks of gestation. *Prenat Diagn.* 1999;19:637–641.

40. Wallny TA, Schild RL, Fimmers VA, Hansmann ME, Schmidt O. The fetal spinal canal—A three dimensional study. *Ultrasound Med Biol.* 1000;25:1329–1333.

41. Garjian KV, Pretorius DH, Budorick NE, Cantrell CJ, Nelson TR. Fetal skeletal dysplasia: Three-dimensional US: Initial experience. *Radiology.* 2000;214: 77–23.

42. Yanagihara T, Hata T. Three-dimensional sonographic visualization of fetal skeleton in the second trimester of pregnancy. *Gynecol Obstet Ivest.* 2000;49:12–16.

43. Pretorius DH, Nelson TR. Prenatal visualization of cranial sutures and fontanelles with three-dimensional ultrasonography. *J Ultrasound Med.* 1994;13: 871–876.

44. Merz E, Ballman F, Weber G. Volume scanning in the evaluation of fetal malformations: A new dimension in prenatal diagnosis. *Ultrasound Obstet Gynecol.* 1995; 5:222–227.

45. Lee A, Deutinger J, Bernaschek G. Three dimensional ultrasound: Abnormalities of the fetal face in surface and volume rendering mode. *Br J Obstet Gynaecol.* 1995;102:302–306.

46. Pretorius DH, House M, Nelson TR, Hollenbach KA. Evaluation of normal and abnormal lips in fetuses: Comparison between three and two dimensional sonography. *AJR Am J Roentgenol.* 1995;165:1233–1237.

47. Pretorius DH, Nelson TR. Fetal face visualization using three-dimensional ultrasonography. *J Ultrasound Med.* 1995;14:349–356.

48. Bonilla-Musoles F, Raga F, Osborne NG, Blanes J. Use of three-dimensional ultrasonography for the study of normal and pathologic morphology of the human embryo and fetus: Preliminary report. *J Ultrasound Med.* 1995;14:757–765.

49. Devonald KJ, Ellwood DA, Griffiths KA, et al. Volume imaging: Three-dimensional appreciation of the fetal head and face. *J Ultrasound Med.* 1995;14:919–925.

50. Pretorious DH, Nelson TR. Fetal face visualization using three dimensional ultrasonography. *J Ultrasound Med.* 1995;14:349–356.

51. Van Mymersch D, Favre R, Gasser B. Use of three-dimensional ultrasound to establish the prenatal diagnosis of Fryns syndrome. *Fetal Diagn Ther.* 1996;11: 335–340.

52. Merz E, Weber G, Bahlmann F, Miric-Tesanic D. Application of transvaginal and abdominal three dimensional ultrasound for the detection or exclusion of malformation of the fetal face. *Ultrasound Obstet Gynecol.* 1997;9:237–243.

53. Hata T, Yonehara T, Aoki S, Manabe A, Hata K, Miyazaki K. Three-dimensional sonographic visualization of the fetal face. *AJR Am J Roentgenol.* 1998; 170:481–483.

54. Hull AD, Pretorius DH. Fetal face: What we can see using two-dimensional and three-dimensional ultrasound imaging. *Semin Roentgenol.* 1998;33:369–374.

55. Lin HH, Liang RI, Chang FM, Chang CH, Yu CH, Yang HB. Prenatal diagnosis of otocephaly using two-dimensional and three-dimensional ultrasonography. *Ultrasound Obstet Gynecol.* 1998;11:361–363.

56. Manabe A, Hata T, Aoki S, et al. Three-dimensional sonographic visualization of fetal facial anomaly. *Acta Obstet Gynecol Scand.* 1999;78:917–918.

57. Kossoff G, Griffiths KA, Warren PS. Real-time quasi-three-dimensional viewing in sonography, with conventional, gray-scale volume imaging. *Ultrasound Obstet Gynaecol.* 1994;4:211.

58. Kossoff G, Griffiths KA, Kadi AP. Transducer rotation: A useful scanning maneuver in three-dimensional ultrasonic volume imaging. *Radiology.* 1995;195:870.

CHAPTER
TEN

Ethical Dimensions in the Management of Pregnancies Complicated by Fetal Brain Anomalies

Frank A. Chervenak
Laurence B. McCullough

Ethics is an essential dimension of the management of pregnancies complicated by fetal brain anomalies. This chapter provides an overview of the principles of obstetric ethics and addresses the important issue of when the fetus is a patient. With this background, we analyze the ethical and clinical dimensions of the obstetric management options for pregnancies complicated by fetal brain anomalies. These management options include aggressive management, abortion, termination of pregnancy during the third trimester, and nonaggressive management. Finally, cephalocentesis, with its complex ethical dimensions, is considered.

PRINCIPLES OF OBSTETRIC ETHICS

Ethics

Ethics should be distinguished from morals or morality. Ethics is the disciplined study of morality. Morality concerns both right and wrong behavior, i.e., what one ought and ought not do, and good and bad character, i.e., virtues and vices. The fundamental question that ethics addresses is "What ought morality to be?" This question involves two further questions: "What ought our behavior to be?" and "What virtues ought to be cultivated in our moral lives?" Ethics in obstetric practice deals with the same questions, focusing on what morality ought to

be for obstetricians.[1] The purpose of asking these questions is to constantly improve the morality of health care professionals.

The bedrock for what morality ought to be in clinical practice for centuries has been the obligation to protect and promote the interests of the patient.[2] However, this general ethical obligation must be made more specific if it is to be clinically useful. This can be accomplished by identifying and exploring the implications of two perspectives in terms of which the patient's interests can be understood: that of the physician and that of the patient.[1]

Beneficence and Respect for Autonomy

The oldest of these two perspectives on the interests of patients in the history of Western medical ethics is a rigorous clinical perspective. Based on scientific knowledge, shared clinical experience, and a careful, unbiased evaluation of the patient, the physician should identify those clinical strategies that will most likely serve the health-related interests of the patient as well as those that will not do so. The health-related interests of the patient include preventing premature death and preventing, curing, or at least managing disease, injury, handicap, or unnecessary pain and suffering. These matters are constitutive of any patient's health-related interests as a function of the competencies of medicine as a social institution. The identification of a patient's interests is not a function of the personal or subjective outlook of a particular physician, but rather of rigorous clinical judgment about the patient's condition.

The ethical principle of beneficence structures obstetric clinical judgment about the interests of the patient because it obliges the physician to seek the greatest balance of clinical goods over harms in the consequences of the physician's behavior for both the pregnant woman and the fetal patient. On the basis of rigorous clinical judgment, the obstetrician should identify those clinical strategies that are expected to result in the greater balance of clinical goods, i.e., the protection and promotion of health-related interests, over clinical harms, i.e., impairment of those interests.

The principle of beneficence in obstetrics must be very carefully distinguished from the ethical principle of nonmaleficence, commonly known as *primum non nocere* or *first, do no harm.*[2] Contrary to the belief of many physicians, *primum non nocere* does not appear in the Hippocratic Oath or in the texts that accompany the oath. Instead, the principle of beneficence was the primary consideration of the Hippocratic writers.[3]

There are good reasons to be skeptical about the clinical adequacy of *primum non nocere* as a basic principle of obstetric ethics. Virtually all medical interventions involve unavoidable risks of harm. If *primum non nocere* were the basic principle of obstetric ethics, virtually all of obstetric practice would be unethical. *Primum non nocere* is therefore essentially superseded in obstetric ethics by the principle of beneficence. The latter is sufficient to alert the physician to those circumstances in which a clinical intervention has the potential to harm a patient. When a clinical intervention is, *on balance,* harmful to a patient, it should not be used. That is, *primum non nocere,* as a corollary of beneficence, makes it obligatory not to act in a way that is *only* harmful. Strong, for example, has argued that in medical ethics, there is a powerful beneficence-based prohibition against killing.[4] This is obviously of direct relevance to the ethical evaluation of cephalocentesis in beneficence-based clinical judgment, as we shall see below.

The physician's perspective on the interests of the patient is not the only legitimate perspective on those interests. The perspective of the *patient* on the patient's interests is equally worthy of consideration by the physician.[1] Each patient has developed a set of values and beliefs according to which she is surely capable of making judgments about what will and will not protect and promote her interests. It is a commonplace that in other aspects of her life the pa-

tient regularly makes such judgments concerning matters of considerable complexity, e.g., choosing a professional calling, rearing children, entering into contracts, or writing a will of property. Despite the complexity of these decisions, she is rightly assumed to be competent to make them, with the burden of proof on anyone who would challenge her decision-making capacity.

The same is true of health care decisions made by the pregnant woman. She must be assumed by her obstetrician to have the decision-making capacity to determine which clinical strategies serve her interests and which do not. In making such judgments it is important to note that the pregnant woman will use values and beliefs that can range far beyond the scope of health-related interests, e.g., religious beliefs or beliefs about how many children she wants to have. Beneficence-based clinical judgment, because it rests on the competencies of medicine, has no competence to assess the worth or meaning to the patient of the patient's non–health-related interests. These are matters solely for the patient to determine. Those values and beliefs help shape the patient's perspective on her interests.

The ethical significance of this perspective is captured by the ethical principle of respect for autonomy. This principle obligates the physician to respect the integrity of the patient's values and beliefs, to respect her perspective on her interests, and to implement only those clinical strategies authorized by her as the result of the informed consent process unless there is some overriding, well-established objection to doing so.

Respect for autonomy is thus put into clinical practice by the informed consent process. This process is usually understood to have three elements: (1) disclosure by the physician to the patient of adequate information about the patient's condition and its management, (2) understanding of this information by the patient, and (3) a voluntary decision by the patient to authorize or refuse clinical management.[5]

There are obviously beneficence-based and autonomy-based obligations to the pregnant patient.[1] The obstetrician's perspective on the pregnant woman's interests provides the basis for beneficence-based obligations owed to her. Her own perspective on those interests provides the basis for autonomy-based obligations owed to her. Because of an insufficiently developed central nervous system, the fetus cannot meaningfully be said to possess values and beliefs. Thus, there is no basis for saying that a fetus has a perspective on its interests. There can therefore be no autonomy-based obligations to any fetus.[1,6,7] Hence, the language of fetal rights has no clinical application in obstetric ethics, despite its popularity in public and political discourse. Obviously, the physician has a perspective on the fetus' health-related interests and the physician can have beneficence-based obligations to the fetus, *but only when the fetus is a patient.* Because of its importance for obstetric ethics generally and the ethics of destructive procedures in obstetrics, the topic of the fetus as patient requires careful consideration.

THE FETUS AS PATIENT

The concept of the fetus as patient has recently developed, largely as a consequence of developments in fetal diagnosis and management strategies to optimize fetal outcome,[8–12] and has become widely accepted.[13–15] This concept has considerable clinical significance because, when the fetus is a patient, directive counseling, i.e., recommending a form of management, for fetal benefit would seem appropriate, and when the fetus is not a patient, nondirective counseling, i.e., offering but not recommending a form of management, would seem appropriate. However, these apparently straightforward roles for directive and nondirective counseling are often difficult to apply in actual obstetric practice because of uncertainty about when the fetus is a patient. One approach to resolving this uncertainty would be to argue that the fetus is or is not a patient by virtue of personhood,[4,16] or some other form of independent moral status.[17–19] We show here that this approach fails to resolve the uncertainty and we therefore defend an alternative approach that does resolve the uncertainty.

The Independent Moral Status of the Fetus

One approach for establishing whether or not the fetus is a patient has involved attempts over many centuries to show whether or not the fetus has independent moral status. Independent moral status for the fetus means that one or more characteristics that the fetus is thought to possess in and of itself, and therefore independently of the pregnant woman or any other factor, generate and thus ground obligations to the fetus on the part of the pregnant woman and her physician.

A striking variety of characteristics have been nominated for this role in the history of the debate on the moral status of the fetus, including moments of conception, implantation, central nervous system development, quickening, and birth.[20–23] It should come as no surprise that, given the variability of proposed characteristics, there have been and are markedly varied views about when the fetus acquires independent moral status. Some take the view that the fetus has independent moral status from the moment of conception or implantation.[24,25] Others believe that independent moral status is acquired in degrees, thus resulting in "graded" moral status.[17,19] Still others hold, at least by implication, that the fetus never has independent moral status so long as it is in utero.[18]

Despite a continuing and voluminous theological and philosophical literature on this subject stretching over more than 2000 years, there has been no closure on a single authoritative account of the independent moral status of the fetus.[26,27] This is not surprising because, given the absence of a single methodology that would be authoritative for all of the markedly diverse theological and philosophical schools of thought involved in this endless debate, closure is impossible. For closure to ever be possible, debates about such a final authority within and between theological and philosophical traditions would have to be resolved in a way that is satisfactory to all. This is an inconceivable event. It is best, therefore, to abandon futile attempts to understand the fetus as patient in terms of the independent moral status of the fetus and to turn to an alternative approach that reliably identifies ethically distinct senses of the fetus as patient and their clinical implications for obstetric practice.

Beneficence-Based Obligations to the Fetus

This alternative approach begins with the recognition that being a patient does not require that one possesses independent moral status. Rather, being a patient means that one can benefit from the applications of the clinical skills of the physician. Put more precisely, a human being without independent moral status is properly regarded as a patient when two conditions are met: when a human being (1) is presented to the physician (2) for the purpose of applying clinical interventions that are reliably expected to be efficacious, in that they are reliably expected to result in a greater balance of good over harm for the human being in question.[1,15]

The authors have argued elsewhere that beneficence-based obligations to the fetus exist when the fetus can later achieve independent moral status.[1] That is, the fetus is a patient when the fetus is presented for medical interventions, whether diagnostic or therapeutic, that reasonably can be expected to result in a greater balance of good over harm for the fetus now and/or in its future. The ethical significance of the concept of the fetus as patient, therefore, depends on links that can be established between the fetus and achieving independent moral status in the future.

One such link is viability. Viability is not, however, an intrinsic property of the fetus, because viability must be understood in terms of both biologic and technological factors.[14,27,28] It is only by virtue of both factors that a viable fetus can exist ex utero and then achieve independent moral status. Moreover, these two factors do not exist as a function of the autonomy of the pregnant woman. When a fetus is viable, i.e., when it is of sufficient maturity that it can survive into the neonatal period and later achieve independent moral status, given the availability of the requisite technological support, and when it is presented to the physician, the fetus is a patient. The viable fetus is a patient when the pregnant woman presents herself to a physician or a hospital or clinic for obstetric services.

Viability exists as a function of biomedical and technological capacities, which are different in different parts of the world. As a consequence, there is, at the present time, no worldwide, uniform gestational age to define viability. In the United States, the authors believe that viability presently occurs at approximately 24 weeks of gestational age.[29] It follows directly from this sense of the fetus as patient that destructive procedures on the at-term fetal patient, cephalocentesis in particular, must be ethically justified, a task to which we turn in the next section.

The only possible link between the previable fetus and the child it can become is the pregnant woman's autonomy. This is because technological factors cannot result in the previable fetus' becoming a child. This is simply what *previable* means. The link, therefore, between a fetus and the child it can become, when the fetus is previable, can be established only by the pregnant woman's decision to confer the status of patient on her previable fetus. The previable fetus, therefore, has no claim to the status of being a patient independently of the pregnant woman's autonomy. The pregnant woman is free to withhold, confer, or, having once conferred, withdraw the status of patient on or from her previable fetus according to her own values and beliefs. The previable fetus is presented to the physician solely as a function of the pregnant woman's autonomy. This has important ethical implications for a range of ethical issues in obstetrics, including antenatal diagnosis and abortion.[23]

Management Options for Pregnancies Complicated by Fetal Brain Anomalies

Before viability, the management of a pregnancy complicated by fetal brain anomalies is ethically straightforward. The pregnant woman is free to withhold or withdraw the moral status of patient

from any previable fetus, including that with brain anomalies. When such an anomaly is detected, counseling should therefore be rigorous and nondirective. The woman should be given the choice between continuing her pregnancy to viability, and thus to term, or terminating her pregnancy. If the woman elects an abortion, it should be performed or an appropriate referral should be made. If the woman elects to continue her pregnancy, she should be apprised about decisions that will need to be made later.[1]

After viability, aggressive management is the ethical standard of care. By *aggressive management* we mean optimizing perinatal outcome by utilizing effective antepartum and intrapartum diagnostic and therapeutic modalities.

One important exception to aggressive management is termination of pregnancy after fetal viability. This exception applies when there is (1) certainty of diagnosis and either (2a) certainty of death as an outcome of the anomaly diagnosed or (2b) in some cases of short-term survival, certainty of the absence of cognitive developmental capacity as an outcome of the anomaly diagnosed.[1] When these criteria are satisfied, recommending a choice between nonaggressive management and termination of pregnancy is justified. Anencephaly is a classic example of a fetal brain anomaly that satisfies these criteria.

A second exception to aggressive management is nonaggressive management. This exception applies when there is (1) a very high probability, but sometimes less than complete certainty, about the accuracy of the diagnosis and either (2a) a very high probability of death as an outcome of the anomaly diagnosed or (2b) survival with a very high probability of severe and irreversible deficit of cognitive developmental capacity as a result of the anomaly diagnosed.[2] When these two criteria apply, both aggressive and nonaggressive management can be justified, from which it follows that a choice between aggressive or nonaggressive management, but not termination, can be recommended. Holoprosencephaly is a classic example of a fetal brain anomaly that satisfies these criteria.

A third important and ethically complex exception to aggressive management is cephalocentesis during the third trimester.

Cephalocentesis for Intrapartum Management of Hydrocephaly

Cephalocentesis is the drainage of an enlarged head, which is due to hydrocephaly.[30] Fetal hydrocephaly is due to obstruction of cerebrospinal flow and is diagnosed by such sonographic signs as dilatation of the atrium or body of the lateral ventricles.[31] In the third trimester macrocephaly often accompanies the ventriculomegaly. In addition, sonography can diagnose hydrocephaly in association with gross abnormalities suggestive of poor prognosis, for example, hydranencephaly, microcephaly, encephalocele, alobar holoprosencephaly, or thanatophoric dysplasia with cloverleaf skull.[31] In the absence of defined anatomic abnormalities, however, diagnostic imaging is, at the present time, unable to predict the outcome. Although cortical mantle thickness can be measured with ultrasound, its value as a prognostic index is not established.[31]

Cephalocentesis should be performed under simultaneous ultrasound guidance so that needle placement into the cerebrospinal fluid is facilitated. An 18-gauge needle is used with collapse of the cranial bones, the end point of this procedure. Enough fluid is drained to permit reduction of the skull diameters so that passage through the birth canal is possible.[32,33]

Cephalocentesis is a potentially destructive procedure. Perinatal death following cephalocentesis has been reported in over 90% of the cases.[30] The sonographic visualization of intracranial bleeding during cephalocentesis, and the demonstration of this hemorrhage at autopsy, further emphasize the morbid nature of the procedure. However, if decompression is performed in a controlled manner, the mortality may be reduced.[34]

Because fetal hydrocephaly is the product of varied etiologies having varied outcomes, ethical analysis must be carried out by respecting the heterogeneity of this condition.[31] Therefore, we consider clinical management strategies for two extremes of the continuum between isolated fetal hydrocephaly and fetal hydrocephaly with severe associated abnormalities (those incompatible with postnatal survival or those characterized by the virtual absence of cognitive function). We then consider fetal hydrocephaly with milder associated abnormalities as a middle ground on the continuum (Fig. 10–1). The proposed analysis of each of these situations takes place in the following steps. First, we identify the beneficence-based and autonomy-based obligations of the physician to the pregnant woman and the fetal patient. Second, we identify the conflicts that can occur among these obligations. Third, we weigh these obligations against each other in an attempt to arrive at a balance among conflicting obligations to guide clinical judgment and intervention.

Isolated Fetal Hydrocephaly

We begin the clinical and ethical analysis of isolated fetal hydrocephaly by noting that there is considerable potential for normal, sometimes superior, intellectual function in fetuses with even extreme, isolated hydrocephalus.[9–11,35] However, as a group, infants with isolated hydrocephaly experience a greater incidence of mental retardation and early death than the general population. In addition, associated anomalies may go undetected, and a fetus may be incorrectly diagnosed as having isolated hydrocephaly.[32,36] One thing is clear in obstetric ethics: a viable at-term fetus with isolated hydrocephaly is a fetal patient.

There are compelling ethical reasons, well founded in beneficence, for concluding that contin-

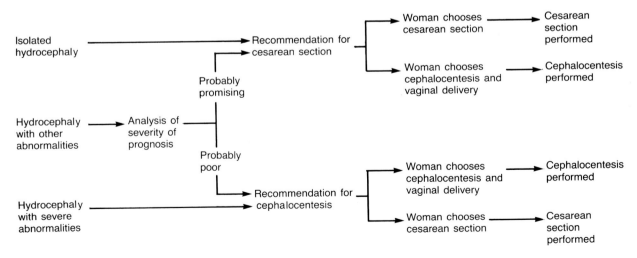

Figure 10–1. Management strategies for resolution of conflicts in the intrapartum management of hydrocephaly with macrocephaly.

uing existence of fetuses with isolated hydrocephaly is in their interest. Beneficence directs the physician to avoid mortality and morbidity for the fetal patient. Beneficence also directs the physician to clinical interventions that ameliorate handicapping conditions such as mental retardation. The probability of mental retardation does not diminish the interests of the fetal patient with isolated hydrocephaly in continuing existence because (1) it is impossible to predict which fetuses with isolated hydrocephaly will have mental retardation and (2) the degree of mental retardation cannot be predicted in advance.

In light of this ethical analysis of the interests of the at-term fetal patient, the beneficence-based obligation of the physician caring for the fetus is to recommend strongly and to obtain the woman's informed consent to perform a cesarean delivery because this clinical intervention clearly involves the least risk of mortality, morbidity, and handicap for the fetus compared with cephalocentesis to permit subsequent vaginal delivery. Even when performed under maximal therapeutic conditions (i.e., under sonographic guidance), cephalocentesis cannot reasonably be regarded as protecting or promoting the interests of the fetal patient with isolated hydrocephaly. This procedure is followed by a high rate of perinatal mortality, fetal heart rate deceleration, and pathological evidence of intracranial bleeding.[32,36] As a consequence, cephalocentesis cannot reasonably be construed as an ethically justifiable mode of management, insofar as it is inconsistent with beneficence-based obligations to avoid increased mortality and morbidity risks for the fetal patient. Cephalocentesis, used with a destructive intent, is altogether antithetical to the beneficence-based prohibition against killing.

Complete ethical analysis requires that beneficence-based obligations to the fetal patient be balanced against beneficence-based and autonomy-based obligations to the pregnant woman. First, the physician has a beneficence-based obligation to avoid performing a cesarean delivery because the possibility of morbidity and mortality for the woman is higher than that associated with vaginal delivery. Respect for autonomy obligates the physician to undertake only those interventions or forms of treatment to which the woman has given voluntary, informed consent. Informed consent is grounded in an autonomy-based right of the pregnant woman to control what happens to her body. In particular, the woman has the right to authorize or refuse operative interventions—those that are, as well as those that are not, consistent with the physician's beneficence-based obligations.[1]

We are now in a position to consider the full complexity of the management of the fetal patient with isolated hydrocephaly: beneficence-based and autonomy-based obligations to the pregnant woman, as well as beneficence-based obligations to her fetus, must be considered. If, with informed consent, the woman authorizes cesarean delivery, there is no conflict among these obligations. The autonomy-based obligation to act on informed consent overrides the beneficence-based obligations to the pregnant woman that were identified earlier.

By contrast, her physician faces a significant conflict, indeed, a genuine moral dilemma, if the woman refuses cesarean delivery. Two clinical interventions, each with substantial ethical justification in beneficence-based and autonomy-based clinical judgment, can be used in intrapartum management. On the one hand, the physician has an autonomy-based obligation to the pregnant woman to perform cephalocentesis followed by vaginal delivery. On the other hand, cephalocentesis violates beneficence-based obligations to the fetal at-term patient. This conflict should be resolved in favor of the beneficence-based obligations to the fetal patient. These obligations properly override beneficence-based and autonomy-based obligations to the woman, because the harm to the fetal patient is final, namely, death, and will occur with high probability. Moreover, if the fetal patient survives (death is not guaranteed by cephalocentesis), it is likely to be more damaged due to intracranial hemorrhage than if cesarean delivery is performed. Morbidity and mortality of the pregnant woman are both minimal and therefore risks that she should be willing to accept to protect the fetal patient's interest.[1] Such ethical conflict should be prevented by employing the preventive ethics strategies of informed consent as an ongoing dialogue, negotiation, and respectful persuasion and by making proper use of ethics committees.[1,37]

If these preventive ethics strategies fail and the pregnant woman continues to refuse cesarean delivery, the physician confronts tragic circumstances. If neither cesarean delivery nor cephalocentesis is performed, the woman is at risk for uterine rupture and death, and the fetal patient is also at risk for death. This logic of beneficence-based obligations is to avoid such total and irreversible harm. Therefore, we believe that because of the grave nature of possible consequences for the woman and her fetus, because of the dangers for the woman of performing a surgical procedure on a resistant patient, and because of the pitfalls of attempted legal coercion, the physician should act on beneficence-based obligations to the woman in such an extreme circumstance. In addition, to fail to respect an unwavering, voluntary, and informed refusal of a cesarean delivery would count as a fundamental assault on the woman's autonomy. The fetal patient is at high risk for death under either alternative. The woman's death, at least, can be avoided. Serious beneficence-based obligations to the fetal patient on the part of both the physician and the pregnant woman will probably be violated and a needless death will most probably result, however, by performing a cephalocentesis. Herein lies the tragedy of these circumstances. To avoid this tragedy, redoubled efforts of preventive ethics should be undertaken. In the experience of one of the authors (F.A.C.), carefully explaining the fact that cephalocentesis does not guarantee death and may produce a worse outcome is very powerfully persuasive. In those rare cases in which this effort at respectful persuasion fails, cephalocentesis should be performed in the least destructive way possible or an appropriate referral should be made.

Hydrocephaly With Severe Associated Abnormalities

Some abnormalities that occur in association with fetal hydrocephaly are severe in nature for the child afflicted with them. We define *severe abnormalities* as those that are either (1) incompatible with continued existence, e.g., bilateral renal agenesis or thanatophoric dysplasia with cloverleaf skull; or (2) compatible with survival in some cases but result in virtual absence of cognitive function, e.g., trisomy 18 or alobar holoprosencephaly.[32,38] Because there is no available intervention to prevent postnatal death in the first group, beneficence-based obligations of the physician and the pregnant woman to attempt to prolong the life of the fetal patient are nonexistent. No ethical theory and no version of obstetric ethics based on beneficence and respect for autonomy obligate the physician to attempt the impossible. For the second group, beneficence-based obligations of the physician and the pregnant woman to sustain the life of the fetal patient are minimal because the handicap imposed by the abnormality is severe. In these cases the potential for cognitive development—and therefore the achievement of other "good" for the child, e.g., relationships with others—are virtually absent. Such fetuses are fetal patients to which there are owed only minimal beneficence-based obligations.

In these circumstances the woman is therefore released from her beneficence-based obligations to the at-term fetal patient to place herself at risk, because no significant good can be achieved by cesarean delivery for the fetal patient or the child it

will become. There remain only the autonomy-based and beneficence-based obligations of the physician to the pregnant woman. After the preceding analysis of these obligations, we conclude that the physician's overriding moral obligations are to the pregnant woman's voluntary and informed decision about the use of cephalocentesis.

Because there are no weighty beneficence-based obligations to the fetus in such clinical and ethical circumstances, the physician may justifiably recommend a choice between cesarean delivery and cephalocentesis to enable vaginal delivery. Cesarean delivery permits women who wish to do so to have a live birth and satisfy religious convictions or help with the grieving process. A cesarean delivery performed in this clinical setting is best viewed as an autonomy-based maternal indication. The strategy of offering a choice also avoids the potential negative consequences of cesarean delivery for maternal health. Because the prognosis for infants with hydrocephaly associated with severe anomalies is poor, we believe that intrapartum fetal death resulting from cephalocentesis would not be a tragic outcome, as it might be in the death of a fetal patient with isolated hydrocephaly.

Hydrocephaly With Other Associated Anomalies

On the continuum between the extreme cases of isolated hydrocephaly and hydrocephaly with severe associated abnormalities, there are cases of hydrocephaly associated with other abnormalities with varying degrees of impairment of cognitive physical function. They range from hypoplastic distal phalanges to spina bifida to encephalocele.[8,32] Because these conditions have varying prognoses, it would be clinically inappropriate, and thus ethically misleading, to treat this third category as homogeneous. Therefore, we propose a working distinction between different kinds of prognoses. The first we call "probably promising," by which we mean that there is a significant possibility that the child will experience cognitive development with learning disabilities and physical handicaps that perhaps can be ameliorated to some extent. The second we call "probably poor." By this we mean that there is only a limited possibility for cognitive development because of learning disabilities and physical handicaps that cannot be ameliorated to a significant extent. We propose these definitions as tentative, so they are subject to revision as clinical and ethical investigation of such associated anomalies continues. As a consequence, our ethical analysis of these two categories cannot be carried out as fully or extensively as those in the previous two sections. In essence, we propose that the clinical continuum in these cases is paralleled by an ethical continuum or progressively less weighty, beneficence-based obligations to the fetus. Such at-term fetuses are indeed fetal patients.

When the prognosis is probably promising, e.g., isolated arachnoid cyst, there are serious beneficence-based obligations to the fetal patient. However, they are not necessarily on the same order as those that occur in cases of isolated hydrocephaly. (It has been suggested that any associated anomaly may increase the possibility of a poor outcome.[32] Therefore, in such cases with a prognosis of "probably promising," we propose that the physician recommend cesarean delivery, although perhaps not as vigorously as in cases of isolated hydrocephaly. A pregnant woman's informed refusal of cesarean delivery should be respected.

In cases in which the prognosis, even though uncertain, is probably poor, e.g., encephalocele, beneficence-based obligations to the fetal patient are less weighty than those owed to the fetal patient with a promising prognosis. These cases, then, ethically resemble those of hydrocephaly with severe anomalies, with the proviso that some, albeit limited, benefits can be achieved for the fetal patient by cesarean delivery and aggressive perinatal treatment. Nonetheless, the physician may, in these cases, justifiably accept an informed voluntary decision by the woman for cephalocentesis followed by vaginal delivery. However, the physician cannot assume an advocacy role for such a decision with the same level of ethical confidence that he or she can in cases of hydrocephaly associated with severe anomalies.

SUMMARY

Ethics is an essential dimension of the obstetric management of pregnancies complicated by fetal brain anomalies. This chapter has provided an ethical framework for obstetric ethics and practical guidance, based on this framework, for the management of these pregnancies. In our view, managing pregnancies complicated by fetal brain anomalies without careful attention to their ethical dimension is clinically inappropriate.

REFERENCES

1. McCullough LB, Chervenak FA. *Ethics in Obstetrics and Gynecology.* New York: Oxford University Press; 1994.

2. Beauchamp TL, Childress JF. *Principles of Biomedical Ethics.* 3rd ed. New York: Oxford University Press; 1989.

3. Hippocrates; Jones WHS, trans. *Epidemics i:xi.* Loeb Classical Library, vol 147. Cambridge, Mass: Harvard University Press; 1923.

4. Strong C. Ethical conflicts between mother and fetus in obstetrics. *Clin Perinatol.* 1987;14:313–328.

5. Faden RR, Beauchamp TL. *A History and Theory of Informed Consent.* New York: Oxford University Press; 1986.

6. Chervenak FA, McCullough LB. Perinatal ethics: A practical method of analysis of obligations to mother and fetus. *Obstet Gynecol.* 1985;66:442–446.

7. Chervenak FA, McCullough LB. Does obstetric ethics have any role in the obstetrician's response to the abortion controversy? *Am J Obstet Gynecol.* 1990;163: 1425–1429.

8. Lorber J, Zachary RB. Primary congenital hydrocephalus: Long-term results of controlled therapeutic trial. *Arch Dis Child.* 1968;43:516.

9. Raimondi AJ, Soare P. Intellectual development in shunted hydrocephalic children. *Am J Dis Child.* 1974;127:664.

10. McCullough DC, Balzer-Martin LA. Current prognosis in overt neonatal hydrocephalus. *J Neurosurg.* 1982;57:378.

11. Sutton LN, Bruce DA, Schut L. Hydranencephaly versus maximal hydrocephalus: An important clinical distinction. *Neurosurgery.* 1980;6:35.

12. Rubin RC, Hochwald G, Liwnicz B, et al. The effect of severe hydrocephalus on size and number of brain cells. *Dev Med Child Neurol.* 1972;14:118.

13. Harrison MR, Golbus MS, Filly RA. *The Unborn Patient.* Orlando, Fla: Grune & Stratton; 1984.

14. Fletcher JC. The fetus as patient; ethical issues. *JAMA.* 1981;246:772–773.

15. Chervenak FA, McCullough LB. The fetus as patient: Implications for directive versus nondirective counseling for fetal benefit. *Fetal Diagn Ther.* 1991;6:93–100.

16. Engelhardt HT Jr. *The Foundations of Bioethics.* New York: Oxford University Press; 1986.

17. Dunstan GR. The moral status of the human embryo. A tradition recalled. *J Med Ethics.* 1984;10:38–44.

18. Elias S, Annas GJ. *Reproductive Genetics and the Law.* Chicago: Year Book Medical Publishers; 1987.

19. Evans MI, Fletcher JC, Zador IE, et al. Selective first-trimester termination in octuplet and quadruplet pregnancies: Clinical and ethical issues. *Obstet Gynecol.* 1988;71:289–296.

20. Curran CE. Abortion: Contemporary debate in philosophical and religious ethics. In: Reich WT, ed. *Encyclopedia of Bioethics.* New York: Macmillan; 1978: 17–26.

21. Chervenak FA, McCullough LB. Ethical challenges in perinatal medicine: The intrapartum management of pregnancy complicated by fetal hydrocephalus with macrocephaly. *Semin Perinatol.* 1987;11:232–239.

22. Noonan JT, ed. *The Morality of Abortion.* Cambridge, Mass: Harvard University Press; 1970.

23. Hellegers AE. Fetal development. *Theol Stud.* 1970; 31:3–9.

24. Noonan JT. *A Private Choice. Abortion in America in the Seventies.* New York: Free Press; 1979.

25. Bopp J, ed. *Restoring the Right to Life: The Human Life Amendment.* Provo, Utah: Brigham Young University; 1984.

26. Callahan S, Callahan D, eds. *Abortion: Understanding Differences.* New York: Plenum Press; 1984.

27. *Roe v Wade,* 410 US 113 (1973).

28. Fost N, Chudwin D, Wikker D. The limited moral significance of fetal viability. *Hastings Cent Rep.* 1980;10: 10–13.

29. Hack M, Fanaroff AA. Outcomes of extremely-low-birth-weight infants between 1982 and 1988. *N Engl J Med.* 1989;321:1642–1647.

30. Chervenak FA, Romero R. Is there a role for fetal cephalocentesis in modern obstetrics? *Am J Perinatol.* 1984;1:170–173.

31. Chervenak FA, Isaacson G, Campbell S. *Anomalies of the Cranium and Its Contents. Textbook of Ultrasound in Obstetrics and Gynecology.* Boston: Little, Brown; 1993:825–852.

32. Chervenak FA, Berkowitz RL, Tortora M, et al. Management of fetal hydrocephalus. *Am J Obstet Gynecol.* 1985;151:933–937.

33. Clark SL, DeVore GR, Platt LD. The role of ultrasound in the aggressive management of obstructed labor secondary to fetal malformations. *Am J Obstet Gynecol.* 1985;152:1042–1044.

34. Birnholz JC, Frigoletto FD. Antenatal treatment of hydrocephalus. *N Engl J Med.* 1981;104:1021.

35. Lorber J. The results of early treatment on extreme hydrocephalus. *Med Child Neurol.* 1968;16(suppl):21.

36. Nyberg DA, Mack LA, Hirsch J, et al. Fetal hydrocephalus: Sonographic detection and clinical significance of associated anomalies. *Radiology.* 1987;163: 187.

37. Chervenak FA, McCullough LB. Clinical guides to preventing ethical conflicts between pregnant women and their physicians. *Am J Obstet Gynecol.* 1990;162: 303–307.

38. Chervenak FA, McCullough LB. An ethically justified, clinically comprehensive management strategy for third-trimester pregnancies complicated by fetal anomalies. *Obstet Gynecol.* 1990;75:311–316.

CHAPTER ELEVEN

Neurosonography of the Infant: The Normal Examination

Harris L. Cohen
Netta M. Blitman
Julian Sanchez

Before the tremendous advances in the analysis of the fetal brain became a reality, much work was done in the ultrasonographic analysis of the neonatal brain. The exchange of neurosonographic experience and technique among those imagers who assess the fetus, those who assess the neonate, and those who assess the intracranial contents of both groups has allowed great strides in analyzing what can be imaged, providing clinicians with the information necessary to assess, diagnose, and treat their patients.

Over the last 15 years, greater clinical experience, improvements in technology and technique, broader availability of Doppler- and color Doppler-capable transducers, and expansion of the evaluated patient populations to include both the younger fetus and the child beyond the age of fontanelle closure have led to continued progress in neurosonographic diagnosis. This chapter reviews the current state of the art in evaluating the normal neonatal brain by ultrasound, with some mention of its use beyond that age.

HISTORICAL BACKGROUND

Ultrasonography (US) has aided in analysis of the intracranial contents since Leksell's use, in 1956, of A-mode US to define the midline of the brain.[1] A-mode intracranial analysis was used in some institutions, into the late 1970s (and before the ready availability of computed tomography [CT]), to study the adult brain. A single spike on an oscilloscope was assumed to define the midline structures of the brain. The spike obtained by placing a transducer on the right temporal bone could be compared with that obtained when the transducer was placed on the left temporal bone. Discrepancies in spike position were thought to be evidence of a shift of midline structures. This was a rudimentary tool that did not allow imaging of the intracranial contents.[1,2]

Contact B-mode scanning was used by some physicians in the late 1970s to create gray-scale images of the intracranial contents. Acoustic mismatch between the transducer and the skull as well as the rounded skull shape limited the usefulness of this modality.[3–5]

It was not until the 1980s, with the availability of real-time imaging[6,7] and popularization of the midline soft tissue opening between the frontal and parietal bones—the anterior fontanelle—as an ultrasonographic window,[8,9] that neurosonography or neuroultrasound (NUS) began to be used extensively in neonates. Use of the anterior fontanelle allowed the sound beam to bypass the bony calvaria (Fig. 11–1) and readily penetrate the brain. The degradation of the ultrasound beam, even when passing through the thin neonatal skull bone, could be avoided. Transfontanelle scanning also allowed for the use of high-frequency transducers, which have excellent near-field resolution. Although high-

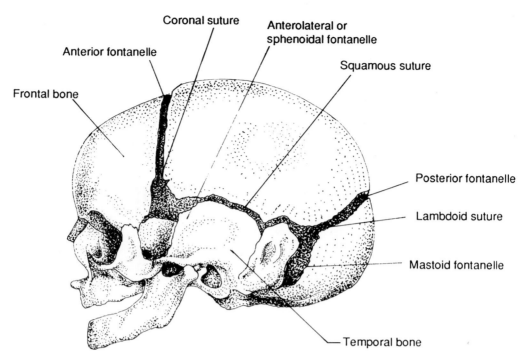

Figure 11–1. Ultrasound windows to the brain. Drawing of the neonatal calvaria in the sagittal plane. Open sutures, as noted here, and the posterior fontanelle can be and have been used in attempts at improved neurosonographic imaging. The anterior fontanelle was the first, and remains the most popular, calvarial opening, allowing high-frequency transducers to bypass the bony calvaria.

frequency transducers do not allow as much penetration as do lower-frequency transducers, their use proved to be nonproblematic because the distance the beam had to travel in assessing the intracranial contents of the infant is limited, particularly in the premature infant. Real-time units use a transducer attached to the ultrasound machine by flexible wiring, rather than the rigid-arm attachment of contact scanners, which had made changes in beam angulation difficult. With a flexible cord the examiner could make rapid changes in transducer positioning and subtle changes in its angulation and could thus make a fast and easy complete assessment of the intracranial contents, despite the necessity of examining many of these patients within their isolettes and, quite often, while attached to respirators.

Neurosonography, using real-time imaging and the anterior fontanelle as an ultrasonographic window, soon supplanted CT as the initial method of infant brain imaging. Where intracranial evaluations by CT once required balancing the clinical condition and clinical need of the patient against the risk of moving a sick premature infant from the neonatal intensive care unit to a CT scanner, NUS allowed effective imaging earlier in the patient's course, while using portable equipment in the controlled environment of the patient's isolette.[10] The absence of radiation exposure, particularly for repeat examinations while the neonate is assessed over his or her neonatal intensive care unit course, the relatively lower cost per examination, the lack of need for contrast agents to help with anatomic evaluation, and the relative ease of neurosonographic performance helped popularize the use of this technique in neonates. The proliferation of neonatal intensive care units and the increased survival rates among premature infants made the ready availability of neonatal NUS a necessity.[11]

The use of NUS in diagnosing hydrocephaly, congenital anomalies, and other clinical problems, particularly intraventricular hemorrhage (IVH) and periventricular leukomalacia, in premature infants has been well documented.[12,13] Although magnetic resonance imaging (MRI) and CT provide a more global view of the intracranial contents, and in the case, particularly with MRI, of providing information such as patterns of myelinization, which cannot be obtained by US, US is a more practical and cost-efficient imaging tool, particularly for the initial examination.[14] Ultrasonography is more adept than CT at imaging the small parenchymal cysts that, as discussed in the section on parasagittal images, can be found in the periventricular areas in patients with periventricular leukomalacia, as well as in the subependymal area in patients with posthemorrhagic or postinfectious cysts. Unlike the case with CT (but like MRI), images can be obtained in several scanning planes.

THE NORMAL EXAMINATION

Approach to Examining the Premature Infant

Examination of the premature infant is most often performed in an isolette. The examiner is gloved and gowned. The infant's anterior fontanelle is palpated. Transducer couplant or gel is placed on the anterior fontanelle to allow good transducer contact without reflection or refraction of the sound beam by air above the skin surface. A high-frequency, preferably 7.5-MHz, transducer is placed on the couplant and the examination is begun. Sector transducers are favored because they allow a wide field of view even with a small acoustic window. Examinations, particularly on unstable premature infants, may be performed through the isolette's portholes as a way of limiting compromise of the controlled atmosphere of the isolette. Angulation of the transducer via the portholes is somewhat limited, particularly with large transducers. For these cases we place the

transducer and the physician's or sonographer's examining arm into the isolette by lifting the isolette cover and closing it over the examining arm. This is intended to decrease heat loss as much as possible. Today, with the availability of pulse oximeters for constant determination of blood oxygen saturation in premature infants, the examiner can readily note whether the infant is having problems during the ultrasound examination. Occasionally, one may note decreasing oxygen saturation levels with transducer pressure on the anterior fontanelle. If this occurs, the examiner should be extremely gentle with transducer placement, just touching the gel placed on the fontanelle, and if decreasing saturation levels persist, he or she should consult the neonatal team for clinical assessment.

Higher-frequency (usually 10-MHz) transducers, with or without a standoff pad, may be used for the evaluation of more superficial structures, such as the superior sagittal sinus (Fig. 11–2) or the subarachnoid space, which may normally be prominent in neonates, particularly premature infants.[15] Prominent subarachnoid spaces may also be evidence of cerebral atrophy.[16] Superficial extra-axial collections, although more readily noted on CT examination, may also be seen using a high-frequency transducer and a standoff pad.

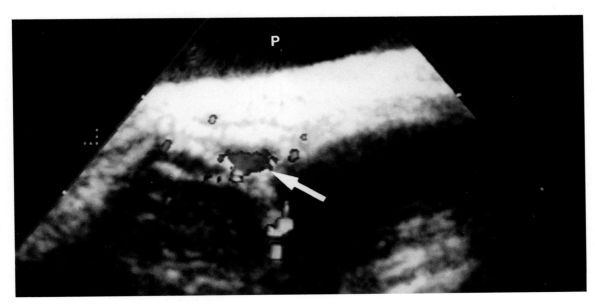
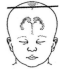

Figure 11–2. Use of a standoff pad to improve near-field resolution. Color Doppler image of the superior sagittal sinus in the transverse (coronal) plane. The letter *P* is in the echopenic image produced by a standoff pad of water-equivalent material. The pad was placed on top of the anterior fontanelle to increase the distance between the transducer and the calvaria and to bypass the near-field artifact that often fills in the most superficial millimeters of an image with echogenicity. In this case the pad allowed excellent resolution of color flow in the superior sagittal sinus *(arrow). (From Cohen and Haller, 1994,[2] with permission.)*

Approach to Examining the Full-Term Infant or the Older Child

Examination techniques are the same for premature and full-term infants. Larger, full-term neonates, particularly those with significant scalp hair, may require the greater penetration provided by a 5-MHz transducer. Older, stable infants, often examined on an outpatient basis as a follow-up to a neonatal problem or because of enlarging head circumferences and a need to rule out hydrocephaly, can be examined on a routine examining table or even in the mother's arms. The anterior fontanelle closes between 9 and 15 months of age.[17] Beyond that point neurosonographic evaluation must be done via a transcranial approach, or another imaging modality, such as CT, must be used.

The Actual Examination

Guidelines for performance of the ultrasound examination of the pediatric brain have been published by both the American Institute of Ultrasound in Medicine (*Standards for Performance of the Ultrasound Examination of the Infant Brain*) and the American College of Radiology. The guidelines request the use of a real-time scanner, a sector or curved linear array transducer, and transducer frequencies of 5 to 7.5 MHz. These guidelines note that adequate documentation is necessary for high-quality patient care requiring hard-copy images in any image format.[18]

The following discussion of the normal examination covers the imaging and information needed to comply with these guidelines. However, the examiner must be aware that imaging, as is the case with all of medicine, remains an art as well as a science and that there are exceptions to every rule. We are fortunate that current ultrasound technology allows us to both view structures while imaging them and angulate the transducer in subtle degrees so as to follow areas of imaging concern, whether or not they are within planes suggested by the guidelines. The following reviews our laboratory's techniques as well as those of others.[2,10,12,17,19]

All examinations should include scanning of the brain on coronal view from front to back and on sagittal view from the periphery of one side to that of the other. Several axioms guide our daily work. No view is sacrosanct. Orthogonal views aid and at times confirm suspected abnormalities. Symmetry suggests, but does not prove, normalcy, i.e., when one can compare the two sides of the brain, for questions regarding brain echogenicity. Comparisons are particularly easy on coronal views in which the brain halves are seen side by side. Alternate approaches and ultrasonographic windows (Fig. 11–1) may allow imaging of structures not seen by the usual anterior transfontanelle approach.

Routine sagittal and parasagittal imaging is performed by viewing the midline of the brain (Fig. 11–3) and then angling the transducer slowly while imaging the right and left sides of the brain from its midline to its periphery at the level of the sylvian fissures, with their contained middle cerebral artery (MCA) tributaries. Routinely, hard-copy images, referred to in the guidelines as "representative" views,[18] are obtained of the midline (Fig. 11–4) itself, as well as right and left paramedian areas through the body of the lateral ventricle and the junction between the head of the caudate nucleus and the body of the thalamus (Fig. 11–5), known as the caudothalamic groove. Hard-copy images are also taken of any abnormality or area of imaging concern. Fetal neurosonography emulates that of the neonate. This enables comparison of the sonographic pictures taken from the fetus and later from the neonate for purposes of follow-up.

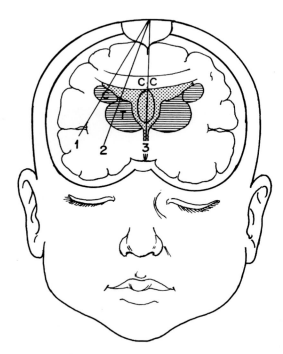

Figure 11–3. Median and paramedian ultrasound planes. Schematic drawing of the neonatal calvarium in the coronal plane. Examples are shown of three possible planes that can be obtained by varying transducer angulation, in this case, on the right side of the brain. Plane I extends through the brain to the lateral sulcus at its periphery, plane II runs between the head of the caudate nucleus (C) and the thalamus (T), and plane III runs through the midline. CC, Corpus callosum.

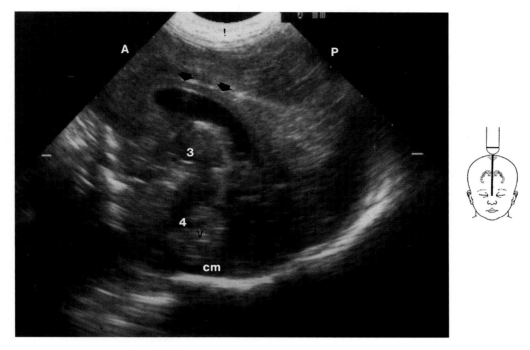

Figure 11–4. Normal image in the median plane. Standard sagittal images place the patient's anterior (A) on the reader's left and the patient's posterior on the right. The *arrows* point to the corpus callosum. The gyral pattern is not seen to be prominent in this young (28-week) premature infant. An exclamation point has been placed in the near-field artifactual echogenicity. The echogenic cerebellar vermis (V) is posterior and the echoless cisterna magna (cm) is inferior to the fourth ventricle (4). 3, Third ventricle.

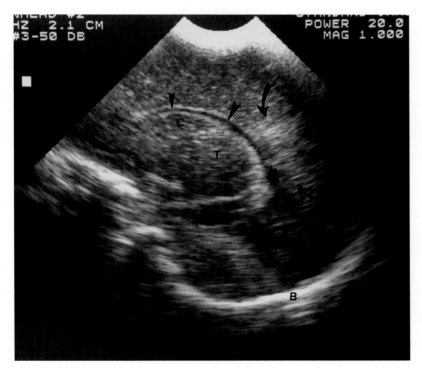

Figure 11–5. Normal paramedian image, left of the median. The straight *arrow* points to the echogenic choroid in the atrium of the lateral ventricle. The *small arrowhead* points to the anterior horn, and the larger one indicates the body of the left lateral ventricle. The *curved arrows* are within the periphery of the normally echogenic peritrigonal white matter. C, Head of the caudate nucleus; T, thalamus; B, bone at the base of the skull.

Information Obtained from Sagittal Views

The median view allows one to image the crescentic corpus callosum, the largest of the medial interhemispheric commissures, just above the cavum septum pellucidum. The corpus callosum is classically described as hypoechoic compared to normal brain parenchyma, although it may be isoechoic, particularly in the very young premature infant. The corpus callosum is definitively more echogenic than the echoless fluid of the cavum septum pellucidum (Fig. 11–6), which may more correctly be termed the cavum septi pellucidi (CSP), in that this potential fluid space lying between the anterior horns of the lateral ventricles is situated between two septi or leaves of the septum pellucidum. Pathologists note a CSP in 100% of newborn premature infants, with a decreasing incidence to 6 months of age. This structure is not imaged as often in routine head US, but certainly is more often seen in the premature infant and may disappear in the first 2 months of life. Babcock and Farrugia[20] reported imaging a CSP in 42% of newborns and 62% of premature newborns. Knowledge of the presence of this normal structure prevents confusion with a high-riding third ventricle.[12,19,20] Often, one may see a more posterior extension of the septum pellucidum

as the cavum vergae. Occasionally, there may be a still more posterior inferior fluid-filled area, said to be consistent with the cavum velum interpositum and to be separated from the cavum vergae by a septation.[17]

Superiorly, the corpus callosum is surrounded by the more echogenic pericallosal sulcus, in which lie the pericallosal arteries. The pericallosal sulcus, in turn, is surrounded by the more cephalad and superior cingulate gyrus. The cingulate gyrus and the more superficial or cephalad gyri course in a direction relatively parallel to that of the corpus callosum and not extending to the third ventricle. (See also Chapter 2.) These gyri, as is true of all gyri, are echopenic compared to the echogenic sulci separating them (Fig. 11–7). As can be noted with somewhat more difficulty in the fetus, the gyral/sulcal pattern of the brain becomes more prominent and more complex, particularly on the midline views of the medial portion of the brain, as gestational age increases. Dorovini-Zis' classic pathology images (Fig. 11–8) show these differences for various gestational ages, with a relatively featureless pattern at 22 weeks maturing into the typical adult pattern at 40 weeks.[21] Knowledge of postmenstrual age may aid in the identification of cases of agyria, with little ev-

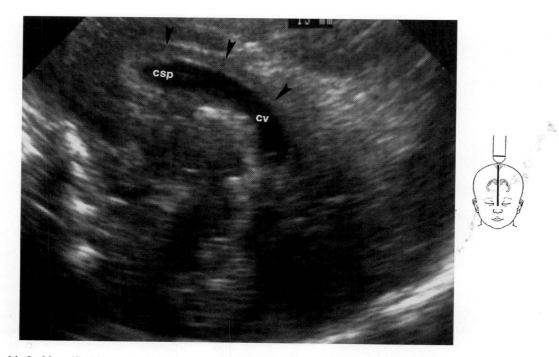

Figure 11–6. Magnified image of the corpus callosum in the median plane. The *arrowheads* point to the corpus callosum, which is superior to the echoless cavum septi pellucidi (csp), which extends posteriorly as the cavum vergae (cv). The exact point at which the cavum septi pellucidi ends and the cavum vergae begins cannot be determined by ultrasonography. The *arrow* points to the fourth ventricle, anterior to the cerebellar vermis.

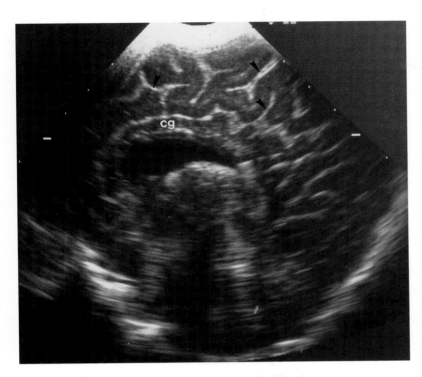

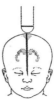

Figure 11–7. Gyri and sulci in the median view. The *arrowheads* point to echogenic sulci. The sulci, with their contained vessels, separate the more echopenic gyri of the brain. This infant's gyri and sulci were very prominent because he was full term and incidentally had a thin calvaria secondary to osteogenesis imperfecta. cg, Cingulate gyrus.

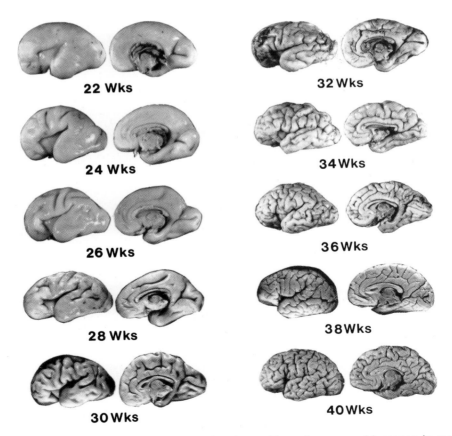

22 Wks

24 Wks

26 Wks

28 Wks

30 Wks

32 Wks

34 Wks

36 Wks

38 Wks

40 Wks

Figure 11–8. Changes in gyri with increasing gestational age. There is a normal increase in gyral number and branching with increasing gestational age, as demonstrated by these pathology specimens. *(From Dorovini-Zis, 1977,[21] with permission.)*

idence of gyri. Gyral/sulcal pattern identification may aid in determination of the gestational age of a newborn.[22,23] Branches of the anterior cerebral artery run within the midline sulci and may be seen to pulsate within them. These vessels can be imaged with color Doppler imaging (CDI) (Fig. 11–9).

Inferior to the corpus callosum and the CSP is the third ventricle, which can be seen, occasionally with difficulty, on the median section. It is certainly seen readily in the face of ventriculomegaly, with its characteristic anterior recesses. The circular solid structure that may be seen within it represents the massa intermedia.[17]

The choroid plexus may be seen as an echogenic structure in the roof of the third ventricle. This echogenicity may extend caudally through the aqueduct. Infratentorially, a triangular echoless area consistent with the fourth ventricle is seen anterior to the characteristically echogenic vermis of the cerebellum (Fig. 11–4). Good technique requires the examiner to have the entire brain imaged on the screen, from the point of transducer placement to the echogenic calvaria at the base of the brain.

Paramedian Images

The key paramedian views are those of the lateral ventricles and their nearby structures. Each lateral ventricle can be evaluated for its frontal portion, body, atrial or trigonal portion, and temporal and occipital portion (Fig. 11–10). Some areas of the lateral ventricles, particularly the occipital horns, may not be readily imaged when there is no hydrocephalus. In most instances the entire lateral ventricle may be seen in one parasagittal plane, although, especially if the ventricular system is dilated, portions of it may be imaged with subtle angulation to the right or left of the body of the lateral ventricle. Usually, one must move the transducer slightly to the periphery of one side of the anterior fontanelle and image across to the contralateral lateral ventricle to obtain a satisfactory image.[23] The oval head of the caudate nucleus can be seen meeting the circular thalamus at the thin, echogenic caudothalamic groove (Fig. 11–11). By 32 weeks of gestation, this is the region of residual germinal matrix that is the potential site of subependymal hemorrhage and, if extending into the ventricle, IVH.

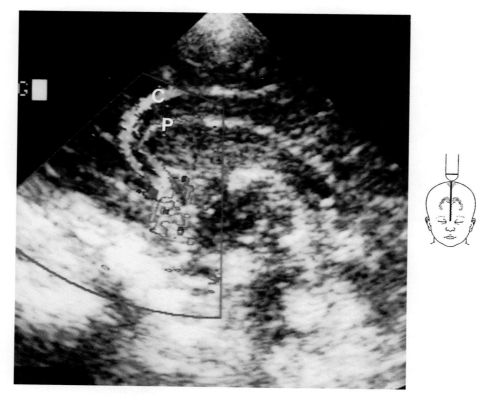

Figure 11–9. Color Doppler image of the anterior cerebral artery branches in the sagittal plane, slightly to the right of the midline. Color Doppler signal, indicating movement in relation to the transducer, is obtained from anterior cerebral artery branch vessels imaged in the anterior half of the brain. P, Pericallosal arterial artery; C, callosomarginal artery.

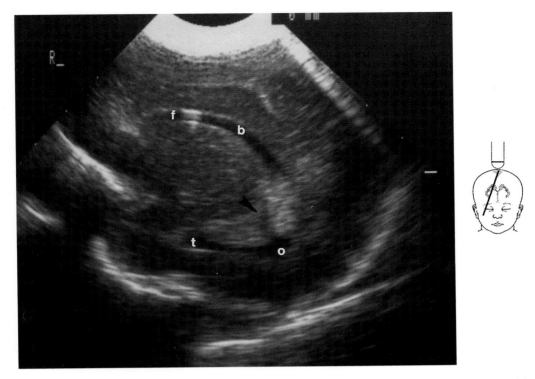

Figure 11–10. A normal lateral ventricle in a right paramedian plane. The *arrowhead* points to the choroid plexus in the atrium of the lateral ventricle. f, Anterior horn; b, body; o, proximal portion of the posterior horn; t, inferior horn of the lateral ventricle.

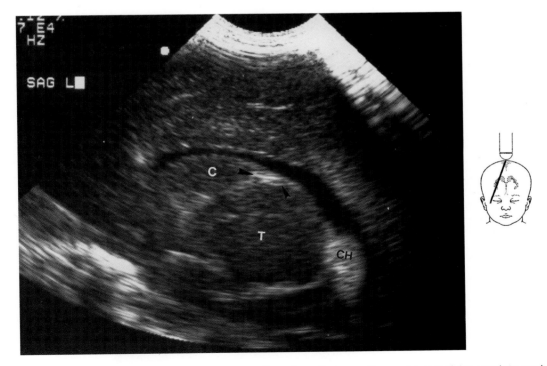

Figure 11–11. Caudothalamic groove in a left paramedian plane. Between the oval head of the caudate nucleus (C) and the round thalamus (T) is a small area of echogenicity representing the caudothalamic groove *(arrowheads),* an area that represents the remaining germinal matrix region in premature infants beyond 32 weeks of gestational age. CH, Choroid plexus.

Lateral ventricular size is assessed on both parasagittal and coronal views. Ventriculomegaly is assessed by most sonologists by gestalt rather than by specific measurements. Normal ventricles are largest at the atrium. Lateral ventricles may normally be somewhat asymmetrical, with the left ventricle slightly larger than the right one and the posterior horns more prominent than the anterior horns. Asymmetry is more common in premature infants, probably because of a relatively less well-developed cerebral cortex than in full-term infants. Narrowed, slitlike ventricles (Fig. 11–12), once believed to be definitive evidence of cerebral edema, can be seen in many normal infants, particularly in the frontal horns. Clinical findings or other abnormal features must be noted before considering narrow ventricles as abnormal.[24,25]

Running along the floor and within each body of the two lateral ventricles is the choroid plexus. Each lateral ventricle's choroid plexus is homogeneously echogenic and tubular with a smooth border. The choroid plexus extends from the foramen Monro to the atrium of the lateral ventricle, where it is largest in dimension, and then curves anteroinferiorly, extending into the inferior horn tip of the lateral ventricle. The choroid plexus does not extend into the posterior horn of the lateral ventricle or anterior to the foramen interventriculare (Monro), egress to the third ventricle. As noted in the discussion of midline images, the choroid runs within the roof of the third ventricle. It is also present within the roof of the fourth ventricle but cannot be imaged sonographically. The highly echogenic choroid may simulate the image of IVH in its earliest stages after fibrin deposition and before clot retraction and lysis. The examiner must therefore be wary of what appears to be choroid either in the occipital horn or, more importantly, anterior to the position of the foramen interventriculare, i.e., in the anterior horns. A particularly thickened area of choroid should be considered with suspicion.

In the search for possible periventricular leukomalacia or posthypoxic encephalopathy on parasagittal views, a key area to analyze is the periventricular area, particularly about the ventricular trigone. The physician must be cautious against making a diagnosis of abnormality when noting the normally prominent echogenicity of the peritrigonal white *matter*.[26] Use of the orthogonal coronal views and a search for asymmetry of the two sides of the brain as evidence of true pathology are useful. Follow-up examinations can be confirmatory.[27]

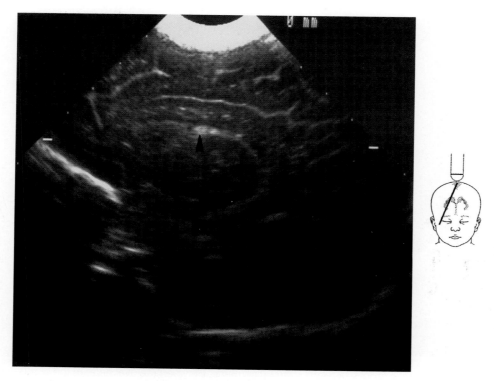

Figure 11–12. Slitlike ventricles in a sagittal plane. Neonatal ventricles may be normal and slitlike. No ventricle is seen in a plane similar to that used for the patient imaged in Figure 11–11. This infant was normal. A number of years ago some authorities suggested that slitlike ventricles were evidence of cerebral edema. This can occasionally be the case. The *arrowhead* indicates the caudothalamic groove.

In the far periphery of the brain, one may note the MCA tributaries pulsating in the sylvian fissure.

Coronal Images

Routine imaging in a coronal plane consists of a 90-degree turn of the transducer in the anterior fontanelle. The transducer is angled slowly from anterior to the frontal horns, at the level of the orbits, to posterior, at the level of the occipital horns, tentorium and cerebellum, and cerebello-medullary cistern (cisterna magna) to view the entire brain (Fig. 11–13). Hard-copy images are taken of the frontal horns. At this site, one can note whether the ventricular size is normal or there is ventricular dilatation, as well as analyze for the presence of the corpus callosum. One can note the interhemispheric fissure, which is normally a thin, echoless line, bordered by two vertical, echogenic lines and looking like an anchor. The echogenic lines represent the medial surfaces of the two frontal lobes as they abut anterior to the corpus callosum. Brain atrophy causing volume loss will allow subarachnoid space fluid to be seen in the medial aspect between the frontal horns and no anchor sign will be imaged. Prominent extra-axial

spaces, however, can sometimes be seen in normal patients in the first years of life (Fig. 11–14).

Somewhat more posterior angulation of the transducer allows imaging of the body of the lateral ventricles (Fig. 11–15), an image of which should be taken as hard copy. Further posterior angulation will show the occipital lobes and the subtentorial cerebellar hemispheres, cerebellar vermis, and cisterna magna. At any level in the coronal portion of the study, one may angle the transducer to the extreme right or left. This allows one to image the periphery of the brain and allows assessment for possible extra-axial collection. This evaluation, however, is limited with more cranial (toward the vertex) planes. Coronal views allow the comparison of parenchymal echogenicity of the right and left halves of the brain. This will hopefully allow ready assessment of the increased echogenicity of hemorrhage or the increased parenchymal echogenicity of brain edema or infarction. At the brain periphery, on coronal view, is the Y-shaped lateral sulcus (Fig. 11–16), in which the branches of the MCA tributaries can be seen to pulsate on real-time imaging and may be insonated by duplex or color Doppler scans. The choroid plexus has the same appearance on coronal views as on sagittal views: a tubular echogenic mass within each lateral ventricle. The benefit of a coronal plane is that each can be compared to its contralateral mate. The fact that the echogenicity of the normal choroid plexus is the same as that of relatively acute IVH is noteworthy, and contralateral comparisons of echogenicity and shape aid in making the diagnosis. Cysts may be seen in the choroid plexus of neonates, as in the fetus. They are incidentally imaged in 3% of neonates.[2,27] There is no clinical significance to the imaging of choroid plexus cysts in the neonate. This finding has not been associated with abnormal karyotypes in neonates, as it has in 6% of the 1 in every 100 to 200 fetuses in which it has been discovered.[2]

The normal lateral wall of the ventricular body hugs the choroid plexus (Fig. 11–15). Significant distances between the choroid and the lateral ventricular wall may suggest ventriculomegaly.

Alternate Windows to the Brain: Improved Technique

Soon after the introduction of the anterior fontanelle as an ultrasonographic window, other sutural openings, such as the metopic suture, found between the frontal bones, and the posterior fontanelle, were used to evaluate the intracranial contents.[27,28] Use of the posterior fontanelle as an ultrasonographic window (Fig. 11–17) is particularly helpful in analyzing the infratentorial contents. A 1994 report from New Zealand suggested improved diagnosis of IVH by ad-

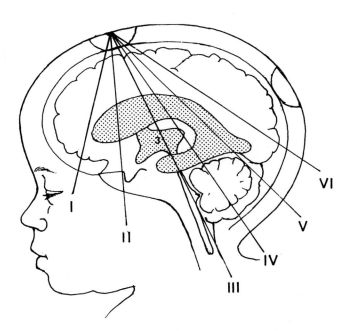

Figure 11–13. Normal coronal planes of head ultrasonography. Schematic drawing in the sagittal view. The correct examination technique in the coronal plane requires angulation of the transducer, placed at the anterior fontanelle, from the front to the back of the skull, so as to image as much of the intracranial contents as possible. This drawing shows six possible planes. Plane I goes through the orbits anterior to the frontal horn. Plane III goes through the third ventricle (3), and plane VI goes through the atrium of the lateral ventricle.

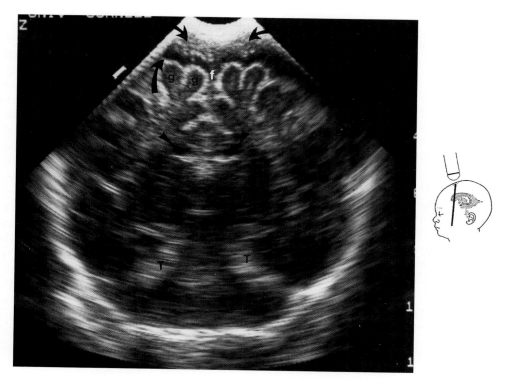

Figure 11–14. Prominent extra-axial space in a coronal plane, with angulation through the anterior horns *(arrowheads).* Normally, the brain borders are not well seen. In this case the anterior horn gyri (g) are imaged, indicating a fluid collection *(curved arrows)* between the brain and the calvaria. This may be due to a pathological extra-axial collection, but in most instances, particularly when symmetrical, this reflects the normal prominent extra-axial space of the premature infant. There is slight separation of the interhemispheric fissure (f). T, Tentorium cerebelli.

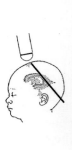

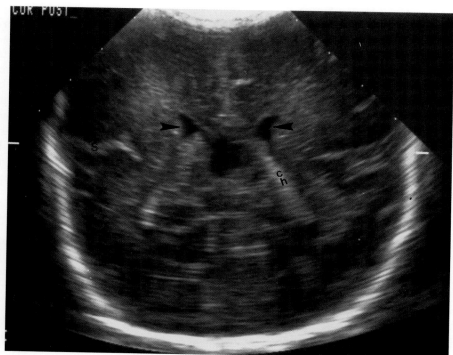

Figure 11–15. Normal coronal view showing moderate posterior angulation (plane V). The choroid plexus (ch) is seen in each lateral ventricle. No choroid is seen in the anterior portion of the lateral ventricle *(arrowheads),* in what is therefore a portion of the anterior horns anterior to the foramen Monro. Note that the lateral ventricular wall normally hugs the choroid, proving that there is no ventriculomegaly. S, Sylvian fissure.

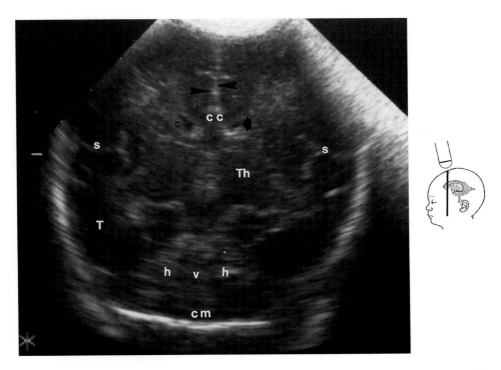

Figure 11–16. Frontal horns of the lateral ventricles in a coronal plane (plane IV). Various normal structures are seen. The *arrowheads* point to the interhemispheric fissure. The *arrow* indicates the left anterior horn. The normal corpus callosum (cc) appears more echopenic than the surrounding parenchyma but more echogenic than the echoless anterior horns. The somewhat echogenic head of the caudate nucleus (c) hugs the lateral aspect of the anterior horn and should not be mistaken for hemorrhage. Th, Left thalamus; s, sylvian fissure (note Y shape); h, cerebellar hemisphere; v, cerebellar vermis; cm, cisterna magna.

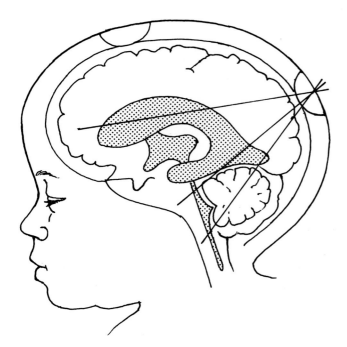

Figure 11–17. Posterior fontanelle planes. Schematic drawing in the sagittal view and planes obtained with coronal angulation through the fontanelle. The posterior fontanelle may be used as an ultrasonographic window. Views may be taken in the coronal or sagittal plane.

ditional analysis of the occipital horn for the presence or absence of hemorrhage (Fig. 11–18) not seen on routine anterior fontanelle imaging by using a posterior fontanelle approach.[29,30] However, as with any change in an imaging method or technique, one needs to become aware of potential simulators of pathology. One group has reported imaging echogenicity within the posterior thalami of normal patients examined with the posterior fontanelle approach (Fig. 11–19). Yet, the thalami appeared normal using the anterior transfontanelle approach. They theorized that this was due to an anisotropic effect (prominent echogenicity seen where linear aligned structures such as neural fibers are imaged by an ultrasound beam perpendicular to them).[31]

Foramen magnum views have been used to image the displaced structures within the spinal canal of patients with Chiari malformation. Placing the transducer just caudal and medial to the mastoid process allows improved imaging of posterior fossa structures.[2,31]

Transcranial Ultrasound

As long ago as 1983, Mercker and collaborators[33] described a lateral approach to the calvarium to note extra-axial collections. Transcranial ultrasound allows good visualization of the brain stem and the basilar artery in the interpeduncular cistern by imaging in a plane parallel to the canthomeatal line.[34] Transcranial ultrasound relies on low-frequency transducers (often 2 or 3 MHz) to penetrate the thinner, squamous portion of the temporal bone after fontanelle closure[35] (Fig. 11–20) and may be used to assess for hydrocephaly or IVH even earlier, if use of the fontanelle is

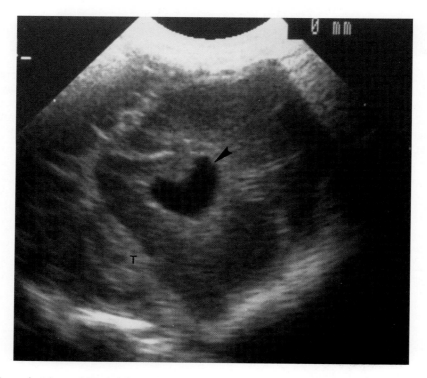

Figure 11–18. Normal atrium of the left lateral ventricle in a coronal plane (angled to the left), using the posterior fontanelle. The atrium of the left lateral ventricle *(arrowhead)* is well imaged just above the tentorium (T). On occasion, the atrium and the posterior horns of the lateral ventricle may be better imaged using a posterior fontanelle approach.

Figure 11–19. Posterior fontanelle approach simulating thalamic pathology. **A.** Right parasagittal plane. Posterior fontanelle approach. Echogenicity is seen in the thalamus *(arrows),* anterior to the choroid. It simulates hemorrhage or other abnormality. **B.** Right parasagittal plane. Anterior fontanelle approach. On this view, the thalamus is normal. The focal area of increased echogenicity is not seen. The neonate was normal. The increased echogenicity seen on posterior fontanelle approach is thought to be due to an anisotropic effect from the ultrasound beam being exactly perpendicular to the neural fibers at the site of increased echogenicity. The direction of the beam using the anterior fontanelle approach is more parallel to the imaged area and no anisotropic effect is seen. *(From Schlesinger, Munden, and Hayman, 1999,[31] with permission.)*

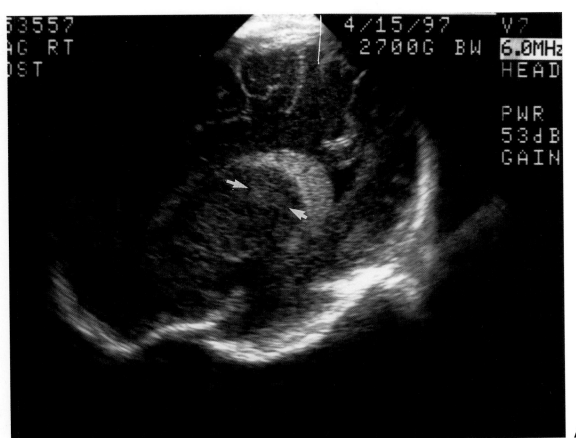
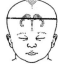

A

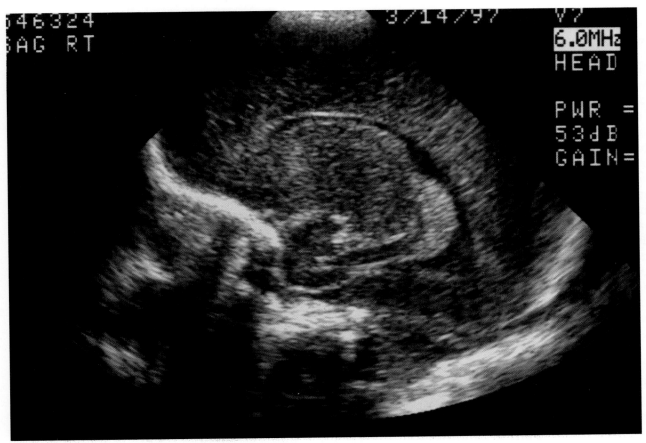
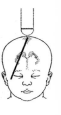

B

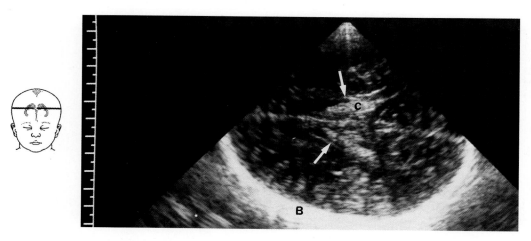

Figure 11–20. Transcranial ultrasonogram in a coronal view. A 2-MHz transducer was placed on the squamous portion of the left temporal bone in this 13-month-old with questionably enlarged head circumference and closed fontanelles. The ventricles are normal in size and the lateral ventricular wall *(arrows)* hugs the choroid plexus (c). The near field is the left side, the side the transducer was placed on. The low-frequency transducer was able to penetrate the entire calvaria to the right side, showing gyri and sulci at the right brain's periphery, as well as through-transmission beyond the right calvaria (B), giving it a falsely thickened appearance.

precluded by, e.g., a local intravenous site.[2] We have used the transcranial approach most often in children that we have followed up over a long period for hydrocephalus and treated hydrocephaly or in children in whom the families espouse a particular fear of radiation exposure. Sound penetration and the image field of view become more limited with time. We certainly do not suggest the use of ultrasound on a routine basis after fontanelle closure.

A recent improvement in transcranial imaging of neonates has been the use of the mastoid fontanelle as an imaging portal. The mastoid fontanelle is located at the junction of the posterior parietal, temporal, and occipital bones. The transducer is positioned approximately 1 cm posterior to the ear and 1 cm above the tragus. Imaging through the mastoid fontanelle allows better visualization of the midbrain and the contents of the posterior fossa than does traditional anterior tranfontanelle imaging. This approach allows the use of higher frequency transducers than does traditional transcranial ultrasound. The method has proven particularly helpful in assessing posterior fossa and cerebellar hemorrhage as well as deep venous sinus thrombosis and basal cistern subarachnoid hemorrhage due to the closer proximity of the transducer to these regions.[36]

Newer Technologies: Doppler and Color Doppler Imaging

The use of duplex and color Doppler in the intracranial assessment of pediatric patients has aided diagnosis and provided a tool for use with regard to normal and abnormal physiological information that has not yet been fully realized. Unlike earlier work with continuous-wave and pulsed-wave Doppler systems that provided a spectral pattern but no image, current duplex US equipment allows the examiner to obtain a spectral pattern and a simultaneous image, hence the term *duplex* imaging (Fig. 11–21). Color Doppler imaging (CDI) systems provide a rapid means of identifying flow and flow direction with machinery that assigns color to flow direction and variable color brightness to different flow velocities.[37,38] More exacting placement of the Doppler sample volume can be accomplished.[40] Duplex Doppler imaging and CDI of the neonate, like in the fetus, child, and adult, have allowed the rapid differentiation between postdestructive or congenital cysts in the brain and the cystic or tubular vascular structures found in intracranial arteriovenous malformations such as the vein of Galen aneurysm.[41]

Normal Vascular Findings Using Doppler

Mitchell and coworkers,[41] using the anterior and anterolateral fontanelles as ultrasonographic windows, were able to image the basilar, internal carotid, anterior (Fig. 11–9), and middle cerebral arteries in all patients in a group of 53 healthy full-term infants examined by CDI. The vertebral, posterior cerebral, superior cerebellar, and posterior communicating arteries were seen in most of these infants.[41] The internal cerebral vein, great cerebral vein (vein of Galen), and the superior sagittal (Fig. 11–2) and straight sinus can also be routinely imaged by CDI.

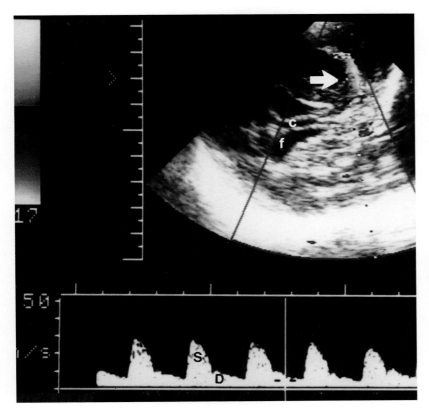

Figure 11–21. Color and duplex Doppler images using a transcranial approach in an axial plane. The transducer, placed on the left side of the skull, shows the left middle cerebral artery with color flow in it. Red denotes normal flow direction toward the calvaria. A Doppler spectrum (lower half of image) shows continual systolic (S) or diastolic (D) flow (markings always above a baseline of 0 cm/sec flow, on the vertical axis) throughout the cardiac cycle, consistent with the normal low-resistance flow of the normal brain's arterial circulation. f, Right anterior horn; c, cavum septi pellucidi.

Angled sagittal views can show the MCA branches in the lateral sulcus. Coronal views, with variable angulation, allow imaging of at least the anterior half of the circle of Willis as well as the thalamostriate arteries (Fig. 11–22).[42]

Transcranial Doppler imaging performed through the thinner, squamous portion of the temporal bone is an excellent method of imaging the circle of Willis vessels. It is particularly well suited for the imaging and insonation of the MCA in its echogenic fissure (Fig. 11–21) because of the more parallel relationship between the transducer and the MCA. The almost 90-degree relationship of the MCA to a transducer placed in the anterior fontanelle limits obtained physiological information since, according to the Doppler equation, frequency shifts from flowing red blood cells approach 0 as the incident angle of the beam approaches 90 degrees.[2,35,42]

Intracranial Vascular Flow Patterns: Arteries and Veins

Normal intracranial arterial spectral flow patterns are low resistance in type, indicating that vascular flow to the brain occurs throughout the cardiac cycle, in systole as well as throughout diastole (Fig. 11–23). The resistance index (RI) (peak systolic flow

velocity [PSV] minus end-diastolic flow velocity [EDV] divided by PSV) and the pulsatility index (PI) (PSV minus EDV divided by time-average velocity [TAV], with TAV determined by the area under the flow velocity curve) are used to measure systolic/diastolic flow relationships.[2,39] There is a linear increase in all flow velocities with advancing gestational age and with increasing patient weight but no significant changes in RI or PI, although a small decrease has been noted by some authors in comparing premature and full-term infants.[39,42] The PSV and the EDV have been determined for the major supratentorial arteries, with RIs ranging between 0.5 and 0.8.[42] Although flow volume determination requires knowledge of the cross-sectional area of the intracranial arteries that cannot be determined by US, brain perfusion studies have shown a good correlation between perfusion and mean flow velocities.[39] Cardiac status is reflected in the intracranial Doppler signals with retrograde diastolic flow in significant ductus arteriosus, truncus arteriosus, or aortic insufficiency as well as in the low PSV in left ventricular outlet obstruction and the high PSV in coarctation of the aorta.

Winkler and Helmke[44] have described three main venous flow patterns that are variably found in the intracranial venous system. A bandlike ve-

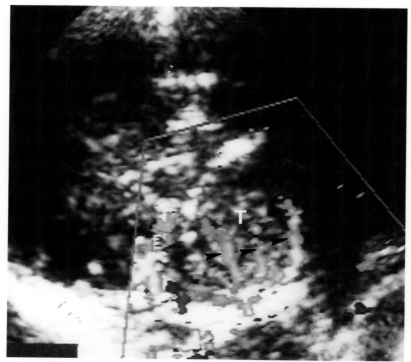

Figure 11–22. Color Doppler image of the thalamostriate vessels in a coronal plane. Thalamostriate arteries *(arrowheads)* are noted in the color Doppler box placed over the left thalamus (T). These are normal vessels but are the same vessels that calcify in patients with mineralizing vasculopathy.

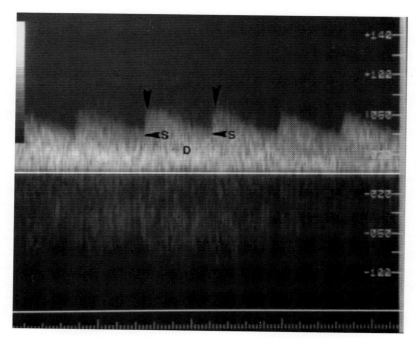

Figure 11–23. Low-resistance arterial flow expressed by Doppler spectral pattern. The spectral pattern was created by insonation of a right middle cerebral artery. The beginning of systole is marked by the *horizontal arrowhead.* The *vertical arrowhead* indicates peak systole. D indicates in diastole. Flow, reflected as the spectral pattern, is continuously above the 0 cm/sec baseline during both systole and diastole. High-resistance systems, such as the external carotid artery, which feeds the face but not the brain, usually show little or no flow (and the spectral pattern remains at the baseline) during diastole.

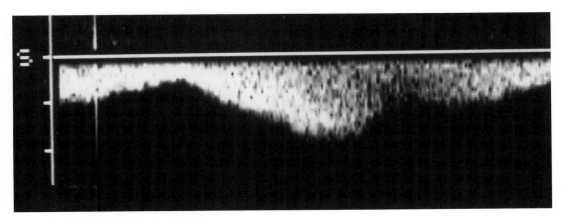

Figure 11–24. Normal venous spectra. This spectrum, obtained from a normal superior sagittal sinus, shows it to be sinusoidal, changing with respiratory motion and synchronous with the patient's pulse. This is the most common form of normal venous flow in the brain. The direction of flow in this case is below the baseline, indicating flow away from the transducer.

nous spectrum is seen in 59% of the great cerebral veins (Galen), while 46% of the straight sinus flows are sinusoid and synchronous with the pulse (Fig. 11–24) and a small percentage of normal veins show an intermittent pulsation pattern in which no signal is obtained at points along the spectrum. This intermittent pattern, seen in only 3% of the straight sinuses in normal infants, was commonly seen in severely ill premature infants, indicating reduced venous volume flow. An irregular biphasic spectrum is typical of venous flow within such intracranial arteriovenous malformations as the great cerebral vein (Galen) aneurysm.[2,44]

ACKNOWLEDGMENTS

We thank Dr. Susan Rachlin for help with the preparatory stages of this chapter.

REFERENCES

1. Leksell L. Echoencephalography: Detection of the intracranial complications following head injury. *Acta Chir Scand.* 1956;110:301–315.
2. Cohen HL, Haller J. Advances in perinatal neurosonography. *AJR.* 1994;163:801–810.
3. Shkolnik A. B-mode scanning of the infant brain. A new approach. Case report. Craniopharyngioma. *J Clin Ultrasound.* 1975;3:229–231.
4. Garrett W, Kossoff G, Jones R. Ultrasonic cross-sectional visualization of hydrocephalus in infants. *Neuroradiology.* 1975;8:279–288.
5. Lees R, Harrison R, Sims T. Gray scale ultrasonography in the evaluation of hydrocephalus and associated abnormalities in infants. *Am J Dis Child.* 1978;132:376–378.
6. London D, Carroll B, Enzmann D. Sonography of ventricular size and germinal matrix hemorrhage in premature infants. *AJR.* 1980;135:559–564.
7. Babcock D, Han B. The accuracy of high resolution real-time ultrasonography of the head in infancy. *Radiology.* 1981;139:665–676.
8. Dewbury K, Aluwihare A. The anterior fontanelle as an ultrasound window for study of the brain: A preliminary report. *Br J Radiol.* 1980;53:81–84.
9. Ben-Ora A, Eddy L, Hatch G, et al. The anterior fontanelle as an acoustic window to the neonatal ventricular system. *J Clin Ultrasound.* 1980;8:65–67.
10. Cohen HL, Ziprkowski M. New diagnostic insights in pediatric neurosonography. *Diagn Imaging.* 1991;13:142–146, 215.
11. Grant E, Richardson J. Infant and neonatal neurosonography—Technique and normal anatomy. In: Taveras J, ed. *Radiology Diagnosis–Imaging–Intervention.* Philadelphia: JB Lippincott; 1994;3:1–7.
12. Babcock D, Han B. *Cranial Ultrasonography of Infants.* Baltimore: Williams & Wilkins; 1981.
13. Grant E. Neurosonography: Periventricular leukomalacia. In: Grant E, ed. *Neurosonography of the Preterm Neonate.* New York: Springer-Verlag, 1986: 69–84.
14. Hyman LA, McArdle CB, Shah Y. Neonatal brain. In: Hyman LA, Hinck VC, eds. *Clinical Brain Imaging. Normal Structure and Functional Anatomy.* St. Louis: Mosby–Year Book; 1992:45–51.
15. Kleinman P, Zito J, Davidson R, et al. The subarachnoid spaces in children: Normal variation in size. *Radiology.* 1983;147:455–457.
16. Fischer A, Aziz E. Diagnosis of cerebral atrophy in infants by near-field cranial sonography. *Am J Dis Child.* 1986;140:774–777.
17. Siegel M. Brain. In: Siegel M, ed. *Pediatric Sonography.* New York: Raven Press; 1991:9–62.
18. American Institute of Ultrasound in Medicine (AIUM) Standards for performance of the ultrasound examination of the infant brain. Lawrell, MD: AIUM; 1999.

19. Rumack C, Johnson M. *Perinatal & Infant Brain Imaging. Role of Ultrasound & Computed Tomography.* Chicago: Year Book Medical Publishers; 1984.

20. Farrugia S, Babcock D. The cavum septi pellucidi: Its appearance and incidence with cranial ultrasonography in infancy. *Radiology.* 1981;139:147–150.

21. Dorovini-Zis K. Gestational development of brain. *Arch Pathol Lab Med.* 1977;101:192–195.

22. Woaxen N, Gilbertson V. Cortical sulcal development seen on sonography: Relationship to gestational parameters. *J Ultrasound Med.* 1986;5:153–156.

23. Teele R, Share J. *Ultrasonography of Infants and Children.* Philadelphia: WB Saunders; 1991.

24. Siegel M, Shackleford G, Perlman J, et al. Hypoxic–ischemic encephalopathy in term infants: Diagnosis and prognosis evaluated by ultrasound. *Radiology.* 1984;152:395–399.

25. Horbar J, Leahy K, Lucey J. Ultrasound identification of lateral ventricular asymmetry in the human neonate. *J Clin Ultrasound.* 1983;152:67–69.

26. DiPietro M, Brody B, Teele R. Peritrigonal echogenic "blush" on cranial sonography: Pathologic correlates. *AJR.* 1986;146:467–471.

27. Reibel T, Nasir R, Weber K. Choroid plexus cysts: A normal finding on ultrasound. *Pediatr Radiol.* 1992; 22:410–412.

28. Yousefzadeh D, Naidich T. Ultrasound anatomy of the posterior fossae in children: Correlation with brain sections. *Radiology.* 1985;156:353–361.

29. Zieger M, Dorr U, Schulz R. Pediatric spinal sonography. Part II: Malformations and mass lesions. *Pediatr Radiol.* 1988;18:105–111.

30. Anderson N, Allan R, Darlow B, et al. Diagnosis of intraventricular hemorrhage in the newborn: Value of sonography via the posterior fontanelle. *AJR.* 1994; 163:893–896.

31. Schlesinger AE, Munden M, Hayman L. Hyperechoic foci in the thalamic region imaged via the posterior fontanelle: A potential mimic of thalamic pathology. *Pediatr Radiol.* 1999;29:520–523.

32. Sudakoff G, Montazemi M, Rifkin M. The foramen magnum: The underutilized acoustic window to the posterior fossa. *J Ultrasound Med.* 1993;4:205–210.

33. Mercker J, Blumhagen J, Brewer D. Echographic demonstration of extracerebral fluid collections with the lateral technique. *J Ultrasound Med.* 1983;2: 265–269.

34. Helmke K, Winkler P, Kock C. Sonographic examination of the brain stem area in infants. An echographic and anatomic analysis. *Pediatr Radiol.* 1987;17: 1–6.

35. Seibert J, Glasier C, Lethiser R, et al. Transcranial Doppler using standard duplex equipment in children. *Ultrasound Q.* 1990;8:167–196.

36. Buckley K, Taylor G, Estroff J, et al. Use of the mastoid fontanelle for improved sonographic visualization of the neonatal midbrain and posterior fossa. *AJR.* 1997;168:1021–1025.

37. Foley WD, Erickson S. Color Doppler flow imaging. *AJR.* 1991;156:3–13.

38. Seibert J, Miller S, Kirby R, et al. Cerebrovascular disease in symptomatic and asymptomatic patients with sickle cell anemia: Screening with duplex transcranial Doppler US—Correlation with MR imaging and MR angiography. *Radiology.* 1993;189:457–466.

39. Deeg K, Rupprecht TH. Pulsed Doppler sonographic measurement of normal values for the flow velocities in the intracranial arteries of healthy newborns. *Pediatr Radiol.* 1989;19:71–78.

40. Koven M, Cohen HL, Goldman M. Case of the day 2. Fetal intracranial avm presenting as enlarged cardiac chamber. *J Ultrasound Med.* 1992;11:177.

41. Mitchell D, Merton D, Mirsky P, et al. Circle of Willis in newborns: Color Doppler imaging of 53 healthy full-term infants. *Radiology.* 1989;172:201–205.

42. Taylor G. Current concepts in neonatal cranial Doppler sonography. *Ultrasound Q.* 1992;9:223–244.

43. Deeg K, Paul R, Rupprecht TH, et al. Pulsed Doppler sonographic measurement of flow velocities in the anterior cerebral arteries of infants with hydrocephalus in comparison to a healthy control group. *Monatsschr Kinderheilkd.* 1988;136:85–94.

44. Winkler P, Helmke K. Duplex-scanning of the deep venous drainage in the evaluation of blood flow velocity of the cerebral vascular system in infants. *Pediatr Radiol.* 1989;19:79–90.

CHAPTER TWELVE

Neurosonography of the Infant: Diagnosis of Abnormalities

Harris L. Cohen
Netta M. Blitman

The previous chapter on neurosonography in the infant (Chapter 11) discussed normal neurosonographic technique and findings. Once it is known what *normal* is, the examiner can go about the task of evaluating the abnormal. Key to analyzing an infant's neurosonogram for abnormality is knowledge of what intracranial abnormalities and conditions can be and are assessed by ultrasonography and what their typical sonographic findings are.

Unlike fetal neurosonography, in assessing the calvaria and its contents, the examiner is no longer aided by the amniotic fluid surrounding the fetal head. The neonatal sonologist, on the other hand, does not have to deal with such difficulties of fetal assessment as decreased amniotic fluid, unusual fetal lie, or a low-lying fetal head that may be assessed only with the aid of transvaginal or transperineal techniques. The neonatal sonologist also benefits from the greater ease in obtaining alternate imaging studies, if necessary, to assess areas of concern beyond the scope of ultrasonography. Obviously, the use of these modalities may be limited by the patient's clinical condition.

Much of the information used in the analysis of congenital abnormalities crosses the "barrier" between fetal and neonatal life. There are areas of diagnostic information that become less important with birth, such as the assessment for myelomeningocele. Use of the, at times, subtle intracranial "banana" and calvarial "lemon" signs, linked to myelomeningocele by their association with the Chiari type II malformation, is no longer necessary when the

myelomeningocele itself can be noted clinically.[1-3] There are diagnostic abnormalities that are relatively unique to neonatal life and neonatal neurosongraphy. They become extremely important in postnatal intracranial evaluation. These include subependymal and intraventricular hemorrhage (IVH) in the premature infant and asphyxia in the full-term infant.

This chapter discusses current uses of sonography in the assessment of abnormalities of the neonatal brain.

HYDROCEPHALY

Hydrocephaly is the most common congenital anomaly of the brain in those who survive fetal life. It consists of ventricular dilatation in the presence of increased cerebrospinal fluid (CSF) pressure. Hydrocephaly is usually due to congenital obstruction at the level of the aqueduct of Sylvius, the CSF pathway between the third and fourth ventricles. Other sites of obstruction may occur anywhere along this pathway, which begins at the predominant CSF production site, the choroid plexus of the lateral ventricles, and ends at the sites of CSF absorption thought to be predominantly the pacchionian granulations or arachnoid villi within the subarachnoid space at the vertex of the brain. From there, the CSF enters the venous system via the dural and venous sinuses (see Fig. 2–75). The cerebral ventricles may also be dilated on the basis of decreased absorption at the pacchionian granulations or, in rarer instances, because of increased CSF production by a choroid plexus papilloma.[4,5]

The pathway for CSF within the brain is from the lateral ventricles to the third ventricle via the interventricular foramina (Monro), through the aqueduct (Sylvius), into the fourth ventricle, and either out the median foramen (Magendie) into the cisterna magna or exiting via either lateral foramen (Luschka) into the basilar cisterns. Eighty percent of CSF flow then continues in the cisternal system, eventually flowing over the cerebral convexities, whereas 20% enters the spinal subarachnoid space, eventually also entering the cerebral subarachnoid space (see Fig. 2–75). Obstructive hydrocephaly is divided into two categories: communicating hydrocephaly, in which the obstruction or area of decreased absorption is at a point beyond the ventricular system, and noncommunicating hydrocephaly, in which the obstruction is at a point (e.g., aqueductal obstruction) within the ventricular system.[4–6]

Congenital hydrocephaly is an important diagnosis in the neonate. It may be suspected from or may already have been diagnosed by prenatal ultrasonography. The majority of these patients are unfortunate, in that 70% have an associated central nervous system (CNS) or non-CNS visceral anomaly. Even when treated, only 38% will have normal cognitive function.[5,7] Hydrocephaly and other intracranial abnormalities should certainly be searched for in any neonate born with an enlarged head, prominent separation of the cranial sutures, or a full fontanelle, or with clinical signs of neurological abnormality. The most common causes beyond aqueductal stenosis are myelomeningocele (with associated Arnold–Chiari malformation), communicating hydrocephaly, and, to a lesser extent, Dandy–Walker malformation. Less common causes of hydrocephaly in the newborn are postinflammatory, usually from intrauterine infection by cytomegalovirus (CMV) or toxoplasmosis, posthemorrhagic, in the unusual cases of intrauterine IVH, or from masses, which may be vascular, such as the vein of Galen "aneurysm" (actually an arteriovenous malformation), or, rarely, neoplastic.[8,9]

The diagnosis of hydrocephaly is of great concern in the initial and follow-up examinations of premature infants with IVH. Clinical suspicion may be aroused by a neonate whose head circumference is growing beyond what is expected from the growth charts. Occasionally, the normal "catch-up" growth in a premature infant may cause concern, as may infants with unusual head shapes. Evaluation of the parent's head shape may ease concern. However, sonography using an anterior fontanelle approach can allow the sonologist a quick and easy intracranial assessment.

Sonographic Findings in Congenital Hydrocephaly

Ventricular enlargement usually indicates hydrocephaly. Dilatation of the individual lateral ventricles may best be determined by paramedian views (Fig. 12–1). The sagittal (median) view allows evaluation of dilatation of the third or the fourth ventricle. However, it is a coronal view (Fig. 12–2), using anterior-to-posterior angulation, that allows comparison of both lateral ventricles for enlargement, as well as the ability to note dilatation of the temporal horn tips and the third and fourth ventricles. Ventriculomegaly may also be seen on an *ex vacuo* basis from brain atrophy or dysgenesis. Associated findings of widening of the interhemispheric fissure or prominent extra-axial spaces, noted by imaging the peripheral borders of the brain, suggest dilatation on the basis of decreased parenchyma. Some patients may have evidence of hydrocephaly and brain atrophy at the same time.[10] Hydrocephaly may be asymmetrical. Most sonologists read neonatal ventriculomegaly by a gestalt that is developed over time, rather than by using any actual measurements. As with the fetus, there are visual clues for neonatal ventriculomegaly. The observation of a prominent amount of CSF lateral to the choroid plexus suggests ventricular enlargement because the lateral ventricular wall typically hugs the choroid plexus, with little, if any, CSF seen between the two. In significant ventriculomegaly, with the patient's head examined on its side, the choroid plexus, on the dependent side, hangs down into the CSF-filled lateral ventricle but does not touch the ventricular wall.[11,12] Ballooning of the superolateral angles of the frontal horns or dilatation of the posterior horns may be early signs of hydrocephaly.[10] Often, the atrium of the lateral ventricle is the first area to be noted as dilated, particularly on paramedian images. Suspicion of ventriculomegaly should be confirmed by serial head circumference measurements and with follow-up head ultrasonographic examinations as clinically warranted.

In aqueductal stenosis only the third and lateral ventricles are dilated. The fourth ventricle is normal in size. In cases of communicating hydrocephaly (Fig. 12–2), all of the ventricles are dilated.

Neurosonography may demonstrate fenestrations (Fig. 12–3) of one or both leaves of the septi pellucidi in cases of untreated hydrocephaly. These fenestrations may increase in size and number over time. Their recognition prevents confusion with congenital absence of the septum pellucidum, often associated with other neuroanatomic abnormalities.[11,13]

Hydrocephaly can affect the Doppler spectra. There is a decrease in forward diastolic flow (i.e., an

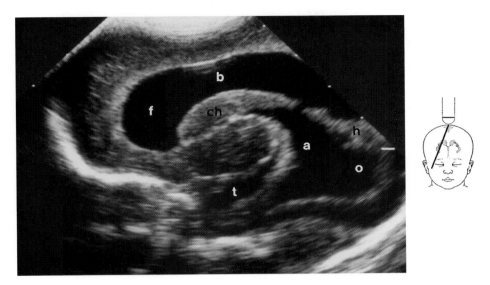

Figure 12–1. Ventricular dilatation shown in a right paramedian plane. Significant dilatation of the right lateral ventricle is noted in this newborn with posthemorrhagic hydrocephalus. Choroid plexus (ch) and residual hemorrhagic clot (h) are noted within the ventricle. f, anterior horn; b, body; a, atrium; o, posterior horn; t, inferior horn tip of the ventricle.

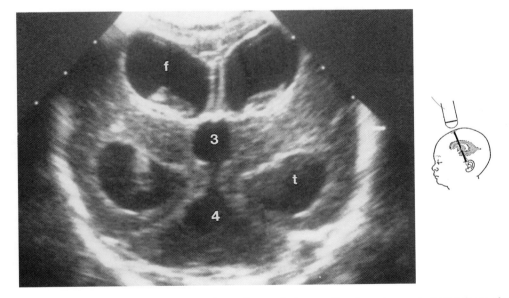

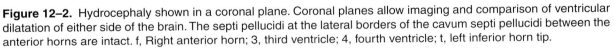

Figure 12–2. Hydrocephaly shown in a coronal plane. Coronal planes allow imaging and comparison of ventricular dilatation of either side of the brain. The septi pellucidi at the lateral borders of the cavum septi pellucidi between the anterior horns are intact. f, Right anterior horn; 3, third ventricle; 4, fourth ventricle; t, left inferior horn tip.

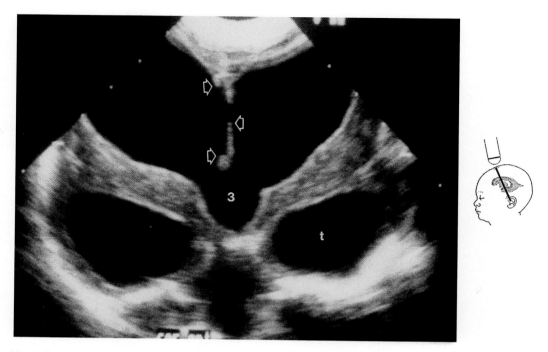

Figure 12–3. Fenestrated septi pellucidi shown in a coronal plane. Breaks *(arrows)* are noted in the usually intact echogenic lines of the septi pellucidi of this 8-week-old infant born with moderate hydrocephaly. Only the edges of the right septum remain. These fenestrations can be seen to increase in size and number in cases of untreated and worsening hydrocephaly. This phenomenon may eventually lead to an image that may be misinterpreted as congenital absence of the septi pellucidi. t, Left inferior horn tip; 3, third ventricle.

increase in resistance index [RI] and pulsatility index) with severe hydrocephaly.[14–16] The pulsatility index determined by transfontanelle or transcranial Doppler imaging decreases as diastolic flow improves with effective ventricular shunting.[17–18] Hemodynamic response to graded compression by the ultrasound transducer on the fontanelle has been used as a noninvasive method to predict hydrocephaly. Some investigators have suggested that Doppler analysis during fontanelle compression can help select out hydrocephalic infants who will benefit from shunt placement. Graded fontanelle compression results in a statistically significant increase in the RI of infants with hydrocephaly and cerebral edema, but is associated with little, if any, increase in RI in healthy infants.[19,20]

Ultrasonography can be used to help the neurosurgeon guide the placement of ventricular shunt devices. Follow-up examinations can note the effectiveness of the shunt procedure by making sure that the ventricles are not enlarging from their immediate postshunting sizes. Occasionally, extra-axial collections, such as subdural hematomas, can occur as a complication of the rapid decompression of the ventricular system by a shunting procedure and may be imaged by ultrasonography, although, typically,

computed tomography (CT) is a better method for imaging this problem.[10,21]

After closure of the anterior fontanelle, transcranial ultrasonography using the thin, squamous portion of the temporal bone and a low-frequency (e.g., 2-MHz) transducer for maximal penetration may allow continued analysis of ventricular size (Fig. 12–4), particularly in children being followed up by serial examinations.[11,17] Certainly, if the necessary information can no longer be obtained by ultrasonography, the clinician should obtain it via another imaging modality, usually CT.

CHIARI TYPE II MALFORMATION

In the 1890s, Chiari described four types of malformation, each representing a different and unrelated anomaly of the hindbrain. Today some authorities do not include his type III, a form of cervical cephalocele with downward displacement of the entire cerebellum into a large cervical spina bifida, or type IV, consisting of severe cerebellar hypoplasia, in the modern grouping of Chiari malformations. The Chiari type I malformation is best evaluated by magnetic resonance imaging (MRI), with which the diagnosis can be made by noting the cerebellar ton-

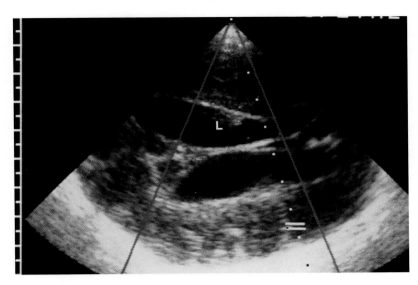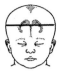

Figure 12–4. Hydrocephaly, shown using the transcranial approach in an axial plane. The transducer is on the left side of the calvarium. This 11-month-old child's hydrocephaly had been followed by ultrasonography (US), and despite a small, closing anterior fontanelle, his parents requested an attempt at US to avoid a computed tomography examination. A low-frequency (2-MHz) transducer was used. The lateral ventricles are well imaged and mild to moderate ventricular dilatation is noted. L, Left lateral ventricle.

sils and the inferior cerebellum (but not the medulla or the fourth ventricle) in a low position, protruding below the foramen magnum. As discussed, the diagnosis of a type II malformation, associated with myelomeningocele, is of great concern in fetal life because it allows the diagnosis of myelomeningocele despite limited imaging of the fetal spine.[22,23] The sonographic diagnosis of a type II malformation is somewhat more difficult, but is also less necessary, in the neonate.

Sonographic Findings in Chiari Type II Malformation

Patients with Chiari type II malformation may be noted to have a small posterior fossa, best seen on sagittal images, due to the downward displacement of the brain stem and the inferior cerebellum into the upper cervical canal. This displacement effaces the cisterna magna.[22] An anteroposterior measurement of 2 mm or less[24] for the echoless cisterna magna is suggestive of effacement, although this analysis is somewhat more difficult in neonates. Most cases of Chiari type II malformation are associated with hydrocephaly. Colpocephaly (Fig. 12–5), the nonspecific finding of greater dilatation of the posterior portion of the lateral ventricles compared to the anterior portion, may be seen on coronal or sagittal view. The ventriculomegaly is thought to be due to stretching and narrowing of the aqueduct (Sylvius), which occurs with the downward displacement of cerebral

structures. Occasionally, ventriculomegaly does not develop until after repair of the myelomeningocele. Anterior and inferior pointing of the frontal horns in a "bat wing" appearance, on coronal view, and a large massa intermedia in the dilated third ventricle, on sagittal view (Fig. 12–5), have been described, as has an unusually large and lobulated choroid plexus.[4,10,25,26]

These sonographic images are usually obtained via the anterior fontanelle approach. The posterior fontanelle can be used occasionally for better evaluation of infratentorial structures.[11] Foramen magnum views have been described for improved imaging of the displaced structures within the spinal canal. These views are not easy to obtain, especially if the patient is confined to an isolette. A technique has been described in which the transducer is placed just caudal and medial to the mastoid process, allowing improved imaging of the posterior fossa structures.[27,28]

DANDY-WALKER COMPLEX AND THE ENLARGED CISTERNA CEREBELLO-MEDULLARIS (MAGNA)

A cerebello-medullary cistern (cisterna magna) larger than 10 mm may be a normal variant, but anomalies such as the dilated fourth ventricle of communicating hydrocephaly or a retrocerebellar arachnoid cyst must be considered.

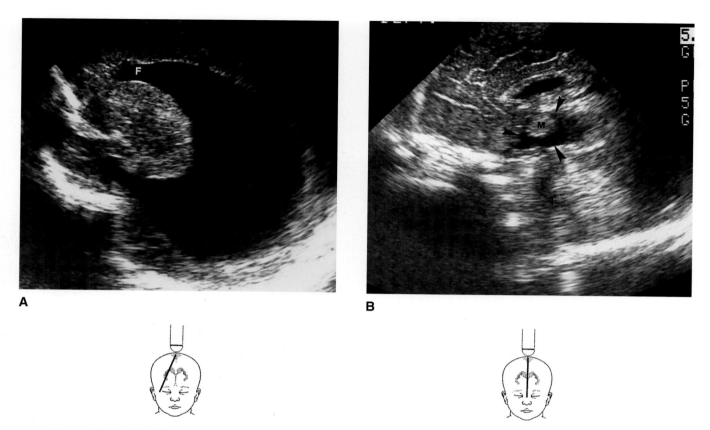

Figure 12–5. Chiari II type malformation. **A.** Colpocephaly shown in a right paramedian plane. This newborn with repaired myelomeningocele and hydrocephaly has colpocephaly, a disproportionate dilatation of the posterior portion of the ventricular system compared to the anterior portion, which may be seen in Chiari type II and other malformations. F, anterior horn. **B.** Large massa intermedia shown in the median view. A prominent massa intermedia (M) is seen in the dilated third ventricle *(arrowheads)*. Effacement of the cisterna magna by the downward displacement of infratentorial structures is responsible for the inability to image the cisterna magna. 4, Fourth ventricle.

The key grouping of anomalies to be wary of when noting a posterior fossa cyst is the Dandy–Walker complex. The complex includes the classic Dandy–Walker malformation, the Dandy–Walker variant, and the mega–cisterna magna.[29] Each is associated with defective development of the roof of the fourth ventricle and is often associated with other intracranial anomalies. Among these are the midline abnormalities of agenesis of the corpus callosum (ACC) and holoprosencephaly, as well as migrational disorders such as schizencephaly and posterior cephaloceles.[22]

In the classic Dandy–Walker malformation (Fig. 12–6), there is a large posterior fossa cyst, which represents severe dilatation of the fourth ventricle because of atresia of the ventricle's lateral and median apertures, respectively Luschka and Magendie. The cyst extends from the area of the fourth ventricle posteriorly to the occiput because of the associated aplasia or hypoplasia of the vermis of the cerebellum. The cerebellar hemispheres are compressed and displaced laterally by the "cyst" or the dilated fourth ventricle. The increased posterior fossa volume is responsible for a higher than normal tentorium (Fig. 12–7). Hydrocephaly is usually, but not necessarily, seen at birth. If it is not seen at birth, the condition develops soon afterward.[1,30–32]

The Dandy–Walker variant consists of mild hypoplasia of the vermis, usually its inferior aspect, and less severe dilatation of the fourth ventricle, as well as a lesser increase in posterior fossa volume. Dandy–Walker variant occurs twice as often as the classic Dandy–Walker malformation but is more difficult to diagnose by ultrasonography. Estroff's group reported that among 17 cases of fetuses with Dandy–Walker variants, 24% had ventriculomegaly, 47% had extra-CNS abnormalities, and 9% had abnormal karyotypes.[29,33] Obviously, the diagnosis is an important one to make; it is even more significant antenatally.

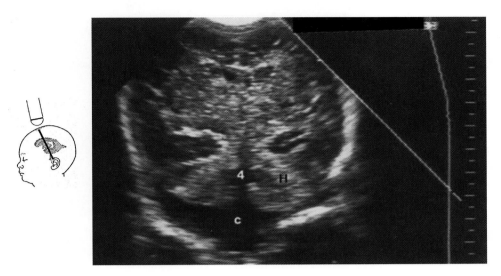

Figure 12–6. Dandy–Walker malformation shown in a coronal plane. A prominent cystic area (c) is seen posteriorly in the region of this newborn's cisterna magna. The cystic area, representing cerebrospinal fluid in an obstructed fourth ventricle, can be seen extending to the more anterior portion of the fourth ventricle (4) via a defect in the cerebellar vermis, which is part of the anomaly. There was no significant ventriculomegaly at this time, but hydrocephaly developed a few weeks later. H = left cerebellar hemisphere.

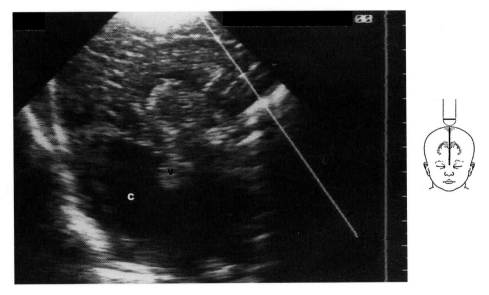

Figure 12–7. Enlarged posterior fossa in Dandy–Walker malformation, shown in a sagittal plane. (The image is not in standard display, in that the anterior portion of the brain is to the reader' right.) The tentorium *(arrows)* is lifted superiorly by the large subtentorial cyst (c), which takes up much of the volume of this enlarged posterior fossa. v, Dysgenetic vermis.

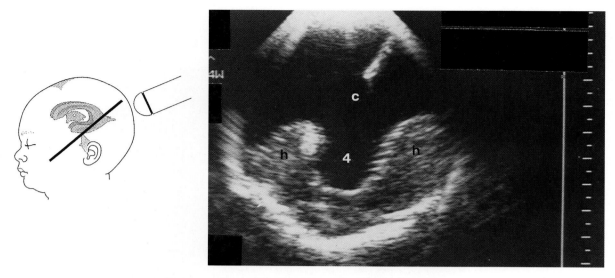

Figure 12–8. Posterior fontanelle approach in diagnosing the classic Dandy–Walker malformation, shown in a coronal plane. Use of the posterior fontanelle for brain assessment is most helpful in evaluating the posterior structures of the brain and subtentorial contents. This is particularly true with the Dandy–Walker abnormality. In this image the subtentorial "cyst" (c) is the first area imaged below the posteriorly placed tranducer. Inferiorly on the image, and therefore anteriorly in the brain, is the laterally displaced cerebellar hemispheres (h). The cyst extends to the anterior portion of the fourth ventricle (4) because of absence of the dysgenetic cerebellar vermis.

The mega–cisterna magna is the most common form of the Dandy–Walker complex, representing 54% of cystic posterior malformations. Sonographically, the abnormality is usually limited to an isolated enlarged cisterna magna of 10 mm or greater. There may be variable enlargement of the posterior fossa, and the cerebellar vermis is intact. Ventriculomegaly is unusual. Where once this entity was thought to be a benign variation, the mega–cisterna magna has been linked to aneuploidy, particularly trisomy 18.[29]

Again, routine anterior fontanelle imaging is most commonly used. This is perhaps the best entity to also evaluate using a posterior fontanelle approach (Fig. 12–8).

AGENESIS OF THE CORPUS CALLOSUM

The corpus callosum is the largest of the median interhemispheric commissures allowing communication between the two halves of the brain. As the cerebral hemispheres grow laterally and posteriorly, the corpus callosum develops upwardly and from front to back. The most anterior or rostral section, the rostrum, develops first, followed by the development of the genu, the trunk, and the splenium of the corpus callosum. Knowledge of this normal anterior-to-posterior development sequence (despite the fact that an anterior portion of the genu actually develops at the same time or later than the splenium) allows one

the ability to differentiate cases of callosal abnormality as primary callosal dysgenesis or secondary dysgenesis from partial or complete destruction of the corpus callosum after normal development. In cases of primary callosal dysgenesis, the portions of the imaged corpus callosum conform to the normal anterior to posterior development sequence. In cases of secondary dysgenesis, what is seen of the corpus callosum does not conform to the normal sequence. If only the posterior corpus callosum is seen, for example, that suggests that the absent anterior portion is due to secondary dysgenesis. Early vascular or inflammatory insults before the 12th postmenstrual week are thought to be the cause of primary callosal agenesis[4,5] (see also Chapter 5).

Agenesis of the corpus callosum may be an isolated anomaly; but in many cases (80% in one series[35]) there are associated anomalies. These may include anomalies such as polymicrogyria and cortical heterotopia (which are best evaluated by MRI) and septo-optic dysplasia, as well as encephalocele, aqueductal stenosis, midline intracerebral lipoma (Fig. 12–9), interhemispheric arachnoid cyst, hydrocephaly, Dandy–Walker cyst, and Chiari type II malformation (which may be diagnosed by ultrasonography).[4,32] Clinical symptomatology is usually based on the associated cerebral anomaly. The abnormality is usually sporadic in its occurrence and is of unknown etiology. There have been reported cases associated with trisomies 8, 13 through 15, and 18.[34,35]

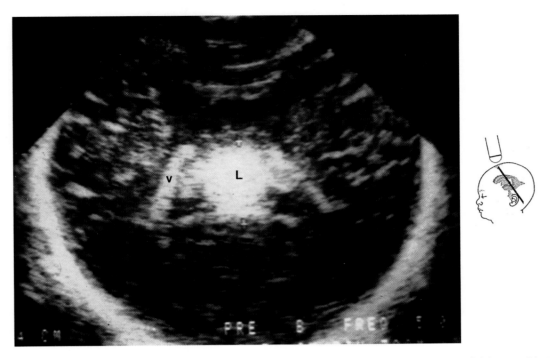

Figure 12–9. Intracerebral lipoma. The typical homogeneously echogenic image of a lipoma (L) is noted between the lateral ventricles of a full-term newborn. Lipomas are one of several midline abnormalities associated with age-nesis of the corpus callosum. There is no ventriculomegaly. Tumor masses, benign or malignant, are not at all common in neonates, and are best seen with the global imaging afforded by computed tomography. They can be imaged by ultrasound, particularly if the echogenicity is not isoechoic with the surrounding normal brain parenchyma. v, Right lateral ventricle.

The normal corpus callosum, as discussed in Chapter 5, should be readily imaged on median views, superior to the cavum septi pellucidi, and on coronal views, anterosuperior to the anterior horns and inferior and posterior to the interhemispheric fissure. There are several classic sonographic findings of complete ACC in neonates. In the coronal plane one can note marked separation of the anterior horns and bodies of the lateral ventricles. The lateral ventricles run parallel to each other (Fig. 12–10). In the absence of this normal dorsal median structure, the third ventricle may be seen in a high-riding position, between, rather than inferior to, the separated anterior horns, creating what has been described as a "Viking's helmet" or "bull's head" configuration. Colpocephaly may be noted. The sulci and the gyri, in the absence of the corpus callosum, run perpendicular (Fig. 12–11) to the third ventricle, rather than paralleling it and the pericallosal sulcus, as they do in a normal patient. This radial pattern of the gyri is known as the sunburst sign and is thought to be pathognomonic of complete ACC.[4,35–37]

An exact antenatal or neonatal sonographic diagnosis of partial ACC is more difficult than that for complete ACC, but has been reported.[38] Magnetic resonance imaging may allow a more ready diagnosis.

HOLOPROSENCEPHALY

Holoprosencephaly occurs when there is incomplete or absent cleavage of the primitive forebrain or prosencephalon into the cerebral hemispheres (the telencephalon) and the individual thalami and hypothalami (the diencephalon). The result is an abnormal continuity of gray and white matter across the midline, seen best with MRI. The abnormal cleavage that leads to holoprosencephaly occurs in the fourth to eighth weeks of fetal life, at about the same time that the fetal face develops, hence the common association of holoprosencephaly with midline facial anomalies of variable severity, including cleft lip and cleft palate as well as cyclopia. The more severe forms of facial anomalies are usually associated with the more severe forms of holoprosencephaly, but this is not always the case, and patients with severe holoprosencephaly may have essentially normal facies. There is always hypotelorism and usually microcephaly. There may be

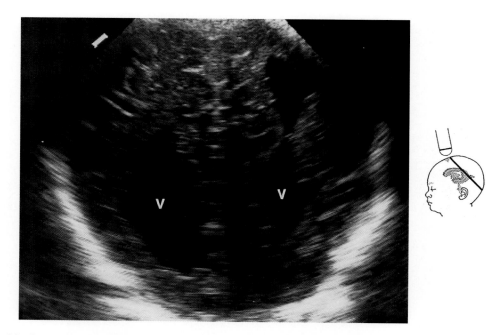

Figure 12–10. Agenesis of the corpus callosum shown in coronal view. The lateral ventricles (V) run parallel to each other because of a lack of central tethering caused by absence of the midline corpus callosum. There was incidental colpocephaly.

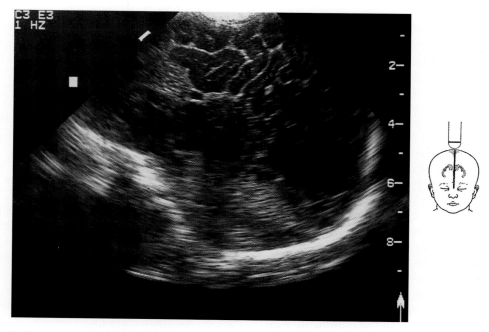

Figure 12–11. Sunburst sign in agenesis of the corpus callosum (ACC), shown in a sagittal plane in the medial surface of brain. Many of the gyri and sulci run in a radial pattern, intersecting the area where the corpus callosum would be, rather than running parallel to it. This is a well-known finding in ACC. 3, Area of the third ventricle; g, gyrus.

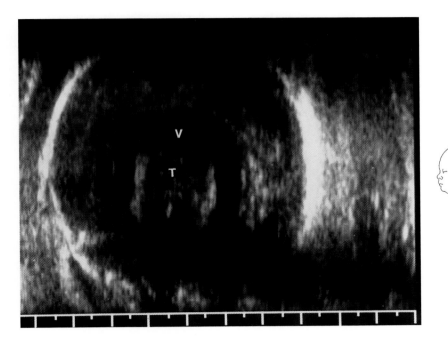

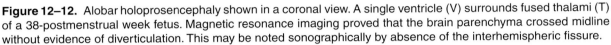

Figure 12–12. Alobar holoprosencephaly shown in a coronal view. A single ventricle (V) surrounds fused thalami (T) of a 38-postmenstrual week fetus. Magnetic resonance imaging proved that the brain parenchyma crossed midline without evidence of diverticulation. This may be noted sonographically by absence of the interhemispheric fissure.

an association with various trisomies, including trisomies 13 through 15 and 18.[4,22,32]

There are various forms of holoprosencephaly. The most severe form is alobar holoprosencephaly, which represents complete failure to form separate cerebral hemispheres. In the less severe semilobar form the posterior portion of the hemispheres develops partially, and in the least severe lobar holoprosencephaly the hemispheres are almost separate, except for minor anteroinferior connections.[4,11,22,39]

Sonographically, patients with alobar holoprosencephaly have no corpus callosum, falx, or interhemispheric fissure. There is a thin, pancakelike primitive cerebrum in the anterior or posterior skull incompletely covering a single monoventricle (Fig. 12–12). The single monoventricle often has a horseshoe shape, in part because of an associated ballooning of the roof of the third ventricle in the form of a dorsal cyst or sac. The thalami are fused. The semilobar form of holoprosencephaly shows more cerebral tissue and a smaller univentricle on ultrasonography. Lobar holoprosencephaly is a difficult ultrasonographic diagnosis, with near-normal cerebral hemispheres and thalami. The anterior horns and the lateral ventricles may appear somewhat closer than normal. This, in combination with an absent septum pellucidum, has been thought to

be responsible for the sometimes reported image of squared anterior horns[4,11,22,32] (see also Chapters 5 and 11).

HYDRANENCEPHALY

Hydranencephaly is thought to be due to antenatal occlusion of both internal carotid arteries,[32,40,41] although there have been cases linked to early toxoplasmosis or CMV infection.[5] Whatever the cause, the result is the massive destruction and resorption of the cerebral cortex, hemispheric white matter, and basal ganglia and their replacement by thin-walled sacs in the frontal, parietal, and temporal lobes that appear echoless and without surrounding brain parenchyma on ultrasonography. There may be difficulty in differentiating the sonographic image of hydranencephaly from severe hydrocephaly (Fig. 12–13). However, in severe hydrocephaly, which can be treated with ventricular shunting, a thin rim of cerebral tissue, peripheral to the cystic spaces, may be noted. A midline or off-midline, relatively complete falx may be seen in patients with hydranencephaly. The posterior lobe and the brain stem as well as paired thalami, fed from the basilar artery, remain intact and normal in appearance, as do the infratentorial contents of the

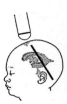

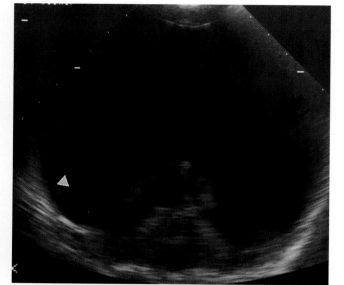

Figure 12–13. Hydrocephaly simulating hydranencephaly, shown in the coronal plane. Severe hydrocephaly in this newborn of 34 postmenstrual weeks' simulates hydranencephaly, except for imaging the choroid plexus (ch) and a small amount of supratentorial brain parenchyma at the calvarial periphery *(arrowhead).*

brain.[11,18,32] Often, the inferior medial aspects of the temporal and frontal lobes are preserved.[5] The evolution of the brain destruction of hydranencephaly[41] and that of the brain clefts of schizencephaly[42] have been reported in fetal examinations. Apparently, these changes do not evolve further after birth.

DISEASES OF PREMATURITY

Subependymal and Intraventricular Hemorrhage

Spontaneous intracranial hemorrhage is a common phenomenon in premature infants. Although some of these infants may suffer subdural or subarachnoid hemorrhage, which, in any event, is difficult to note with ultrasonography, subependymal hemorrhage (SEH) and IVH of germinal matrix (GM) origin are the most common types of spontaneous intracranial hemorrhage and the most common intracranial abnormality in premature infants, particularly those weighing less than 1500 g at birth or born at 32 postmenstrual weeks or earlier.[11,32] The incidence, which Papile and associates[43] noted in 1978 in as many as 44 of 100 premature infants weighing less than 1500 g, continues to be quoted as high as 25% to 40% compared to an incidence of 2% to 4% among full-term infants.[10] These hemorrhages can be a cause of serious morbidity and mortality, and their diagnosis, which can be made quite readily by neurosonography, is the most frequent reason, along with periventricular leukomalacia in the somewhat older premature infant, for neonatologists to request neurosonography in the intensive care unit.

The GM is an area of spongioblasts and neuroblasts that eventually develops into neurons and glial cells that will migrate to the cerebral cortex and the basal ganglia. Until the 12th week of fetal life, the GM can be found above the caudate nucleus, in the floor of the entire lateral ventricle, extending from the anterior to the inferior horn. With time this area regresses, so that by 32 postmenstrual weeks, the GM is found only along the ventricular surface of the caudate nucleus and at its border with the thalamus, the caudothalamic groove.[10,44,45]

The GM contains a rich supply of fragile, thin-walled blood vessels with little connective tissue support. These vessels are sensitive to increased arterial blood pressure, which may occur in the pressure-passive brains of premature infants who receive preferential cerebral arterial flow in the presence of hypercapnia caused by hypoxia or ischemia or who have increased venous pressure as a result of myocardial failure or pneumothorax. Increased pressure in these fragile vessels leads to vascular rupture and hemorrhage in the GM area.[10,11] This hemorrhage may extend locally, most often into the ventricular system, and far less often into the caudate or the thalamus.

Acute IVH is homogeneously echogenic. In fact, hemorrhage, immediately after its occurrence, is echoless and is not recognizable by ultrasonography. Relatively immediate fibrin deposition allows its identification as an echogenic mass. The echogenicity of acute hemorrhage is similar to that of the choroid plexus. Knowledge that the normal choroid plexus is not present in the posterior horns of the lateral ventricles or in the anterior horns anterior to the interventricular foramina (Monro) allows hemorrhage in these locations to be differentiated from choroid plexus. The classification of these hemorrhages is essentially unchanged from that proposed by Papile and collaborators in 1978.[43] The grading system has some limitations, however, in that it does not take into account the uncommon extension of hemorrhages into the thalamus, often associated with a poor prognosis, or hemorrhage in the cerebellum, which can occur but may be technically difficult to diagnose sonographically. Hemorrhage limited to the subependymal area has been labeled grade I SEH (Fig. 12–14). Extension of the hemorrhage into a normal-sized or minimally dilated lateral ventricle is labeled grade II IVH. The presence of IVH in a dilated lateral ventricle is labeled grade III IVH (Fig. 12–15).

New concepts have developed with regard to grade IV IVH (Fig. 12–16), in which there is hemorrhage in a dilated ventricle and increased echogenicity of nearby periventricular white matter. The parenchymal component of the grade IV hemorrhage was once considered to be due to a direct extension of hemorrhage from the ventricular system into the brain parenchyma, with the inevitable development of a porencephalic cyst (Fig. 12–17).[11,23,46,47] The current theory, based on pathology studies and the fact that associated intraparenchymal hemorrhage (IPH) is typically found sonographically 2 days (usually day 4 of life) after the identification of IVH (days 1 to 2), suggests that some other event occurs, rather than direct extension of hemorrhage.[48,49] Volpe[48] has linked the large IVH and the somewhat later development of IPH to increased pressure on the periventricular venous system leading to venous congestion and subsequent ischemia and hemorrhagic infarction. The medullary veins in the periventricular white matter converge at the ventricular angle, forming the terminal vein in the subependymal area. Hemorrhage may obstruct venous return and may lead to hemorrhagic infarction or reperfusion injury, which appears echogenic, in a watershed region after a period of cerebral hypoperfusion.[48,50] One institution reported a 2% to 3% incidence of this venous infarction among premature infants of less than 35 weeks' gestation.[11,51] The incidence of IPH associated with IVH is increased among patients requiring emergency cesarean section, possibly complicating complications of labor leading to its development.[11,49,50]

In the sonographic examination the search for GM hemorrhage requires the use of both sagittal and coronal views (orthogonal projections). The ex-

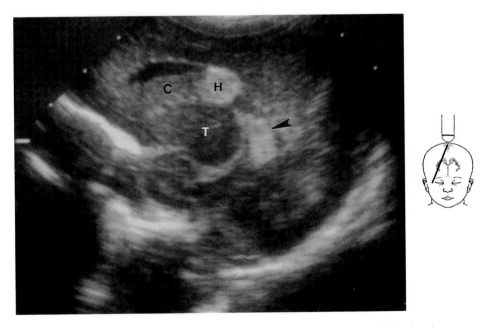

Figure 12–14. Subependymal hemorrhage shown in a right parasagittal plane. A circular, homogeneously echogenic mass consistent with acute hemorrhage (H) is noted at the caudothalamic groove of this 3-day-old of 32 postmenstrual weeks. The hemorrhage is subependymal, or grade I, in type, since it is seen limited to the region of the caudothalamic groove, i.e., between the head of the caudate nucleus (C) and the thalamus (T). The *arrowhead* indicates the normal choroid plexus, which has an echogenicity identical to that of acute hemorrhage.

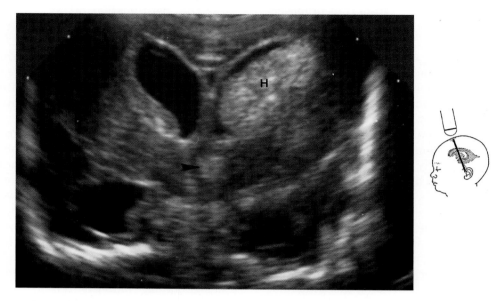

Figure 12–15. Grade III intraventricular hemorrhage shown in a coronal plane. There is a large clot (H) in a dilated left anterior horn of this 7-day-old of 29 postmenstrual weeks. Subtle heterogeneity of the clot's echogenicity suggests that it is subacute in age. The *arrowhead* indicates a small amount of hemorrhage in the third ventricle.

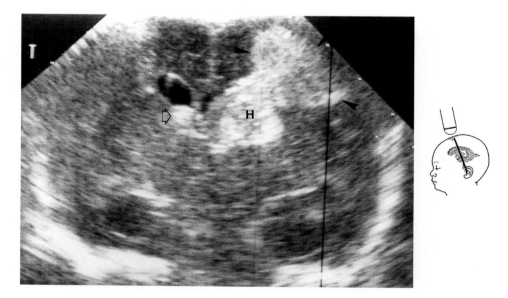

Figure 12–16. Grade IV intraventricular hemorrhage shown in a coronal plane. An acute hemorrhagic clot (H) is noted filling the left lateral ventricle's anterior horn and apparently extending into the left frontal brain *(arrowheads)*. A small amount of clot is also noted in the right anterior horn *(small arrow)*. Intraventricular hemorrhage associated with involvement of nearby brain parenchyma is characteristic of grade IV intraventricular hemorrhage.

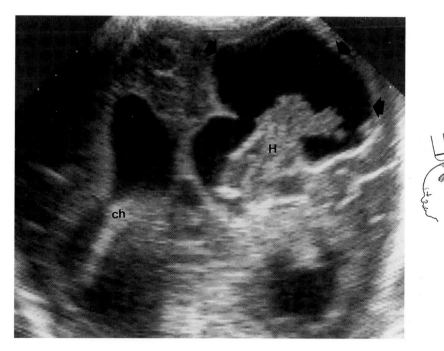

Figure 12–17. Porencephalic cyst shown in a coronal plane. This 4-week-old premature infant, who had a grade IV hemorrhage in the first week of life, is now noted to have an aging clot (H) (noted by decreased echogenicity and retraction from the ventricular walls) and ventricular dilatation. The clot extends from the dilated anterior horn of the left lateral ventricle into a porencephalic cyst *(arrows)*. This cystic area, communicating with the ventricle, developed as a result of breakdown of an echogenic area of periventricular white matter involvement noted during the first week of life. ch, Choroid plexus.

aminer should look for any asymmetry, but particularly for the presence of a well-defined area of increased echogenicity inferior or inferior and lateral to the floor of the anterior horns and in the area of the head of the caudate nucleus, indicative of SEH (Fig. 12–14). Intraventricular hemorrhage is diagnosed by noting a filling in of a portion of the ventricular system with echogenic material (Fig. 12–15). The sonologist may sometimes have difficulty in differentiating a prominent SEH from grade II IVH because of a lack of ventricular dilatation. Follow-up examinations may be needed to clear up this point. The fact that both grade I and II lesions typically have a far better prognosis than grade III and IV lesions makes the immediate differentiation of SEH from grade II IVH not absolutely necessary.

Sonographic diagnosis is easier when the ventricles are dilated, as they are in grades III and IV hemorrhage. Again, the sonologist should look for asymmetry, in this case, of the intraventricular contents, although hemorrhages may often be seen as bilateral and symmetrical. The acute, homogeneously echogenic clot may be adjacent to the choroid plexus and may blend in with its similar echogenicity pattern. Comparison with the contralateral choroid for any irregularity in shape may suggest a clot within the ventricle. As the clot ages over a few weeks and as it evolves toward complete dissolution, it retracts in size, its central echogenicity decreases (Fig. 12–18), and differentiation from the normal choroid plexus becomes easier. Occasionally, one may note residual increased echogenicity of the ventricular ependyma for several weeks after an IVH.[5,10] A 1994 report suggested an improved diagnosis of IVH in the posterior horn, a dependent portion of the lateral ventricle in a supine neonate, by using a posterior fontanelle as well as an anterior fontanelle approach.[52]

One third to one half of IPHs can be diagnosed on the first day of life. Intraventricular hemorrhage occurs more often in those with SEH within the first 6 hours of life. Nine of every 10 hemorrhages will have occurred by the sixth day of life. Hemorrhages that first occur after this are often subependymal and not intraventricular. It has therefore been suggested that unless there is an urgent clinical concern requiring immediate neurosonography, a first

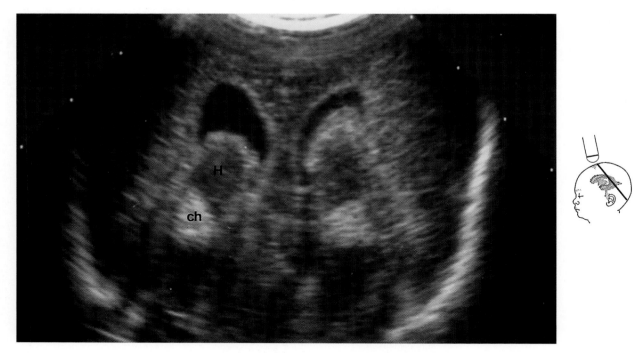

Figure 12–18. Asymmetry of the choroid plexus echogenicity in a patient with intraventricular hemorrhage, shown in a coronal plane. This 4-week-old premature infant is noted to have moderate ventriculomegaly and apparent heterogeneous choroid plexus (ch) echogenicity. This heterogeneity is due to older echopenic intraventricular hemorrhage (H) adjacent to the normally homogeneously echogenic choroid.

scan should be performed during days 4 to 7 of life.[10,53–55]

After IVH, hemorrhagic material may block the aqueduct (Sylvius) or the arachnoid villi and lead to ventricular dilatation, which often resolves. Severe hemorrhage, however, may lead to a secondary hydrocephaly due to obliterative arachnoiditis, often developing at the cisterna magna, which may block CSF flow from the fourth ventricle and may lead to an unrelenting hydrocephaly that requires shunting.[5] The development of this secondary hydrocephaly is a poor prognostic sign with regard to normal development.[8] It is suggested that a 1- to 2-week follow-up ultrasonographic examination be performed after the initial diagnosis of IVH to rule out the possibility of posthemorrhagic hydrocephaly. Evaluations during this period will help note the development or absence of periventricular leukomalacia.[5,44,53–55]

Subependymal hemorrhages often disappear within days to weeks. Some undergo central liquefaction, resulting in a subependymal cyst (Fig. 12–19) that can be imaged for up to 1 year. These cysts have no clinical significance, but cannot be differentiated from the incidental, postinfectious, or other subependymal cysts discussed later in this chapter.[10,11]

Histologically, porencephaly is a focal cavity within the brain, having a smooth wall and minimal surrounding glial reaction. It is thought to be the result of brain destruction before the 26th gestational week and to be due to the limited capacity of the fetal brain for astrocyte proliferation. Encephalomalacia, on the other hand, is noted as a shaggy-walled cavity with considerable glial reaction (astrocyte proliferation) and is often the result of a brain insult in later gestation or a perinatal or postnatal event. In patients who have grade IV IVH, the development of the echoless porencephaly or the septated echopenic to echoless area of encephalomalacia may be related to the timing of the brain insult as well as the individual premature infant's response to that insult. Not all neonatal intraventricular hemorrhage has a subependymal origin. Choroid plexus hemorrhage was once thought to be a common cause for intraventricular hemorrhage. It is now thought to be an unusual cause. It is said to occur more often in full term infants and is thought to be due to elevated venous pressures from asphyxia or mechanical causes.

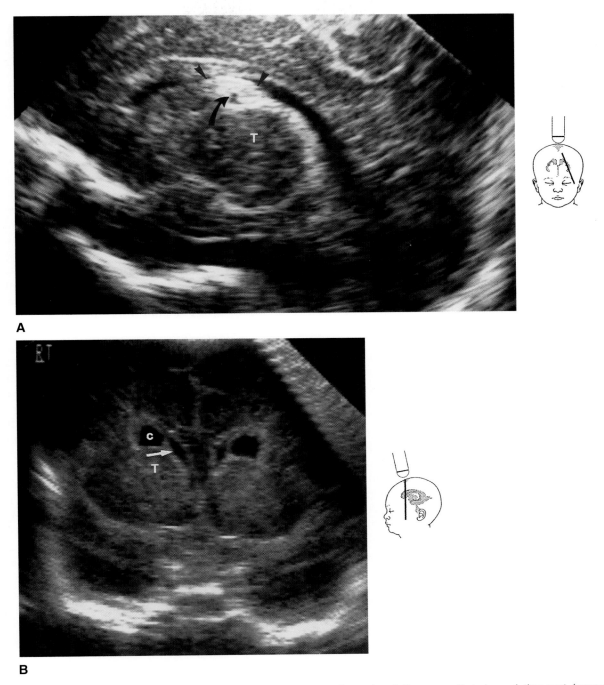

Figure 12–19. Subependymal cyst. **A.** Early cyst development shown in a left parasagittal plane. A tiny cyst *(arrow)* is seen developing within the subependymal hemorrhage *(arrowheads)* of a 3-week-old premature infant. T, Thalamus. **B.** Older cysts shown in a coronal plane. Subependymal cysts within the area of the caudate nucleus. The *arrow* points to the nondilated right anterior horn. As the clot of a subependymal hemorrhage resolves, a residual cyst may develop and can be seen sonographically for up to 1 year. These cysts have no clinical significance. T, Right thalamus; c, right subependymal cyst.

CEREBELLAR HEMORRHAGE

Cerebellar hemorrhage is a type of intraparenchymal hemorrhage that occurs in premature infants. Cerebellar hemorrhage is diagnosed far less commonly than germinal matrix hemorrhage in preterm infants. The actual presence of cerebellar hemorrhage may be underdiagnosed because it is said to be found in 10% to 25% of very low birth weight infants at autopsy.[57] Difficult delivery was identified as a predisposing factor in 70% to 85% of infants with posterior fossa hemorrhage.[58] In light of this fact, neonates with prolonged or precipitous labors or those with trauma from forceps or breech deliveries are thought to be at greater risk for cerebellar hemorrhage. Theoretically, this may be on the basis of stretching of the tentorium and/or falx with subsequent laceration often occurring at the tentorial junction with the falx. This is thought to be the mechanism for subdural hemorrhage in infants. Hemorrhage may, obviously, be due to actual injury to the cerebellum itself.[58,59]

Cerebellar hemorrhages are otherwise seen most frequently in patients on extracorporeal membrane oxygenation (ECMO). The pathogenesis of these hemorrhages is not clear. Potential theoretical causes include hypoxic episodes with resulting endothelial damage and bleeding, at least in part, due to impaired autoregulation of cerebral blood flow.

Hemorrhages appear in the cerebellum on US as hemorrhages do in other areas of the brain. Acute hemorrhage after fibrin deposition is homogeneously echogenic. As time goes on, hemorrhages evolve and the ultrasonographic mass becomes more heterogeneous (Fig. 12–20) and eventually, hypoechoic. There may be loss of definition of the cerebellum and fourth ventricle on the median view of such patients. Bulas[58] also reported tentorial elevation in four of five and hydrocephaly developing in five of five infants studied with cerebellar hemorrhage after ECMO. Use of the posterior fontanelle or transcranial imaging via the posterolateral (mastoid) fontanelle (see Chapter 11) have improved the imaging of the cerebellum for

hemorrhage.[57] These techniques place the transducer closer to the subtentorial pathology than does the classic anterior fontanelle approach.

PERIVENTRICULAR LEUKOMALACIA AND PERIVENTRICULAR CYSTS

Perhaps the most significant pathological injury to the brain of premature infants during neonatal life is periventricular leukomalacia. This is an ischemic abnormality thought to be responsible for later development of spastic diplegia and prominent intellectual deficits.[60] It is due to necrosis of the cerebral white matter at arterial border zones (watershed areas).[55] Most commonly occurring in the optic radiation at the trigone of the lateral ventricle and/or in the cerebral white matter just lateral to the anterior horns (Fig. 12–21), periventricular leukomalacia was first identified by CT in 1978.[61] An early description of its sonographic appearance was published in 1983.[62]

In the acute phase, periventricular leukomalacia (PVL) can be imaged as well defined areas of hyperechogenicity. Usually, these are seen anterolateral or lateral to the anterior horns and superior or posterior or lateral to the atria of the lateral ventricles. The difficulty in making a definitive diagnosis of PVL during this acute (echogenic) phase is that neonates normally have somewhat prominent echogenicity in the periventricular brain parenchyma imaged on coronal views of the bodies of the lateral ventricles. There is also normal increased echogenicity in the parasagittal images of the peritrigonal areas of newborns due to a physiologic anisotropic effect of the ultrasound beam on normal white matter at this site.[63] These areas of normal increased echogenicity include the classic areas of PVL involvement we have described in the previous paragraph. The ultrasound diagnosis of PVL is eased within 2 to 3 weeks, when the echogenic areas of involvement become cystic and several periventricular or peritrigonal cystic areas or cavities can be seen. Normal echogenic areas do

Figure 12–20. Cerebellar hemorrhage. Neurosonographic examination. **A.** Transfontanelle study through the anterior fontanelle. Coronal plane, level of bodies of lateral ventricles. Posteriorly and slightly to the left of midline, within the subtentorial brain parenchyma, i.e., the left cerebellum, is a cystic structure (arrowhead). On this view alone, one might consider an arachnoid cyst or an abnormal blood vessel among several possibilities in this 20-day-old premature infant. The anterior horns (arrow points to left) are somewhat prominent but the remainder of the lateral ventricles are normal in size. **B.** Transcranial view through the mastoid fontanelle. Patient is left side up. The cystic area seen on coronal view is part of a complex area that has a prominent echogenic (arrow) component. This proved to be a subacute cerebellar hemorrhage with the echoless component being related to clot dissolution. This patient did not have a history of ECMO. (Images courtesy of Dorothy Bulas, MD, Children's Hospital Medical Center, Washington, DC.)

not become cystic. Therefore, "tincture of time" can be used to make a definitive diagnosis of PVL versus normal echogenicity in those infants who cannot be moved to MR for corroboration.[64] The cysts and cavities are seen as encephalomalacia develops. Eventually, gliosis fills in the affected areas. After gliosis fills the cysts in, the US images of the affected brain will look normal.

Early images of periventricular echogenicity may resemble those of the normal brain, but within 2 to 3 weeks the more readily diagnosed periventricular cysts can be seen (Fig. 12–22). Periventricular leukomalacia is said to occur because of the premature infant's pressure-passive blood pressure (remaining constant despite hypotension) and the limited vasodilatory adjustment of the periventricular blood vessels, even in the presence of hypoxemia or hypotension.[53] Periventricular leukomalacia has been well documented in association with

obvious perinatal problems, but has also been seen in newborns without them. In one study of seven neonates born with periventricular cysts but showing no evidence of ventriculomegaly, areas of abnormally echogenic brain parenchyma, evidence of intrauterine infection, or history of illicit drug use by the mother, each showed mild neurological deficits, which partially or completely resolved in six of them by 1 year of age, suggesting that the cysts were due to relatively small in utero hemorrhagic events.[10,66]

HYPOXIA AND ISCHEMIC INJURY

Ischemic injury, which affects full-term infants more often than premature infants, is seen to a more global extent on CT. It can, however, be diagnosed sonographically (Fig. 12–23). Increased echogenicity within the brain parenchyma is usually seen in an

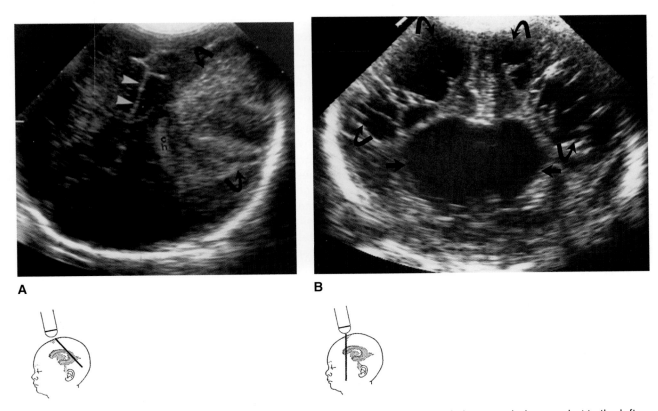

A   **B**

Figure 12–23. Ischemic abnormalities. **A.** Cerebral infarction shown in a coronal plane, angled somewhat to the left. An area of increased echogenicity is noted *(curved arrows)* in the area of distribution of the left middle cerebral artery in this 10-day-old of 38 postmenstrual weeks with a history of birth asphyxia. The findings of cerebral infarction were confirmed by computed tomographic examination. The *arrowheads* indicate an interhemispheric fissure. ch, Left choroid plexus. **B.** Cystic encephalomalacia shown in a coronal plane. Cystic areas *(curved arrows)* are noted in the brain parenchyma anterior and lateral to the hydrocephalic anterior horns *(straight arrows)*. The patient was a 3-week-old full-term infant who suffered from perinatal anoxia. There is incidental absence, from fenestration, of the septi pellucidi, probably on the basis of long-term hydrocephaly.

arterial distribution and is most often due to occlusion of the middle cerebral artery. Echogenicity beyond the areas of distribution of individual arterial vessels may be due to (less frequent) venous infarctions. The increased echogenicity may be due to cerebritis, the edema of ischemic infarction, or the hemorrhage of hemorrhagic infarction. The sonographic diagnosis, which is aided by imaging the associated loss of gyral–sulcal interfaces or slitlike ventricles from mass effect (which may also be seen in normal patients), is easiest when involvement is unilateral and parenchymal asymmetry can be imaged. Decreased vascular pulsations, on the abnormal side, have been reported on real-time sonographic imaging. Infrequently, there may be hypoxia or ischemia of the basal ganglia, particularly the thalami, noted as bilateral increased echogenicity of these structures. Ischemic brain injury can be due to many causes, particularly hypoxia/anoxia, infection, and embolism. The increased echogenicity of the involved areas may resolve and return to normal, or cavitation or necrosis as well as asymmetrical ventricular dilatation may develop in the involved areas.[10,11,67]

Hemorrhagic and ischemic cerebral infarctions have been reported in the full-term offspring[10,67] and periventricular subependymal cysts,[68] and subependymal hemorrhage has been reported in both the premature and full-term offspring of maternal cocaine users.[69] The subependymal or GM area's active proliferating cells have large energy and oxygen demands, and the area is therefore very susceptible to hypoxic/ischemic injury.[70,71] The subependymal cysts and periventricular cystic areas occurring in these patients may be due to cocaine's induction of placental vasoconstriction with resultant fetal ischemia or may be related to a direct effect on fetal cerebral arteries.[11,72]

For additional data please refer also to Chapters 4 and 16.

IN UTERO AND POSTNATAL INFECTION

Of less importance than the evaluation of intracranial congenital anomalies, GM hemorrhage, or ischemic injury, but still within the capabilities of neonatal neurosonography, is the analysis of intracranial contents for evidence of in utero or postnatal infection (see also Chapter 16).

The most common causes of intrauterine infection are the TORCH (toxoplasmosis, other, rubella, CMV, and herpes) organisms. Most of these infections are caused by the transplacental passage of the organism from mother to fetus during pregnancy. The major exception to this are herpes simplex infections, which are, in 75% of the cases, due to herpes simplex virus type 2, which infects the maternal genital tract. In these cases the infection is acquired at birth as the infant passes through the birth canal.[10] These typically later occurring infections result in more limited sonographic findings when examining the neonate by ultrasonography.

Infections of the intracranial contents may lead to meningitis, encephalitis, ventriculitis, or a combination of all three. The classic sonographic evidence of intrauterine infection is periventricular calcification (Fig. 12–24), most often noted in, but not exclusive to, CMV or toxoplasmosis infection. More severe infections often show more diffuse intraparenchymal calcifications. These periventricular or parenchymal calcifications are imaged as echogenicities, with or without shadowing. One must note, however, that significant in utero and postnatal bacterial, viral, and fungal infections can occur, have serious sequelae, and yet may show no sonographic abnormality.[11]

All intracranial infections, whether acquired prenatally, at birth, or postnatally, may also cause ventricular dilatation and may show intraventricular echoes or strands, periventricular cavitation, irregularity of the ependymal surface, cystic degeneration of brain parenchyma, or abscess development.[10,11]

The widespread use of broad-spectrum antibiotics and prolonged hyperalimentation with indwelling catheters have led to increased candidal infections in premature infants. Although renal obstruction by candidal bezoars is a more common sonographic finding,[73] a few cases of CNS involvement have been reported, although far fewer than would be suggested by the 64% prevalence of candidal ependymitis and small abscesses of the brain reported during the autopsy of such infants.[11,74,75]

Huang and colleagues[76] have described small rimlike microabcesses with hypoechoic centers and irregular echogenic borders, usually occurring bilaterally and found at the cerebral gray–white matter junction, in the periventricular white matter and in the basal ganglia as characteristic of candidiasis of the brain parenchyma. These microabscesses may coalesce into larger masses. Findings of candidal infection of the ventricular system is, as already noted, nonspecific with findings typical of any ventriculitis, including irregularity of the ventricular walls and intraventricular stranding and debris.

A sonographic finding, related to infection, that has been reported in recent years is that of mineralizing vasculopathy. This finding of single (Fig. 12–25) or multiple linear or punctate bright echo-

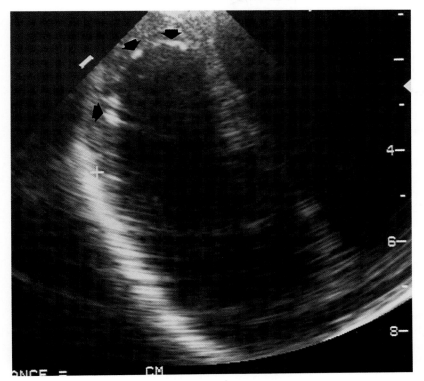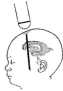

Figure 12–24. Periventricular calcification shown in a coronal plane, angled to the right. The *arrows* point to calcification in the wall of a dilated right lateral ventricle. These calcifications were due to an intrauterine cytomegalovirus infection.

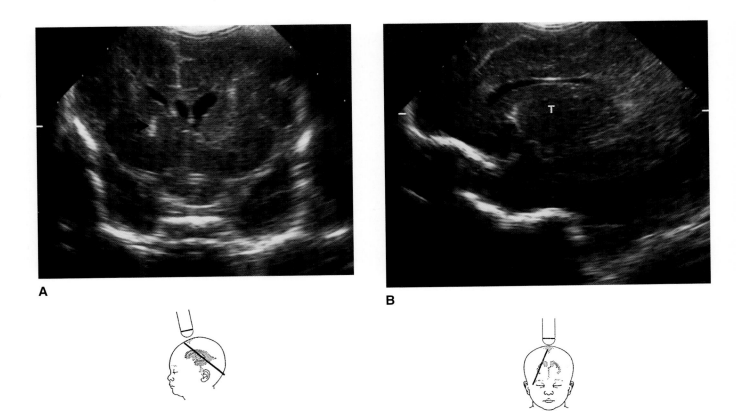

A

B

Figure 12–25. Mineralizing vasculopathy. **A.** Coronal plane. The *arrow* points to a single linear calcification in the right thalamus of a newborn with a history of intrauterine TORCH infection (see text). **B.** Right parasagittal plane. The *arrow* points to a branching calcification in the thalamus (T) of a newborn with a history of intrauterine TORCH infection. Sonographically, mineralizing vasculopathy may consist of single or multiple punctate or linear calcifications. The linear echogenicities represent calcification of the walls of thalamostriate arteries that run in the thalami.

genicities in the thalami of neonates is nonspecific and has been associated with intrauterine infections such as CMV, rubella, syphilis, and bacterial meningitis as well as karyotype abnormalities without infection and intrauterine exposure to cocaine and other drugs.[30,77,78] Histologically, the linear echogenicities are perforating medium-sized arteries with thick hypercellular walls and amorphous basophilic deposits.[77,78] Questions about the significance of this sonographic finding persist, with one study of 15 cases of mineralizing vasculopathy showing no disease specificity. Two patients had CMV, five had human rotavirus infection, and others had a variety of clinical problems. Mineralizing lenticulostriate vasculopathy seems unrelated to a delay in neurodevelopmental progress.[11,79]

We have already noted that subependymal cysts are a sequela of SEH in infants as well as a consequence of maternal cocaine use. Subependymal cysts may also be evidence of germinolysis due to intrauterine infection, especially when noted in the first week of life, in neonates without evidence of SEH or IVH. Such cysts may be seen in older neonates as a consequence of ventriculitis or as part of the Zellweger (cerebrohepatorenal) syndrome. To make matters more confusing, subependymal cysts have been reported in neonates without evidence of hemorrhagic or viral disease.[11,69,71,80,81]

Sonography is limited in the evaluation of meningitis. Echogenic sulci or convolutional marking have been reported as evidence of pus or fluid between the sulci. Babcock and Han described increased echogenicity of the normally echopenic gyri as evidence of acute gyral infarcts.[30,82,83]

USE OF DUPLEX AND COLOR DOPPLER IMAGING IN NEONATES

The vast majority of sonographic imaging of the neonate does not involve Doppler evaluation. Certainly, if a cystic mass is seen, both duplex and color Doppler imaging allow rapid differentiation between a blood vessel with contained vascular flow and an area of brain destruction. There has been some interesting investigative work in recent years using Doppler in the neonatal intensive care unit. As clinical experience grows and with the greater availability of Doppler on portable ultrasonography machines, the clinical utility of this modality and its findings may be better understood. The normal intracranial arteries are of low resistance and therefore show flow throughout the entire cardiac cycle, in both systole and diastole. Classically, patients are assumed to be having clinical difficulty when diastole is low and therefore the RI (peak systolic velocity minus end-diastolic velocity/peak systolic velocity) is high. The average RI in healthy newborns is 75 $\pm$ 10[84] Seibert and coworkers,[17] using transcranial Doppler sonography, showed that in cerebral edema flow may be so decreased that there is reversal of diastolic flow. In recent reports Seibert and others have shown that, in fact, too high a diastolic flow in neonates, specifically, an RI of less than 60, can also be associated with poor neurodevelopmental outcome (Fig. 12–26).[85] One must note, however, that intracranial vascular spectral patterns may reflect extracranial as well as intracranial physiology. Retrograde flow can be noted in diastole in cases of significant ductus arteriosus or aortic insufficiency. A low peak systolic velocity is noted in association with obstruction of the left ventricular outlet; high peak systolic velocity in coarctation of the aorta.[11]

Doppler imaging has been used in the analysis of intracranial vascular flow in neonates who have undergone ECMO. The ECMO procedure for neonates with severely impaired lung function shunts deoxygenated blood from the hypoxic infant to an external membrane for oxygenation. The blood is then returned to the arterial circulation. The right jugular vein and common carotid artery are cannulated for this procedure and eventually are ligated. These infants may develop cerebral infarctions, venous thrombosis, and, because they are heparinized for the procedure, intracerebral, including cerebellar, hemorrhages that may be difficult to diagnose sonographically because the heparinization makes them hypoechoic.[10,11] Mitchell and collaborators[86] used Doppler imaging to assess the collateral pathways of flow to the right hemisphere immediately after the procedure and usually involving, in part, retrograde flow through the right anterior cerebral artery via the circle of Willis, and the eventual return to antegrade flow through the right carotid artery.

Venous spectral signal is almost always seen throughout the normal infant's cardiac cycle, often with variation in its peak related to respiration. A pattern of intermittent venous signal, with flow absent in portions of the spectra, is commonly seen in severely ill premature infants and indicates reduced venous flow.[18,87]

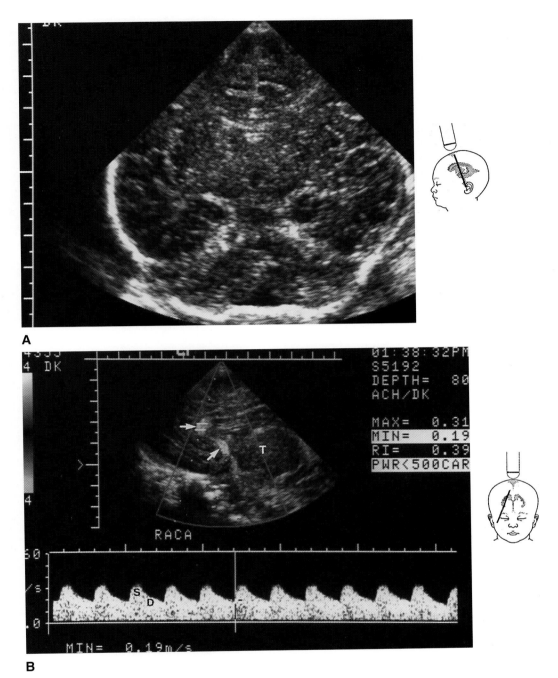

Figure 12–26. High diastolic flow (low resistance index) associated with poor neurodevelopmental outcome. **A.** Head ultrasonogram in a coronal plane. The echogenicity of the brain parenchyma of this full-term neonate with a history of asphyxia appears normal. The anterior horns are not imaged and may be slitlike, which is a finding in normal patients as well as in patients with cerebral edema. **B.** Triplex (color and duplex) Doppler image in a right parasagittal plane. Black and white hard copy. The upper half of the image shows color vascular flow, identified by an echogenic tube (arrows), the right anterior cerebral artery, running anterior and superior to the thalamus (T). The two parallel lines within the artery are at the point of duplex Doppler insonation. The Doppler spectral pattern in the lower half of the image shows high systolic (S) and diastolic (D) flow, consistent with an abnormally low resistance index of 0.39. Resistance indices below 0.60 are associated with poor developmental outcome.

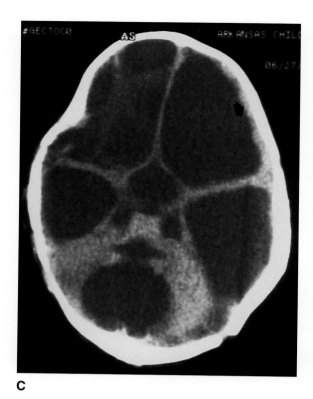

C

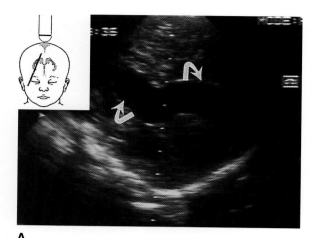

A

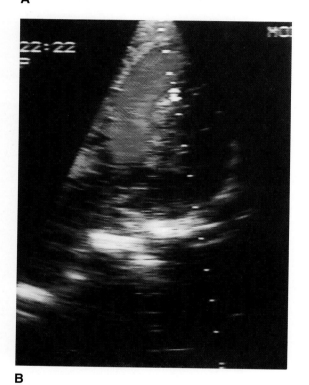

B

Figure 12–26. continued. C. Computed tomography of the head in an axial view. A scan performed in this patient 6 months later showed massive loss of cerebral tissue, as noted by low-density areas throughout the anterior two thirds of the brain, and a small amount of peripheral brain tissue *(arrow). (From Stark and Seibert, 1994,[76] with permission.)*

VEIN OF GALEN AND OTHER ARTERIOVENOUS MALFORMATIONS

The key condition in which duplex and color Doppler techniques have a major clinical impact and make a quick and ready diagnosis by Doppler is the intracerebral arteriovenous malformation, particularly the so-called vein of Galen aneurysm (Fig. 12–27), which may be more correctly referred to as a galenic arteriovenous malformation (AVM). These malformations are thought to be due to a failure of embryonic arteriovenous shunts to be replaced by capillaries. Their persistence in late fetal and neonatal life creates prominent shunting of arterial blood into the cerebral deep venous system. The vein of Galen becomes dilated either primarily as part of an arteriovenous fistula fed directly from the carotid or basilar artery or secondarily because another arteriovenous malformation, fed usually by the posterior cerebral circulation, shunts significant amounts of blood from itself to the vein of Galen.[10,11] The cystic dilated vein of Galen is usually seen superior to the

Figure 12–27. Vein of Galen aneurysm. Color Doppler diagnosis. **A.** Gray-scale image of the posterior half of the calvarium, shown in the median plane. This image, taken from a videotape, shows a tubular cystic structure *(arrows)* in the posterior portion of a full term newborn's brain. **B.** Color Doppler image in a coronal/oblique plane. The tubular structure filled with color, proving its vascular nature. This was a vein of Galen "aneurysm" or arteriovenous malformation.

quadrigeminal plate cistern and posterior to the third ventricle. On coronal view it is often imaged between the lateral ventricles, often obstructing them and causing hydrocephaly. The dilated vessels of these abnormalities are imaged as tubular and cystic structures at the vein of Galen and other regions of the brain. In fact, on occasion, an arach-

noid cyst may morphologically simulate a tubular AVM on US examination.[88] Color Doppler will image vascular flow in the AVM, whereas no flow will be noted in the arachnoid cyst. The typical spectral pattern of an AVM is irregular and biphasic.[11] Associated dilatation of feeding and draining intracranial vessels as well as extracranial neck vessels may

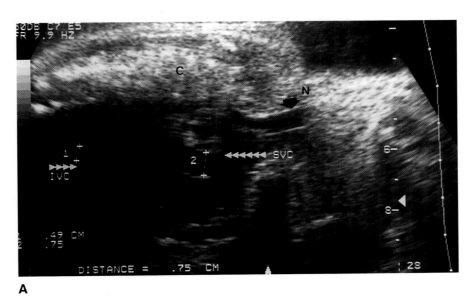

A

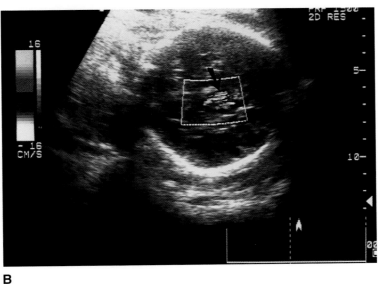

B

Figure 12–28. Intracerebral arteriovenous malformation diagnosis in a fetus. **A.** Dilated neck vessels shown in a coronal plane through the right neck (N) and chest (C), with the image positioned as if the fetus were lying on his left side. The superior vena cava (SVC) and the right carotid artery *(arrow)* are dilated in this fetus, referred in the third trimester for cardiac evaluation because of a possible dilated right atrium. **B.** Intracranial arteriovenous malformation. Color Doppler image in an axial plane. Black and white hard copy. Color Doppler filled in *(arrow)* a cystic area noted within the fetal brain, near the area of the vein of Galen, proving it to be vascular. The Doppler spectra showed the biphasic, to-and-fro signal of an arteriovenous malformation. The dilatation of the neck vessels was due to increased vascular flow to the brain. After birth the patient proved to have an extensive intracranial arteriovenous malformation that was not limited to the vein of Galen.

be seen. Findings of cardiomegaly or jugular vein distention in a fetus may be due to the increase in vascular flow of an intracranial AVM. In such cases, one should carefully image the brain parenchyma to note any abnormal vasculature (Fig. 12–28), and confirm the diagnosis[89–91] (see also Chapter 4).

The number of feeding vessels of an intracranial arteriovenous malformation and their origin, usually pial and branching off the middle cerebral artery, are often readily determined by color Doppler imaging of the fetus or neonate.[14,92] This information aids preoperative and postembolization assessment of these malformations.[93] Doppler can also help in monitoring hemodynamic changes during and after embolotherapy of vein of Galen aneurysms. A spectral pattern of arterialized venous flow noted after the procedure, suggests the persistence of a hemodynamically significant arteriovenous fistula despite imaging evidence of obliteration of large arterial feeders[94] Color Doppler has been able to denote improved flow to uninvolved portions of the brain after treatment as well as show changes in the caliber and flow through feeder vessels that have not been embolized.[88]

SUMMARY

We have reviewed the most prominent uses of neurosonography in the neonate and their findings. Neurosonographic is a helpful tool in imaging abnormalities of the premature and full-term infant's brain. It allows the analysis and confirmation of antenatal findings as well as the diagnosis of conditions specific to neonatal life. At the very least, it serves as a triaging tool for other neuroradiological imaging modalities.

REFERENCES

1. Cohen HL, Haller JO, Gross B. Diagnostic sonography of the fetus: A guide to evaluation of the neonate. *Pediatr Ann.* 1992;21:87–99.
2. Nyberg D, Mack L, Hirsch J, et al. Abnormalities of fetal cranial contour in sonographic detection of spina bifida: evaluation of the "lemon" sign. *Radiology* 1988; 167:387–392.
3. Benacerraf B, Stryker J, Frigoletto J Jr, et al. Abnormal US appearance of the cerebellum (banana sign). Indirect sign of spina bifida. *Radiology.* 1989;171: 151–153.
4. Babcock D. Cranial sonography: Congenital anomalies. *Clin Diagn Ultrasound.* 1989;24:1–24.
5. Barkovich AJ. *Pediatric Neuroimaging.* 2nd ed. New York: Raven; 1995.
6. Rumack C, Johnson M. Hydrocephalus. In: Rumack CM, Johnson ML, eds. *Perinatal and Infant Brain Imaging: Role of Ultrasound and Computed Tomography.* Chicago: Year Book Medical Publishers, 1984: 155–174.
7. Rousseau GL, McCullough DC, Joseph AL. Current prognosis in fetal ventriculomegaly. *J Neurosurg.* 1992;77:551–552.
8. Volpe JJ. *Neurology of the Newborn.* 2nd ed. Philadelphia: WB Saunders; 1987.
9. Fogarty K, Cohen HL, Haller JO. Sonography of fetal intracranial hemorrhage: Unusual causes and a review of the literature. *J Clin Ultrasound* 1989;17: 366–370.
10. Siegel M. Brain. In: Siegel M, ed. *Pediatric Sonography.* 2nd ed. New York: Raven Press; 1994:29–101.
11. Cohen HL, Haller J. Review. Advances in perinatal neurosonography. *AJR.* 1994;163:801–810.
12. Cardoza J, Filly R, Podrasky A. The dangling choroid plexus: A sonographic observation of value in excluding ventriculomegaly. *AJR.* 1988;151:767–770.
13. Cohen HL, Haller J, Pollack A. Ultrasound of the septum pellucidum: Recognition of evolving fenestrations in the hydrocephalic infant. *J Ultrasound Med.* 1990;9:377–383.
14. Deeg K, Rupprecht T. Pulsed Doppler sonographic measurement of normal values for the flow velocities in the intracranial arteries of healthy newborns. *Pediatr Radiol.* 1989;19:71–78.
15. Taylor G. Current concepts in neonatal cranial Doppler sonography. *Ultrasound Q.* 1992;9:223–244.
16. Seibert J, McCowan T, Chadduck W, et al. Duplex pulsed Doppler US versus intracranial pressure in the neonate: Clinical and experimental studies. *Radiology.* 1989;171:155–159.
17. Seibert J, Glasier C, Lethiser R, et al. Transcranial Doppler using standard duplex equipment in children. *Ultrasound Q.* 1990;8:167–196.
18. Winkler P, Helmke K. Duplex-scanning of the deep venous drainage in the evaluation of blood flow velocity of the cerebral vascular system in infants. *Pediatr Radiol.* 1989;19:79–90.
19. Taylor GA, Madsen JR. Neonatal hydrocephalus: Hemodynamic response to fontanelle compression—Correlation with intracranial pressure and need for shunt placement. *Radiology.* 1996;201:685–689.
20. Westra SJ, Lazareff J, Curran JG, et al. Transcranial Doppler ultrasonography to evaluate need for cerebrospinal fluid drainage in hydrocephalic children. *J Ultrasound Med.* 1998;17:561–569.
21. Shackleford G. Neurosonography of hydrocephalus in infants. *Neuroradiology.* 1986;28:452–462.
22. Byrd S, Naidich T. Common congenital brain anomalies. *Radiol Clin North Am.* 1988;26:755–772.
23. Harwood-Nash DC, Fitz CR. *Neuroradiology in Infants and Children.* St. Louis: CV Mosby; 1976.
24. Goldstein R, Podrasky A, Filly R, et al. Effacement of the fetal cisterna magna in association with myelomeningocele. *Radiology.* 1989;72:409–413.
25. Babcock D, Han B. Cranial sonographic findings in meningomyelocele. *AJR.* 1981;136:563–569.

26. Netanyahu I, Grant E. Prominent choroid plexus in meningomyelocele: sonographic findings. *AJNR.* 1986; 7:317–321.

27. Yousefzadeh D, Naidich T. Ultrasound anatomy of the posterior fossae in children: Correlation with brain sections. *Radiology.* 1985;156:353–361.

28. Sudakoff G, Montazemi M, Rifkin M. The foramen magnum: The underutilized acoustic window to the posterior fossa. *J Ultrasound Med.* 1993;4:205–210.

29. Laing F, Frates M, Brown D, et al. Sonography of the fetal posterior fossa: False appearance of mega–cisterna magna and Dandy–Walker variant. *Radiology.* 1994;192:247–251.

30. Knutzon RK, McGahan J, Salamat M, et al. Fetal cisterna magna septa: A normal anatomic finding. *Radiology.* 1991;180:799–801.

31. Benacerraf B. Fetal central nervous system anomalies. *Ultrasound Q.* 1990;8:1–42.

32. Hayden CK, Swischuk LE. *Pediatric Sonography.* 2nd ed. Baltimore: William & Wilkins; 1992.

33. Estroff J, Scott M, Benacerraf B. Dandy–Walker variant: Prenatal sonographic features and clinical outcome. *Radiology.* 1992;185:755–758.

34. Ettlinger G. Agenesis of the corpus callosum. In: Bruyn V, ed. *Handbook of Clinical Neurology.* Amsterdam: Elsevier/North-Holland; 1977;30:285–297.

35. Rosenthal C, Cohen HL. Diagnostic challenge: Agenesis of the corpus callosum. *J Diagn Med Sonogr.* 1987; 3:101–102.

36. Atlas S, Skolnik A, Naidich T. Sonographic recognition of agenesis of the corpus callosum. *AJR.* 1985;145: 167–173.

37. Babcock DS. The normal, absent and abnormal corpus callosum: Abnormal findings. *Radiology.* 1984;151: 449–453.

38. Lockwood C, Ghidini A, Aggarwal R, et al. Antenatal diagnosis of partial agenesis of the corpus callosum: A benign cause of ventriculomegaly. *Am J Obstet Gynecol.* 1988;159:184–186.

39. Chervenak F, Isaacson G, Hobbins J, et al. Diagnosis and management of fetal holoprosencephaly. *Obstet Gynecol.* 1984;63:115–121.

40. Crome L, Sylvester PE. Hydranencephaly (hydrencephaly). *Arch Dis Child.* 1958;33:235–245.

41. Green M, Benacerraf B, Crawford J. Hydranencephaly: US appearance during in utero evolution. *Radiology.* 1985;156:779–780.

42. Klingensmith W, Cioffi-Ragan D. Schizencephaly: Diagnosis and progression in utero. *Radiology.* 1986; 159:617–618.

43. Papile L, Burstein J, Burstein R, et al. Incidence and evolution of subependymal and intraventricular hemorrhage: A study of infants with birth weights less than 1500 gm. *J Pediatr.* 1978;92:529–534.

44. Rumack C, Johnson M. Intracranial hemorrhage. In: Rumack CM, Johnson ML, eds. *Perinatal and Infant Brain Imaging: Role of Ultrasound and Computed Tomography.* Chicago: Year Book Medical Publishers; 1984:117–153.

45. Hay T, Rumack C, Horgan J. Cranial sonography: Intracranial hemorrhage, periventricular leukomalacia, and asphyxia. *Clin Diagn Ultrasound.* 1989;24:25–42.

46. Grant E, Borts F, Schellinger D, et al. Real-time ultrasonography of neonatal intraventricular hemorrhage and comparison with computed tomography. *Radiology.* 1981;139:687–691.

47. Grant E. Neurosonography: Germinal matrix-related hemorrhage. In: Grant E, ed. *Neurosonography of the Pre-term Neonate.* New York: Springer-Verlag; 1986: 33–68.

48. Volpe JJ. Intraventricular hemorrhage in the premature infant—Current concepts: Part I. *Ann Neurol.* 1989;25:3–11.

49. Takashima S, Mito T, Ando Y. Pathogenesis of periventricular white matter hemorrhages in preterm infants. *Brain Dev.* 1986;8:25–30.

50. Perlman J, Rollins N, Burns D, et al. Relationship between periventricular intraparenchymal echodensities and germinal matrix–intraventricular hemorrhage in the very low birth weight neonate. *Pediatrics.* 1993;91:474–480.

51. Allan W, Riviello J Jr. Perinatal cerebrovascular disease in the neonate. Parenchymal ischemic lesions in term and preterm infants. *Pediatr Clin North Am.* 1992;39:621–650.

52. Anderson N, Allan R, Darlow B, et al. Diagnosis of intraventricular hemorrhage in the newborn: Value of sonography via the posterior fontanelle. *AJR.* 1994; 163:893–896.

53. Hecht ST, Filly RA, Callen PW, et al. Intracranial hemorrhage: Late onset in the preterm neonate. *Radiology.* 1983;149:697–699.

54. Partridge JC, Babcock DS, Steichen JJ, et al. Optimal timing for diagnostic cranial ultrasound in low-birth-weight infants: Detection of intracranial hemorrhage and ventricular dilatation. *J Pediatr.* 1983;102: 281–287.

55. Rumack CM, Manco-Johnson ML, Manco-Johnson MJ, et al. Timing and course of neonatal intracranial hemorrhage using real-time ultrasound. *Radiology.* 1985;154:101–105.

56. Babcock D. Cranial sonography of the infant. In: Ball W, ed. *Pediatric Neuroradiology.* Philadelphia: Lippincott-Raven; 1997:37–54.

57. Merrill JD, Piecuch RE, Fell SC, et al. A new pattern of cerebellar hemorrhages in preterm infants. *Pediatrics.* 1998;102:E62.

58. Bulas DI, Taylor GA, Fitz CR, et al. Posterior fossa intracranial hemorrhage in infants treated with extracorporeal membrane oxygenation: Sonographic findings. *AJR.* 1991;156:571–575.

59. Volpe JJ. Neonatal intracranial hemorrhage. Pathophysiology, neuropathology, and clinical features. *Clin Perinatol.* 1977;4:77–102.

60. Banker B, Larroche J. Periventricular leukomalacia of infancy. *Arch Neurol.* 1962;7:32–50.

61. DiChiro G, Armitsu T, Pellock J, et al. Periventricular leukomalacia related to neonatal anoxia: Recognition

by computed tomography. *J Comput Assist Tomogr.* 1978;2:352–355.

62. Grant E, Schellinger D, Richardson J, et al. Echogenic periventricular halo: Normal sonographic findings or neonatal cerebral hemorrhage. *AJNR.* 1983;4:43–46.

63. DiPietro M, Brody B, Teele R. Peritrigonal echogenic "blush" on cranial sonography. Pathologic correlates. *AJR.* 1986;146:467–471.

64. Yang R, Cohen HL. Posthemorrhagic hydrocephalus and periventricular leukomalacia. In: Cohen HL, Sivit C, eds. *Fetal and Pediatric Ultrasound: A Case-Based Approach.* New York: McGraw Hill; (in press).

65. Volpe JJ. Current concepts of brain injury in the premature infant. *AJR.* 1989;153:243–251.

66. Sudakoff G, Mitchell D, Stanley C, et al. Frontal periventricular cysts on the first day of life: A one year clinical follow-up and its significance. *J Ultrasound Med.* 1991;10:25–30.

67. Hernanz-Schulman M, Cohen W, Geneiser N. Sonography of cerebral infarction in infancy. *AJR.* 1988;150:897–902.

68. Cohen HL, Sloves J, DeMarinis P, et al. Subependymal germinal matrix cysts in full term neonates with intrauterine cocaine exposure. *J Clin Ultrasound.* 1994;22:327–333.

69. Dogra V, Menon P, Poblate J, et al. Neurosonographic imaging of small–for–gestational age neonates exposed and not exposed to cocaine and cytomegalovirus. *J Clin Ultrasound.* 1994;22:93–102.

70. Kim M, Elyaderani M. Sonographic diagnosis of cerebroventricular hemorrhage in utero. *Radiology.* 1982;142:479–480.

71. Shaw C, Alvord E. Subependymal germinolysis. *Arch Neurol.* 1974;31:374–381.

72. Zorzi C, Angonese I. Subependymal pseudocysts in the neonate. *Eur J Pediatr.* 1989;148:462–464.

73. Cohen HL, Haller J, Schechter S, et al. Renal candidiasis of the infant: Ultrasound evaluation. *Urol Radiol.* 1986;8:17–21.

74. Kirpekar M, Abiri M, Hilfer C, et al. Ultrasound in the diagnosis of systemic candidiasis (renal and cranial) in very low birth weight premature infants. *Pediatr Radiol.* 1986;16:17–20.

75. Bozynski M, Naglie R, Russel E. Real-time ultrasonographic surveillance in the detection of CNS involvement in systemic candida infection. *Pediatr Radiol.* 1986;16:235–237.

76. Huang CC, Chen CY, Yang HB, et al. Central nervous system candidiasis in very low-birth-weight premature neonates and infants: US characteristics and histopathologic and MR imaging. *Radiology.* 1998;209:49–56.

77. Teele R, Hernanz-Schulman M, Sotrel A. Echogenic vasculature in the basal ganglia of neonates: A sonographic sign of vasculopathy. *Radiology.* 1988;169:423–427.

78. Ben-Ami T, Yousefzadeh D, Backus M, et al. Lenticulostriate vasculopathy in infants with infection of the central nervous system: Sonographic and Doppler findings. *Pediatr Radiol.* 1990;20:575–579.

79. Weber K, Riebel T, Nasir R. Hyperechoic lesions in the basal ganglia: An incidental sonographic finding in neonates and infants. *Pediatr Radiol.* 1992;22:182–186.

80. Mito T, Ando Y, Takeshita K, et al. Ultrasonography and morphologic examination of subependymal cystic lesions in maturely born infants. *Neuropediatrics.* 1989;20:211–214.

81. Shen E, Huang Y. Subependymal cysts in normal neonates. *Arch Dis Child.* 1985;60:1072–1074.

82. Babcock DS, Han BK. Sonographic recognition of gyral infarction in meningitis. *AJR.* 1985;144:833–836.

83. Han BK, Babcock DS, McAdams L. Bacterial meningitis in infants: Sonographic findings. *Radiology.* 1985;154:645–650.

84. Seibert J, McCowan T, Chadduck W, et al. Duplex pulsed Doppler US versus intracranial pressure in the neonate: Clinical and experimental studies. *Radiology.* 1989;171:155–159.

85. Stark J, Seibert J. Cerebral artery Doppler ultrasonography for prediction of outcome after perinatal asphyxia. *J Ultrasound Med.* 1994;13:595–600.

86. Mitchell D, Merton D, Graziani L, et al. Right carotid artery ligation in neonates: Classification of collateral flow with color Doppler imaging. *Radiology.* 1990;175:117–123.

87. Graves V, Duff T. Intracranial arteriovenous malformations: Current imaging and treatment. *Invest Radiol.* 1990;25:952–960.

88. Haugland G, Cohen HL, Arachnoid cyst simulating vein of Galen aneurysm. In: Cohen HL, Sivit C, eds. *Fetal and Pediatric Ultrasound: A Case-Based Approach.* New York: McGraw Hill; (in press).

89. Koven M, Cohen HL, Goldman M. Case of the day 2. Fetal intracranial AVM presenting as enlarged cardiac chamber. *J Ultrasound Med.* 1992;11:177.

90. Ishimatsu J, Yoshimura O, Tetsuou M, et al. Evaluation of an aneurysm of the vein of Galen in utero by pulsed and color Doppler ultrasonography. *Am J Obstet Gynecol.* 1991;164:743–744.

91. Comstock C, Kirks J. Arteriovenous malformations—Locations and evolution in the fetal brain. *J Ultrasound Med.* 1991;10:361–365.

92. Taylor G, Walker L. Intracranial venous system in newborns treated with extracorporeal membrane oxygenation: Doppler US evaluation after ligation of the right jugular vein. *Radiology.* 1992;183:453–456.

93. Westra S, Curran J, Duckwiler G, et al. Pediatric intracranial vascular malformations: Evaluation of treatment results with color Doppler US (work in progress). *Radiology.* 1993;186:775–783.

94. Dean LM, Taylor GA. The intracranial venous system in infants: Normal and abnormal findings on duplex and color Doppler sonography. *AJR.* 1995;164:51–56.

CHAPTER THIRTEEN

Ultrasonography of the Neonatal Spine

Madhuri Kirpekar
Harris L Cohen

High-resolution sonography has become a popular technique for the elucidation of abnormalities of the spinal cord of infants. Its most important role is in identifying the low-lying tethered spinal cord. Initial studies[1,2] using B-mode sonography were somewhat limited. The development of both real-time sonography and high-frequency transducers, as well as the limited ossification of the vertebral column, has resulted in the current ability to image fine anatomic detail of the neonatal vertebral column and its contents. The objective of spinal sonography in these patients is to image the entire spinal cord and attempt to evaluate the location of the conus medullaris. A careful search is made for the presence of abnormalities of the soft tissues and the thecal sac. An attempt is also made to evaluate cord pulsatility.

TECHNIQUE AND NORMAL ANATOMY

The neonate is placed in a prone position. The knees may be flexed or a small pillow may be placed under the abdomen to decrease the normal lumbar lordosis and maximize transducer contact with the vertebral column. It may be necessary to elevate the infant's head so that the lumbosacral spine is in a position inferior to that of the cervical and thoracic spine. This is done to optimize visualization of a subtle lumbosacral meningocele, which may not be imaged when the infant is in a true prone position but may be seen when distended by cerebrospinal fluid (CSF), filling it in this more dependent position.

It is important to localize vertebral body levels on the infant's back in order to establish the location (i.e., the vertebral level) of the conus medullaris. After the conus is localized sonographically, the infant's back may be marked with a radiopaque item (e.g., a paper clip). Plain films can then be used to definitively position the distal cord with regard to the vertebral bodies. Some examiners rely on physical findings to determine the vertebral body level. The lowest thoracic vertebral body (T12) can be identified by tracing the lowest rib medially. The fifth lumbar vertebral body (L5) may be identified by a line connecting the two iliac wings. The second lumbar vertebral body (L2) may be identified by a line connecting the lowest palpable rib on each side.[3]

Imaging is performed using the highest possible frequency transducer—usually either 5- or 7.5–MHz linear array (although a 10-MHz transducer can be used)—that provides adequate penetration. It may, at times, be necessary to use a standoff pad to establish adequate skin contact. The purpose of the standoff pad is also to place the region of interest into the focal range to better visualize the skin surface as well as the underlying superficial subcutaneous tissues. Cord visualization is optimal in the neonate and the infant due to the presence of thinner bones and lesser amounts of soft tissues. The application of spinal sonography is limited in older children, especially in those in whom there is a greater degree of vertebral body ossification. This is particularly true if the patient suffers from kyphoscoliosis. Patients with this disease have very

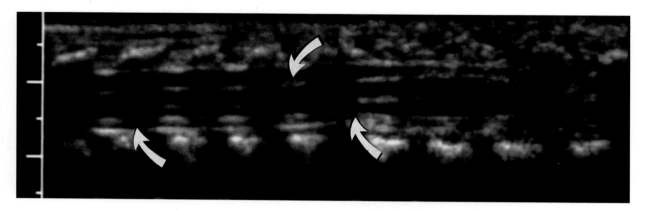

Figure 13–1. Normal longitudinal section of the thoracolumbar spine. Note the echogenic anterior and posterior borders of the cord, as defined by *arrows.*

narrow sonographic windows, resulting in poor visualization of the spinal canal.

The spinal cord is scanned in its entirety in the sagittal and axial planes. Sometimes a parasagittal approach with about 15 degrees of medial angulation may be necessary in the older child. Sonographic imaging begins with evaluation of the cervical spine. The helpful bony landmarks identifying the upper cervical vertebrae are the *clivus* and the posterior rim of the *foramen magnum.* Slight flexion of the neck may be needed to identify the upper cervical spine and maintain adequate transducer contact. On sagittal imaging the spinal cord is easily recognized as a hypoechoic tubular structure with echogenic anterior and posterior walls (Fig. 13–1).[3] The bright linear echoes seen along the

walls of the spinal cord represent the *arachnoid* and the *dura mater.* The central echogenic line corresponds to the echo interface at the central end of the *anterior median fissure,* not the central canal, as was initially thought.[4,5] At the level of the upper lumbar vertebral bodies, the spinal cord normally tapers down to the *conus medullaris* (Fig. 13–2). The location of the conus medullaris is then determined. In a large prospective study by DiPietro, it was possible to determine the location of the conus by spinal sonography in 161 of 163 normal children. DiPietro examined patients ranging in age from 4 days to 13 years and 5 months. The conus did not extend caudally beyond the superior aspect of L3 in any of these patients. Sagittal imaging of the cord is completed by visualization of the thin

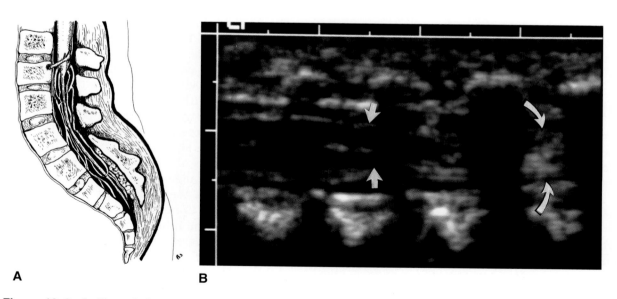

A   **B**

Figure 13–2. A. Normal diagrammatic section of the conus medullaris. **B.** Normal, tapered appearance of the conus medullaris *(solid arrows).* Echogenic linear densities are shown, representing the nerve *(open arrows)* roots.

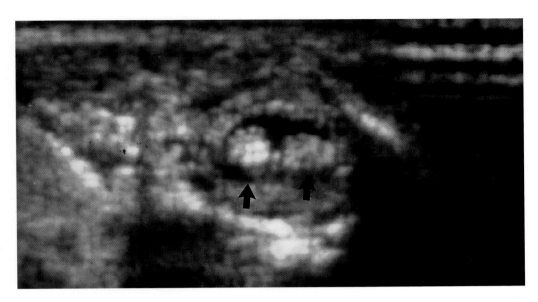

Figure 13–3. Normal transverse section at the level of the sacral nerve roots. Note the normal columnization (arrows).

linear echogenicities of the nerve roots that form the *cauda equina*.[7] These nerve roots may form columns, which then descend into the *sacral canal* (Fig. 13–3). It is important to try to assess normal rhythmic pulsations of the cauda equina. These pulsations, which are best noted on real-time examination, may be dampened in patients with a tethered cord. The *filum terminale* appears as a somewhat echogenic midline echo that separates from the nerve roots as it extends posteriorly in the canal (Fig. 13–4). Pathological thickening of the filum has been observed in certain types of spinal

dysraphism, particularly the tethered cord syndrome.[8] The thecal (dural) sac ends at about the level of S2. On axial images, the normal spinal cord is imaged as a somewhat ovoid hypoechoic structure in the cervical spine.[9] It becomes rounded (Fig. 13–5) and progressively larger in diameter from the thoracic to the lumbar region, finally tapering into the conus medullaris. The complete spinal sonographic examination should include evaluation of the soft tissues as well as the vertebral bodies about the spinal cord.[3] Vertebral abnormalities such as a *hemivertebra* may be seen. These findings

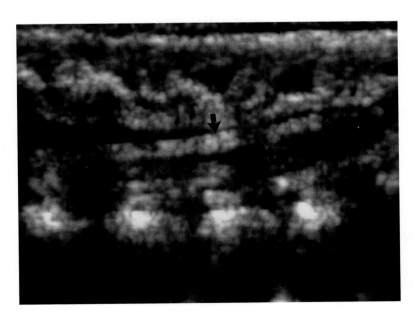

Figure 13–4. Normal median longitudinal image at the level of the sacral spine. The filum terminale represents the thicker echogenic linear density coursing posteriorly. It measures only 1.5 mm in this example. (*Arrows* define the anterior and posterior margins of the filum.)

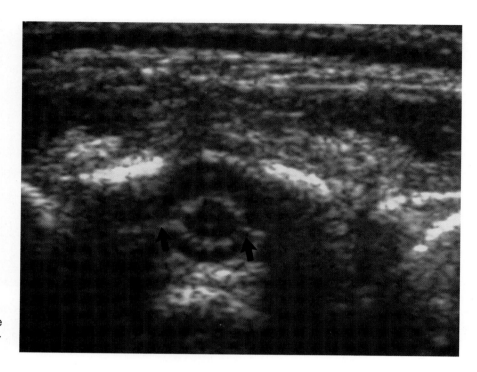

Figure 13–5. Normal appearance of the spinal cord in a transverse plane. (*Arrows* define the transverse ligament.)

may be confirmed by obtaining appropriate plain films. Soft tissue abnormalities that may be imaged include the presence of echogenic dermal sinus tracts as well as soft tissue masses of variable echogenicity. Due to the high association of urinary tract pathology with spinal anomalies as well as an association of urinary tract infection in patients with *myelomeningocele,* we also include one longitudinal and one transverse image of each kidney.[9] This helps to determine the presence or absence of kidneys within the renal beds and allows evaluation of renal size, dilatation of the collecting system, and, to a lesser extent, renal scarring (better determined by nuclear medicine examination).

CLASSIFICATION OF SPINAL MALFORMATIONS

Spinal dysraphism is a general term used to describe malformations of the spine. This term encompasses any anomaly that results from incomplete midline closure of fetal mesenchymal, osseous, or neural tissues. A modification of Derek Harwood-Nash's classification of dysraphism by Byrd and associates[10] divides spinal dysraphism into three categories (Table 13–1).

The first category includes all patients with a non-skin-covered back mass, including myelomeningocele and myelocele (Fig. 13–6). This group has also been termed *spina bifida aperta,* or *open spina bifida.* The second group consists of patients with a clinically obvious back mass with associated skin covering. The major malformations in this group are lipomyelomeningocele, myelocystocele, and meningocele (Fig. 13–7). This category of anomalies has also been referred to as *spina bifida cystica.* The third category of spinal dysraphism includes patients without an associated back mass, termed *occult spinal dysraphism.* These patients have spinal defects that are covered with skin and have no exposed neural tissue or visible cystic masses.

TABLE 13–1. CLASSIFICATION OF COMMON TYPES OF SPINAL DYSRAPHISM

Spinal dysraphism associated with a non–skin covered back mass (spina bifida aperta)
Myelomeningocele
Myelocele
Spinal dysraphism associated with a skin-covered back mass (spina bifida cystica)
Lipomyelomeningocele
Myelocystocele
Meningocele (posterior)
Occult spinal dysraphism (spina bifida occulta)
Diastematomyelia
Dorsal dermal sinus
Tight filum terminale
Anterior sacral meningocele
Lateral thoracic meningocele
Hydromyelia
Split notochord syndrome
Syndrome of caudal regression

After Byrd et al[10]

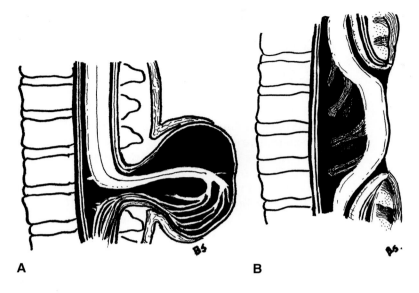

Figure 13–6. Non-skin-covered back mass. **A.** Myelomeningocele. The sac contains herniated meninges, nerve roots, and portions of the spinal cord. **B.** Myelocele. The spinal cord completely fills the sac.

The Neonate with Occult Spinal Dysraphism

The bulk of spinal sonography examinations are performed for the evaluation of occult spinal dysraphism.[8,11] This heterogeneous group of malformations is the most common type of spinal dysraphism. They include meningocele, dorsal dermal sinus, spinal lipoma, hydromyelia, diastematomyelia, and spinal lipoma.

Occult spinal dysraphism is believed to be due to incomplete fusion of the neural tube with a resultant spectrum of anomalies that have a skin covering with no exposed neural tissues. The neurological manifestations vary. They include motor and sensory deficits of the lower extremities, gait disturbances, bowel and bladder dysfunction, clubfeet, and

scoliosis.[12–14] Cutaneous abnormalities may be clinically evident prior to any neurological manifestations. These include the presence of a subcutaneous lipoma, hair tuft, sinus tract, dimple, hemangioma, and pigmented nevi (Fig. 13–8).

The most common indication for spinal sonography is for the evaluation of the patient with a dimple. A prospective study[15] was performed on neonates with dorsal cutaneous stigmata to ascertain which cutaneous stigma is more closely associated with spinal dysraphism. The study involved 180 cases of dimples. Of these, 160 were simple dimples (midline, within 2.5 cm of the anus, and no cutaneous stigmata). None of the infants with simple dimples had spinal dysraphism. Of atypical dimples,

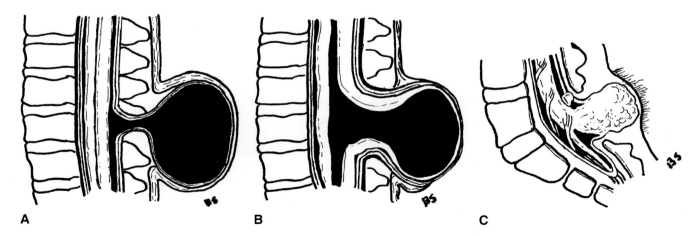

Figure 13–7. A. Meningocele. A herniated sac contains only the dura mater, the arachnoid, and CSF. **B.** Myelocystocele. Portions of the cord as well as a dilated central canal herniate into the sac. **C.** Lipomyelomeningocele. A herniated sac contains the cord as well as a fatty mass contiguous with the subcutaneous tissues. The cord is usually cleft and fixed by the fatty mass.

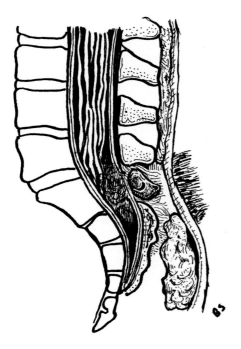

Figure 13–8. Spina bifida occulta. Cutaneous abnormalities include hair tuft, subcutaneous lipoma, and others.

23% had some form of spinal dysraphism. Hence, the factors that increase the likelihood of occult spinal pathology include atypical dimples, dimples seen in combination with other lesions, hemangiomas, upraised lesions such as subcutaneous masses, hairy patches, skin tags, or multiple cutaneous stigmata. Most dimples occur at the sacrococcygeal region. Those below the gluteal cleft have little clinical significance. The majority of patients with low-lying dimples have shallow pilonidal dimples. The result of spinal sonography in this group of patients is usually normal. A small percentage of patients with dimples have a *pilonidal sinus*. The pilonidal sinus (Fig. 13–9) is an epithelium-lined tube that extends from the skin surface to the dorsal surface (periosteum) of the coccyx. These sinuses do not communicate with the spinal canal. Although they are usually asymptomatic, they may, on rare occasion, become infected. Sonographically, they appear as a wide echogenic band that traverses the sonolucent fat plane of the subcutaneous tissues to extend to the periosteum of the coccyx.

This entity should be differentiated from the dermal sinus. The dorsal dermal sinus results from an embryological segmental adhesion between the cutaneous and the neural ectoderm. This adhesion persists as an epithelium-lined tube that connects the spinal canal to the skin. The pilonidal sinus usually takes a caudad course, in contrast to the dermal

sinus, which takes a cephalad course. Clinical differentiation of these two entities may be accomplished by cephalad retraction of the skin near the dimple. In the case of the pilonidal sinus, where the tract is coursing inferiorly, the dimple will seem to deepen. Conversely, a superiorly directed tract of a dermal sinus will become shallower as the skin is retracted. Dorsal dermal sinuses occur most commonly in the lumbosacral area, followed by the occipital region. These sinuses can terminate in the subcutaneous tissues, the dura mater, or the spinal cord, or, as occurs in 60% of the patients, within an epidermoid or dermoid cyst in the spinal canal (Fig. 13–10). When the dermal sinus terminates in the spinal canal, the spinal cord is usually tethered. The sinus may be demonstrated on either sagittal or axial scans as either an echogenic sonolucent tract[1,8] extending from the skin to the spinal cord. The intraspinal extent of the tract may be difficult to demonstrate via sonography, and the more global imaging modalities of computed tomography or magnetic resonance imaging may be necessary.[16,17]

Spinal cord tethering refers to abnormal fixation of the cord. It may be the result of a multitude of pathological causes.[18] These include a mass (such as an intraspinal lipoma) or an osseous, fibrous, or cartilaginous septum (associated with diastematomyelia). The cord may also be abnormally fixed by fibrous or fatty infiltration of the filum terminable. Sonographic findings that suggest a tethered cord include a low-lying conus medullaris, atypical shape of the conus tip, dorsal positioning of the cord, dampened cord motion at the site of tethering, and a thickened echogenic filum (Fig. 13–11).[19,20] It is important not only to recognize this entity, but also to determine its etiology. Early diagnosis and treatment can prevent the cord schema that develops secondary to traction on the cord during the longitudinal growth of the child. Progressive neurological, urologic, and orthopedic deterioration may occur if this entity is left untreated.

Diastematomyelia is a complex malformation characterized by clefting of the spinal cord by a bony, fibrous, or cartilaginous spur (Fig. 13–12). This results in segmental duplication of the cord with the formation of two hemicords. Each hemicord contains a central canal and one set of ventral and dorsal nerve roots. In 50% of the cases, the two hemicords share a single dural tube. In the remaining 50%, separate dural sacs envelop the hemicords. The two hemicords typically reunite below the cleft, with the conus lying in an abnormally low position. Vertebral body abnormalities are seen in the majority of patients. There is a strong female predominance. A variety of skin lesions mark the site of the defect. The

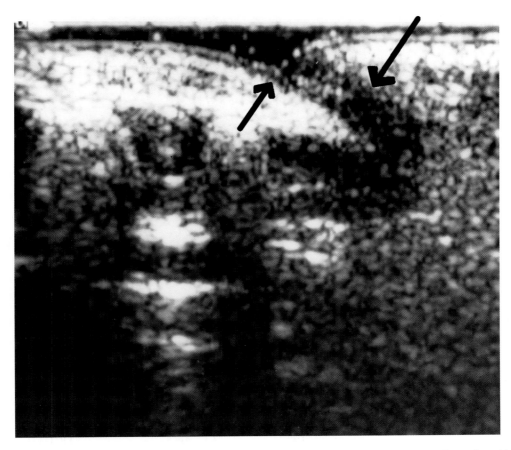

Figure 13–9. Pilonidal sinus. Longitudinal image demonstrating the linear tract emanating from the skin and extending to the periosteum of the coccyx *(arrows).*

cutaneous manifestations include tufts of hair (hypertrichosis), dimples, subcutaneous lipomas, vascular malformations or hemangiomatous discoloration, and/or congenital dermal sinus. As many as 50% of patients have hypertrichosis. This entity is frequently associated with vertebral malformations. A large percentage of patients have a congenital scoliosis. Two distinct clinical syndromes may occur. The first is unilateral in which one hypoplastic lower extremity is enervated by a hypoplastic segment of the cord. In this entity there is hypotonia and weakness of predominantly one extremity. In a second syndrome, the patient has weakness and spasticity of both lower extremities with resultant awkward gait. There is incontinence of the bladder and rectum. There is often atrophy of the leg muscles and skeletal deformities of the feet. These findings are often slowly progressive over a period of several months or years. Two theories have been proposed for the pathogenesis of these clinical syndromes. The first is that the bony spur impales the cord. This results in differential growth of the vertebral column and the spinal cord. There is stretching of the cord above its point of fixation. An alternative theory is that progressive neurological damage results form trauma and traction at the spur during head and neck flexion in the child. The acquired neurological deficits may be reversible. Prophylactic surgery with removal of the bony spur for the infant is indicated to prevent the development of neurologic sequelae. Surgical removal of the bony spur allows the cord to become freely mobile. The sonographic[21,22] appearance is characteristic, with the depiction of two distinct hemicords, each containing a central canal. (Fig. 13–13) Sonography may not be helpful when there is associated severe scoliosis and laminar fusion.[16]

The Skin-Covered Back Mass

Sonography of spinal dysraphism associated with a skin-covered back mass[23] is useful not only for evaluation of the primary entity but also for evaluating the known associated spinal cord anomalies. The key entities to consider are lipomyelomeningocele, myelocystocele, and meningocele (Fig. 13–6). The meningo-

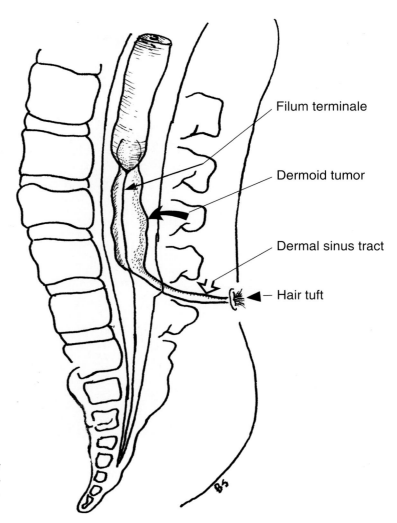

Filum terminale

Dermoid tumor

Dermal sinus tract

Hair tuft

Figure 13–10. Dorsal dermal sinus. The *long arrow* represents the filum terminale; *curved arrows,* a dermoid tumor; *open arrow,* a dermal sinus tract; *arrowhead,* a hair tuft.

cele is a herniated sac of meninges containing CSF without neural contents. This appears as a sonolucent mass associated with widening of the spinal canal (Fig. 13–14). The mass may change in size with Valsalva's maneuver. There is a rare association with other spine anomalies. The myelocystocele is a herniated sac that contains an abnormally low spinal cord with a tethered cord. The cystic mass within the myelocystocele is actually the dilated distal portion of the central canal. There is an association of myelocystocele with sacral agenesis and hydromyelia.

Lipomyelomeningocele consists of a skin-covered back mass that contains fat, neural tissue, CSF, and meninges. The spinal cord is usually tethered and is cleft dorsally. The lipomatous portion of the mass grows into the cleft. Lipomyelomeningocele usually appear sonographically as large homogeneously echogenic masses that extend from the subcutaneous tissues into the spinal canal (Fig. 13–14). Conus is not present in these patients. Lipomyelomeningocele are usually associated with large bony defects as well as segmentation anomalies of the vertebral bodies. Hydromyelia may also be present. This entity should be distinguished from a lipomyelocele, in which the cord is usually seen within the canal and may be displaced anteriorly by an echogenic mass that may grow into the cord. The homogeneously echogenic mass represents the lipoma.

The Non-Skin-Covered Back Mass

The two major anomalies of the group of non-skin-covered back masses are the myelomeningocele and the myelocele. Sonographic imaging of the non-skin-covered back mass is not necessary, as the surgery is not altered by the imaging findings and the pathology is clinically obvious. A relative contraindication to sonographic imaging is the risk of contamination of the sac with resultant infection of the subarachnoid space.

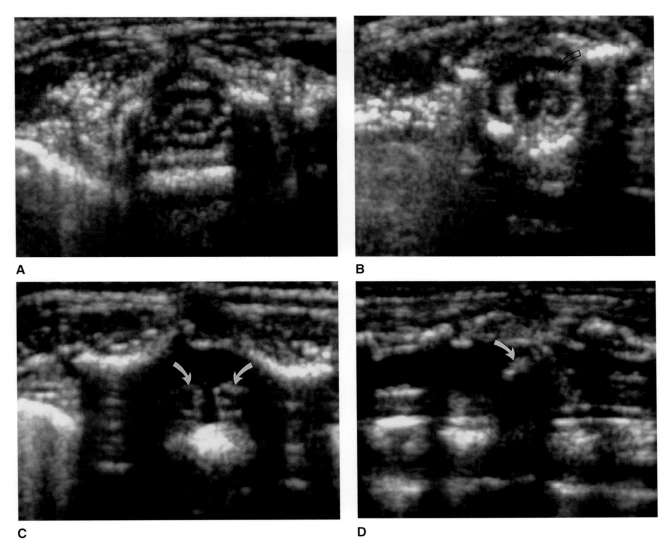

Figure 13–13. A. Multiple sequential transverse sections in a patient with diastematomyelia showing the normal transverse appearance of the cord. **B.** Region where the cord becomes split. **C.** Two distinct hemicords *(arrows)*. **D.** The arrow defines the body longitudinal section showing a bony spur, which caused the clefting of the cord.

Sonography may have a role in the evaluation of the repaired myelomeningocele. Postsurgically ultrasound may be helpful in the elucidation of spinal cord malformations associated with myelomeningocele. Diastematomyelia has been reported to occur in as many as 30% to 41% of the patients with myelomeningocele.[16,23] Sonography may also play a role in the evaluation of postoperative complications such as hydrosyringomyelia (*hydromyelia* refers to dilatation of the spinal canal; *syringomyelia,* to a cavity within the cord). Sonography may also be used to follow up epidermoids and lipomas to look for an increase in their size. Postsurgical neurological deterioration may occur in patients with repaired myelomeningocele, secondary to scar-induced tension on the spinal cord with resultant tethered cord syndrome.[24] Schumacher and collaborators[7] have proposed using M-mode sonography for identifying patients who are at risk for secondary tethered cord syndrome. They have observed the lack of normal physiological movements due to tension on the cord, an observation that can also be readily made with real-time imaging. Other sonographic observations[16] suggesting spinal cord tethering include fixation of the cord against the posterior wall of the canal and the absence of CSF behind the cord at the point of tethering.

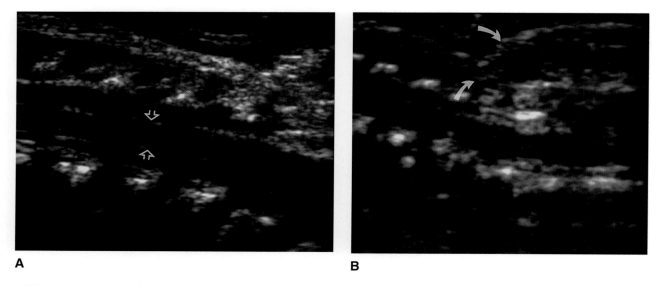

A   B

Figure 13–14. A. Longitudinal image showing the relatively normal appearance of the cord (*arrows*) above a bony defect. **B.** A large lipomatous mass is seen infiltrating and fixing the cord.

SUMMARY

Sonography plays an important role in imaging of the spine and its contents even after birth. It can be used to analyze the various forms of spinal dysraphism. Its use in intraoperative and postoperative spinal cord and vertebral column spine evaluation is still evolving. Its key role is in the analysis of spinal cord position and anatomy in an attempt to avoid a delayed diagnosis and the future morbidity of a tethered cord.

At this time, two-D ultrasound equipment is being used to evaluate the pediatric spine. Recently, three-D ultrasound is being performed to image the fetal spine and to evaluate it for complex malformations (see Chapter 9). It has been the experience of most authors that three-D sonography is superior to two-D for the evaluation of fetal anomalies (see Chapter 14). Often in the experience of the authors, the reconstructed three-D image was not as helpful as being able to view and to manipulate simultaneously the three orthogonal planes. Multiplanar imaging improved the understanding of complex anomalies. A future role is seen for three-D sonography for the evaluation of the pediatric spine.

REFERENCES

1. Naidich TP, Fernbach SK, McLone DG, et al. Sonography of the caudal spine and back: Congenital anomalies in children. *AJNR*. 1984;5:221–234.

2. Miller JH, Reid BS, Kemberling CR. Utilization of ultrasound in the evaluation of spinal dysraphism in children. *Radiology*. 1982;143:737–740.

3. Gusnard DA, Naidich TP, Yousefzadeh DK, et al. Ultrasonic anatomy of the normal neonatal and infant spine: Correlation with cryomicrotome sections and CT. *Neuroradiology*. 1986;28:493–511.

4. St. Amour TE, Rubin JM, Dohrmann GJ. The central canal of the spinal cord: Ultrasonic identification. *Radiology*. 1984;152:767–769.

5. Nelson MD Jr, Sedler JA, Gilles FH. Spinal cord central echo complex: Histoanatomic correlation. *Radiology*. 1989;170:479–481.

6. DiPietro MA. The conus medullaris: Normal US findings throughout childhood. *Radiology*. 1993;188:149–153.

7. Schumacher R, Kroll B, Schwarz M, et al. M-mode sonography of the caudal spinal cord in patients with meningomyelocele. *Radiology*. 1992;184:263–265.

8. Korsvik HE, Keller MS. Sonography of occult dysraphism in neonates and infants with MR imaging correlation. *Radiographics*. 1992;12:297–306.

9. Kawahara H, Andou Y, Takashima S, et al. Normal development of the spinal cord in neonates and infants seen on ultrasonography. *Neuroradiology*. 1987:29:50–52.

10. Byrd SE, Darling CF, McLone DG. Developmental disorders of the pediatric spine. *Radiol Clin North Am*. 1991:29:711–752.

11. Tortori-Donati P, Cama A, Rosa ML, et al. Occult spinal dysraphism: Neuroradiological study. *Neuroradiology*. 1990;31:512–522.

12. Anderson FM. Occult spinal dysraphism: A series of 73 cases. *Pediatrics*. 1975;55:826–835.

13. Hall DE, Udvarhelyi GB, Altman J. Lumbosacral skin lesions as markers of occult spinal dysraphism. *JAMA.* 1981;246:2606–2608.

14. Powell KR, Cherry JD, Hougen TJ, et al. A prospective search for congenital dermal abnormalities of the craniospinal axis. *J Pediatr.* 1975;87:744–750.

15. Kriss VM, Desai S. Occult spinal dysraphism in neonates: Assessment of high-risk cutaneous stigmata on sonography. *AJR.* 1998:171:1687–1692.

16. Naidich TP, Radkowski MA, Britton J. Real-time sonographic display of caudal spinal anomalies. *Neuroradiology.* 1986;28:146–161.

17. Barkovich AJ, Edwards MSB, Cogen PH. MR evaluation of spinal dermal sinus tracts in children. *AJR.* 1991;156:791–797.

18. Merx JL, Bakker-Niezen SH, Thijssen HOM, et al. The tethered spinal cord syndrome: A correlation of radiological features and preoperative findings in 30 patients. *Neuroradiology.* 1989;31:63–70.

19. Raghavendra BN, Epstein FJ, Pinto RS, et al. The tethered spinal cord: Diagnosis by high-resolution real-time ultrasound. *Radiology.* 1983;149:123–128.

20. Zieger M, Dorr U, Scultz RD. Pediatric spinal sonography. Part II: Malformations and mass lesions. *Pediatr Radiol.* 1988;18:105–111.

21. Kirpelcar M. Diastematomelia In: Cohen HL, Sivit CJ. Fetal and Pediatric Ultrasound. A casebook approach. McGraw-Hill. New York 2001. (in press)

22. Raghavendra BN, Epstein FJ, Pinto RS, et al. Sonographic diagnosis of diastematomyelia. *J Ultrasound Med.* 1988;7:111–113.

23. Glasier CM, Chadduck WM, Leithiser RE Jr, et al. Screening spinal ultrasound in newborns with neural tube defects. *J Ultrasound Med.* 1990;9:339–343.

24. Nelson MD Jr, Bracchi M, Naidich TP, et al. The natural history of repaired myelomeningocele. *Radiographics.* 1988;8:695–706.

25. Braun IF, Raghavendra BN, Kricheff II. Spinal cord imaging using real-time ultrasound. *Radiology.* 1983; 147:459–465.

26. Garcia CJ, Keller MS. Intraspinal extension of paraspinal masses in infants: Detection by sonography. *Pediatr Radiol.* 1990;20:437–439.

27. Jequier S, Cramer B, O'Gorman AM. Ultrasound of the spinal cord in neonates and infants. *Ann Radiol.* 1985;28:225–231.

28. Kangarloo H, Gold RH, Diament MJ, et al. High-resolution spinal sonography in infants. *AJR.* 1984; 142:1243–1247.

29. Scatliff JH, Kendall BE, Kingsiey DPE, et al. Closed spinal dysraphism: Analysis of clinical, radiological and surgical findings in 104 consecutive patients. *AJR.* 1989;152:1049–1057.

30. Zieger M, Dorr U. Pediatric spinal sonography. Part 1: Anatomy and examination technique. *Pediatr Radiol.* 1988;18:9–13.

31. Riccabona M, Johnson D, Pretorius DH, Nelson TR. Three dimensional ultrasound: Display modalities in the fetal spine and thorax. *Eur J Radiol.* 1996;22: 141–145.

32. Mueller GM, Weiner CP, Yankowitz J. Three-dimensional ultrasound in the evaluation of fetal head and spine anomalies. *Obstet Gynecol.* 1996:88:372–378.

CHAPTER FOURTEEN

Three-Dimensional Neonatal Neurosonography

Michael L. Manco-Johnson
Gary Thieme
Darleen Cioffi-Ragan

In the late 1970s and early 1980s, neonatal neurosonography became a well-established tool to diagnose the presence and determine the degree of intracranial hemorrhage (ICH) in the premature infant.[1–3] It has also been shown to be accurate in the diagnosis of other acquired and congenital brain malformations.[4–7]

The open anterior fontanel offers easy access to the neonatal brain and until that acoustic window closes (at about 6 months of age), it allows clinically useful ultrasound imaging. Two-dimensional (2D) sonography of the newborn brain often requires 20 to 30 minutes to perform, exposing the sometimes severely ill neonate to potentially significant hazards. It was hoped that three-dimensional (3D) volume acquisitions would supply adequate diagnostic information and significantly decrease the examination time, thus exposing the neonate to less stress.[8–9] It was found that 3D volume acquisitions can indeed yield diagnostic information similar to a conventional 2D study with a shorter examination time, which may be less than 5 minutes. For some diagnostic problems, the 3D technique provides even more information than the standard 2D technique.[8,9]

Conventional 2D imaging of the neonatal brain is accomplished by real-time scanning with a hand-held transducer. As the operator orients the transducer in coronal and sagittal planes through the anterior fontanelle, a series of representative pictures at different locations of the brain anatomy can be obtained. Interpretation and reporting are based upon this selected set of images. Questions with regard to the clinical quality of the examination are answered by a subsequent follow-up examination session to acquire additional views. This 2D imaging technique is greatly dependent on the operator recognizing normal and abnormal anatomy during the examination and documenting the findings with a sufficiently large set of images to enable the sonologist to establish the correct diagnosis. As with other imaging modalities obtained by 2D techniques, the operator or the sonologist must reconstruct mentally the successive sections and planes to gain spatial information of the three-dimensional organ.

TECHNIQUE OF THREE-DIMENSIONAL NEUROSONOGRAPHY

The 3D volumetric imaging of the neonatal brain described in this chapter was accomplished by using the Medison Voluson 530 system (Medison America, Inc. Cypress, CA) and a specialized transducer that mechanically sweeps the image plane through a predetermined angle (e.g., 90 degrees) and records images at fixed angular increments (e.g., every 2 degrees) in a digital fashion. The spatial relationships among the individual image planes of the 3D volume data set constitute a comprehensive representation of the sonographic features of the brain. The 3D method minimizes operator-dependent gaps in the information set inherent to the hand operated acquisition method typical of 2D traditional imaging. To maximize image detail, high-resolution mode and slow-sweep speeds are used. The digital data set is saved as polar coordinates so that it can be recalled, examined, and interpreted offline. The data can also be saved in Cartesian format. Orthogonal sets of images in any desired plane throughout the 3D volume can be generated. In addition to the standard sagital and coronal planes traditionally obtained through the anterior fontanelle, the brain can be viewed in axial and oblique planes, which can not be obtained by conventional 2D imaging through the anterior fontanelle. The volume can be recalled, reconstructed, and examined at a convenient time or sent to another specialist by electronic means. The operator can generate as many views as are needed for the diagnosis.

TECHNIQUE OF THREE-DIMENSIONAL IMAGING

The following procedure is specific to the **Medison Voluson 530D** equipment used to generate the images in this chapter. The neonatal probe (S-VNA 5-8) is used in the **program 1** setting. The groove on the transducer probe is oriented toward the right of the head when placed on the anterior fontanel in a coronal plane. The **B-mag** magnification control adjusts image size, so that the entire brain is included in the cranial–caudal field of view with the focal zones evenly spaced within this field of view. While imaging the region of the third ventricle, the time gain control (TGC) and gain is set for optimal resolution using the **resolution** mode. Selecting the **volume mode,** the **volume-angle (sweep angle)** is set to include the largest area of the full anterior–posterior depth of the brain in the sagital plane. Then the **B-angle volume-box** size (angle) and position are adjusted so that the entire width of the brain is included in the coronal plane and is symmetrically positioned (centered) in the volume box. The **slow** acquisition time (speed) is used to maximize image plane density during the acquisition phase and to optimize the spatial resolution during off-line processing. To start the acquisition process, the **volume-start** button or the **freeze** button is activated to begin the volume mode sweep. Once the volume data is acquired and the images in the three boxes appear on the monitor, the examiner should scroll through the multiplanar images from anterior to posterior and left to right to

determine if all of the brain is imaged and the quality of the picture is adequate.

Similar to conventional 2D imaging, proper labeling of the right and the left side as well as the anterior and the posterior direction of images displayed from the 3D volume data set is crucial for accurate localization of the anatomy and pathology. The rendering software changes the labeling automatically as new viewing planes are generated from the stored 3D data volume set. In other words, the orientation labels follow the anatomy as the orthogonal image planes are rotated.

To correctly label the scan orientation during a volume acquisition in the coronal plane, refer to the **plane ID** section and select the **cranial** key. Only that key should be high-lighted. The **anterior** key is the default selection and should be in the off position. Only the **cranial** key should be high-lighted as the transducer is on the cranium (top of the skull). Next, **rotate** key should be activated to indicate **R (right);** this will be correct only if the groove on the transducer is facing the right side of the neonate's head. Subsequently, the image will be correctly orientated at all times after the above information is entered correctly.

If a volume acquisition is performed in the sagital plane, the groove of the transducer should point toward the front of the head (anterior). The subsequent steps are similar to those outlined for the volume acquisition in the coronal plane; however, labeling the scan orientation is different. After activating the **plane ID** window the **cranial** key should again be selected. Only that key should be high-lighted; and the default **anterior** key should be turned off. Next, the **rotate** should be turned to **A (anterior)** as the transducer groove is now facing anterior on the baby's head. All images should now have the correct orientation labels as the multiplanar projections are manipulated.

The 3D method minimizes dependence on the operator recognizing the pathology and obtaining the needed views at the time of the examination. Performance of the 3D examination, still requires a level of technical skill that is similar to the conventional 2D examination. Compared to a conventional 2D examination, the acquisition time for the 3D examination is brief (typically 5 seconds or less). It is possible to immediately view the 3D data obtained at the ultrasound system console and determine if the data set is technically adequate. For the conventional 2D examination, the time required to obtain a complete image set may range from 15 minutes to 20 minutes. The individual images must be recorded on a hard copy as the examination progresses and cannot be viewed online. In addition, viewing the sagital plane requires an additional acquisition and repositioning of the transducer. The acquisition of an axial plane requires even more time and must be performed through the temporal bone.

Interpretation time for a 3D examination at a diagnostic workstation can be similar to or shorter than a conventional 2D examination if the volume set is surveyed for pathology in the multiplanar mode and key views are saved in a digital DICOM archive. A complete set of 2D images (similar to a conventional examination) can be obtained from the 3D set during the interpretation phase by selecting the coronal, then the sagital and finally, the axial view box and acquiring hardcopies or storing each image while scrolling through the brain from front to back, side to side, and from top to bottom. At times, reviewing the 3D volume set may take longer, due to the fact that a large amount of information can be extracted from the volume set using the orthogonal planes and rendering some views in 3D "slabs."

In theory, spatial resolution for the displayed 2D images is optimal for only the original plane in which the acquisition of the 3D volume set was performed. This is due to the fact that additional imaging planes must be interpolated using averaging from lateral beam width and slice thickness information, which degrade spatial resolution for those planes. When imaging through the neonate's anterior fontanel, coronal plane and sagital plane acquisitions are possible. Theoretically, images displayed in the coronal plane will have the best resolution when acquired in the coronal plane; images displayed in the sagital plane from coronally acquired data will have slightly degraded resolution. Similarly, images displayed in sagital planes will have the best resolution when acquired in the sagital plane; images displayed in coronal planes from sagitally acquired data will have slightly degraded resolution. Despite this, with respect to our practical experience, we have not noticed any significant difference in resolution in any sagital and coronal images regardless of the plane of acquisition. This was untrue in the axial plane (C-plane), which is oriented perpendicular to the original beam axis and is heavily interpolated by slice thickness (interpolated) information. As expected, the authors have observed significantly degraded spatial resolution for axial images, especially for the near field and the far field depths (outside of the focal zone). These observations probably hold true also for the 3D fetal transfontanelle neuroscan.

The applications of 3D volume ultrasound imaging include assessing for extent of intracranial hemorrhage, detection of periventricular leukomalacia, assessing the degree and the cause of ventriculomegaly, and, of course, evaluation of congenital malformations of the brain. The indications, therefore, are similar to those of conventional 2D ultrasound imaging.

NORMAL BRAIN ANATOMY

First, the normal neonatal brain anatomy seen by 3D transfontanelle ultrasound imaging is presented. This allows the reader to have a reference for comparison to pathological scans.

The relationship of the cavum septi pellucidi and cavum vergae with respect to the corpus callosum, lateral ventricles, caudate nuclei, and thalami is shown in Figure 14–1. The center point of rotation for each set of orthogonal images is marked by a white dot. Figure 14–1A is the originally acquired coronal image through the interhemispheric fissure (mid-line) demonstrating the small lateral ventricles on either side of the central fluid filled cavum septi pellucidi (white marker dot). In the sagitally displayed image (Fig. 14–1B), the full length of the cavum septi pellucidi and cavum vergae is seen (white marker dot), with the corpus callosum being the thin curved band of tissue that drapes over the cavum from front to back. The axially displayed section (Fig. 14–1C) shows the full length of the lateral ventricles on either side of a small amount of the cavuum septi pellucidi (white marker dot). By tilting the coronal image plane in Figure 14–1A, and moving the center point of rotation (white marker dot) over to the left caudate nucleus, the multiplanar image set in Figure 14–2 is obtained. This allows the left lateral ventricle with its three horns to be seen in a sagital plane (Fig. 14–2B). This view was described in Chapter 9 and called the "three-horn view." As the coronal image is tilted and the center of rotation is in the left caudate region, the axially displayed image (Fig. 14–2C) is sectioned below the bodies of the lateral ventricles and only a portion of the left anterior horn and right and left atrium are visualized. The coronally acquired image and the displayed sagital image follow normal 2D imaging convention. For the displayed axial plane, the anterior and posterior ends are flipped with the anterior or front of the face down (Fig. 14–2C).

When the 3D volume data is acquired in the sagital plane, the sagital image is viewed in the standard orientation (Fig. 14–3A) and the right and left sides of the coronally displayed image are flipped (Fig. 14–3B). Also, the displayed axial view is

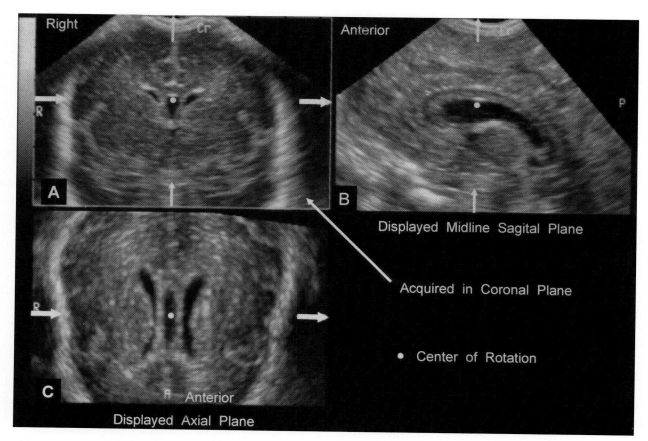

Figure 14–1. This multiplanar image set shows normal brain anatomy that is centered on the cavum septi pellucidi. The 3D volume data is acquired in the coronal plane **(A)**. The sagital image **(B)** and the axial image **(C)** are reconstructed at right angles to the coronal plane. The *white marker dot* marks the center of rotation for the orthogonal set of images and represents the common point of intersection of these planes. For the sagital view, the anterior and posterior directions conform to standard convention. For the axial view, the convention is reversed such that the posterior end is at the top and the anterior end is at the bottom. The top of the head or cranial aspect (Cr) is toward the top of the image in the coronal and sagital view and the right (R) side of the brain is on the left of the image in the coronal and axial view.

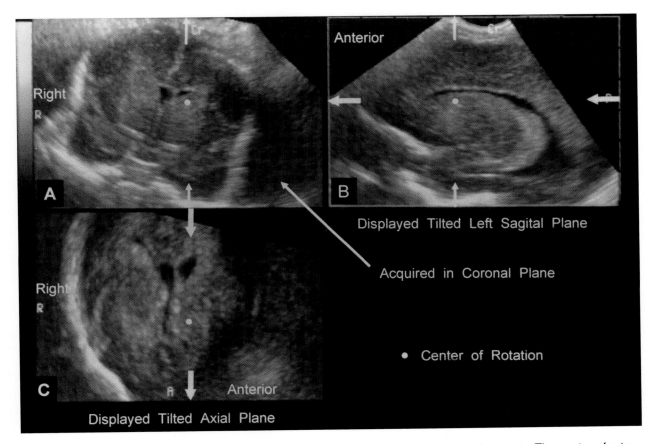

Figure 14–2. This 3D volume data is acquired in the coronal plane **(A)** in this normal neonate. The center of rotation *(white marker dot)* is moved into the left caudate nucleus and the coronal image is rotated counter-clockwise around the point of rotation until the length of the left lateral ventricle is brought into view in its entirety in the sagital reconstruction **(B).** The axial plane **(C)** tilts such that the body of the left and right lateral ventricles is not seen. The common point of reference is the center point of rotation represented by the white marker dot.

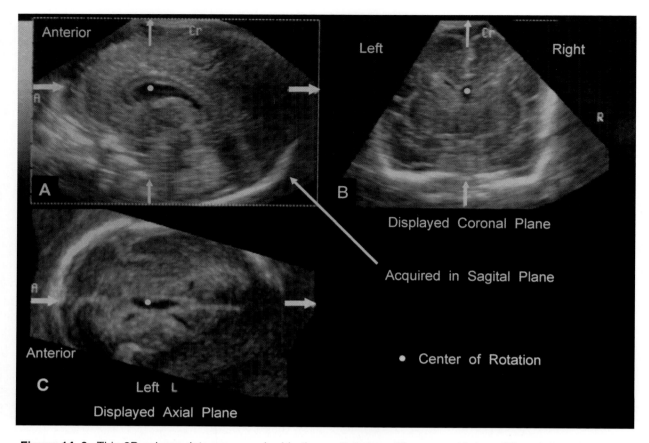

Figure 14–3. This 3D volume data was acquired in the sagital plane. The coronal image **(B)** and the axial image **(C)** are reconstructed at right angles to the sagital plane. The *white dot* marks the center of rotation for the orthogonal set of images and represents the common point of intersection of these planes through the middle of the cavum septi pellucidi. The left and right sides of the coronal view are reversed from the standard right–left convention as this data set was acquired in the sagital plane. The axial view **(C)** is turned on its side with the right side of the head toward the top of the image and the anterior (frontal) aspect of the head to the left of the image.

now positioned on its side (Fig. 14–3C) with the face to the left. Because the proper labeling of the acquired volume has been performed, the anatomic relationships are correctly labeled on the displayed views regardless of their orientation. The importance of proper labeling of the data set at the time of the examination cannot be over emphasized.

The images in Figures 14–1, 14–2, and 14–4 were all obtained from one coronal acquisition and then repositioned and photographed. Once the 3D volume data set has been acquired, it is possible to "walk through" (scroll) the entire brain in a coronal, sagital, or axial view. Figure 14–4 is an example of "walking through" the brain in the coronal projection. By high-lighting the top left box (Fig. 14–1A), it is possible to move the center of rotation on the sagital view (Fig. 14–1B) forward until the coronal plane is in front of the cavuum septi pellucidi and

going only through the tips of the anterior horns as shown in Figure 14–4A. Then, by moving the center point on the sagital projection from front to back, multiple scans through the brain in the coronal view can be reviewed and photographed. Of the multiple possible images, only four have been displayed in Figure 14–4. Figure 14–4B is at the level of the cavum septi pellucidi (large broken arrow) and corpus callosum (small arrow). The interhemispheric fissure is well seen and the small third ventricle is below the cavuum. The echogenic lateral sulcus (Sylvian fissure) is seen laterally near the skull bilaterally. Figure 14–4C is more posterior, demonstrating the echogenic choroid plexus at the base of the lateral ventricles bilaterally and Figure 14–4D is even more posterior through the lateral ventricle and echogenic choroid plexus as they dive down to the posterior horns.

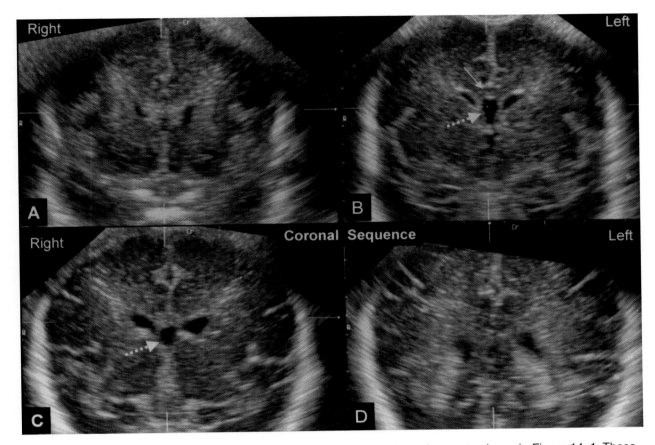

Figure 14–4. Multiple coronal images are displayed from the same normal neonate shown in Figure 14–1. These represent only four of numerous cuts through the brain that are available from the 3D volume data set. The examiner can "walk through" (scroll) the brain from front to back and see the anterior aspects of the anterior horns **(A)**, the cavum septi pellucidi *(broken arrow)*, corpus callosum *(small arrow)*, anterior horns of the lateral ventricles, and third ventricle **(B)**. Slightly more posterior are the bodies of the lateral ventricles with the choroid plexus seen as echogenic structures at the base of the ventricles **(C)** and more posteriorly through the trigone the echogenic choroid plexus is sweeping down toward the posterior horns **(D)**.

PATHOLOGIES OF THE NEONATAL BRAIN

In the remainder of this chapter, examples of 3D ultrasound in several important pathologies of the neonatal brain are presented. It is clear to the authors that only a few abnormal scans can be included. It is our hope, however, that by the use of these examples, a general understanding of the importance of 3D neonatal brain scanning can be achieved.

INTRACRANIAL HEMORRHAGE

Intracranial hemorrhage (ICH) occurs frequently in premature infants below 32 weeks of gestational age[3,7,10,11–14] and usually starts in the germinal matrix in the subependymal area near the base of the lateral ventricles. Four grades of ICH are used to describe increasing severity of the bleed. Grade I ICH is when the hemorrhage is confined to the germinal matrix and is called sub-ependymal hemorrhage (SEH). Grade II is present when the bleed extends into the lateral ventricle itself, but no ventriculomegaly has occurred. Hemorrhage into the ventricle causes ventriculitis, therefore the ventricles often enlarge. When ventriculomegaly in the presence of a hemorrhage is seen, it is considered a grade III ICH. If the bleeding extends into the brain parenchyma, it is regarded as a grade IV ICH. Fresh hemorrhages are echogenic on ultrasound; however, within a few weeks they may become cystic, as the clot is removed by macrophages. This then appears as an echo free area of porencephaly within the brain.

INTRACRANIAL HEMORRHAGE GRADE I

The 3D ultrasound examination in Figure 14–5 shows a left sided grade I germinal matrix hemorrhage (small arrow) in the brain of a premature infant. The orthogonal image planes are centered on the left subependymal hemorrhage (SEH) (white marker dot), and the sagittal and axial displays were tilted slightly to better demonstrate the entire length of the left lateral ventricle. The density within the thalamocaudate notch represents the germinal matrix hemorrhage and is seen on all three planes. Although the diagnosis can be made just as easily from conventional 2D images, the multiplanar relationships of the coronal and sagittal planes are unknown and no axial views are available for examination.[8]

INTRACRANIAL HEMORRHAGE GRADE III

Figure 14–6 is a 3D ultrasound examination on a premature infant with bilateral subependymal hemorrhage (SEH) and mild ventriculomegaly. This is a grade III ICH. The sagittal view is through the right lateral ventricle at the level of the SEH and demonstrates dilatation of the posterior horn. The axial view (Fig. 14–6C) demonstrates bilateral SEH in each caudate nucleus.

Figure 14–7 is from another patient with a grade III ICH. The orthogonal views show the spatial relationships of the partially lysed clot within the dilated right lateral ventricle (white marker dot in Fig. 14–7A, B, and C), the hyperechoic clot within the occipital horn (Fig. 14–7B), and the isoechoic clot within the temporal horn (Fig. 14–7A). Also, clot is

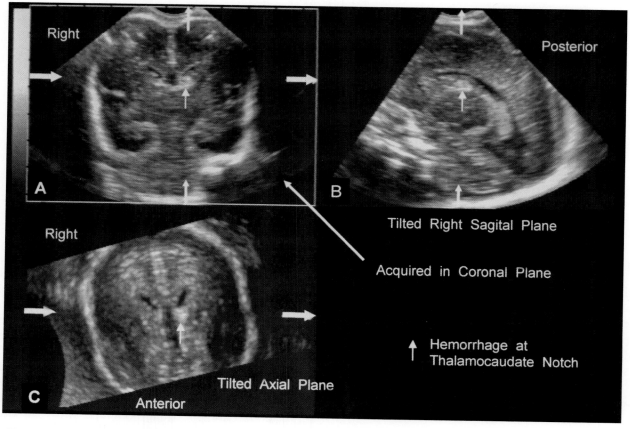

Figure 14–5. This multiplanar image set is centered on the left germinal matrix hemorrhage in this premature infant with grade I intracranial hemorrhage. Orthogonal views demonstrate the relationship of the hemorrhage to the surrounding normal brain anatomy, as seen in the coronal **(A)**, sagittal **(B)**, and axial **(C)** planes. The 3D volume data was acquired in the coronal plane and is presented with a slight tilt on the axial view to lay out the entirety of the left lateral ventricle in the sagittal view.

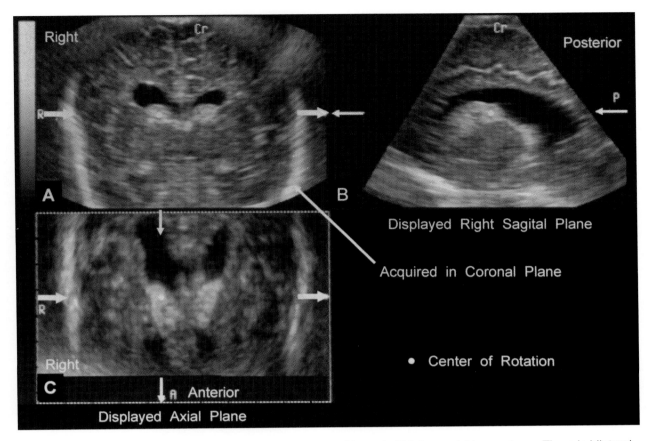

Figure 14–6. Three-Dimensional ultrasound of a neonate with grade III intracranial hemorrhage. There is bilateral SEH, with mild to moderate ventriculomegaly. The center point of rotation *(marker dot)* is placed in the right SEH in the coronal view **(A)** and the sagital **(B)** and axial **(C)** views demonstrate the relationship of that SEH to the right caudate nucleus and right lateral ventricle.

present within the dilated third ventricle (Fig. 14–7A). A complete understanding of the size of the ventricles, the location of the clot, and the absence of intraparenchymal blood can be obtained by scrolling through the coronal, sagital, and axial images.

Occasionally, septations or adhesions can occur within the ventricle secondary to the intraventricular blood and these can be excellently displayed by 3D ultrasound. Figure 14–8 is a 3D study from another child with a grade III ICH demonstrating ventriculomegaly and an adhesion extending from the choroid plexus to the medial wall in the atrium of the left lateral ventricle. The center point of rotation (marker dot) has been placed on the adhe-

sion and it is visualized in all three orthogonal planes.

The strength of the 3D multiplanar display is demonstrated in Figure 14–9 from a patient with a grade III ICH. This baby demonstrated mild ventriculomegaly, with clot lying in the right lateral ventricle. On the sagital projection, a large echogenic structure was noted, which appeared to be within the third ventricle (Fig. 14–9B). By placing the center point of rotation on this structure, it is obvious in the coronal and axial projection, that this structure is the normal massa intermedia traversing between the two thalami, and not a mass lesion or clot.

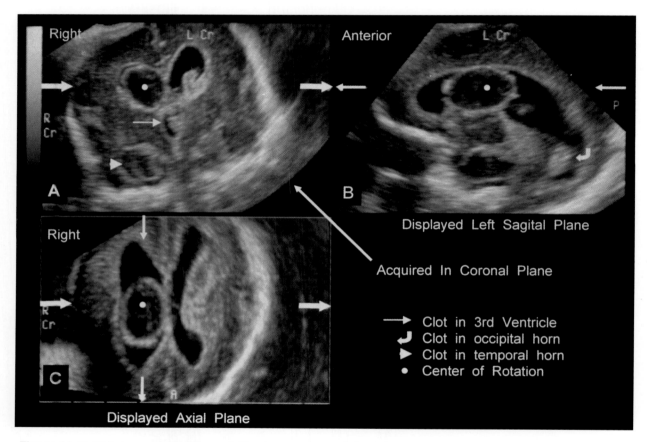

Figure 14–7. This is a coronal 3D acquisition in a premature infant with grade III intracranial hemorrhage. The center point of rotation *(white marker dot)* of the multiplanar image set is centered on the partially lysed clot in the right lateral ventricle. Orthogonal views demonstrate the relationship of the hemorrhage to the surrounding brain anatomy, as seen in the coronal **(A),** sagittal **(B),** and axial **(C)** planes. *Arrows* point to the clots within the third ventricle *(straight arrow),* the posterior horn of the lateral ventricle *(curved arrow),* and inferior horn of the lateral ventricle *(arrowhead).*

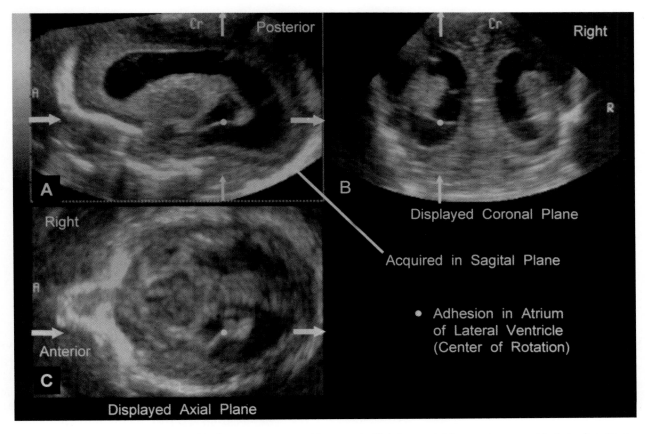

Figure 14–8. This 3D ultrasound is from a neonate with a grade III intracranial hemorrhage and is focusing on a septation or adhesion *(white marker dot)* extending from the choroid plexus to the medial wall of the lateral ventricle seen on all three projections. Adhesions are much more easily appreciated in the 3D images. The ventricles are moderately enlarged.

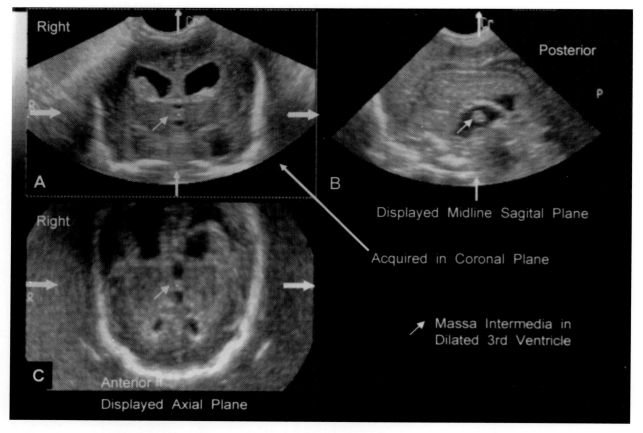

Figure 14–9. Grade III intracranial hemorrhage in neonate with clot lying in the right lateral ventricle **(A).** The massa intermedia *(straight arrow)* is seen within the dilated third ventricle.

INTRACRANIAL HEMORRHAGE GRADE IV

Grade IV ICH is demonstrated in Figure 14–10. There is a large echogenic mass in the left parietal lobe adjacent to the interhemispheric fissure, which extends from the roof of the left lateral ventricle superiorly. The full extent of this hemorrhage can best be appreciated on sagital and axial views (Fig. 14–10A and C). There is also clot in both lateral ventricles and the third ventricle. The multiplanar displays allow a complete understanding of the location and extent of intraparenchymal hemorrhages and have added a great deal to the understanding of brain damage.

Periventricular Leukomalacia

Periventricular leukomalacia (PVL) consists of infarction and necrosis of the periventricular white matter in fetuses or premature infants. This pathology is usually the result of hypotension, severe hypoxia, and ischemia.[4,15,13,14,16,17] Although less common than intracranial hemorrhage, PVL is a much more significant abnormality with nearly universally poor prognosis. The developing spastic diplegia or quadraplegia in neonates diagnosed with PVL is almost always a late sequela with frequent cortical blindness and developmental delays.

The location of PVL is usually between the arterial border zones of the white matter at the frontal–parietal area and at the level of the trigone of the lateral ventricles. Initially, the ultrasound examination in PVL may be unremarkable; however, within 7 to 14 days, the periventricular region becomes echogenic and 2 to 4 weeks following the initial insult, multiple cystic regions develop. Periventricular leukomalacia with its cystic pattern is usually bilateral and often symmetric.

The extent and severity of the periventricular leukomalacia in a neonatal brain is shown in the sequence of images demonstrated in Figure 14–11. This volume set was acquired in the coronal plane. Figure 14–11A is a coronal image through the region of the trigone demonstrating a "swiss cheese" appearance to the brain, with echogenic and echolu-

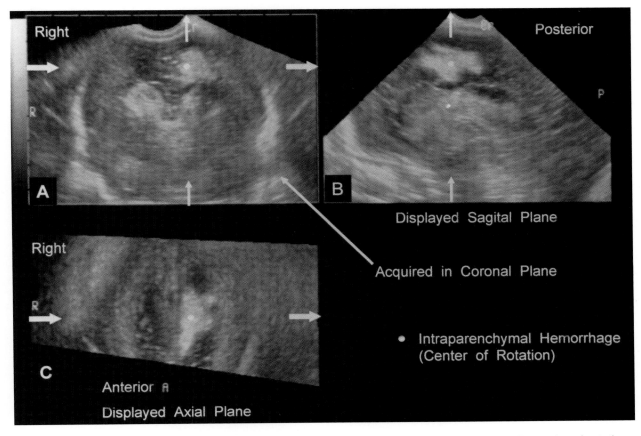

Figure 14–10. This 3D volume data shows features of a grade IV intracranial hemorrhage. The point of rotation *(white marker dot)* of the orthogonal image set is centered on the intraparenchymal hemorrhage within the left frontal lobe to parietal lobe, as seen in the coronal **(A)**, sagital **(B)**, and axial **(C)** planes. The hemorrhage is initially echogenic. The displayed axial plane shows there is no midline shift. There is also clot within both lateral ventricles and the third ventricle. The 3D volume data was acquired in the coronal plane.

cent areas. The cystic areas represent destruction and resorption of brain parenchyma. The level of the coronal plane can be appreciated by the location of the center point of rotation (white marker dot) seen in Figure 14–11B. The sagital and axial reformatted images also demonstrate the significant destruction of the normal brain tissue. This same volume set can also be rendered in a 3D "slab" projection, which brings out the cystic destructive process even more clearly (Fig. 14–12).

For additional data and images the reader is referred to Chapters 4 and 16.

Other Intracranial Abnormalities Imaged by Three-Dimensional Neonatal Neurosonography

In a premature neonate evaluated for possible intracranial hemorrhage, conventional 2D imaging showed a hyperechoic peripheral mass near the frontal–parietal junction in the left cerebral hemi-

sphere (Fig. 14–13). Power Doppler imaging showed a vessel at the lateral margin of the mass. Initial differential diagnosis included focal hemorrhage, neoplasm, and vascular malformation. A magnetic resonance imaging examination (MRI) showed no evidence for a mass. Three-dimensional imaging through this area (Fig. 14–14 and 14–15) revealed the same echogenic focus in the left frontoparietal region. The axial reformatting, however, demonstrated that the mass was located within a sulcus in the left hemisphere and was symmetrically positioned with respect to a normal structure, with a density within the corresponding sulcus of the right hemisphere. These gyri and sulci are seen only in the axial plane, which can be obtained only by rendering from the 3D volume data set. When serial examinations showed no change with time, it was concluded that the density most probably was simply benign subarachnoid tissue occupying space between opposing gyri.

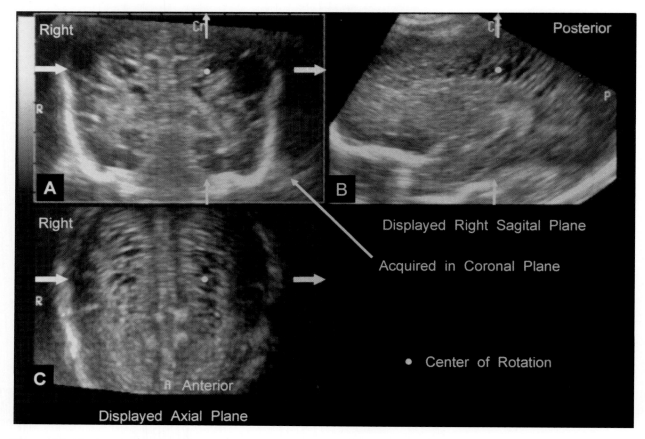

Figure 14–11. A coronal view **(D)** shows periventricular leukomalacia features *(white marker dot)* in this neonatal brain. Small cysts are seen within the hyperechoic periventricular tissues. This abnormality is present bilaterally. The sagital and axial projections demonstrate the full extent of the damage in this baby with perventricular leukomalacia.

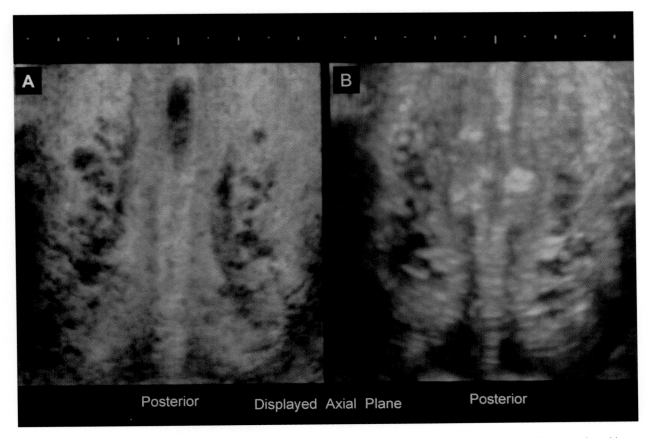

Figure 14–12. The orthogonal images of the 3D volume data have been rotated to produce a surface rendered image of the periventricular leukomalacia in an axial plane. The 3D relief effect or "slab" is generated using a surface rendering technique where the viewer looks down on the axial plane from above. The "holes" in the parenchyma are much more obvious by this 3D rendering.

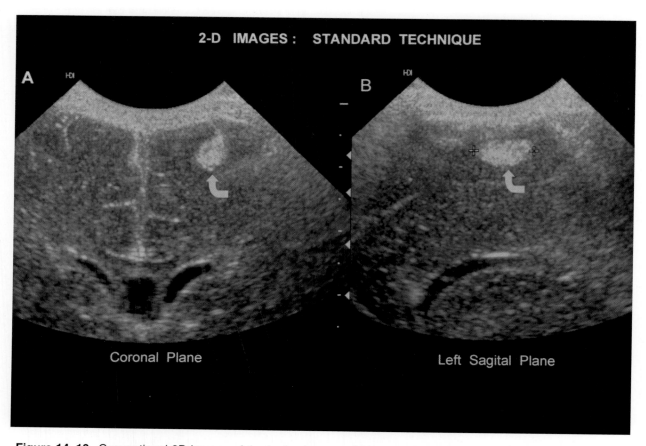

Figure 14–13. Conventional 2D images of the brain show a solid hyperechoic mass near the frontal-parietal junction in the left cerebral hemisphere. A curved arrow points to the mass in the coronal image (A) and the sagital image (B).

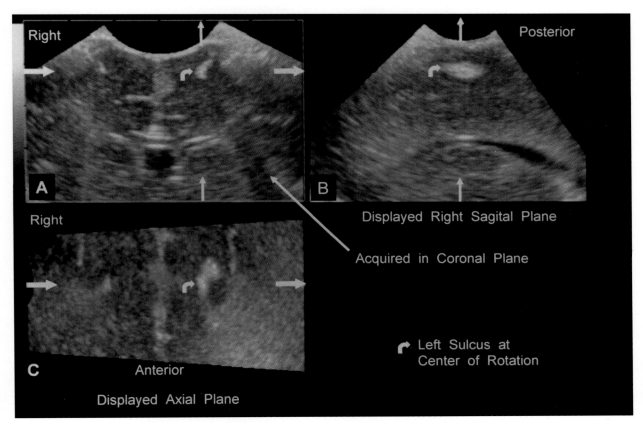

Figure 14–14. Three-dimensional ultrasound through the brain of the neonate shown in Figure 14–13. **(A)** The mass in the left frontoparietal area *(curved arrow)* is seen and the center point of rotation *(white marker dot)* is placed in the mass. The sagital **(B)** and axial **(C)** displayed images show this mass to be in the region of the left sulcus, and most likely represents fat within the sulcus. Figure 14–15 demonstrates the same finding in the right sulcus.

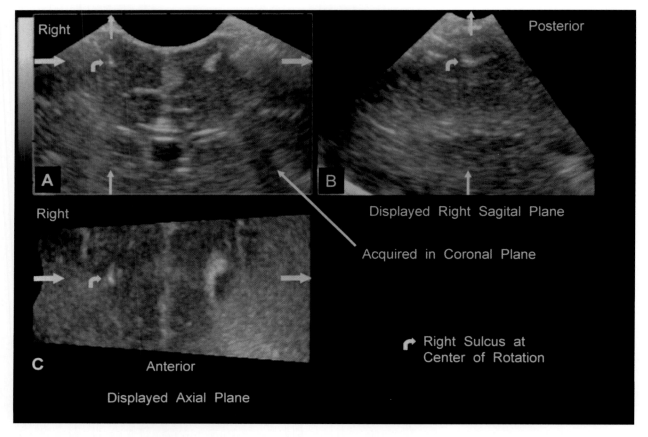

Figure 14–15. Three-dimensional ultrasound centered on a smaller, but similar, density seen in the right sulcus, in the same anatomic location as the "mass" seen in the left frontoparietal region. The axial view best demonstrates the similar bilateral locations and the gyri and sulci features are best seen in the axial reconstruction.

Congenital malformations of the neonatal brain can be imaged adequately by 2D ultrasound[2,3,7,18–22]; however, we feel that better diagnosis may be achieved with 3D neurosonography. Because of the multiplanar capability of 3D ultrasound, it is possible to establish the relationships of the enlarged ventricles and to determine with certainty the presence or absence of the corpus callosum, the interhemisphere fissure, and the vermis of the cerebellum. By using the center point of rotation and moving it to an area of interest in the 3D volume data set, it is possible to refer to these anatomic structures in all three orthogonal planes with a high degree of accuracy that is not possible with conventional 2D neurosonography imaging.

The images in Figures 14–16 and 14–17 illustrate how the 3D technique helps the sonologist to better understand the relationships of the midline brain anatomy in a newborn with agenesis of the corpus callosum and ventriculomegaly. Absence of the corpus callosum is easily appreciated in the coronal and sagital views. The normal corpus callosum is not seen on either the coronal or sagital projections and the third ventricle is elevated to the position the cavum septi pellucidi normally occupies. We know it is the third ventricle because it communicates with the lateral ventricles (Fig. 14–17) and the massa intermedia lies within it (Figs. 14–16 and 14–17). The anatomy of the third ventricle is much easier to understand when it can be related to corresponding locations seen in all three (coronal, sagital, and axial) views. Initially, the center point of rotation is placed in the back of the third ventricle, posterior to the massa intermedia (Fig. 14–16). Next, the center point is placed in front of the massa intermedia and the open foramina between the third and lateral ventricles is seen in the coronal view bilaterally (Fig. 14–17).

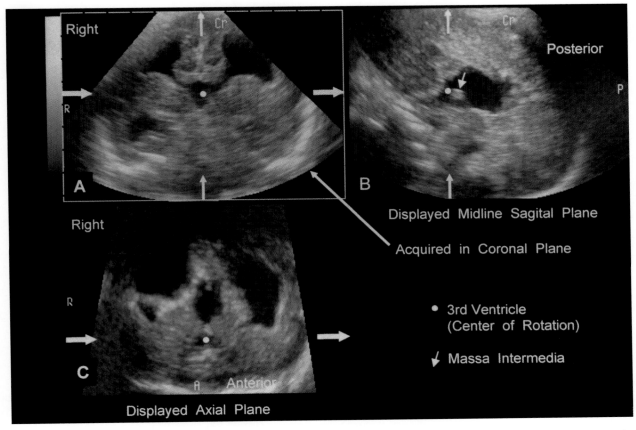

Figure 14–16. This orthogonal image set shows sonographic features of agenesis of the corpus callosum and ventriculomegaly. The anatomy of the third ventricle in axial **(C)** views and coronal **(A)** views is much easier to comprehend when it can be related to corresponding locations seen in sagital views. Initially, the point of rotation *(white marker dot)* is placed in the third ventricle at the level of the interventriclar foramina (Monroe), just anterior to the massa intermedia. The open foramen between the lateral ventricle and the third ventricle is well seen in **(A)**. The interhemisphere fissure is seen above the center point **(A)**, but the normal corpus callosum is absent in the axial **(A)** and sagital **(B)** views. (Compare with Fig. 14–1).

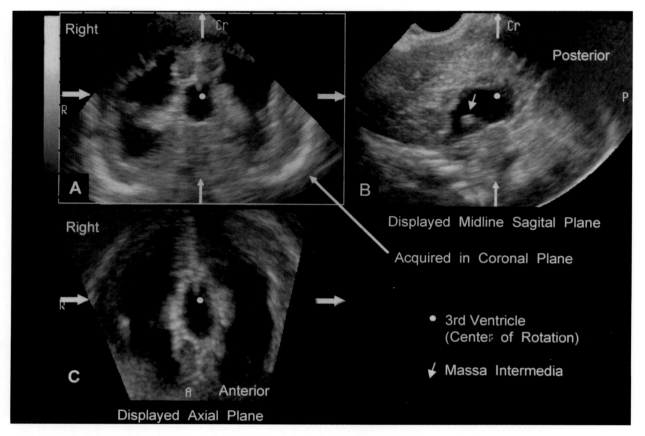

Figure 14–17. From the same orthogonal image set, the location of the back of the third ventricle *(white marker dot)* is identified in all three planes by moving the center point of rotation on the sagittal image to the back of the third ventricle. The massa intermedia *(arrow)* is seen and absence of the corpus callosum is apparent on the coronal and sagital views.

SUMMARY

In this chapter, we have presented a new scanning modality of the neonatal brain using a stored volume data set obtained with the Medison Voluson 530 System. This volume set is obtained and then used to recreate any desired plane with its two additional orthogonal axes. Scrolling and "navigating" within the volume and using the center point of rotation (marker dot) for orientation and localization of structures presents real advantages over the 2D scans.

3D technique can provide a shorter acquisition time and can improve understanding of the pathology through better depiction of the three-dimensional relationships among structures. Diagnostic accuracy has been shown to improve also, since the complete data set is available for the sonologist's review, rather than a limited set of images obtained by the sonographer.[8,9]

The major diagnostic advantage of 3D volume imaging is the ability to view three orthogonal im-

age planes centered at any selected anatomic location. This 3D relationship can be approximated in conventional 2D imaging only by careful, conscious localization of the sagital and coronal planes at the selected sites of pathology (or interest) during real-time scanning. Even though every imaging specialist is able to mentally recreate "swept" 2D images, the viewing in the axial plane relationships is not possible with conventional 2D technique. Furthermore, the conventional 2D image set is a composition of selected representative frozen images that may not necessarily depict the pathology accurately, especially if the pathology was not recognized at the time of the examination. It is true that videotaping the 2D examination potentially can fill the information gap, however, video tape review is time consuming and still-frame image documentation from video tape requires specialized video equipment. Using the 3D imaging system, it is easy to send images from the workstation to the digital storage system or to a printer as the examination is interpreted. Each recorded image set can include the orthogonal three-view orientation image, which shows the relationship of the chosen image planes. Selected enlarged images of any one of the multiplanar slices can also be obtained. In addition, the acquisition of the data is faster and the time involvement of the neonate and the sonographer or sonologist is less with 3D ultrasound compared to the conventional 2D technique. We believe this new and exciting technique will become the primary imaging tool in the neonatal brain.

REFERENCES

1. Johnson ML, Mack LA, Rumack CM, et al. B-mode echoencephalography in the normal and high risk infant. *AJR*. 1979;133:375–381.
2. Johnson ML, Rumack CM. Ultrasonic evaluation of the neonatal brain. *Radiol Clin North Am*. 1980;18: 117–131.
3. Rumack CM, Johnson ML. *Perinatal and Infant Brain Imaging: Role of Ultrasound and Computed Tomography*. Chicago: Year Book Medical Publishers, 1984.
4. Rumack CM, Wilson S, Charboneau JW. Neonatal and infant brain imaging. In *Diagnostic Ultrasound,* 2nd ed. St. Louis: Mosby-Year Book, 1998;1443–1502.
5. Babcock DS. Sonography of the brain in infants: Role in evaluating neurologic abnormalities. *AJR*. 1995; 165:417–423.
6. Cohen HL, Haller JO. Advances in perinatal neurosonography. *AJR*. 1994;163:801–810.
7. Rumack CM, Johnson ML. Neonatal brain ultrasonography. In: Sarti DA, ed. *Diagnostic Ultrasound: Text and Cases,* 2nd ed. Chicago: Year Book Medical Publishers; 1987;1200–1241.
8. Manco-Johnson, ML, Thieme G. Three-Dimensional Ultrasound of the Neonatal Brain. Paper presented at the *Second World Congress on Three-Dimensional Ultrasound*. Las Vegas, October 15, 1999.
9. Thieme G, Manco-Johnson ML, Cioffi-Ragan D. Technique and accuracy of 3D US in Neonatal Neurosonography. Submitted for publication.
10. Taylor GA. New concepts in the pathogenesis of germinal matrix intraparenchymal hemorrhage in premature infants. *AJNR*. 1997;18:231–232.
11. Rumack CM, Manco-Johnson ML, Manco-Johnson MJ, et al. Timing and course of neonatal intracranial hemorrhage using real-time ultrasound. *Radiology*. 1985;154:101.
12. Boal DK, Watterberg KL, Miles S, and Gifford KL et al. Optimal cost effective timing of cranial ultrasound in low birthweight infants. *Pediatr Radiol*. 1995;25: 425–428.
13. Carson SC, Hertzberg BS, Bowie JD, Burger PC. Value of sonography in diagnosis of intracranial hemorrhage and periventricular leukomalacia: A postmortem study of 35 cases. *AJR*. 1990;155:595–601.
14. Barr LL, McCullough PJ, Ball WS, et al. Quanitative sonographic feature analysis of clinical infant hypoxia: A pilot study. *AJR*. 1996;17:1025–1031.
15. Kirks DR, Bowie JD. Cranial ultrasonography of neonatal periventricular/intraventricular hemorrhage: Who, why and when? *Pediatr Radiol*. 1986;16: 114.
16. Grant EG, Schellinger D, Smith Y, et al. Periventricular leukomalacia in combination with intraventricular hemorrhage: Sonographic features and sequelae. *AJNR*. 1986;7:443.
17. Barkovich AJ, Sargent SK. Profound hypoxia in the premature infant: Imaging findings. *AJNR*. 1995;16: 1837–1846.
18. DeMeyer W.: Classification of cerebral malformations. *Birth Defects* 1971;7:78–93.
19. Babcock DS. The normal, absent and abnormal corpus callosum: Sonographic findings. *Radiology*. 1984;151: 450–453.
20. Kier EL, Truwit CL. The normal and abnormal genu of corpus callosum. *AJNR*. 1996;17:1631–1641.
21. Atlas SW, Shkolnik A, Naidich TP. Sonographic recognition of agenesis of the corpus callosum. *AJR*. 1985; 145:167–173.
22. Volpe JJ. Normal and abnormal human brain development. *Clin Perinatol*. 1977;4:3–30.

CHAPTER FIFTEEN

Neurobehavioral Development of the Fetal Brain

Jan G. Nijhuis
Ilse J.M. Nijhuis

Although the anatomy of the fetal brain can reasonably be visualized by ultrasonography and the development of the fetal brain is fairly well understood, not much is known about the functional development of the fetal central nervous system (CNS). The fetal CNS can be regarded as a "black box" that is very difficult to open; in other words, the fetal CNS is rather inaccessible (Fig. 15–1). Because of this inaccessibility of the fetal CNS, it is only possible to measure the output of the CNS, i.e. "fetal behavior." The need to know something about the quality and the activity of the CNS is not only of interest for researchers. In contrast, many times a day an obstetrician is dealing with fetal surveillance and questions about the fetal "condition," which is in fact a question about the quality and the activity of the fetal CNS.

Fetal behavior can be defined as the total of fetal activities as observed or recorded with ultrasonographic equipment. As the fetus has a diurnal rhythm and many activities depend on relation to meals or medication, the study of fetal behavior should be standardized as much as possible. Furthermore, an objective analysis with strict application of techniques[2–5] and the use of valid reference ranges appropriate for the gestation duration are essential. Without them, comparisons with former or future measurements or between groups of patients and studies cannot be made.

In this chapter we discuss several aspects of fetal behavior during the whole of gestation. In the first 20 weeks or so, the fetus can be observed with one ultrasound transducer. In the second half of pregnancy, two scanners are needed to observe the whole fetus, while simultaneously the fetal heart rate pattern (FHRP) can be recorded cardio-tocography. The major problem with the study of fetal behavior is that it is very time consuming. However, the study of fetal behavior is the only possibility to open somewhat the black box, and this is needed when we want to get more insight in the neurodevelopmental pathways of the fetal CNS. Only if normal behavior is completely understood, is it possible to recognize and to understand abnormal behavior before birth. When we have reached that stage, it will perhaps be possible to get more insight in the origin of mental handicaps, which is still a *huge* problem in modern perinatology. This thought by itself is not new; In 1897, Freud postulated that "difficult birth in itself in certain cases is merely a symptom of deeper effects that influenced the development of the fetus."[6]

THE FIRST TRIMESTER

Fetal heart motion is in fact the first activity that can be observed using transvaginal ultrasound. Heart activity can already be observed at a gestational age (menstrual age) of 5 weeks and 5 days. The initial rate of 100 beats per minute (bpm) increases to a mean rate of 167 bpm at 9 weeks, which will then be followed by a gradual decrease (to 156 bpm at 10 to 12 weeks[7] and to a range of 110 to 150 bpm near term). At about 7 to 8 weeks of gestation, one can observe the first "vermicular" movements of

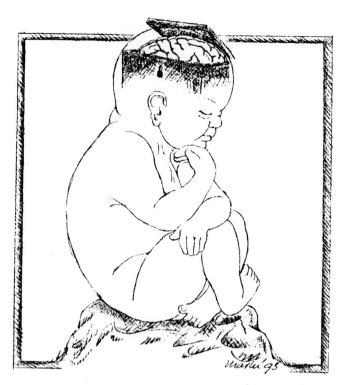

Figure 15–1. Caricature that emphasizes that the fetal central nervous system is, in fact, a "black box" that is very difficult to open.

TABLE 15–1. LIST OF SEVERAL FETAL MOVEMENTS AND THEIR FIRST OCCURRENCE

Fetal Movement	First Occurrence (Postmenstrual Weeks)
Just discernible movement	7–8 weeks
Startle	8–9 weeks
General movement	8–9 weeks
Isolated arm movement	9–10 weeks
Isolated leg movement	9–10 weeks
Head retroflexion	9–10 weeks
Head rotation	10–11 weeks
Hand–face contact	10–11 weeks
Breathing movement	10–11 weeks
Jaw opening	11–12 weeks
Stretch	11–12 weeks
Head anteflexion	12–13 weeks
Yawn	12–13 weeks
Sucking and swallowing	12–13 weeks
Eye movements[27]	16–17 weeks

Adapted from DeVries[15].

the fetus, which will then rapidly be followed by many other movements. De Vries and coworkers described the developmental pathway of fetal movements in a longitudinal study of 12 fetuses of healthy nulliparous women. They reported not only how to describe a particular movement, but also how these movements were performed in terms of speed and amplitude.[9,10] Their classification was based on movements that had been noted previously in low-risk preterm and fullterm infants.[11,12] The first occurrence of the movements described by De Vries and colleagues are summarized in Table 15–1. Their observations were performed using transabdominal ultrasonography, and it is entirely possible that—with the better resolution of transvaginal ultrasonography—some of these movements will already be present at a somewhat younger age. In 1982, De Vries and colleagues also emphasized that most movement patterns vary in amplitude, speed, and force.[9] The character of the movements is not jerky, but rather coordinated and graceful. Of course, startles, hiccups, twitches, and cloni are, more or less by definition, rather jerky. It is not only important how a movement is performed, it is perhaps even more important to know how long fetal activity can be absent. With increasing gestational age, the fetus becomes more capable of demonstrating longer periods

with complete absence of movements. In 1985[13] and 1989,[14] De Vries and coworkers showed that the fetus is continually active during 24 hours and that the fetus does not exhibit long periods of quiescence. The longest period of quiescence varies from about 12 minutes at 8 postmenstrual weeks to 5 to 6 minutes at 17 postmenstrual weeks.[15] We have already postulated that fetal motility can be seen as an expression of the quality of the central nervous system. However, Visser and colleagues, in a study on anencephalic fetuses, demonstrated that in early life normal fetal movements can be present with only few motor neurones present. The quality of the observed movements however, differed dramatically as compared to controls.[16] Similarly, in a case with Fanconi anaemia, De Vries, Laurini, and Visser[17] described qualitatively abnormal fetal motor behavior when the mother reported excessive fetal kicking at 15 weeks of gestation. Postmortem examination after termination at 22 weeks showed a spongy myelinopathy of the CNS. This illustrates what has already been emphasized earlier: for the integrity of the CNS, quality of movements may be of much greater importance than quantity.

THE SECOND TRIMESTER

Only a few studies are available on fetal movement patterns during the second trimester. De Vries and colleagues[13,18] published data up to 22 postmenstrual weeks[19,20]; that studied fetal movements, respectively, from 20 and from 24 postmenstrual weeks onward. During the second trimester of pregnancy, the incidence of body movements gradually decreases and breathing movements increase considerably. The periods of quiescence become longer and eye movements are now clearly visible. The incidence of hiccups, startles, and stretches decreases whereas other movement patterns (jaw movements, hand–face contacts, head movements) show no clear developmental changes.[21] The incidence of movements may vary considerably. At 28 postmenstrual weeks, Roodenburg and associates[19] presented the following ranges and median values based on 1-hour observations: jaw movements 60 to 460, median 300; hand–face contact 30 to 190, median 95; head rotations 20 to 125, median 37; head retroflexions 4 to 29, median 12.

Also the development of rest–activity cycles can be seen, but clear behavioral states are not yet present.[22–24] This can be concluded from studies that show an increased percentage of "association of state variables."[22–25] This means that if one variable is in the "off" condition, the other variable is much more likely to be in the "off" condition than in the "on" condition (e.g. if eye movements are absent, body movements are much more likely to be absent than present). From a developmental point of view, one could say that in the second trimester the development goes on, but there are no new movements that appear for the first time.

THE THIRD TRIMESTER

In the third trimester, the recording of the fetal heart rate pattern (FHRP) becomes increasingly important. Together with the ultrasonographic observations of body movements and eye movements,[26,27] fetal behavior can be readily described. The association of these movements—as already mentioned in

the previous section—increases steadily and in the last weeks of pregnancy, fetal behavior can almost completely be described in terms of behavioral state, [i.e., "constellations of physiological and behavioral variables (e.g., no eye movements, silent heart rate pattern, and absence of body movements) which are stable over time and recur repeatedly, not only in the same infant, but also in similar forms in all infants."][28] The concept of behavioral states has been used as a descriptive categorization of behavior, and also as an explanatory concept in which states are considered to reflect particular modes of nervous activity that modify the responsiveness of the infant.[28] After laying the "groundwork" for the electronic recording of the different physiologic variables to be able to determine fetal behavioral states[29–31]; Timor-Tritsch et al reported in 1978 for the first time on successfully identifying "quiet" and "active" fetal sleep states.[32,33] Fetal movement, breathing, and heart rate pattern (accelerations of the fetal heart rate) were used to determine these behavioral states. At that time one of the most important state determinants, fetal eye movements, was not yet available. The development of ultrasonography, after 1977, made the addition of this variable possible. In 1982, Nijhuis and colleagues[34] were the first to present the definitions of these fetal behavioral states. The definitions were based on the concept of behavioral states in the neonate, but some other criteria had to be used because of the differences between the fetus and the neonate. For example, regularity of breathing can be used as a state criterion in the neonate. This is not the case in the human fetus, because breathing is not continuously present. Because regularity of breathing is state dependant, it can be used as a "state concomitant."[35] With great similarity to Prechtl and coworkers' neonatal states 1 through 4,[28] four fetal behavioral states, 1F through 4F, could be defined (Table 15–2).[36]

TABLE 15–2. COMPARISON OF NEONATAL STATES 1 THROUGH 4 AND FETAL BEHAVIORAL STATES 1F THROUGH 4F

State	Eyes	Body Movements	FHRP[a]	Breathing
1	Eyes closed	Isolated	Not defined	Regular
1F	No eye movements	Isolated	A (see *Figure 15–2*)	Regular (if present)
2	Eyes open	Frequent	Not defined	Irregular
2F	Frequent eye movements	Frequent	B (see *Figure 15–2*)	Irregular (if present)
3	Eyes open	Absent	Not defined	Regular
3F	Frequent eye movements	Absent	C (see *Figure 15–2*)	Not defined
4	Eyes open	Vigorous	Not defined	Irregular
4F	Frequent eye movements	Vigorous	D (see *Figure 15–2*)	Irregular (if present)
5	Vocalization	—	—	—

[a]In the fetus the fetal heart rate pattern (FHRP) is used in combination with presence or absence of body and eye movements and breathing is not a state criterion. In the neonate, *eyes open* or closed is used as a state criterion, in combination with the presence or absence of body movements and the regularity of fetal breathing. A fetal state comparable with state 5 in the neonate (vocalization) has not yet been described.

- **State 1F** (similar to state 1 or "non-REM-sleep" in the neonate): quiescence, which can be regularly interrupted by brief gross body movements, mostly startles. Eye movements are absent. Fetal heart rate pattern (FHRP) A is a stable pattern, with a small oscillation bandwidth and no accelerations, except in combination with a startle.
- **State 2F** (similar to state 2 or "REM-sleep" in the neonate): frequent and periodic gross body movements—mainly stretches and retroflexions—and movements of the extremities. Eye movements are present. FHRP B has a wider oscillation bandwidth and frequent accelerations during movements.
- **State 3F** (similar to state 3 or "quiet wakefulness" in the neonate): gross body movements absent. Eye movements present. FHRP C is stable but with a wider oscillation bandwidth than FHRP A and no accelerations.
- **State 4F** (similar to state 4 or "active wakefulness" in the neonate): vigorous, continual activity including many trunk rotations. Eye movements are present. FHRP D is unstable, with large and long-lasting accelerations, often fused into a sustained tachycardia.

The definitions of both the fetal and neonatal state are summarized and compared in Table 15–2. Figure 15–2 shows examples of FHRP A through D. Behavioral state 3F (quiet wakefulness) occurs less than 5% of the recording time. Because of its low incidence, Pillai and James[37] questioned if this state really existed. In the postmature fetus however, a significant increase of the presence of this state up to 9% has been reported[38] so this may again be an age-related phenomenon.

It is important to emphasize that the existence of states can only be excepted if three requirements are satisfied.

1. A specific combination of variables occurs (e.g. absence of eye movements, absence of body movements and a silent heart rate pattern),
2. Which is stable over time (by definition at least 3 minutes), and
3. If clear state transitions can be recognized in between.

These state transitions should be 3 minutes or shorter.[34]

Of course, the concept of behavioral states allows further insight in the activity of the central nervous system. Examples have been shown in which the association develops somewhat later, e.g., in nulliparous women,[39] in intrauterine growth-retarded human fetuses,[40–42] and also in type-1-diabetic women.[43,44] Van de Pas et al[32] showed that the development of behavioral states continues after 41 weeks of gestation, with an increasing percentage of states 3F and 4F.

The administration of medication to the mother can have an effect on fetal behavior as is shown, for example, by antiepileptic drugs[45] and corticosteroids.[46,47] Abnormal fetal behavior has been described in fetuses of cocaine addicted mothers[48] and in a fetus exposed to maternal alcohol abuse,[49] while temporary changes are found in fetuses whose mothers drank two glasses of white wine.[50] Fetal gender might also be of importance as has been suggested in recent literature.[20,51–53]

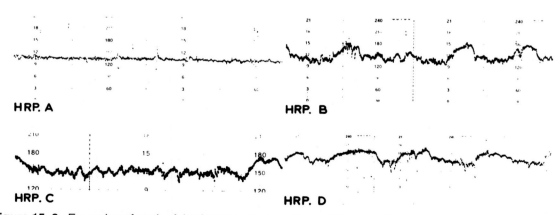

Figure 15–2. Examples of each of the fetal heart rate patterns A through D at a recording speed of 3 cm/min.

TOWARD INTRAUTERINE NEUROLOGIC EXAMINATION

In 1988, Nelson and Ellenberg[54] published data from an extensive NIH-study in which they showed that prepregnancy factors contributed to 13% of the cases of cerebral palsy and pregnancy factors contributed to 34%. This enormous study has never been repeated, but in 1989 Hagberg and Hagberg[55] showed that in Sweden, the incidence of cerebral palsy had not changed during the past years, despite improving obstetric and neonatal care. These types of studies make it very clear that it is absolutely worthwhile to look for possibilities to perform an intrauterine neurologic examination in fetuses at risk for cerebral palsy. But what tools do we have?

Follow-up of One Variable

It is clear that the follow-up of the presence of just one variable (e.g., the presence of body movements) is insufficient. Up to now, the study of fetal behavior has not yet shown that the sensitivity of this study is very promising. Except of course, in extreme cases. Nijhuis and coworkers[56] published a review of cases with fetal brain death in utero which were characterized by an absolutely silent heart rate pattern with a somewhat elevated base line and without decelerations. On the basis of absence of decelerations, hypoxia can be excluded, which may lead to prevention of unnecessary interventions. Furthermore, Tas and Nijhuis[57] published a case with a silent heart rate pattern and the presence of fetal movements, and a case of a reactive heart rate pattern with absence of movements. Clearly, in such cases, a behavioral study will lead to the suspicion of a brain damaged child whereas nothing could have been concluded on the basis of the recording of an isolated variable alone.

The Study of Transitions and Insertions

Arduini and associates were among the first to draw attention to the possibility of studying transitions.[42] It could be the case that a fetus exhibits rather normal states, but that the transitions are abnormal with respect to the sequence of change of variables or with respect to the duration of the transition. Moreover, there might be long periods of no coincidence bounded on both sides by the same behavioral state. These periods have been called insertions.[58,59]

Neurologic Reflexes In Utero

Tas et al showed in 1990[60] and 1993[61] that, from 24 weeks of pregnancy, an intercostal-to-phrenic inhibitory reflex can be elicited in the human fetus. If the examiner compresses the lateral thoracic wall of the fetus during breathing, breathing will stop over a mean period of 13.9 seconds (range 4 to 37) in 1F and 18.3 seconds (range 4 to 48) in 2F. They expected that the absence of breathing would be prolonged in a possible compromised fetus, but they could not demonstrate a significant prolongation in intrauterine growth retarded fetuses.[61]

Fetal Stimulation

The fetus can easily be stimulated. The observation of a startle response to a vibroacoustic stimulus (VAS) has not yet been proven to be the final solution.[62] It has, however, become clear that stimulation should be done under standardized conditions and the behavioral state must be taken into account. As an example, Groome and coworkers[63] tested 96 normal human fetuses between 37 and 41 weeks using a VAS and concluded that the response depended on the prestimulus duration of state 1F. Zimmer and associates[64] showed not only that the fetus responds to speech stimuli, but also that this response is state-dependant.

Fetal Consistency

A remarkable within-subject consistency was found in the fetal behavioral states of fetuses monitored on 3 separate days.[65] Furthermore, the intrafetal differences in fetal heart rate are less than the interfetal differences. The heart rate of the individual fetus is on average 19% to 55% of the total variability between fetuses.[4] This intrafetal consistency is also present in growth-retarded fetuses.[23] For monitoring of trends and/or the detection of small changes, each fetus should be its own control using recordings of standardized duration and appropriate reference ranges.[4]

Quality of Motility

De Vries and coworkers[9] have already emphasized this aspect in the first trimester, but not much attention has been paid to the possibilities in the second half of pregnancy. It could well be the case that, as in the neonate, disturbances of quality are much more important than changes in quantity. It will, however, be rather difficult to create a reliable and reproducable technique.

SUMMARY

In this chapter, we have not really discussed or emphasized the consequences of aspects of fetal behavioral phenomena for fetal monitoring (for overviews, see ref. 30), but rather, looked into the possibilities of getting more insight into the functional neurodevelopment of the human fetal CNS. The study of fetal behavior, behavior-related phenomena, and fetal reflexes has given us a great deal of insight into the developmental pathway of the fetal CNS and the possibilities to create an intrauterine neurologic investigation. In extreme cases, it is clear that dissociation of variables (e.g., a reactive heart rate pattern with absence of body movements) is indicative of a neurologic disturbance. However, it is not yet clear how we might recognize the fetuses with more distinct cerebral damage. For the future, it is crucial that an examiner be aware of normal fetal behavior over the whole duration of gestation and familiar with the background theory behind behavioral observations. Furthermore, it is necessary to be familiar with aspects of neonatal developmental neurology as the neonate is much easier to study and the fetus seems to very comparable with the neonate. Whether we will be able to develop an intrauterine neurologic examination that is sensitive enough to predict which fetus is really at risk and which fetus is not remains to be seen. Finally, as a future perspective, one wishes to reduce and to prevent cerebral handicaps and to reach that goal, we still have a long way to go.

REFERENCES

1. Swaab DF, Honnebier MBOM, Mirmiran M. Development of the central nervous system. In: Nijhuis JG, ed. *Fetal Behaviour, Developmental and Perinatal aspects.* Oxford: Oxford University Press; 1992:75–91.
2. Nijhuis IJM, ten Hof J, Nijhuis JG, et al. Temporal organization of fetal behavior from 24 weeks gestation onwards in normal and complicated pregnancies. *Dev Psychobiol.* 1999;34:257–268.
3. ten Hof J, Nijhuis IJM, Mulder EJH, et al. Quantitative analysis of fetal generalized movements: Methodological considerations. *Early Hum Dev.* 1999;56:57–73.
4. Nijhuis IJM, ten Hof J, Mulder EJH, et al. Numerical fetal heart rate analysis: Nomograms, minimal duration of recording and intrafetal consistency. *Prenat Neonat Med.* 1998;3:314–322.
5. ten Hof J, Nijhuis IJM, Mulder EJH, et al. Sex differences in fetal body movements. Submitted.
6. Freud S. Die infantile Cerebrallämung. In: Nothnagel H, ed. *Specielle Pathologie und Therapie.* Vienna: Holder; 1987:1–327.
7. Heeswijk M van, Nijhuis JG, Hollanders HMG. Fetal heart rate in early pregnancy. *Early Hum Dev.* 1990;22:151–156.
8. Rooth G, Huch A, Huch R. Guidelines for the use of fetal monitoring. *Int J Gynecol Obstet.* 1987;25:159–167.
9. Vries JIP de, Visser GHA, Prechtl HFR. The emergence of fetal behavior. I. Qualitative aspects. *Early Hum Dev.* 1982;7:301–322.
10. Vries JIP de, Visser GHA, Prechtl HFR. The emergence of fetal behavior. III. Individual differences and consistencies. *Early Hum Dev.* 1988;16:85.
11. Prechtl HFR. The neurological examination of the full-term newborn infant, 2nd ed. *Clin Dev Med.* London: Heinemann; 1977:168.
12. Prechtl HFR, Fargel JW. Posture, motility and respiration in low-risk preterm infants. *Dev Med Child Neurol.* 1979;21:3–27.
13. Vries JIP de, Visser GHA, Prechtl HFR. The emergence of fetal behavior. II. Quantitative aspects. *Early Hum Dev.* 1985;12:99.
14. de Vries et al., 1989
15. Vries JIP de. The first trimester. In Nijhuis JG, ed. *Fetal Behaviour, Developmental and Perinatal Aspects.* Oxford: Oxford University Press; 1992:3–17.
16. Visser GHA, Laurini RN, de Vries JIP, Bekedam DJ, and Prechtl HFR. Abnormal motor behavior in anencephalic fetuses. *Early Hum Dev.* 1985;12:173–182.
17. Vries JIP de, Laurini RN, Visser GHA. Abnormal motor behavior and developmental postmortem findings in a fetus with Fanconi anaemia. *Early Hum Dev.* 1994;36:137–142.
18. Vries JIP de, Visser GHA, Mulder EJH, Prechtl HFR. Diurnal and other variations in fetal movement, and heart rate patterns at 20–22 weeks. *Early Hum Dev.* 1987;15:333–348.
19. Roodenburg PJ, Wladimiroff JW, van Es A, Prechtl HFR. Classification, and quantitative aspects of fetal movements during the second half of normal pregnancy. *Early Hum Dev.* 1991;25:19–36.
20. ten Hof J, Nijhuis IJM, Mulder EJH, et al. A longitudinal study of fetal body movements: Nomograms, intrafetal consistency and relationship with the rest–activity cycle. Submitted.
21. Visser GHA. The second trimester. In Nijhuis JG, ed. *Fetal Behaviour, Developmental and Perinatal Aspects.* Oxford; Oxford University Press; 1992:17–26.
22. Drogtrop AP, Ubels R, Nijhuis, JG. The association between fetal body movements, eye movements, and heart rate patterns between 25 and 30 weeks of gestation. *Early Hum Dev.* 1990;23:67–73.
23. Nijhuis IJM, ten Hof J, Mulder EJH, et al. Fetal heart rate in relation to its variation in normal and growth retarded fetuses. *Eur J Obstet Gyneco Reprod Bio.* 2000;89:27–33.
24. Visser GHA, Poelman-Weesjes G, Cohen TMN, Bekedam DJ. Fetal behavior at 30 to 32 weeks of gestation. *Pediat Res.* 1987;22:655–658.
25. Nijhuis JG, Pas M van de. Behavioral states and their ontogeny: Human studies. *Semin Perinatol* 1992;16:206–210.
26. Bots RSGM, Nijhuis, JG, Martin Jr. CB, Prechtl HFR. Human fetal eye movements: Detection in utero by ultrasonography. *Early Hum Dev.* 1981;5:87–94.
27. Birnholz JC. The development of human fetal eye movement patterns. *Science.* 1981;213:679–681.

28. Prechtl HFR, Weinmann HM, Akiyama Y. Organization of physiological parameters in normal and neurologically abnormal infants. *Neuropädiatrie.* 1969;1:101–129.

28a. Prechtl HFR. The behavioral states of the newborn (a review). *Brain Res.* 1974;76:185–212.

28b Swartjes JM, Van Geijn HP, Mantel R, Van Woerden EE, Schoemaker HC. Coincidence of behavioural state parameters in the human fetus at three gestational ages. *Early Hum Dev.* 1990;23:75–83.

29. Timor-Tritsch I, Zador I, Hertz RH, and Rosen MG. Classification of human fetal movement. *Am J Obstet Gynecol.* 1976;126:70–79.

30. Timor-Tritsch I, Zador I, Hertz RH, and Rosen MG. Human fetal respiratory arrhythmia. *Am J Obstet Gynecol.* 1977;127:622–666.

31. Timor-Tritsch IE, Dierker LJ, Zador I, and Rosen MG. Fetal movements associated with fetal heart rate accelerations and decelerations. *Am J Obstet Gynecol,* 1978;131:276–281.

32. Timor-Tritsch IE, Dierker LJ, Hertz RH, et al. Studies of antepartum behavioral state in the human fetus at term. *Am J Obstet Gynecol.* 1978;132:524–531.

33. Rosen MG, Dierker LJ, Hertz RH, and Timor-Tritsch IE. Fetal behavioral states and fetal evaluation. *Clinical Obstet Gynecol.* 1979;22:605–611.

34. Nijhuis JG, Bots RSGM, Martin Jr. CB Prechtl HFR. Are there behavioral states in the human fetus? *Early Hum Dev.* 1982;6:177–195.

35. Nijhuis JG, Martin Jr. CB, Gommers S, Bouws P, Bots RSGM, Jongsma HW. The rhythmicity of fetal breathing varies with behavioural state in the human fetus. *Early Hum Dev.* 1983;9:1–7.

36. Nijhuis JG, ed. Fetal Behaviour, Developmental and Perinatal Aspects. Oxford: Oxford University Press, 1992.

37. Pillai M James D. Are the behavioral states of the newborn comparable to those of the fetus? *Early Hum Dev.* 1990;22:39–49.

38. Pas M van de, Nijhuis JG, Jongsma HW. Fetal behavior in uncomplicated pregnancies after 41 weeks of gestation. *Early Hum Dev.* 1994;40:29–38.

39. Vliet MAT van, Martin Jr. CB, Nijhuis JG, Prechtl HFR. Behavioral states in the fetuses of nulliparous women. *Early Hum Dev.* 1985;12:21–37.

40. Vliet MAT van, Martin Jr CB, Nijhuis JG, et al. The relationship between fetal activity, and behavioral states and fetal breathing movements in normal and growth-retarded fetuses. *Am J Obstet Gynecol.* 1985; 153:582–588.

41. Bekedam DJ, Visser GHA, De Vries JJ, Prechtl HFR. Motor behavior in the growth-retarded fetus. *Early Hum Dev.* 1985;12:155–165.

42. Arduini D, Rizzo G, Caforio L, Romanini C, Mancuso S. Behavioral state transitions in healthy and growth retarded fetuses. *Early Hum Dev.* 1989;19:155–165.

43. Mulder EJH, Visser GHA, Bekedam DJ, and Prechtl HFR. Emergence of behavioral states in fetuses of type-1-diabetic women. *Early Hum Dev.* 1987;15:231–251.

44. Mulder EJH. Diabetic pregnancy. In Nijhuis JG, ed.: *Fetal Behaviour, Developmental and Perinatal Aspects.* Oxford: Oxford University Press; 1992:193–208.

45. van Geijn HP, Swartjes JM, van Woerden EE, Caron FJ, Brons JT, Arts NF. Fetal behavioural states in epileptic pregnancies. *Eur J Obstet Gynecol Reprod Biol.* 1986;21:309–313.

46. Derks JB, Mulder EJH, Visser GHA. The effects of maternal betamethasone administration on the fetus. *Br J Obstet Gynecol.* 1995;102:40–46.

47. Mulder EJH, Derks JB, Visser GHA. Antenatal corticosteroid therapy and fetal behaviour: A randomised study of the effects of betamethasone and dexamethasone. *Br J Obstet Gynecol.* 1997;104:1239–1247.

48. Hume RF, O'Donnell KJ, Stanger CL, Killam AP, Gingras JL. In utero cocaine exposure: Observations of fetal behavioral state may predict neonatal outcome. *Am J Obstet Gynecol* 1989;161:685–690.

49. Mulder EJH, Kamstra A, O'Brien MJ, Visser GHA, Prechtl HFR. Abnormal fetal behavioral state regulation in a case of high maternal alcohol intake during pregnancy. *Early Hum Dev.* 1986;14:321–326.

50. Mulder EJH, Morssink LP, van der Schee T, Visser GHA. Acute maternal alcohol consumption disrupts behavioral state organization in the near-term fetus. *Pediatr Res.* 1998;44:774–779.

51. Dawes NW, Dawes GS, Moulden M, Redman CWG. Fetal heart rate patterns in term labor vary with sex, gestational age, epidural analgesia, and fetal weight. *Am J Obstet Gynecol.* 1999;180:181–187.

52. DiPietro JA, Costigan KA, Shupe AK, Pressman EK, Johnson TRB. Fetal neurobehavioral development: Associations with socioeconomic class and fetal sex. *Dev Psychobiol.* 1998;33:79–91.

53. Hepper PG, Shannon EA, Dornan JC. Sex differences in fetal mouth movements. *Lancet.* 1997;350:1820.

54. Nelson KB, Ellenberg JH. Intrapartum events and cerebral palsy. In: Kubli, F, eds. *Prenatal Events and Brain Damage in Surviving Children.* Heidelberg: Springer Verlag; 1988:139–148.

55. Hagberg B, Hagberg G. The changing panorama of infantile hydrocephalus and cerebral palsy over forty years. A Swedish Survey. *Brain Dev.* 1989;11:368–375.

56. Nijhuis JG, Crevels AJ, Dongen PWJ van. Fetal brain death: The definition of a fetal heart rate pattern and its clinical consequences. *Obstet Gynecol Surv.* 1990; 46:229–232.

57. Tas BAPJ, Nijhuis JG. Consequences for fetal monitoring. In: Nijhuis JG, ed. *Fetal Behaviour, Developmental and Perinatal Aspects.* Oxford: Oxford University Press; 1992:258–269.

58. Groome LJ, Bentz LS, Singh KP. Behavioral state organization in normal human term fetuses: The relationship between periods of undefined state and other characteristics of state control. *Sleep* 1995;18:77–81.

59. Groome LJ, Benanti JM, Bentz LS, Singh KP. Morphology of active sleep–quiet sleep transitions in

normal human term fetuses. *J Perinat Med.* 1996;24: 171–176.

60. Tas BAPJ, Nijhuis JG, Lucas AJ, et al. The inter-costals-to-phrenic inhibitory reflex in the human fetus near term. *Early Hum Dev.* 1990;22:145–149.

61. Tas BAPJ, Nijhuis JG, Nelen W, Willems, E. The inter-costals-to-phrenic inhibitory reflex in normal and in-tra-uterine growth-retarded (IUGR) human fetuses from 26–40 weeks of gestation. *Early Hum Dev.* 1993; 32:177–182.

62. Gagnon R. Fetal behaviour in relation to fetal stimu-lation. In Nijhuis JG ed. *Fetal Behaviour, Developmen-tal and Perinatal Aspects.* Oxford: Oxford University Press; 1992:209–226.

63. Groome LJ, Bentz LS, Singh KP, Mooney DM. Behav-ioral state change in normal fetuses following a single vibro-acoustic stimulus: Effect of duration of quiet sleep prior stimulation. *Early Hum Dev.* 1993;33: 21–27.

64 Zimmer EZ, Fifer WP, Kim Y-I, Rey HR, Chao CR, Mey-ers MM. Response of the premature fetus to stimula-tion by speech sounds. *Early Hum Dev.* 1993;33: 207–215.

65. Groome LJ, Singh KP, Bentz LS, Holland SB, Atter-bury JL, Swiber MJ et al. Temporal stability in the distribution of behavioral states for individual human fetuses. *Early Hum Dev.* 1997;48:187–197.

CHAPTER SIXTEEN

The Role of Infection in the Etiology of Cerebral Palsy

Luís F. Gonçalves
Eli Maymon
Bo Hyun Yoon
Roberto Romero

Cerebral palsy (CP) is a complex of symptoms characterized by the aberrant control of movement or posture that appears in early life and can lead to costly life-long disability.[1] It is a neuromuscular condition only and not necessarily associated with mental retardation.[2] The estimated prevalence of CP ranges from 1.5 to 2.5 per 1000 live births.[3,4] Cerebral palsy was initially described in 1862 by William John Little, a London orthopedic surgeon who coined the term "spastic rigidity" to describe a group of motor disabilities associated with difficult deliveries, perinatal asphyxia, and prematurity.[5] This spastic rigidity implies excessive muscular tonus, increased stretch reflexes, and hyperactive tendon reflexes and, therefore, CP is associated with damage to the upper motor neurons.[2]

Approximately 30 percent of the individuals with CP are mentally retarded and 25 percent are unable to walk, even with assistance.[6,7] Epilepsy is present in one third of the cases. A substantial number of those without cognitive impairment have visual-motor or other learning difficulties.[8] In addition to the obvious emotional suffering for the families of affected individuals, the Advisory Council of the National Institute of Neurological Disorder and Stroke has estimated the annual financial cost of CP in the United States to be approximately $5 billion per year.[9]

In recent years, substantial improvement in the survival rates of very-low-birth-weight (VLBW) infants has been associated with an increase in the rates of CP.[4,10,11] Infection plays a major role in the etiology and pathogenesis of preterm labor.[12] The objective of this chapter is to discuss the evidence linking infection to preterm labor and the subsequent development of CP.

CLASSIFICATION

The predominant characteristic of CP, motor dysfunction, is classified as spastic, dyskinetic, or ataxic. The most common form, spastic CP, is associated with cerebral cortex and pyramidal tract injury, and is characterized by persistent hypertonia, rigidity, frequent contractures, and abnormal curvature of the spine. Dyskinetic CP is characterized by impaired voluntary muscle control resulting in bizarre, twisting motions with exaggerated posturing that is more obvious in the distal extremities. This posturing is predominately associated with kernicterus. Ataxic CP is associated with cerebellar damage and results in abnormal muscle coordination, lack of balance, and lack of position sense.

If all four extremities are affected, CP is classified as quadriplegic and is thought to be caused by diffuse damage to the cortex and pyramidal tracts. This type of CP is characteristic of children who are affected at term. In contrast, diplegic CP is the result of periventricular injury and is more likely to affect the lower extremities. This concept is important because prematurity is associated with periventricular leukomalacia (PVL) and children born prematurely typically present with spastic diplegia. When one side of the body is affected, the CP is classified as hemiplegic and thought to result from brain injury to one cerebral hemisphere from localized hemorrhage or infarction and when only one limb is involved, the CP is classified as monoplegic.

RISK FACTORS

Risk factors for CP are classified according to whether they occur before pregnancy or during the perinatal period.[9] Risk factors occurring before pregnancy include a history of previous fetal wastage, long intervals between menses, and an unusually long (more than 3 years) or short (less than 3 months) interval since the previous pregnancy. Perinatal risk factors include: congenital malformations, twin gestation, fetal growth restriction, abnormal fetal presentation, premature separation of the placenta, birth weight less than 2001 grams, and neonatal ischemic/hypoxic encephalopathy.

ETIOLOGY

Although there is an overall impression among the general public and even among health professionals that the main cause for CP is birth asphyxia and/or trauma, these events account for only 8% to 10% of CP cases.[13] The International Cerebral Task Force recently proposed[14] that all three of the following criteria should be met in order to establish a causal relationship between CP and intrapartum hypoxia: (1) the CP should be of the spastic quadriplegic or dyskinetic type; (2) there should be early onset of severe or moderate neonatal encephalopathy in a neonate born at 34 weeks or later; and (3) there should be evidence of metabolic acidosis in intrapartum fetal, umbilical arterial cord, or very early neonatal blood samples (pH < 7.00 and base deficit ≥12 nmol/L).

In addition to asphyxia and trauma, several conditions have been implicated as possible etiologic factors for CP: central nervous system (CNS) malformations, fetal infection, genetic syndromes, hypothyroidism, radiation exposure, exposure to toxins such as mercury or alcohol, abnormal fetal presentation, cerebral hemorrhage, prematurity, kernicterus, vaccination reaction, and vascular thrombosis. Although in the majority of the cases (more than 75%) a precise etiologic factor may not be recognized,[15] the leading identifiable cause of CP is prematurity.[14] The prevalence of CP at age 3 years is 44 per 1000 for infants born at or before 27 weeks, 21 per 1000 for those born between 28 and 30 weeks, and only 0.6 per 1000 for those delivered at term.[16]

Regardless of etiology, CP is the end result of brain injury. Depending on the timing of the insult, different areas of the brain are selectively affected. During the late second trimester, lesions are more likely to affect the cerebral white matter, which is undergoing myelinization. Later in the third trimester, the basal ganglia and other nonpyramidal motor areas appear to be more vulnerable to injury. Potential pathways leading to cell death include increased production of cytokines and nitric oxide, activation of N-methyl-D-aspartate (NMDA) receptors, and calcium influx.

Theoretically, as certain conditions associated with CP are identified and treated, the proportion of the subtypes of CP should change. For example, the availability of effective treatment and preventive measures against hemolytic disease of the newborn has lead to a decrease in the prevalence of kernicterus and choreoathetosis.[17] In contrast, improvements in perinatal care have led to an increase in the survival rates of VLBW infants and a rise in the proportion of spastic diplegia among cases of CP.[4,15] Ozmen and colleagues[18] described 1873 cases of CP evaluated in Turkey between 1982 and 1989. Because survival of VLBW infants was rare at that time in Turkey, most of the cases occurred in term infants and the most common type of CP was spastic quadriplegia.

CEREBRAL PALSY AND INFECTION

Approximately one third of all babies who subsequently have signs of CP, weighed less than 2500 g at birth. For babies who weigh less than 1500 g at birth, the rate of CP is 25 to 31 times higher than infants with normal weights at term. The most common form of CP affecting premature babies is spastic diplegia.[10] Preterm babies that subsequently develop spastic diplegia have a high rate of PVL.[19–28]

There is strong evidence linking brain injury and infant exposure to perinatal infection.[1,29–32] The general view is that an initiator event (either prepregnancy infection or intrauterine infection) leads to maternal and fetal inflammatory responses that, in turn, contribute to undesirable outcomes such as preterm delivery, intraventricular hemorrhage (IVH), white matter damage (WMD), and neurodevelopment disability (mainly CP).[33] The following topics are discussed to delineate the evidence supporting these concepts.

1. A fetal inflammatory response precedes imminent preterm delivery.
2. Periventricular leukomalacia-associated lesions are associated with spontaneous preterm labor.

3. Chorioamnionitis is associated with an increased risk of CP.
4. There is evidence that infection has a causal relationship with WMD.
5. Fetal cytokinemia is associated with IVH, WMD, and CP.
6. Chorionic and umbilical cord vessel inflammation (fetal vasculitis) is associated with an increased risk for IVH and WMD.

Fetal Inflammatory Response Precedes Imminent Preterm Delivery

Amniotic fluid infection occurs in up to 45% of the infants born at 23 to 26 weeks of gestation and 18% of the infants born at 27 to 30 weeks of gestation.[34] Microbial invasion of the amniotic cavity is present in 10% of patients with preterm labor and intact membranes[35–38] and in 30% of patients with preterm premature rupture of membranes.[39–42] Bacterial footprints have been detected in the amniotic fluid of as many as 60% of patients with preterm labor and intact membranes.[43,44]

In the past, maternal fever was thought to be an early marker of amniotic fluid infection. Recent evidence, however, points out that the fetus becomes infected and develops an inflammatory response before the mother manifests clinical signs of infection and that this fetal inflammatory response precedes preterm delivery. It has been demonstrated by using probes against the Y chromosomes that leukocytes in the amniotic fluid of pregnant women with male fetuses in preterm labor are of fetal origin.[45] In the context of intrauterine infection, microorganisms in the amniotic cavity or the maternal compartment are thought to reach the fetus and elicit an inflammatory response characterized by increased biosynthesis of proinflammatory cytokines.[12,42,46] This systemic fetal proinflammatory cytokine response, in turn, is followed by the onset of spontaneous preterm parturition.[47–52] Romero et al[51] demonstrated that in pregnancies complicated by preterm premature rupture of membranes, an elevated IL-6 concentration in fetal plasma obtained by cordocentesis (> 11 pg/mL) is associated with a shorter cordocentesis-to-delivery interval (median 0.8 days [range 0.1 to 5] versus median 6 days [range 0.2 to 33.6]; $P < .05$), and a higher rate of deliveries within 48 and 72 hours of the procedure (88% versus 29% and 88% versus 35%, respectively; $P < .05$). Importantly, in this study pregnancies with elevated amniotic fluid IL-6 (but normal fetal plasma IL-6) concentrations had similar cordocentesis-to-delivery interval when compared to pregnancies with normal amniotic fluid and fetal plasma IL-6 concentrations (median 5 days, range 0.2 to 33.6 days versus median 7 days, range 1.5 to 32 days). In a subsequent study, Gomez and colleagues[52] showed that elevated IL-6 concentration in the fetal plasma was associated with severe neonatal morbidity (respiratory distress syndrome, proved or suspected neonatal sepsis, IVH, PVL, necrotizing enterocolitis, and bronchopulmonary dysplasia) in pregnancies complicated by preterm labor or premature rupture of the membranes.

Periventricular Leukomalacia Lesions Are Associated with Spontaneous Preterm Labor

The term periventricular leukomalacia (PVL) is used to describe foci of coagulation necrosis of the white matter near the lateral ventricles. PVL is more common in infants born at 28 to 31 weeks. It is nine times more common in babies with documented bacteremia.[24] The brain of preterm infants, especially before 32 postmenstrual weeks, is more vulnerable to white matter lesions triggered by infection, endotoxin, and cytokines. Prior to 32 postmenstrual weeks, oligodendrocyte precursors are undergoing the process of myelogenesis. In addition to this group of cells, endothelial cells of blood vessels, especially those in the supracaudate germinal matrix, are also susceptible to injury. The probable mechanism of damage in this case seems to be the increased synthesis of nitric oxide leading to enhanced production of nitric oxide radicals and cell death.[53]

PVL is often detected at the time of neonatal cranial ultrasonography as either hyperechoic (echodense) or hypoechoic (echolucent) lesions in the periventricular region.[24] Hyperechoic lesions appear early and are thought to represent vascular congestion or hemorrhage (Figs. 16–1 and 16–2). They are followed by the appearance of cystic-like structures (Figs. 16–1 and 16–2) days or weeks later. This reflects the removal of necrotic tissue and replacement by fluid.[54,55] For additional images of PVL see Chapter 4 (Figs. 4–71 and 4–73) and Chapter 14 (Figs. 14–11 and 14–12).

Leviton and Paneth[24] reviewed the long-term outcome of children with ultrasound determined echodense and echolucent parenchymal lesions with regard to the subsequent development of CP. In children with neonatal echodense lesions, the prevalence of CP ranged from 40% to 100%. In children with echolucent lesions, the prevalence was even higher, ranging from 62% to 100%.

Verma and coworkers[56] studied 745 neonates with birth weights ranging from 500 to 1750 g divided in three groups: (1) those born after preterm

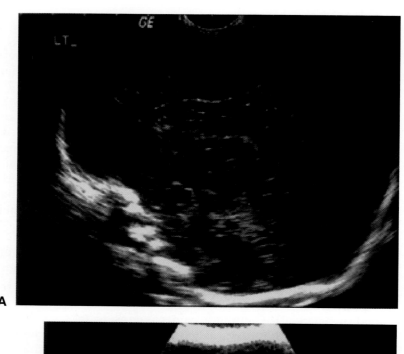

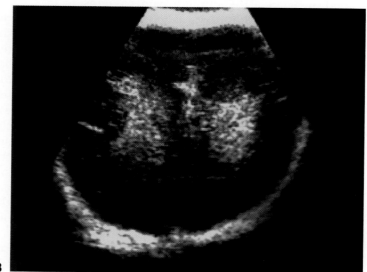

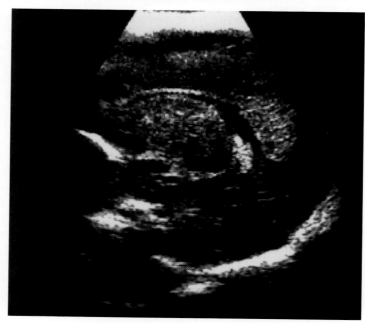

Figure 16–1. Ultrasound images of the fetal brain. **a.** Normal fetal brain, sagittal section. **b.** Coronal view of the fetal brain demonstrating increased periventricular echogenicity. **c.** Sagittal view demonstrating increased periventricular echogenicity.

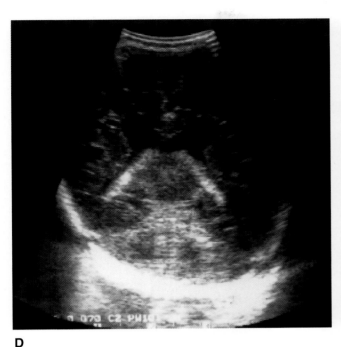
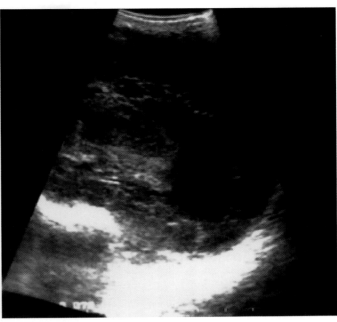

D   **E**

Figure 16–1. continued Ultrasound images of the fetal brain. **d.** Mid-coronal section of the fetal brain with cystic lesions. **e.** Fetal brain, parasagittal section, demonstrating periventricular cystic lesions.

rupture of the membranes (n = 279); (2) infants born after refractory preterm labor with intact membranes (n = 285); and (3) neonates delivered for fetal or maternal indications (n = 181). The incidence of IVH and PVL were significantly higher in babies born after spontaneous preterm labor or premature rupture of the membranes than in those delivered for maternal or fetal indications (group 1 odds ratio 2.29, 95% confidence interval 1.46 to 3.59; group 2 odds ratio 2.97, 95% confidence interval 1.91 to 4.61,). After adjusting for gestational age, birth weight, Apgar scores at 5 minutes, RDS, antenatal steroid usage, and clinical and histologic chorioamnionitis, only the preterm labor group persisted with a significant increase in the odds of abnormal neurosonography (odds ratio 1.89, 95% confidence interval 1.16 to 3.06, P = .01). Clinical chorioamnionitis independently increased the odds of abnormal neurosonography (odds ratio 2.03, 95% confidence interval 1.24 to 3.30, P = .005). In this study, 86.4% (203 of 235) of the fetuses with abnormal neurosonography were born after premature rupture of the membranes or preterm labor. Similar findings were reported by Yoon and colleagues[57] in a study of 172 consecutive preterm births. Among 25 neonates that developed PVL, 21 (84%) were born after the onset of spontaneous preterm labor, either with intact or ruptured membranes.

Chorioamnionitis Is Associated with an Increased Risk of White Matter Damage and Cerebral Palsy

Using data from the Collaborative Perinatal Project, Nelson and Ellenberg,[58] were the first to describe an association between chorioamnionitis and CP. In this study, in low-birth-weight infants, chorioamnionitis increased the risk of CP from 12 per 1000 to 39 per 1000 live births. Similarly, Murphy and associates[29] demonstrated that, in premature infants born before 32 weeks, chorioamnionitis increased the risk of CP from 3% to 17%. Bejar and colleagues[20] found that chorioamnionitis was present in more than half of the preterm infants who developed white matter echolucencies within 3 days after birth. In a cohort of 1228 newborns with birthweight between 500 and 1500 g, Shea and associates[59] found that chorioamnionitis and labor lasting less than 4 hours significantly increased the risk of subsequent development of CP (chorioamnionitis: odds ratio 2.4, 95% confidence interval 1.0 to 5.9; labor lasting more than 4 hours: odds ratio 3.4, 95% confidence interval 1.4 to 7.8). Verma and coworkers[56] reported that clinical chorioamnionitis independently increased the odds of abnormal neurosonography after birth (odds ratio 2.03, 95% confidence interval 1.24 to 3.30). Finally, Alexander and associates[60] demonstrated that when compared to infants born without evidence of chorioamnionitis, low-birth-weight infants born to mothers with chorioamnioni-

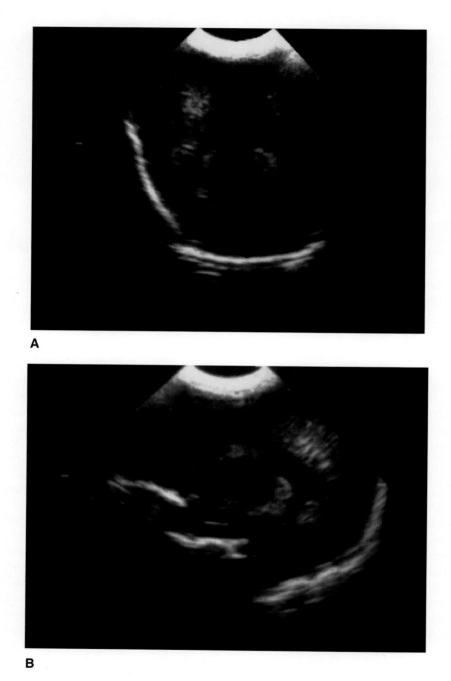

A

B

Figure 16–2. Ultrasound images of the neonatal brain. **a.** Increased echogenicity, coronal view. **b.** Increased periventricular echogenicity, sagittal view.

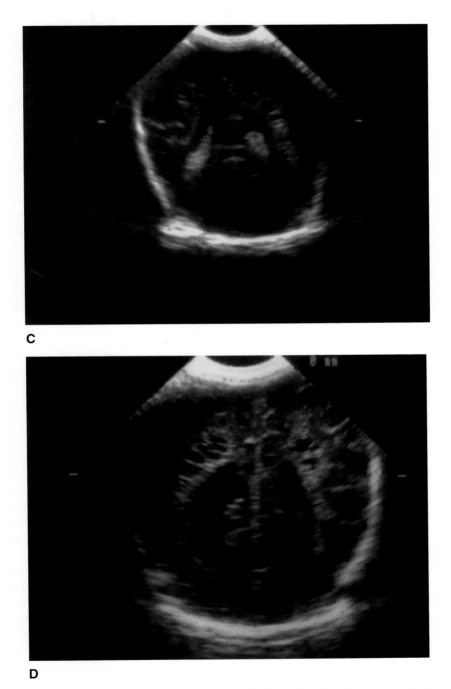

C

D

Figure 16–2. continued Ultrasound images of the neonatal brain. **c.** Cystic lesions, coronal view. **d.** Cystic lesion, mid-coronal view.

tis had approximately three times more risk of neonatal sepsis (odds ratio 2.7, 95% confidence interval 1.03 to 7.1), respiratory distress syndrome (odds ratio 2.7, 95% confidence interval 1.03 to 7.1), seizures in the first 24 hours of life (odds ratio 2.9, 95% confidence interval 1.2 to 6.8), IVH (odds ratio 2.8, 95% confidence interval 1.8 to 4.8) and PVL (odds ratio 3.4, 95% confidence interval 1.6 to 7.3) than those born to mothers without evidence of infection.

Maternal infection has been implicated as a risk factor for CP even in term neonates. Grether and Nelson[1] investigated maternal infection during admission for delivery as a possible risk factor for CP in infants weighing 2500 g or more. In a cohort of 155,636 children of four Northern California counties, 46 children with disabling spastic CP who had no recognized prenatal brain lesions and survived to age 3 years were compared to 378 randomly selected control children. Maternal fever exceeding 38°C in labor or a clinical diagnosis of chorioamnionitis were strongly associated with subsequent development of CP [odds ratio (OR) 9.3, 95% confidence interval (CI) 2.7 to 31.0]. Histological evidence of placental infection was also associated with CP (OR 8.9, 95% CI 1.9 to 40.0). Twenty-two percent of children with CP had one or more indicators of maternal infection. In addition, newborns exposed to maternal infection more often had signs attributed to birth asphyxia: 5 minute Apgar scores below 6 than those unexposed to infection. In addition, they also had a higher frequency of hypotension, need for intubation, neonatal seizures, and clinical diagnoses of hypoxic-ischemic encephalopathy.

Infection Has a Causal Relationship with White Matter Damage

Bejar and coworkers[20] reported that the risk of antenatal WMD was 9.4-fold greater in preterm neonates with purulent amniotic fluid than in those without this finding (75% versus 8%). Verma and colleagues[56] reported that WMD was more common in patients with histologic and clinical chorioamnionitis. Leviton and associates[61] found that bacteremia was five times more common in neonates who had white matter lesions.

To determine if there was a causal relationship between infection and WMD, Yoon and colleagues[31] experimentally induced ascending intrauterine infection with *Escherichia coli* in 31 rabbits. Fourteen controls were inoculated with sterile saline solution. Histologic evidence of brain WMD was identified in 12 fetuses born to 10 *E. coli*-inoculated rabbits but in none of the saline solution group ($P < .05$).

Fetal Cytokinemia Is Associated with Intraventricular Hemorrhage, White Matter Damage, and Long-term Disability

Cytokines are molecules that modulate immune and inflammatory response. They are secreted by lymphocytes and macrophages. Various cytokines, including IL-6, IL-1, IL-8, and tumor necrosis factor (TNF), are elevated in the amniotic fluid of pregnant women with chorioamnionitis (even with infection confined to the amniotic membranes).[33] IL-1 is involved in the modulation of fever, bone resorption and prostaglandin release and stimulates cytokine production by macrophages and T cells. IL-6 induces antibody secretion and is involved in the differentiation of cytotoxic T cells and proliferation of megakaryocytes. IL-8 is produced by macrophages and is responsible for neutrophil and T-cell chemotaxis. TNF-α is involved in the modulation of fever and shock; it activates macrophages and stimulates polimorphonuclear chemotoxin, angiogenesis, and bone resorption. It is cytotoxic to many cells.[62]

Leviton[63] proposed that inflammatory cytokines (TNF-α and IL-1) released during the course of intrauterine infection could play a central role in the pathophysiologic mechanisms of brain WMD. TNF would participate in the pathogenesis of PVL by four different mechanisms: (1) induction of fetal hypotension and brain ischemia;[64] (2) stimulation of the production of tissue factor, which in turn could activate the hemostatic system and contribute to coagulation necrosis of white matter;[65] (3) induction of the release of platelet activating factor, which could act as a membrane detergent causing direct brain damage;[66] and (4) a direct cytotoxic effect of TNF on oligodendrocytes and myelin.[67,68] Subsequently, a series of studies provided support for the hypothesis. First, Yoon and coworkers[57] demonstrated that fetal plasma concentrations of IL-6 were significantly higher in 25 preterm neonates with PVL-associated lesions than in 147 control neonates (median 718, range < 226 to 32,000 pg/mL versus median < 226, range < 226 to 43,670 pg/mL; $P < .00001$). Subsequently, mothers of preterm newborns with brain WMD and CP were shown to have higher concentrations of TNF-α, IL-1β, and IL-6 in the amniotic fluid than those who delivered newborns without WMD.[32] All infants who had CP (8 of 75) had ultrasonographically detectable WMD and elevated amniotic fluid cytokines before birth. In a case-control study using immunohistochemical techniques to determine the antigenic expression of cytokines, Yoon and coworkers compared 17 brain specimens with PVL with 17 controls. TNF-α and IL-6 were expressed more often in cases with PVL when compared to controls [TNF-α: 82% (14 of 17) versus 18% (3 of 17), $P < 0.005$; IL-6: 71% (12 of 17) versus 6% (1 of 17), $P < .005$], mainly in hypertrophic astrocytes and microglia cells situated in and around areas of coagulation necrosis.[69]

Yoon and colleagues[32] proposed a mechanism to explain how inflammatory cytokines could lead to WMD and CP (Fig. 16–3). Microbial invasion of the amniotic cavity, which occurs in approximately 25% of preterm births, would result in congenital fetal infection, stimulating fetal mononuclear cells to produce IL-1 and TNF-α. These cytokines, in turn, would increase the permeability of the blood–brain barrier, facilitating the passage of microbial products and cytokines into the brain. Microbial products would then stimulate the human fetal microglia to produce IL-1 and TNF-α, with subsequent activation of astrocyte proliferation and production of TNF. TNF would damage the oligodendrocyte, which is the cell responsible for the deposition of myelin.

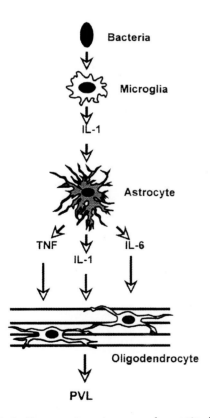

Figure 16–3. Proposed sequence of events leading to periventricular leukomalacia in fetuses with intrauterine infection *(Gomez R, Romero R, et al.: The Role of Infection in Preterm Labor and Delivery in Preterm Labor. Churchill Livinstone Inc.; Elder MG, Romero R, Lamont RF, eds. New York: 1997.)*

Fetal Vasculitis Is Associated with an Increased Risk for Intraventricular Hemorrhage, White Matter Damage, and Cerebral Palsy

In a study of 123 children born prematurely and followed up until the age of 3 years, Yoon and coworkers[70] demonstrated that the odds of developing CP were significantly higher in the presence of funisitis (odds ratio 5.5, 95% confidence interval 1.2 to 24.5), increased amniotic fluid IL-6 (odds ratio 6.4, 95% confidence interval 1.3–33.0), and increased amniotic fluid IL-8 concentrations (odds ratio 5.9, 95% confidence interval 1.1 to 30.7). Among the 14 children in this cohort who subsequently developed CP, all had evidence of WMD, and 11 had evidence of intrauterine inflammation (elevated amniotic fluid cytokines and white blood cell count and were born to mothers with either preterm labor or premature rupture of the membranes). Fifty percent of the children (7 of 14) had positive amniotic fluid cultures. Of note is that histologic chorioamnionitis was associated with subsequent development of CP in univariate analysis. However, after adjusting for gestational age at birth, the association disappeared. These findings suggest that it is the fetal, rather than maternal, inflammatory response that predisposes to CP. Nonetheless, because CP did not develop in 82% (23 of 28) fetuses with documented microbial invasion of the amniotic cavity and in 76% (34 of 45) of those with evidence of intrauterine inflammation, neither infection nor inflammation were considered sufficient causal factors for WMD or CP. It is likely that genes coding for proinflammatory and anti-inflammatory cytokines regulate the intensity of the inflammatory response and, therefore, the host response to infection and tissue injury.[71–74] Genetic factor may control the intensity of the inflammatory response and predispose to CP.

SUMMARY

Intrauterine infection and the fetal inflammatory response are important but not sufficient factors in the pathogenesis of CP. Factors predisposing to brain injury in the setting of intrauterine infection include gestational age, integrity of the blood–brain barrier, vulnerability of the central nervous system, fetal infection, and the nature and intensity of the fetal inflammatory response.[70]

Potential strategies to prevent CP in this population of patients may need to begin in utero.[70] It has been suggested that prenatal exposure to magnesium sulfate could decrease the prevalence of CP in very low birthweight infants, although the evidence is controversial.[75,76,77] Mechanisms of action are speculative and may include: increased threshold and decreased excitability of neuron membranes and muscle cells, thereby increasing cohesiveness and structural integrity of these membranes; decreased excitotoxic effects by suppression of calcium-dependent transmitter release; blockage of the NMDA receptor (activation of which is implicated in excitotoxic mechanisms; changes in free radical levels; nitric oxide synthase; cyclic GMP and endothelins; and regulation of cardiovascular tone and function.[75] However, in a subsequent retrospective study the association between exposure to $MgSO_4$ during labor and a decreased prevalence of CP could not be confirmed.[78,79] Two randomized clinical trials are in progress in the United States and Australia to test this hypothesis. Other strategies that would eventually result in prolongation of pregnancy in patients at risk for preterm labor are under investigation. Among them is a randomized trial examining the effect of cervical cerclage in prolonging pregnancy for patients with a short cervix. The impact of these novel strategies on the prevalence of CP is awaited with interest.

REFERENCES

1. Grether JK, Nelson KB. Maternal infection and cerebral palsy in infants of normal birth weight. *JAMA.* 1997;278:207–211.
2. Gondenberg RL, Nelson KL. Cerebral palsy. In: Chapter 63. In: Creasy RK, Resnick R, eds. Maternal Fetal Medicine, 4th Edition. Philadelphia, PA: W.B. Saunders; 1999:1194–1214
3. Paneth N, Kiely J. The frequency of cerebral palsy: A review of population studies in industrialised nations since 1950. In: Stanley F, Alberman E, eds. *The Epidemiology of the Cerebral Palsies.* Oxford: Blackwell Scientific Publications; 1984:46–56.
4. Stanley FJ, Watson L. Trends in perinatal mortality and cerebral palsy in Western Australia, 1967 to 1985. *BMJ.* 1992;304:1658–1663.
5. Little WJ. On the influence of abnormal parturition, difficult labors, premature birth, and asphyxia neonatorum, on the mental and physical condition of the child, especially in relation to deformities. *Trans Obstet Soc London.* 1861–1862;3:293–344.
6. Evans PM, Evans SJW, Alberman E. Cerebral palsy: Why we must plan for survival. *Arch Dis Child.* 1990;65:1329–1333.
7. Rumeau-Ruquette C, du Mazaubrun C, Mlika A, Dequae L. Motor disability in children in three birth cohorts. *Int J Epidemiol.* 1992;21:359–366.
8. Grether JK, Cummins SK, Nelson KB. The California Cerebral Palsy Project. *Paediatr Perinat Epidemiol.* 1992;6:339–351.
9. Kuban KCK, Leviton A. Cerebral palsy. *N Engl J Med.* 1994;330:188–195.
10. Hagberg B, Hagberg G, Olow I, von Wendt L. The changing panorama of cerebral palsy in Sweden. V. The birth year period 1979–82. *Acta Paediatr Scand.* 1989;78:283–290.
11. Pharoah POD, Cooke T, Cooke RWI, Rosenbloom L. Birthweight specific trends in cerebral palsy. *Arch Dis Child.* 1990;65:602–606.
12. Gomez R, Romero R, Edwin SS, David C. Pathogenesis of preterm labor and premature rupture of membranes associated with intraamniotic infection. *Infect Dis Clin North Am.* 1997;11:135–176.
13. Bakketeig LS. Only a minor part of cerebral palsy cases begin in labour. *BMJ.* 1999;319:1016–1017.
14. MacLennan A. A template for defining a causal relation between acute intrapartum events and cerebral palsy: International Consensus Statement. *BMJ.* 1999;319:1054–1059.
15. Nelson KL, Ellenberg JH. Antecedents of cerebral palsy: Multivariate analysis of risk. *N Engl J Med.* 1986;315:81–86.
16. Cummins SK, Nelson KB, Grether JK, Velie EM. Cerebral palsy in four northern California counties, births 1983 through 1985. *J Pediatr.* 1993;123:230–237.
17. Stanley F. Social and biological determinants of the cerebral palsies. In: Stanley F, Alberman E, eds. *Clinics in Developmental Medicine No 87: The Epidemiology of the Cerebral Palsies.* Lavenham, England: Lavenham Press; 1984:69–86.
18. Ozmen M, Caliskan M, Apak S, et al: Eight-year clinical experience in cerebral palsy. *J Trop Pediatr.* 1993;39:52–54.
19. Weinding AM, Wilkinson AR, Cook J, Calvert AS, Fok TF, Rochefort MJ. Perinatal events which precede periventricular haemorrhage and leukomalacia in the newborn. *Br J Obstet Gynaecol.* 1985;92:1218–1223.
20. Bejar R, Wozniak P, Allard M, et al. Antenatal origin of neurologic damage in newborn infants. I. Preterm infants. *Am J Obstet Gynecol.* 1988;159:357–363.
21. Trounce JQ, Shaw DE, Levene MI, Rutter N. Clinical risk factors and periventricular leucomalacia. *Arch Dis Child.* 1988;63:17–22.
22. Costello AM, Hamilton PA, Baudin J, et al. Prediction of neurodevelopmental impairment at four years from brain ultrasound appearance of very preterm infants. *Dev Med Child Neurol.* 1988;30:711–722.
23. Shortland D, Levene MI, Trounce J, Ng Y, Graham M. The evolution and outcome of cavitating periventricular leukomalacia in infancy: A study of 46 cases. *J Perinat Med.* 1988;16:241–247.
24. Leviton A, Paneth N. White matter damage in preterm newborns—An epidemiologic perspective. *Early Hum Dev.* 1990;24:1–22.
25. Levene MI. Cerebral ultrasound and neurological impairment: Telling the future. *Arch Dis Child.* 1990;65:469–471.
26. Pidcock FS, Graziani LJ, Stanley C, Mitchell DG, Merton D. Neurosonographic features of periventricular echodensities associated with cerebral palsy in preterm infants. *J Pediatr.* 1990;116:417–422.

27. Fazzi E, Lanzi G, Gerardo A, Ometto A, Rondini G. Correlation between clinical and ultrasound findings in preterm infants with cystic periventricular leukomalacia. *Ital J Neurol Sci.* 1991;12:199–203.

28. Graziani LJ, Mitchell DG, Kornhauser M, et al. Neurodevelopment of preterm infants: Neonatal neurosonographic and serum bilirubin studies. *Pediatrics.* 1992;89:229–234.

29. Murphy DJ, Sellers S, MacKenzie IZ, et al. Case-control study of antenatal and intrapartum risk factors for cerebral palsy in very preterm singleton babies. *Lancet.* 1995;346:1449–1454.

30. Nelson KB, Dambrosia JM, Grether JK, Phillips TM. Neonatal cytokines and coagulation factors in children with cerebral palsy. *Ann Neurol.* 1998;44:665–675.

31. Yoon BH, Kim CJ, Romero R, et al. Experimentally induced intrauterine infection causes fetal brain white matter lesions in rabbits. *Am J Obstet Gynecol.* 1997;177:797–802.

32. Yoon BH, Jun JK, Romero R, et al. Amniotic fluid inflammatory cytokines (interleukin-6, interleuin-1b, and tumor necrosis factor-α), neonatal brain white matter lesions, and cerebral palsy. *Am J Obstet Gynecol.* 1997;177:19–26.

33. Damman O, Leviton A. Role of the fetus in perinatal infection and neonatal brain damage. *Curr Opinion Pediatr.* 2000;12:99–104.

34. Watts DH, Krohn MA, Hillier SL, Eschenbach DA. The association of occult amniotic fluid infection with gestational age and neonatal outcome among women with preterm labor. *Obstet Gynecol.* 1992;79:351–357.

35. Duff P, Kopelman J. Subclinical intra-amniotic infection in asymptomatic patients with refractory preterm labor. *Obstet Gynecol.* 1987;69:756–759.

36. Arias F, Rodriquez L, Rayne S, Kraus F. Maternal placental vasculopathy and injection: two distinct subgroups among patients with preterm labor and preterm ruptured membranes. *Am J Obstet Gynecol.* 1993;168:585–591.

37. Romero R, Sirtori M, Oyarzun E, et al. Infection and labor. V. Prevalence, microbiology, and clinical significance of intraamniotic infection in women with preterm labor and intact membranes. *Am J Obstet Gynecol.* 1989;161:817–824.

38. Romero R, Yoon BH, Mazor M, et al. The diagnostic and prognostic value of amniotic fluid white blood cell count, glucose, interleukin-6, and Gram stain in patients with preterm labor and intact membranes. *Am J Obstet Gynecol.* 1993;169:805–816.

39. Garite T, Freeman R. Chorioamnionitis in the preterm gestation. *Obstet Gynecol.* 1982;59:539–545.

40. Romero R, Quintero R, Oyarzun E, et al. Intraamniotic infection and the onset of labor in preterm premature rupture of membranes. *Am J Obstet Gynecol.* 1988;159:661–666.

41. Feinstein S, Vintzileos A, Lodeiro J, Campbell W, Weinbaum P, Nochimson DJ. Amniocentesis with premature rupture of membranes. *Obstet Gynecol.* 1986;68:147–152.

42. Romero R, Yoon BH, Mazor M, et al. A comparative study of the diagnostic performance of amniotic fluid glucose, white blood cell count, interleukin-6, and Gram stain in the detection of microbial invasion in patients with preterm premature rupture of membranes. *Am J Obstet Gynecol.* 1993;169:839–851.

43. Jalava J, Mantymaa ML, Ekblad U. Bacterial 165 rDNA polymerase chain reaction in the detection of intra-amniotic infection. *Br J Obstet Gynaecol.* 1996;103:664–669.

44. Markenson G, Martin R, Foley K, Yancey M. The use of polymerase chain reaction to detect bacteria in amniotic fluid in pregnancies complicated by preterm labor [abstract 100]. *Am J Obstet Gynecol.* 1997;176:S39.

45. Sampson JE, Theve RP, Blatman RN, et al. Fetal origin of amniotic fluid polymorphonuclear leukocytes. *Am J Obstet Gynecol.* 1997;176:77–81.

46. Yoon BH, Romero R, Park JS, et al. Microbial invasion of the amniotic cavity with *Ureaplasma urealyticum* is associated with a robust host response in fetal, amniotic, and maternal compartments. *Am J Obstet Gynecol.* 1998;179:1254–1260.

47. Romero R, Brody DT, Oyarzun E, et al. Infection and labor. III. Interleukin-1: A signal for the onset of parturition. *Am J Obstet Gynecol.* 1989;160:117–123.

48. Romero R, Manogue KR, Mitchell MD, et al. Infection and labor. IV. Cachectin tumor necrosis factor in the amniotic fluid of women with intraamniotic infection and preterm labor. *Am J Obstet Gynecol.* 1989;161:336–341.

49. Romero R, Ceska M, Avila C, Mazor M, Behnke E, Lindley I. Neutrophil attractant/activating peptide-1/interleukin-8 in term and preterm parturition. *Am J Obstet Gynecol.* 1991;165:813–830.

50. Romero R, Mazor M, Munoz H, Gomez R, Galasso M, Sherer DM. The preterm labor syndrome. *Ann N Y Acad Sci.* 1994;734:414–429.

51. Romero R, Gomez R, Ghezzi F, et al. A fetal systemic inflammatory response is followed by the spontaneous onset of preterm parturition. *Am J Obstet Gynecol.* 1998;179:186–193.

52. Gomez R, Romero R, Ghezzi F, Yoon BH, Mazor M, Berry SM. The fetal inflammatory response syndrome. *Am J Obstet Gynecol.* 1998;179:194–202.

53. Johnston MV, Trescher WH, Taylor GA. Hypoxic and ischemic central nervous system disorders in infants and children. *Adv Pediatr.* 1995;42:1–45.

54. DeReuck J, Chattha AS, Richardson EP Jr. Pathogenesis and evolution of periventricular leukomalacia in infancy. *Arch Neurol.* 1982;27:229–236.

55. Tamisari L, Vigi V, Fortini CCC, Scarpa P. Neonatal periventricular leukomalacia: Diagnosis and evolution evaluated by real-time ultrasound. *Helv Paediatr Acta.* 1986;41:399–407.

56. Verma U, Tejani N, Klein S, et al. Obstetric antecedents of intraventricular hemorrhage and periventricular leukomalacia in the low-birth-weight neonate. *Am J Obstet Gynecol.* 1997;176:281.

57. Yoon BH, Romero R, Yang SH, et al. Inteleukin-6 concentrations in umbilical cord plasma are elevated in

neonates with white matter lesions associated with periventricular leukomalacia. *Am J Obstet Gynecol.* 1996;174:1433–1440.

58. Nelson KB, Ellenberg JH. Epidemiology of cerebral palsy. *Adv Neurol.* 1978;19:421–435.

59. Shea TM, Klinepeter KL, Dillard RG. Prenatal events and the risk of cerebral palsy in very low birth weight infants. *Am J Epidemiol.* 1998;147:362–369.

60. Alexander JM, Gilstrap LC, Cox SM, McIntire DM, Leveno KJ. Clinical chorioamnionitis and the prognosis of very low birth weight infants. *Obstet Gynecol.* 1998;91:725–729.

61. Leviton A, Gilles F, Neff R, Yaney P. Multivariate analysis of risk of perinatal telencephalic leucoencephalopathy. *Am J Epidemiol.* 1976;104:621–626.

62. Benett JC. Approach to the patient with immune disease. In: Benett JC, Plum F, eds. *Cecil Textbook of Medicine.* Philadelphia: WB Saunders; 1996:1993–1998.

63. Leviton A. Preterm birth and cerebral palsy: is tumor necrosis factor the missing link? *Dev Med Child Neurol.* 1993;35:553–558.

64. Iida K, Takashima S, Takeuchi Y. Etiologies and distribution of neonatal leukomalacia. *Pediatr Neurol.* 1992;8:205–209.

65. Van der Poll T, Büller HR, ten Cate H, et al. Activation of coagulation after administration of tumor necrosis factor to normal subjects. *N Engl J Med* 1990;322:1622–1627.

66. Camussi G, Bussolino F, Salvidio G, Baglioni C. Tumor necrosis factor cachectin stimulates peritoneal macrophages, polymorphonuclear neutrophils, and vascular endothelial cells to synthesize and release platelet activating factor *J Exp Med.* 1987;166:1390–1404.

67. Selmaj K, Raine CS, Path FRC, Cross AH. Tumor necrosis factor mediates myelin and oligodendrocyte damage in vitro. *Ann Neurol.* 1988;23:339–346.

68. Robbins DS, Shirazi Y, Drysdale BE, Lieberman A, Shin HS, Shin ML. Production of cytokine profile in plasma of baboons challenged with lethal and sublethal *Escherichia coli. Circ Shock.* 1992;33:84–91.

69. Yoon BH, Romero R, Kim CH, et al. High expression of tumor necrosis factor-α and interleukin-6 in periven-tricular leukomalacia. *Am J Obstet Gynecol.* 1997;177:406–411.

70. Yoon BH, Romero R, Park JS, et al. Fetal exposure to an intra-amniotic inflammation and the development of cerebral palsy at the age of three years. *Am J Obstet Gynecol.* 2000;182:675–681.

71. Wilson AG, Symons JA, McDowell TL, McDevitt HO, Duff GW. Effects of a polymorphism in the human tumor necrosis factor-α promoter on transcriptional activation. *Proc Natl Acad Sci U S A* 1997;94:3195–3199.

72. Stuber F, Petersen M, Bokelmann F, Schade U. A genomic polymorphism within the tumor necrosis factor locus influences plasma tumor necrosis factor-α concentrations and outcome of patients with severe sepsis. *Crit Care Med.* 1996;24:381–384.

73. McGuire W, Hill AV, Allsopp CE, Greenwood BM, Kwiatkowski D. Variation in the TNF-α promoter region associated with susceptibility to cerebral malaria. *Nature.* 1994;371:508–510.

74. Monzon-Bordonaba F, Parry S, Holder J, et al. A genetic marker for preterm delivery [abstract]. *J Soc Gynecol Invest.* 1998;5:71A.

75. Nelson KB, Grether JK. Can magnesium sulfate reduce the risk of cerebral palsy in very low birthweight infants? *Pediatrics.* 1995;95:263–269.

76. Hauth JC, Goldenberg RL, Nelson KG, et al. Reduction of cerebral palsy with maternal MgSO4 treatment in newborns weighing 500–1000 g. *Am J Obstet Gynecol.* 1995;172(1, pt 2):419.

77. Schendel DE, Berg CJ, Yeargin-Allsopp M, Boyle CA, Decoufle P. Prenatal magnesium sulfate exposure and the risk of cerebral palsy or mental retardation among very low-birth-weight children aged 3 to 5 years. *JAMA.* 1996;276:1805–1810.

78. Paneth N, Jetton J, Pinto-Martin J, Susser M. Magnesium sulfate in labor and risk of neonatal brain lesions and cerebral palsy in low birth weight infants. The Neonatal Brain Hemorrhage Study Analysis Group. *Pediatrics.* 1997;99:E1.

79. Rouse DJ, Hauth JC, Nelson KG, Goldenberg RL. The feasibility of a randomized clinical perinatal trial: Maternal magnesium sulfate for the prevention of cerebral palsy. *Am J Obstet Gynecol.* 1996;175:701–705.

CHAPTER SEVENTEEN

Fetal and Neonatal Cerebral Circulation

Shimon Degani

Human perinatal brain damage in humans attributed to abnormal labor and delivery was found to be much less common than previously believed.[1] Antenatal intrauterine cerebrovascular events were found to play an important role.[2]

The fetal brain is protected from pressure changes by autoregulation of the cerebral circulation. This mechanism keeps blood flow relatively constant, despite variations in perfusion pressure.[3] The arterial vasculature constricts and dilates in response to the changes in transmural pressure, to prevent brain hypoxia in low pressures and edema in high pressures. Extreme vasodilation can result in damage to the endothelial cells and thus further compromise the vasomotor reactivity.

Animal studies have provided the basic knowledge of the physiological states. The human fetus due to its inaccessibility, could not be studied to the same extent until the introduction of high-resolution ultrasound imaging.

Doppler ultrasound was first used to study cerebral blood flow velocity waveforms in 1979 when Bada and associates[4] studied the anterior cerebral artery through the anterior fontanelle in normal newborns and in those with perinatal asphyxia, cerebrovascular hemorrhage, and growth failure. This technique was later widely applied to further study the newborn and fetal cerebral circulation in health and disease.

ANATOMICAL CONSIDERATIONS

Transcranial Doppler ultrasonography is a technique that allows noninvasive evaluation of the flow pattern of the basal cerebral artery.[5] Using a 2-MHz ultrasound probe in adults, the examiner can generally obtain a reasonably strong Doppler signal in the region of the temporal bone window. This preauricular location allows insonation of the anterior cerebral artery, middle cerebral arteries, and posterior cerebral artery.

The fetal skull, surrounded by amniotic fluid, allows clear flow velocity signals to be obtained from cerebral arteries without the need for special localized windows. Using this technique, Wladimiroff and colleagues[6] carried out Doppler measurements of the human fetal cerebral circulation at the level of the internal carotid artery. This level can easily be obtained on an axial view of the brain stem (Fig. 17–1). Anterior to the cerebral peduncles, on either side of the mid-line, an oblique cross-section of the internal carotid artery can be seen (see Chapter 2).

Some difficulty has been encountered in localizing specific cerebral arteries, due to the size and complexity of the circle of Willis. The circle is a unique form of anastomosis of the main cerebral vessels connected by communicating arteries (anterior and posterior) on both sides and its structure plays a role in pressure equilibrium of cerebral vasculature. Alpers and coworkers[7] stated that almost 50% of all persons studied had anatomical variations of the circle of Willis. Woo and associates[8] reported that, in their experience, it was not possible to determine with absolute certainty whether the Doppler signals were derived from the main trunk of the internal carotid artery or from very proximal parts of the middle cerebral artery.

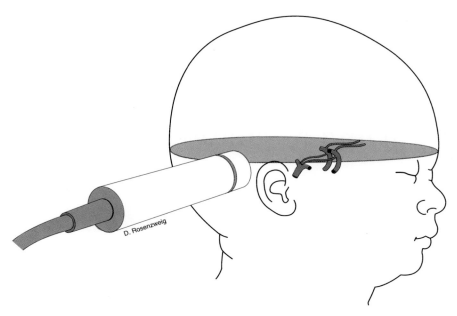

Figure 17–1. Plane of cerebral vessels used for Doppler studies. *(Modified after Degani and colleagues,[143] with permission.)*

The longest branch of the circle of Willis is the *middle cerebral artery,* which runs laterally in the sylvian fissure as a continuation of the intracranial internal carotid artery. It consists of four segments and sends branches to the corpus striatum, internal capsule, and lenticulostriate artery. It continues its cruise posteriorly over the surface of the insula and inferior frontal gyrus,[9] carrying about 80% of blood flow to the hemisphere.[10]

For studying the middle cerebral artery according to anatomical data, Mari and collaborators[11] suggested a plane more caudal to the cerebral peduncles in the section containing the pons and the medulla oblongata and greater paired wings of the sphenoid. It can also be visualized at the level of the cerebral peduncles at its anterolateral border, running anterolaterally towards the lateral edge of the orbit. One can see this artery also on the Midcoronal-2 as well as the Oblique-2 sections (see Chapter 2).

The base of the skull at the level of the temporal and sphenoidal bones is the preferred plane for recording Doppler signals from the anterior and posterior cerebral arteries. The *anterior cerebral artery* flow velocity waveforms can be obtained close to the midline—anterior to the pulsating internal carotid artery—half the distance from the midbrain to the frontal bone. One of the important branches of this artery in the pericallosal artery seen on the Median section (see Chapters 2 and 4) The *posterior cerebral artery* recordings are done at the level of the transverse cerebral fissure on the side of the midbrain.

Using the transabdominal route, a prerequisite for recording cerebral Doppler signals is that the head is not too deeply engaged in the maternal pelvis.[12] Transvaginal scanning of cerebral vessels was recommended by Lewinsky and coworkers.[13] The coronal section obtained by this approach showed separate and easily distinguishable images of these arteries because the internal carotid arteries are located medially and inferiorly to the corresponding middle cerebral arteries. With the use of a transfontanelle approach in the newborn, detection of flow is easily obtained from the anterior cerebral artery, where it curves around the corpus callosum.[14] In most studies of the fetal cerebral circulation, Doppler-derived data are gained from the middle cerebral artery and internal carotid artery due to the ease of obtaining recordings. Few studies have reported on data collected from other cerebral vessels, i.e., the anterior and posterior cerebral arteries.[15–17] To correlate fetal with neonatal cerebral flow data, the same vessels should be studied.[18,19]

TECHNICAL CONSIDERATIONS AND DOPPLER CRITERIA

Detection of vessels is based on visualization of pulsatile flow velocity waveforms with duplex systems or by using color flow imaging.[20] Transducers with carrier frequencies of 2.5, 3.5, and 5 MHz are usually used, the sample gate not exceeding 3 to 4 mm. This allows clear flow velocity signals without interference from other nearby vessels. A high-pass filter of 50 to 150 Hz is applied to remove signals originating from slow-moving tissues in the path of the Doppler beam. The angle of insonation is kept as small as possible, and the low-power output mode should be used throughout the study. For standard conditions, all samples are taken with subjects in the semirecumbent position and during fetal apnea because high-amplitude fetal breathing modulates the blood flow.[21]

For calculation of qualitative Doppler indices, velocity waveforms are recorded and peak velocity, end-diastolic velocity, and mean maximum velocity are measured. Three to five consecutive waveforms are analyzed and the results are averaged. Using these Doppler variables, the pulsatility index (PI), defined as the difference between the peak systolic and end-diastolic values divided by the mean maximum flow velocity,[22] can be calculated. Substantial interobserver agreement and intraobserver repeatability were found for cerebral vessels studied.[23,24] Other qualitative parameters may be determined, but are less frequently used: the ratio of peak systolic to maximum end-diastolic velocity (S/D ratio), the resistance index (R; the difference between peak systolic and end-diastolic velocities divided by the peak systolic and velocity), and cerebral index (peak systolic velocity minus S/D ratio).[25] Ratios of qualitative parameters in other fetal vessels are also in use: the ratio of RI in the fetal common carotid artery, to the RI in the umbilical artery, as described by Arabin and associates,[26] or the ratio between the cerebral RI and the placental RI, as described by Arbeille and colleagues.[17] The use of color flow imaging enables accurate measurement of the angle of vessel insonation to determine absolute mean blood flow velocity values in intracranial vessels.[27]

The venous circulation of the fetal brain can be identified by color Doppler. Recently,[28] the ultrasound–anatomical correlates were established for the venous blood flow in the fetal brain, and the reference values for flow velocity waveforms in the transverse sinus were documented. Power Doppler improves the sensitivity of detection of the presence of flow, when compared with conventional color Doppler velocity imaging. Fetal intracerebral arteries and veins which could not have been imaged by the transabdominal approach were demonstrated using a combination of transvaginal sonography and power Doppler flow mapping.[29]

Normal Fetuses

The intracranial circulation becomes visible as early as the 8th postmenstrual week of the pregnancy:

arterial pulsation can be detected on an axial view of the embryonic skull. In a study by Kurjak and coworkers using transvaginal ultrasound, the visualization rate of pulsation on the base of the skull increased from 50% at the 8th to 83% at the 10th postmenstrual week.[30] From the 11th week onward, it became a constant finding. It is very difficult to distinguish blood flow between the various cerebral arteries because the distances are in a range of a few millimeters or even less. The waveform signal profile at this gestational age is characterized by the absence of an end diastolic component.

During the third trimester, continuous flow is present throughout the cardiac cycle in the internal carotid artery, confirming the existence of a low peripheral vascular resistance in the fetal brain.[31] Flow velocity waveforms from the fetal middle cerebral artery are highly pulsatile, and the presence of end-diastolic frequencies becomes more common with advancing gestation.[27] Thus, end-diastolic frequencies were present in 75% of fetuses at 18 to 25 postmenstrual weeks, and in all fetuses examined after 34 postmenstrual weeks.[27]

The PI of the middle cerebral artery was found to be higher than that for either the internal carotid or the proximal anterior cerebral artery.[11] Hata and coworkers[32] found the RI of the posterior cerebral artery to be lower than that of the middle and and anterior cerebral arteries.

These differences emphasize the need for an exact definition of the vessel that is being insonated and could be caused by different resistances in various portions of the cerebral circulation. In vitro examination of the contractile properties of the common carotid artery in the fetal lamb has shown that this vessel has less dilating capacity in response to hypoxia than do the intracranial arteries.[33] However, in cross-sectional studies, mean blood flow velocities in the common carotid artery increased throughout pregnancy in contrast to aortic velocities, which tend to decrease toward the end of pregnancy. The PI in the aorta remains constant, whereas in the common carotid artery it falls steeply after 32 postmenstrual weeks.[34] A significant decrease in the PI was also observed in the middle cerebral artery, especially after 36 postmenstrual weeks (Table 17–1).[35–37] These results suggest that with advancing gestation, there is redistribution of the fetal circulation, with decreased impedance to flow to the fetal brain, presumably to compensate for the progressive decrease in fetal blood pO_2. In studies of the middle cerebral artery in the second trimester,[38–40] an increasing PI was found until the late second trimester, followed by a decline in the third trimester. Mari and Deter[40] attributed the low PI values at the beginning and end of pregnancy

TABLE 17–1. PULSATILITY INDEX OF THE MIDDLE CEREBRAL ARTERY IN NORMAL FETUSES AS A FUNCTION OF GESTATIONAL AGE: REGRESSION EQUATIONS

Authors	Regression Equation	r^2	References
Van den Wijngaard and colleagues	PI = −3.44 + 0.36 × GA − 0.006 × GA²	—	49
Arstrom and colleagues	PI = 5.13 − 0.09 × GA	0.52	177
Arduini and Rizzo	PI = 0.006 + 0.144 × GA − 0.003 × GA²	0.52	38
Mari and Deter	PI = 1.97 + 0.327 × GA − 0.006 × GA²	0.45	40

PI, Pulsatility index; GA, gestational age; r^2, coefficient of determination.
After Marsal and colleagues, 1994,[67] with permission.

to increased metabolic requirements and, therefore, lower cerebral vascular impedance to blood flow.

Studies of waveforms recorded from the fetal internal carotid artery demonstrated that the PI remains fairly constant during the last trimester of pregnancy, and only during the last 4 weeks does there seem to be a slight decrease.[27] Reference resistance indices of fetal middle cerebral artery were established in a large and minimally selected population attending a single clinic.[41] Cerebral vascular resistance decreases constantly up to postmenstrual week 42.[42]

In a longitudinal study, fetal and neonatal cerebral blood flow velocities were assessed in the middle cerebral artery in 40 uncomplicated pregnancies during the third trimester and in 22 neonates born from these pregnancies (Table 17–2).[18] Peak systolic, temporal mean, and end-diastolic flow velocities increased during the third trimester and were significantly higher from 36 postmenstrual weeks on, as compared to values obtained at 28 postmenstrual weeks, suggesting an increase in actual blood flow. The PI and RI of the middle cerebral artery did not differ significantly during this period. Immediately after birth, flow velocities decreased significantly and remained lower during the first 5 postnatal days compared to fetal values. The PI and RI of the middle cerebral artery tended to decrease during the first

postnatal day, but stabilized afterward. These alterations in cerebral blood flow in the transition from the fetal to the neonatal state are explained by local rather than central cardiovascular changes, mainly the local effect of oxygen on peripheral vessels.[43] Doppler flow studies in twins without growth retardation or discordance demonstrated changes throughout pregnancy similar to those in singletons.[44,45]

PHYSIOLOGICAL VARIABLES AFFECTING CEREBRAL BLOOD FLOW IN NORMAL PREGNANCY

The physiological changes to cerebral blood flow in normal pregnancy are summarized in Table 17–3.

Fetal Heart Rate

An inverse correlation was found between fetal heart rate and PI in the middle cerebral artery of fetuses with heart rate decelerations[46] and with tachycardia secondary to ritodrine infusion.[47] Within the normal range of fetal heart rate, Doppler indices did not alter significantly.

Fetal Breathing Movements

High-amplitude fetal breathing movements modulate flow velocity waveforms in the fetal internal

TABLE 17–2. REFERENCE VALUES FOR DOPPLER INDICES OF CEREBRAL VESSELS IN THE THIRD TRIMESTER OF PREGNANCY

Vascular Index	26 to 27 Weeks*	40 Weeks*	References
Common carotid artery pulsatility index	2.13 ± 0.11	1.89 ± 0.07	34
Internal carotid artery pulsatility index	1.63 ± 0.35	1.31 ± 0.41	30
Middle cerebral artery			
Pulsatility index	2.30 ± 0.48	1.82 ± 0.38	27
Systolic/diastolic ratio	6.89 ± 1.48	4.23 ± 0.67	8
Resistance index	0.93 ± 0.049	0.68 ± 0.087	32
Mean velocity (cm/sec)	5.3 ± 2.3	11.3 ± 3.1	27
Anterior cerebral artery resistance index	0.83 ± 0.05	0.79 ± 0.04	175
Posterior cerebral artery resistance index	0.73 ± 0.05	0.70 ± 0.06	175

After Degani and colleagues,[178] with permission.
*Postmenstrual weeks.

TABLE 17–3. CHANGES IN IMPEDANCE CRITERIA (PULSATILITY AND RESISTANCE INDICES) IN FETAL CEREBRAL ARTERIAL VASCULATURE SECONDARY TO VARIOUS PHYSIOLOGICAL AND NONPHYSIOLOGICAL STATES IN PREGNANCY

State	Impedance					References
	Internal Carotid Artery	Middle Cerebral Artery	Anterior Cerebral Artery	Posterior Cerebral Artery	Mean Blood Velocity	
Gestational age	↓	N/↓	↓	↓↓	↑	27, 30, 34, 36, 44, 45
↑ Fetal heart rate	↓	—	—	—	—	47
↓ Fetal heart rate	↑	—	—	—	—	46, 47
Fetal breathing movement	↑/↓	—	—	—	—	48
Fetal behavior stage 2F	↓	—	—	—	—	50
Plasma glucose concentration	↑	↓/↑[a]	—	—	—	51, 52, 54
Fetal head compression	↑	↑	—	—	—	55
Uterine contractions	↑/N	↑/↓	—	—	—	58–60
Fetal anemia	↑/N	↑/N	—	—	↑	62, 63
Oligohydramnios	↑	↑	—	—	—	56, 82–86
Growth retardation	↓↓	↓↓/↓	↓	↓	↑	6, 8, 11, 13, 17, 25, 27, 40
Fetal hydrocephaly	↑	↑/N/↓	—	—	—	106–108
Arteriovenous malformation	—	↓	—	—	—	112–113
↑ P_{CO_2}	↓	↓	—	—	—	129, 130
↓ P_{CO_2}	↓	↓	—	—	↑	6, 27

↑, Increased; ↓, decreased; N, normal.
[a] Depending on fetal behavior stage.
After Degani and colleagues,[178] with permission.

carotid artery.[48] This is similar to findings in the umbilical artery and vein and fetal descending aorta where changes in PI ranging from −25% to +30% have been observed.[21] It is recommended, therefore, that cerebral flow velocity waveforms should be recorded under a standardized condition, e.g., fetal apnea.

Fetal Behavioral States

Nijhuis and coworkers described behavioral states in the human fetus from 36 weeks on.[49] Based on changes in fetal heart rate patterns, fetal body movements, and eye movements, four states were defined. Doppler flow velocity waveforms recorded from the fetal internal carotid artery in normal pregnancies at 37 to 38 weeks of gestation during fetal behavioral states 1F (quiet sleep) and 2F (active sleep) demonstrated a significant reduction of the PI in state 2F compared to that in state 1F.[50] This reduction of PI was not related to heart rate only, and could be demonstrated at standardized heart rate. Increased oxygen demand during fetal activity is followed by increased cerebral blood flow, reflecting autoregulation. It is suggested that fetal neurological development expressed by the emergence of fetal behavior is associated with specific hemodynamic adaptation (see Chapter 15).

Plasma Glucose Concentration

We found a significant positive correlation between maternal plasma glucose concentration and the PI of the internal carotid artery.[51] Similar changes were demonstrated in the fetal middle cerebral artery after glucose challenge test.[52] In preterm infants, hypoglycemia was found to be associated with an increase of cerebral blood flow.[53] This may be a compensatory mechanism to maintain glucose supply to the brain. An indirect effect, mediated through induced changes in behavioral state, was suggested by others.[54]

Fetal Head Compression

The increase in the PI of flow velocity waveforms from the middle cerebral artery was found to be associated with maternal abdominal pressure, even from the ultrasound transducer,[55] oligohydramnios,[56] polyhydramnios,[57] or to uterine contractions during labor.[58] Fetal head compression was suggested as the underlying mechanism of these changes. End-diastolic flow velocities are reduced and in some cases reverse diastolic flow is seen.

Transvaginal Doppler assessment of the fetal middle cerebral artery could not confirm a change in peripheral resistance in the fetal cerebral vascular bed during the first stage of normal labor.[59,60] The growing list of internal and external variables affecting cerebral circulation emphasizes the need for strict standards in study design.

Labor and Delivery

Fetal aortic blood flow was demonstrated to be increased with progress of labor.[54] The umbilical circulation seems to remain unaffected by uterine contractions.[62,63] However, conflicting results are reported on changes in fetal cerebral vascular resistance during and between contractions. Yagel and collaborators[60] found a reduction of 40% in vascular resistance in the fetal middle cerebral artery during labor. Their hypothesis suggests a protective mechanism to prevent fetal cerebral hypoxia.

During contractions increased PI values were found in the fetal internal carotid artery,[58] but no difference was found in the anterior cerebral artery[64] and middle cerebral artery.[59] The varying results may be related to other variables (e.g., the intensity of the contractions, the fetal head position and station, or the degree of molding of the skull).

In pregnancies complicated by preterm labor with intact membranes, significantly reduced PI values from the middle cerebral artery were recorded when compared to fetuses delivered later or to normal reference limits for gestation.[65]

The mode of delivery does not seem to influence cerebral blood flow velocities in healthy term newborns.[66] Decompression of the fetal head during vaginal delivery may influence cerebral blood flow. Marsal and coworkers[67,68] found a very high cerebral blood flow velocity and low resistance values at the moment of birth. Ipsiroglu and associates,[69] in a study of infants delivered by cesarean section, reported the highest blood velocities among infants after prolonged and difficult delivery of the head.

PATHOLOGICAL PREGNANCIES

Fetal Anemia

In neonatal polycythemia, partial plasma-exchange transfusion improves cerebral hemodynamics; the exchange procedure results in significantly decreased hematocrit, viscosity, and PI.[14]

Vyas and colleagues[70] found mean blood flow velocity in the fetal middle cerebral artery to be increased with anemia. The blood flow velocity in red-cell-isoimmunized pregnancies was not related to fetal blood PO_2, and the relation of increased velocity to anemia was not affected by the PI; therefore, these authors suggest that the hyperdynamic circulation is a consequence of decreased blood viscosity.[71] Increased peak systolic velocity in the middle cerebral artery was found to be reliable in detecting anemia

in pregnancies complicated by maternal blood group immunization.[72] Intravascular transfusion to correct anemia was not associated with a significant difference in the PI values of cerebral vessels when measured 1 day after the procedure.[37] In fact, the PI was reduced significantly immediately after transfusion, but returned to pretransfusion levels by the following day.[15] These data suggest that the PI cannot be used as an indicator of fetal anemia.

Elevated Placental Resistance and Growth Retardation

The fetoplacental circulation is a low-resistance system in which downstream flow continues throughout the cardiac cycle. The effects of elevated placental resistance on diastolic blood flow in the main fetal arteries were studied by Fouron and associates.[73] Placental resistance was mechanically increased in exteriorized lambs by tightening a string inserted into an exposed section of umbilical cord around the vein. Doppler flow velocity waveforms were measured over the cord through an acoustic bag. Compression of the umbilical vein continued until retrograde diastolic flow was observed in the umbilical artery.

The patterns of diastolic flow observed after compression were as follows: descending aorta and aortic arch, retrograde; ascending aorta, bidirectional; and cephalic aorta, forward. These were quite different from their respective baseline patterns. The appearance of reverse diastolic flow in the umbilical artery[74] indicates, first, that the lowest vascular resistance in the fetal circulatory network is no longer at the placental but at the cerebral level; and second, that preplacental blood with low oxygen content from the descending aorta and pulmonary artery is being shifted towards the brain.

Loss of end-diastolic velocities in the fetal aorta and/or umbilical artery was observed by Arabin and collaborators[75] in 30 of 137 high-risk pregnancies, indicating a high downstream impedance. All the fetuses were growth-retarded, and the observations of absent end-diastolic velocities were made nearly 8 days before pathological cardiotocographic findings. In nine cases, the ratio of the blood flow volume in the common carotid artery to that of the fetal aorta could be determined. The values were significantly increased compared to values of undisturbed pregnancies, demonstrating a redistribution of fetal blood flow in favor of the cerebral circulation.

Failure of the physiological invasion of myometrial spiral arteries by cytotrophoblast in the second trimester and the development of acute atherosis are phenomena associated with higher vascular resistance of the feto-placental vasculature.[76]

Animal experiments have suggested that fetal growth retardation is associated with reduced umbilical and placental blood flow and increased distal resistance.[77,78] Under experimental conditions in animal models during hypoxia, the redistribution of cardiac output and increased peripheral vascular resistance, with the aim of maintaining cerebral blood flow, resulted in the "brain-sparing" effect.[43,79] This phenomenon (Figs. 17–2 and 17–3) has been suggested as the pathophysiological mechanism for asymmetrical growth retardation in the human fetus, and is characterized by relative sparing of the brain with respect to body weight. This reflex of centralization of the fetal circulation has already been established in fetal hypoxia.[27,80] Maximum reduction in PI was found when the fetal pO_2 was 2 to 4 standard deviations below the normal mean for gestation. When the oxygen deficit was greater, there was a tendency for the PI to rise, and this presumabley reflected the development of brain edema.[27] Compensatory redistribution is regulated by more than one mechanism; hypoxemia, alone or with hypercapnia, is responsible for cerebral vascular responses.[81]

In growth-retarded pregnancies, pulsatility in all of the major intracranial arteries was significantly reduced compared with normal pregnancy, suggesting participation in a brain-sparing effect in the presence of chronic fetal hypoxia.[6,8,11,13,17,25,27,40,82–92] Antenatally raised ratios were found to be associated with poor obstetric outcome (i.e., fetal death and severe growth retardation).[93] Therefore, the brain-sparing effect is suggested as a mechanism to prevent fetal brain hypoxia, rather than as a sign of impending brain damage.

Several studies have proposed Doppler criteria involving intracranial vessels to predict small-for-date (SGA) neonates. We analyzed published data concerning these criteria for which sensitivity and specificity could be determined.[94] The predictive values were computed using Bayes' theorem, based on an SGA prevalence rate of 10%. Intracranial vessels had positive predictive values ranging between 49% and 66%. The use of a lower prevalence rate in Bayes' formula would decrease the positive predictive value of all parameters.

Conflicting findings preclude the clinical use of cerebral Doppler alone as predictor of growth retardation. For example, McCown and Duggan[95] found in 28 SGA fetuses a highly significant association between an abnormal internal carotid artery waveform and a poor outcome; this was particularly pronounced at a gestational age of less than 34 weeks, when the sensitivity, specificity and predictive values were all 100%. On the other hand, in a study of 44 cases of IUGR with eight perinatal deaths,

Wladimiroff and colleagues[96] found no correlation between the indicators of fetal well-being (i.e., Apgar score at 1 min, FHR patterns, umbilical arterial pH) and the internal carotid artery PI. This group[20] considered the end velocities in the anterior and middle cerebral artery to be the most sensitive parameters discriminating between small for gestational age fetuses and control fetuses but found the umbilical artery PI to be the best indicator for the SGA fetus.

Maternal hyperoxygenation has been suggested for treatment of growth-retarded and hypoxic fetuses.[97,98] No effect was observed on placental RIs, but flow waveforms were modified in cerebral arteries.[99] Such a positive response was found to be a good prognostic factor, in contrast to the poor prognosis associated with a negative test response, which may indicate gross placental failure such that fetal PO_2 cannot be improved.[100,101]

Twin Discordance

The value of Doppler waveform analysis in the surveillance of twin fetuses was assessed by us in a prospective longitudinal study.[45] Measurements of indices from the internal carotid and umbilical arteries gave an overall sensitivity in prediction of an SGS fetus of 58% and a positive predictive value of 71%. These data were not as sensitive and specific as our earlier data.[44] However, Doppler changes preceded ultrasound diagnosis of growth retardation by a mean interval of 3.7 weeks and demonstrated greater specificity and sensitivity. A combination of these parameters improved sensitivity to 84% and may complement real-time ultrasonography for the early diagnosis of abnormal growth in twin pregnancies. Rizzo and coworkers[102] found different trends in Doppler serial recordings according to the underlying mechanism of growth defect. Gaziano and colleagues[103] studied fetal growth and blood flow distribution in diamniotic monochorionic compared with dizygotic (diamniotic/dichorionic) twins. They found that diamniotic/monochorionic twins from the lower birth weight group more often show blood flow redistribution compared with dizygotic twins of similar low birth weight. Placental vascular connections and the attendant hemodynamic changes in this group probably account for this difference. Brain sparing events occurred commonly without clinical twin-to-twin transfusion syndrome.

Ventriculomegaly and Increased Intracranial Pressure

In adults, the volume of blood, spinal fluid, and brain tissue in the cranium at any time must be relatively constant (Monro–Kellie doctrine).[104] During

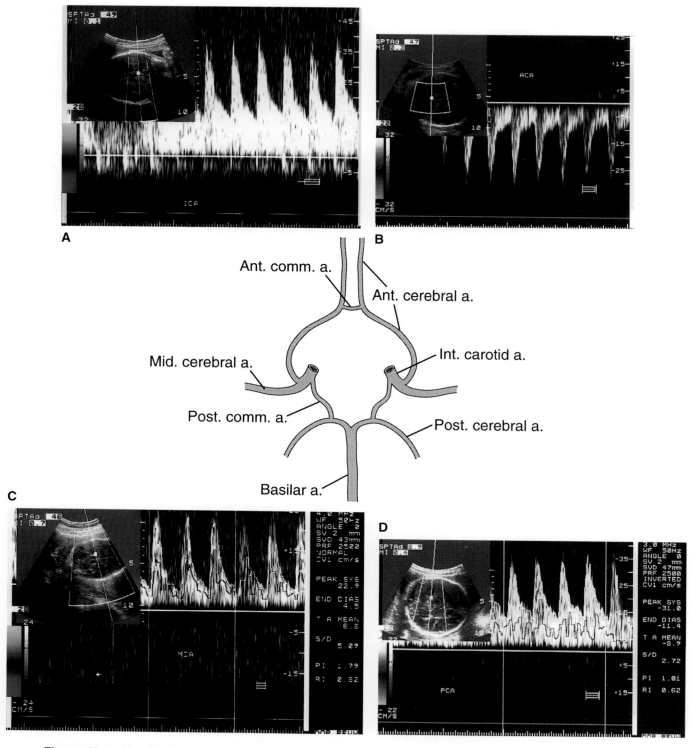

Figure 17–2. Doppler frequency spectra from arteries of the circle of Willis with normal flow velocities and pulsed waveforms. **A.** Internal carotid artery. **B.** Anterior cerebral artery. **C.** Middle cerebral artery. **D.** Posterior cerebral artery.

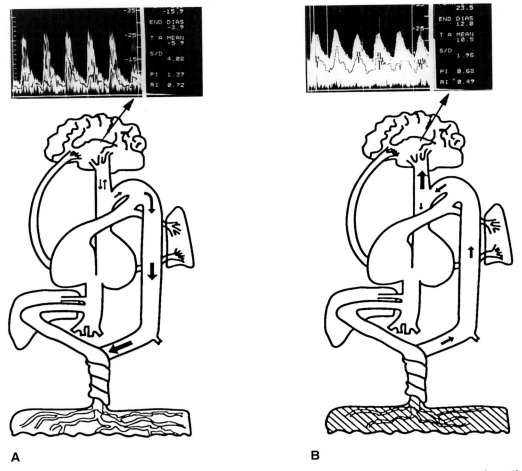

Figure 17–3. Schematic drawing of fetal diastolic flow distribution and flow velocity waveforms from the middle cerebral artery in the presence of normal **(A)** and increased **(B)** placental resistance.

fetal life, the fontanelles and the open skull sutures enable better adaptation to increased intracranial volume. Hill and Volpe[105] found ventriculomegaly to be a more critical factor than intracranial pressure in the pathogenesis of the impaired flow in infantile hydrocephaly.

The effect of ventriculomegaly on cerebral pulsatile flow was studied by us in four hydrocephalic fetuses.[106] The PI in the internal carotid artery showed progressive elevation, proportional to the developing ventriculomegaly.

Van den Wijngaard and associates[107] presented data on nine fetuses with bilateral symmetrical hydrocephaly and four with unilateral hydrocephaly. An elevated internal carotid artery PI was demonstrated in five cases. The fetal outcome was poor: only one infant seemed to be developing normally at 1 year of age. However, in contrast to reports on elevated PI, according to Kirkinen and colleagues,[108] blood flow patterns seem to differ individually from case to case. Normal, increased, and decreased veloc-

ity waveform indices could be measured. The discrepancies in results may be related to different pathophysiological mechanisms of hydrocephaly.

Posterior fossa subdural hematoma was diagnosed antenatally by Ben-Chetrit and associates[109] in a fetus at 30 weeks of gestation. Doppler studies of the middle cerebral artery showed an abnormally high resistance pattern with reverse end diastolic flow reflecting high intracranial pressure; associated quadriplegia was noted during ultrasound assessment. Color Doppler energy imaging (power Doppler) may help in the diagnosis of intracranial hemorrhage.[110] Another case of cerebral intraparenchymal hemorrhage[111] allowed the authors to analyze the evolution of cerebral Doppler abnormalities but the modifications in Doppler velocimetry could not be predicted.

The underlying disorder and the presence of other malformations rather than cerebral blood flow measurements, are of greater prognostic value regarding brain damage in fetuses with hydrocephaly.

Arteriovenous Malformations

A cerebral cystic structure in the median plane with turbulent flow pattern within the lesion and decreased cerebral vascular resistance is typical of an arteriovenous malformation.[112–114] An aneurysm of the vein of Galen may lead to cardiac failure and nonimmune hydrops fetalis.[113,115] Fetuses without evidence of hydrocephaly or signs of cardiac insufficiency were followed and treated postnatally by embolization.[116–118] Very high volume blood flow in the draining prosencephalic vein were measured in two cases by Goelz and colleagues.[119] The huge shunting of blood flow in this vein was associated with the development of severe encephalomalacia and progressive heart failure of both fetuses.

PHARMACOLOGICAL ASPECTS

Various drugs administered to the mother during pregnancy are reported to affect cerebral blood flow.

Ritodrin infusion for premature uterine contractions was associated with significantly decreased waveform indices in the middle cerebral and renal arteries. There was no change in the indices of the umbilical artery.[47]

Magnesium supplementation during pregnancy, particularly in cases of preterm labor, was found to be associated with a decrease in vascular resistance, both in the umbilical artery and in the fetal middle cerebral artery.[120]

Indomethacin for preterm labor or polyhydramnios resulted in constriction of the ductus arteriosus in 11 of 13 fetuses, within 48 h of therapy.[121] In the fetuses that manifested both ductal constriction and tricuspid insufficiency, the PI of the middle cerebral artery decreased significantly.[121] In another randomized controlled trial,[122] indomethacin did not significantly affect cerebral blood flow. If antenatal indomethacin in preterm fetus increases the risk of intraventricular hemorrhage, it would appear to be by another mechanism.

Prostaglandin E_2 administered intracervically for preinduction cervical ripening was found to be associated with increased pulsatility in cerebral artery.[123]

Nifedipine therapy for preterm labor had no influence on Doppler criteria of either fetal or uteroplacental circulation.[124]

Betamethasone administration causes a transient but considerable reduction in fetal body and breathing movements and in fetal heart rate variation. No significant changes occurred in the PI of uterine arteries, umbilical arteries, fetal aorta and renal artery, and fetal cerebral arteries, suggesting

that the change is not mediated through fetal hypoxemia.[125]

Nicotine injections induced vasoconstriction on the umbilical and cerebral arteries of ovine fetuses and were associated with poor perinatal outcome.[126]

Extradural anesthesia (e.g., with bupivacaine) had no detrimental effects on the uteroplacental and fetal circulation in the uncomplicated pregnancy when maternal hypotension was avoided with rapid prehydration.[127]

Oxygen administration to the mother was followed by increase of maternal PO_2, which raised the pressure difference in PO_2 across the placenta.[97,98] Fetal PO_2 increased if it was below the normal range. Oxygen administration had no effect on placental RIs, but modified the waveforms in cerebral arteries.[99] Maternal oxygenation results in velocity waveform changes that that suggest an increase of cerebral vascular resistance and a redistribution of blood from the brain to the vascular beds supplied by the ascending aorta.[100,101] Absent or reversed end-diastolic velocity in the aortic isthmus appears to be an early sign of blood redistribution in SGA fetuses.[128]

Carbon dioxide is also an important determinant of cerebral blood flow. Inhalation of a prepared gas mixture with 2% to 3% carbon dioxide or increased PCO_2 in patients undergoing controlled hyperventilation selectively caused a decrease in resistance in the fetal cerebral circulation.[129,130]

Nitrous oxide inhalation.[131] Both maternal and fetal cerebral vascular resistance were decreased by 30% nitrous oxide inhalation. No adverse effects to mother or fetus have been demonstrated in clinical practice. However, preterm fetuses are susceptible to intracranial hemorrhage, and the cerebral hyperemia by nitrous oxide might increase the risk of hemorrhage in these fetuses. From animal experiment it is known that nitric oxide (NO) influences cerebral vascular tone both in the normal fetus and in the hypoxemic fetus.[132] Prostaglandins are important in facilitating the full expression of NO-induced vasodilation.

FETAL DISTRESS

The significant alterations in cerebral flow velocity and PI in fetal hypoxemia and acidemia suggest the use of Doppler criteria to detect imminent fetal distress in complicated pregnancies. Combinations of Doppler parameters from various vessels may be used.

1. The cerebro-umbilical Doppler ratio (the ratio between the PI of the middle cerebral artery and the PI of the umbilical

artery) is usually constant during the last 10 weeks of gestation.[133] Using a single cut-off value, it was found to provide a better predictor for adverse perinatal outcome than the PI of either artery alone. The predictive value of the ratio in diagnosing SGA newborns was 70%, compared to 54.4% for the middle cerebral artery and 65.5% for the umbilical artery.

2. Serial measurement of mean velocity of the fetal descending thoracic aorta is the best fetal parameter identifying prolonged pregnancy at increased risk for perinatal complications,[134] but the velocity ratio of the fetal common carotid artery to the fetal descending thoracic aorta had the highest predictive capacity for the SGA pregnancy complicated by fetal distress.[80]

Arduini and colleagues[135] reported on Doppler studies from fetal vessels preceding the onset of late decelerations in growth-retarded fetuses. Maximum vasodilatation in cerebral arteries was reached 2 weeks before the onset of antepartum late fetal heart rate decelaration, whereas significant changes in the peripheral and umbilical vessels occurred close to the onset of abnormal fetal heart rate patterns. Weiner and coworkers[136] reported on abnormal fetal heart rate pattern in fetuses with absent end-diastolic velocity in the umbilical artery when the middle cerebral artery begins to lose its compensatory dilation.

In another preliminary report, pathological fetal heart rate changes were associated with changes in diastolic flux to the brain; in one case the change was biphasic, returning to basic levels, and was interpreted as possible loss of cerebrovascular autoregulation.[137] Hypoxemia at delivery appeared to be better recognized by the fetal velocity waveform of the middle cerebral artery than by the fetal heart rate analysis.[138]

The response of the ovine fetus to umbilical cord compression with variable-type heart rate deceleration were studied by Richardson and coworkers.[139] Although cerebral oxidative metabolism appeared to be well maintained during moderate to severe variable deceleration, the need to increase fractional oxygen extraction and the redistribution of blood flow from carcass tissue may contribute to an accumulation of lactic acid both within the brain and systemically when such an insult occurs repeatedly.

High perinatal mortality has been reported in association with the finding of absent end-diastolic flow velocity in the umbilical artery. In these cases, abnormal end-diastolic umbilical venous pulsation in the cord is a late and ominous sign of a severely compromised fetus,[140] whereas abnormal blood flow velocimetry in the middle cerebral artery might be an earlier sign of fetal hypoxia, with a better prognosis. Visualization of the fetal coronary blood flow in severe uteroplacental insufficiency was suggested as a preterminal event.[141,142]

In prolonged pregnancy[143,144] resistance in the middle cerebral artery did not change abruptly when gestation exceeded 287 days. Doppler studies in pregnancies with preterm prelabor amniorrhexis[145] demonstrated that microbial invasion of the amniotic cavity and fetal bacteremia are not associated with detectable changes in fetal circulation and oxygenation.

FETAL DEATH

Reverse end-diastolic flow in the middle cerebral artery may be an ominous sign and was suggested as one of the terminal hemodynamic events preceding fetal death.[146] In the majority of cases the cause of the observed phenomenon remains unknown, but an increase in pressure in the right ventricle and possible tricuspid regurgitation should be considered.[147] Few reports on the terminal patterns of the fetal cerebral blood velocity have been published.[146–150] Two pregnant women with hypertension and early severe IUGR and one with lupus anticoagulants showed decreasing PI on follow-up examinations. Increased impedance to flow was found in Doppler measurements obtained close to fetal death. This pattern may reflect a phase of decompensation with loss of the brain sparing phenomenon. Preterminal brain edema has been suggested on the underlying cause of this effect which has been noted in studies on monkey fetuses deprived of oxygen.[2] Heart rate pattern with loss of long- and short-term variability with or without decelerations is suggestive of severe brain impairment and described after fetal decerebration.[151]

Cerebral Blood Flow in Neonatal Period

Using the anterior fontanelle as an acoustic window, the anterior cerebral artery can be easily insonated in the neonate. The artery curves around the corpus callosum (where it is called the pericallosal artery), running along the longitudinal fissure from anterior to posterior. The pulsed Doppler has enabled investigation of other major cerebral vessels.

Cerebral autoregulation continues to play a role in the neonatal period as in fetal life. The ability of the brain to maintain constant perfusion in varying perfusion pressures was demonstrated in newborn experimental animals.[152] Investigations of the pattern of cerebral flow velocity waveforms in the first week of life in healthy full-term newborns showed initial decrease in cerebral blood flow velocity[68,153] followed by stabilization and subsequent increase.[154,155] The early changes can be attributed to fall of pO_2. A linear increase in cerebral blood flow velocity with increasing postnatal age has been reported.[154,155]

Perinatal Asphyxia

Different pathologic brain tissue changes are reported after perinatal asphyxia in the very preterm infant (33 postmenstrual weeks or less) compared to the more mature newborn. Based on a different blood perfusion pattern in the brain, peri-intraventricular hemorrhage is a common event in the very preterm infant. After 33 postmenstrual weeks, parenchymal hemorrhages or infarctions with or without cerebral edema are the typical manifestations of hypoxic-ischemic encephalopathy. Cerebral arterial blood supply is predominantly directed to basal ganglia at the early stage and to the white matter later. Bada[4] found that infants who experienced perinatal asphyxia and subsequent periventricular hemorrhage demonstrated a lower PI of the anterior cerebral artery prior to hemorrhage, followed by high indices at the occurance of hemorrhage indicating vasospasm. A fluctuating pattern of flow velocity waveform was found in extension of peri-intraventricular hemorrhage.[156] In term infants after acute, near-total intrauterine asphyxia at the end of labor, imaging studies documented a consistent pattern of injury in subcortical brain nuclei, including thalamus, basal ganglia, and brainstem. In contrast, the cerebral cortex and white matter were relatively spared.[157] This clinical and imaging syndrome is in contrast with that seen in more prolonged but less severe intrauterine asphyxia, in which shunting of blood flow from the nonbrain organs to the brain and from cerebral hemispheres to the thalamus and brainstem renders organs other than the brain and cerebral hemispheres most vulnerable.

In full-term perinatally asphyxiated infants, decreased PI was found,[158] compared with a control group. These hemodynamic changes were positively correlated with hypoxic-ischemic encephalopathy. Low PI values in first days were predictive of adverse outcome.

Growth Retarded Newborns

Cerebral autoregulation has been shown to be disturbed in hypoxic,[159] hypercarbic, and hypocar-

bic[160,161] human neonates. Chronic intrauterine hypoxia is an important cause of fetal growth retardation. Continuation of the fetal situation of the lower cerebrovascular resistence was demonstrated in SGA infants.[162–164] Changes in arterial carbon dioxide tension result in changes of cerebral blood flow.[160,161] Extreme elevation decreased cerebrovascular resistance and transmural pressure in the capillaries to the point of germinal matrix hemorrhage. Severe hypocarbia induced by hypoventilation can result in ischemic and periventricular leukomalacia in preterm infants.

Various Clinical Conditions in the Neonate

The awake state was found to be associated with increased cerebral blood flow velocity compared to quiet or active sleep.[165]

A patent ductus arteriosus influences cerebrovascular resistance, causing an increase in RI.[166,167] Delayed closure was reported in neonate after preinduction intracervical prostaglandin E_2 administration.[168] Closure of the ductus arteriosus by indomethacin is associated with decrease in mean cerebral blood flow velocity, these changes were suggested as a marker of increased risk of peri-intraventricular hemorrhage.[169–171] In neonatal hydrocephaly an abnormally high RI was described, returning to normal values after drainage.[105,170]

Changes in Doppler indices that were found to reflect changes in systemic blood pressure were described in neonates with endotracheal suction,[172] pneumothorax,[173] seizures,[173] apnea, and bradycardia.[174]

SUMMARY

Data collected from Doppler velocity recordings using both spectral and color Doppler mode, confirm the fundmental aspects of the fetoplacental circulation. Changes in placental vascular resistance, cardiac contractibility, vessel compliance, and blood viscosity alter the normal dynamics of fetal cerebral circulation. These data have improved the understanding of the regulatory mechanisms involved in fetal cerebral hemodynamic events. Reference values have been established for the main cerebral vessels. During the last trimester in normal pregnancies, the values of Doppler waveform indices decrease in all main cerebral vessels. After birth, vascular resistance decreased and stabilized later. Cerebral autoregulation persists from fetal to postnatal life, with low waveform indices in cerebral vessels of growth-retarded fetuses and neonates. The low indices indicate decreased cerebrovascular resistance representing the redistribution of flow—the brain-sparing effect.

Clinical application of the simple and noninvasive Doppler technique remains incompletely defined. Flow velocity changes in cerebral vessels are major components of Doppler evaluation; management of the SGA age fetus may be aided by study of waveforms from these vessels. Combined parameters recorded from different vascular beds may provide support for the diagnosis of significant hemodynamic changes and are of prognostic value in predicting fetal outcome.

REFERENCES

1. Nelson KB, Leviton A. How much of neonatal encephalopathy is due to birth asphyxia? *Am J Dis Child.* 1991;145:1325–1331.

2. Myers RF, de Courtney-Myers GM, Wagner KR. Effects of hypoxia on fetal brain. In: Beard RW, Nathanielaz PW, eds. *Fetal Physiology and Medicine.* London: Butterworths; 1984;419–436.

3. Edvinsson I, Mackenzie ET, McCullock J. *Cerebral Blood Flow and Metabolism.* New York: Raven Press; 1993:40–56.

4. Bada HS, Hajjar W, Chua C, et al. Noninvasive diagnosis of neonatal asphyxia and intraventricular hemorrhage by Doppler ultrasound recording of flow velocity in basal cerebral arteries. *J Neurosurg.* 1979; 57:769–774.

5. Asalid R, Markwalder TM, Normes H. Noninvasive transcranial Doppler ultrasound recording of flow velocity in basal cerebral arteries. *J Neurosurg.* 1982; 57:769–774.

6. Wladimiroff JW, Tonge HM, Stewart PA. Doppler ultrasound assessment of cerebral blood flow in the human fetus. *Br J Obstet Gynaecol.* 1986;93:471–475.

7. Alpers BJ, Berry RG, Paddison RM. Anatomical studies of the circle of Willis in normal brain. *Arch Neurol Psychiatr.* 1959;81:409–418.

8. Woo JK, Liang ST, Lo RS, et al. Middle cerebral artery Doppler flow velocity waveforms. *Obstet Gynecol.* 1987;70:613–616.

9. Asalid R. *Transcranial Doppler Sonography.* New York: Springer-Verlag; 1986:42–56.

10. Miller DJ, Bill BA. Cerebral blood flow variations with perfusion pressure and metabolism. In: Wood JH, ed. *Cerebral Blood Flow.* New York: McGraw Hill; 1987:119–131.

11. Mari G, Moise KJ, Deter RL, et al. Doppler assessment of the pulsatility index in cerebral circulation of the human fetus. *Am J Obstet Gynecol.* 1989;160: 698–703.

12. Arbeille PH, Tranquart F, Benson M, et al. Visualization of the fetal circle of Willis and intracerebral arteries by color-coded Doppler. *Eur J Obstet Gynecol Reprod Biol.* 1989;32:195–198.

13. Lewinsky RM, Farine D, Ritchie JWK. Transvaginal Doppler assessment of the fetal cerebral circulation. *Obstet Gynecol.* 1991;78:637–640.

14. Bada HS, Korones SB, Kolni HW, et al. Partial plasma-exchange transfusion improves cerebral hemodynamics in symptomatic neonatal polycythemia. *Am J Med Sci.* 1986;291:157–163.

15. Mari G, Moise KJ, Deter RL. Flow velocity waveforms of the umbilical and cerebral arteries before and after intravascular transfusion. *Obstet Gynecol.* 1990;75:584–589.

16. Mirro R, Gonzalez A. Perinatal anterior cerebral artery Doppler flow indexes: Methods and preliminary results. *Am J Obstet Gynecol.* 1987;156:1227–1231.

17. Arbeille P, Roncin A, Berson M, et al. Exploration of the fetal cerebral blood flow by duplex Doppler-linear, assay system in normal and pathological pregnancies. *Ultrasound Med Biol.* 1987;13:329–337.

18. Meerman RJ, Van Bel F, Van Zuiten PH, et al. Fetal and neonatal cerebral blood velocity in the normal fetus and neonate. *Early Hum Dev.* 1990;24:209–217.

19. Raju TN. Cerebral Doppler studies in the fetus and newborn infant. *J Pediatr.* 1991;119:165–174.

20. Noordam MJ, Heydanus R, Hop WC, et al. Doppler color flow imaging of fetal intracerebral arteries and umbilical artery in the small for gestational age fetus. *Br J Obstet Gynaecol.* 1994;101:504–508.

21. Marsal K, Lindblad A, Lingman G, et al. Blood flow in the fetal descending aorta: Intrinsic factors affecting fetal blood flow, i.e., fetal breathing movements and cardiac arrhythmia. *Ultrasound Med Biol.* 1984;10:339–349.

22. Gosling RG, King DH. Ultrasound angiology. In: Marcus AW, Adamson L, eds. *Arteries and Veins.* Edinburgh: Churchill-Livingstone; 1975:61–75.

23. Fong K, Ryan ML, Cohen H, et al. Doppler velocimetry of the fetal middle cerebral and renal arteries: Interobserver reliability. *J Ultrasound Med.* 1996;15: 317–321.

24. Alcazar JL. Intraobserver variability of pulsatility index measurements in three fetal vessels in the first trimester. *J Clin Ultrasound.* 1997;25:366–371.

25. Arbeiile P, Body G, Saliba E, et al. Fetal cerebral circulation assessment by Doppler ultrasound in normal and pathological pregnancies. *Eur J Obstet Gynecol Reprod Biol.* 1988;29:261–273.

26. Arabin B, Mohnhaupt A, Becker R, et al. Comparison of the prognostic value of pulsed Doppler blood flow parameters to predict SGA and fetal distress. *Ultrasound Obstet Gynecol.* 1992;2:272–278.

27. Vyas S, Nicolaides KH, Bower S, et al. Middle cerebral artery flow velocity waveforms in fetal hypoxaemia. *Br J Obstet Gynaecol.* 1990;97:797–803.

28. Laurichesse-Delmass H, Grimaud O, Moscoso G, et al. Color Doppler study of the venous circulation in the fetal brain and hemodynamic study of the cerebral transverse sinus. *Ultrasound Obstet Gynecol.* 1999;13:34–42.

29. Pooh PK, Aono T. Transvaginal power Doppler angiography of the fetal brain. *Ultrasound Obstet Gynecol.* 1996;8:417–421.

30. Kurjak A, Predonic M, Kupesic S, et al. Transvaginal color Doppler study of middle cerebral blood flow in

early normal and abnormal pregnancy. *Ultrasound Obstet Gynecol.* 1992;2:424–428.

31. Wladimiroff JW, Van den Wijngaard JAGW, Degani S, et al. Cerebral and umbilical arterial blood flow velocity waveforms in normal and growth-retarded pregnancies. *Obstet Gynecol.* 1987;69:705–709.

32. Hata K, Hata T, Makihara K, et al. Fetal intracranial arterial hemodynamics assessed by color and pulsed Doppler ultrasound. *Int J Gynecol Obstet.* 1991;35:139–145.

33. Gilbert RD, Pearce W, Ashwal S, et al. Effects of hypoxia on contractility of isolated fetal cerebral arteries. *J Dev Physiol.* 1990;13:199–203.

34. Bilardo CM, Campbell S, Nicolaides KH. Mean blood velocities and flow impedance in the fetal descending thoracic aorta and common carotid artery in normal pregnancy. *Early Hum. Dev.* 1988;18:213–221.

35. Ferrazi E, Gementi P, Bellotti M, et al. Doppler velocimetry: Critical analysis of umbilical cerebral and aortic reference values. *Eur J Obstet Gynecol Reprod Biol.* 1991;38:189–196.

36. Satoh S, Kojanagi T, Hara K, et al. Developmental characteristics of blood flow flow in the middle cerebral artery in the human fetus in *utero,* assessed using the linear assay-pulsed Doppler method. *Early Hum Dev.* 1988;17:195–203.

37. Veille JC, Hanson R, Tatum K. Longitudinal quantitation of middle cerebral artery blood flow in normal human fetuses. *Am J Obset Gynecol.* 1994;169:l393–1398.

38. Arduini D, Rizzo G. Normal values of pulsatility index from fetal vessels: A cross sectional study on 1556 healthy fetuses. *J Perinat Med.* 1990;18:165–172.

39. Van den Wijngaard JAGW, Groenenberg IAI, Wladimiroff JW, et al. Cerebral Doppler ultrasound of the human fetus. *Br J Obstet Gynecol.* 1989;96:845–849.

40. Mari G, Deter RL. Middle cerebral artery flow velocity waveforms in normal and small-for-gestational-age fetuses. *Am J Obstet Gynecol.* 1992;166:1262–1270.

42. Jaeren H, Funk A, Goetz M, et al. Development of quantitative Doppler indices for uteroplacental and fetal blood flow during the third trimester. *Ultrasound Med Biol.* 1996;22:823–835.

43. Peeters LLH, Sheldon RE, Jones MD, et al. Blood flow to fetal organs as a function of arterial oxygen content. *Am J Obstet Gynecol.* 1979;135:637–646.

44. Degani S, Paltiely Y, Lewinsky R, et al. Fetal internal carotid artery flow velocity time waveforms in twin pregnancies. *J Perinat Med.* 1988;16:405–409.

45. Degani S, Gonen R, Shapiro I, et al. Doppler flow velocity waveform analysis in fetal surveillance of twins: A prospective longitudinal study. *J Ultrasound Med.* 1992;11:537–541.

46. Mari S, Moise KJ Jr, Deter RL, et al. Fetal heart rate influence on the pulsatility index in the middle cerebral artery. *J Clin Ultrasound.* 1991;19:149–153.

47. Rasanen J. The effect of ritodrine infusion on fetal myocardial function and fetal hemodynamics. *Acta Obstet Gynecol Scand.* 1990;69:487–492.

48. Wladimiroff JW, Van Bel F. Fetal and neonatal cerebral blood flow. *Semin Perinatol.* 1987;11:335–346.

49. Nijhuis JG, Prechtl HFR, Martin CB Jr. Are there behavioral states in the human fetus? *Early Hum Dev.* 1982;6:177–195.

50. Van Eyck J, Wladimiroff JW, van den Wijngaard J.A, et al. The blood flow velocity waveform in the fetal internal carotid and umbilical artery: Its relation to fetal behaviour in normal pregnancy at 37–38 weeks. *Br J Obstet Gynaecol.* 1987;94:736–741.

51. Degani S, Paltiely Y, Gonen R, et al. Fetal internal carotid artery pulsed Doppler velocity waveforms and maternal plasma glucose levels. *Obstet Gynecol.* 1991;7:379–381.

52. Pardo J, Orvieto N, Rabinerson D, et al. Fetal middle cerebral and umbilical artery flow assessment after glucose challenge test. *Int J Gynecol Obstet.* 1999;65:255–259.

53. Pryds O, Greisen G, Friis-Hansen B. Compensatory increase of CBF in preterm infants during hypoglycemia. *Acta Peadiatr Scand.* 1988;77:632–637.

54. Gillis S, Conners G, Potts P, et al. The effect of glucose on Doppler flow velocity waveforms and heart rate pattern in the human fetus. *Early Hum Dev.* 1992;30:1–10.

55. Vyas S, Campbell S, Bower S, et al. Maternal abdominal pressure alters fetal cerebral blood flow. *Br J Obstet Gynaecol.* 1990;97:740–742.

56. Van den Wijngaard JAGW, Wladimiroff JW, Reuss A, et al. Oligohydramnios and fetal cerebral blood flow. *Br J Obstet Gynaecol.* 1988;95:1309–1311.

57. Mari G, Wasserstrum N, Kirshon B. Reduction in the middle cerebral artery pulsatility index after decompression of polyhydramnios in twin gestation. *Am J Perinatal.* 1992;9:381–384.

58. Fendel H, Funk A, Jorn J. Cerebral blood flow during labor. *Z Geburtsh Perinatol.* 1990;194:272–274.

59. Maesel A, Lingman G, Marsal K. Cerebral blood flow during labor. *Z Geburtsh Perinatol.* 1992;194:272–274.

60. Yagel S, Anteby E, Levy Y, et al. Fetal middle cerebral artery blood flow during normal active labour and in labour with variable decelerators. *Br J Obstet Gynaecol.* 1992;99:483–485.

61. Lindblad A, Berman J, Marsal K. Obstetric analgesia and fetal aortic blood flow during labour. *Br J Obstet Gynaecol.* 1987;94:306–311.

62. Fleischer A, Anyaegbumam AA, Schulman H, et al. Uterine and umbilical artery velocimetry during normal labor. *Am J Obstet Gynecol.* 1987;157:40–43.

63. Brar HS, Platt ID, De Vore GR, et al. Qualitative assessment of maternal uterine and fetal umbilical artery blood flow and resistance in laboring patients by Doppler velocimetry. *Am J Obstet Gynecol.* 1988;158:952–956.

64. Mirro R, Gonzalez A. Perinatal anterior cerebral artery Doppler flow indexes: Methods and preliminary results. *Am J Obstet Gynecol.* 1987;156:1227–1231.

65. Rizzo G, Capponi A, Arduini D, et al. Uterine and fetal blood flows in pregnancies complicated by preterm labor. *Gynecol Obstet Invest.* 1996;42:163–166.

66. Shuto H, Yashuhara A, Sugimoto T, et al. Longitudinal determination of cerebral blood flow velocity in neonates with the Doppler technique. *Neuropediatrics.* 1988;18:218–221.

67. Marsal K, Gunmarsson G, Ley DR, et al. Cerebral circulation in the perinatal period. In: Kurjak A, Chervenak FA, eds. *The Fetus as a Patient.* New York: Parthenon; 1994:4.

68. Maesel A, Sladkevicius P, Valentin L, et al. Fetal cerebral blood flow velocity during labor and the early neonatal period. *Ultrasound Obstet Gynecol.* 1995;4:372–376.

69. Ipsiroglu OS, Stockler S, Hausler MCH, et al. Cerebral blood flow velocities in the first minutes of life. *Eur J Pediatr.* 1993;152:269–271.

70. Vyas S, Nicolaides KH, Campbell S. Doppler examination of the middle cerebral artery in anemic fetuses. *Am J Obstet Gynecol.* 1990;162:1066–1068.

71. Mari G, Moise KJ Jr, Deter RL, et al. Flow velocity waveforms of the vascular system in the anemic fetus before and after intravascular transfusion for severe red blood cell alloimmunization. *Am J Obstet Gynecol.* 1990;162:1060–1064.

72. Mari G, Adrignolo A, Abuhamed AZ, et al. Diagnosis of fetal anemia with Doppler ultrasound in the pregnancy complicated by maternal blood group immunization. *Ultrasound Obstet Gynecol.* 1995;5:400–405.

73. Fouron JC, Teyssier G, Maroto E, et al. Diastolic circulatory dynamics in the presence of elevated placental resistance and retrograde diastolic flow in the umbilical artery: A Doppler echographic study in lambs. *Am J Obstet Gynecol.* 1991;164:195–203.

74. Fouron JC, Teyssier G, Shalaby L, Lessard M, et al. Fetal central blood flow alterations in human fetus with umbilical artery reversed diastolic flow. *Am J Perinatol.* 1993;10:197–207.

75. Arabin B, Siebert M, Jimenez E, et al. Obstetrical characteristics of a loss of end-diastolic velocities in the fetal aorta and/or umbilical artery using Doppler ultrasound. *Gynecol Obstet Invest.* 1988;25:173–180.

76. Khong TY, De Wolf F, Robertson WB, et al. Inadequate maternal vascular response to placentation in pregnancies complicated by small for gestational age infants. *Br J Obstet Gynaecol.* 1986;93:1049–1059.

77. Clap JF, Szeto HH, Larrow R, et al. Umbilical blood flow response to embolization of the uterine circulation. *Am J Obstet Gynecol.* 1980;138:60–67.

78. Creasy RK, Barret T, De Swiet M, et al. Experimental intrauterine growth retardation in the sheep. *Am J Obstet Gynecol.* 1972;112:566–573.

79. Berman RE, Less MH, Peterson EN, et al. Distribution of the circulation in the normal and asphyxiated fetal primate. *Am J Obstet Gynecol.* 1970;108:956–969.

80. Bilardo CM, Nicolaides KH, Campbell S. Doppler measurements of fetal and uteroplacental circulations: Relationship with umbilical venous blood gases measured at cordocentesis. *Am J Obstet Gynecol.* 1990;162:115–120.

81. Akalin Sel T, Nicolaides KH, Peacock J, et al. Doppler dynamics and their complex interrelation with fetal oxygen pressure, carbon dioxide pressure and pH in growth retarded fetuses. *Obstet Gynecol* 1994;84:439–444.

82. Kirkinen P, Muller R, Huch R, et al. Blood flow velocity waveforms in human fetal intracranial arteries. *Obstet Gynecol.* 1987;70:617–621.

83. Lingman G, Marsal K. Noninvasive assessment of cranial blood circulation in the fetus. *Biol Neonate.* 1989;56:129–135.

84. Veille JC, Cohen I. Middle cerebral artery blood flow in normal and growth-retarded fetuses. *Am J Obstet Gynecol.* 1990;162:391–396.

85. Degani S, Paltiely Y, Lewinsky R, et al. Fetal blood flow velocity waveforms in pregnancies complicated by intrauterine growth retardation. *Isr J Med Sci.* 1990;26:250–254.

86. Campbell S, Vyas S, Nicolaides KH. Doppler investigation of the fetal circulation. *J Perinat Med.* 1991;19:21–26.

87. Arbeille P. Fetal arterial Doppler—IUGR and hypoxia. *Eur J Obstet Gynecol Reprod Biol.* 1997;75:51–53.

88. Loy GL, Lin CC, Chien EK, et al. Cerebral and umbilical vascular resistance response to vibroacustic stimulation in growth restricted fetuses. *Obstet Gynecol.* 1997;90:947–952.

89. Yoshima S, Masuzaki H, Miura K, et al. Fetal blood flow redistribution in term intrauterine growth retardation and postnatal growth. *Int J Gynecol Obstet.* 1998;60:3–8.

90. Forouzan I, Tian ZY. Fetal middle cerebral artery blood flow velocities in pregnancies complicated by intrauterine growth restriction and extreme abnormality in umbilical artery Doppler velocity. *Am J Perinatol.* 1996;13:139–142.

91. Bahado-Singh RO, Kovanci E, Jeffres A, et al. The Doppler cerebroplacental ratios and perinatal outcome in intrauterine growth restriction. *Am J Obstet Gynecol.* 1999;180:750–756.

92. Harrington K, Carpenter RG, Nguyen M, et al. Changes observed in Doppler studies of the fetal circulation in pregnancies complicated by preeclampsia or the delivery of a SGA baby. I. Cross sectional analysis. *Ultrasound Obstet Gynecol.* 1995;6:19–28.

93. Scherjon SA, Smolders-De-Haas H, Kok JH, et al. The "brain-sparing" effect: Antenatal cerebral Doppler findings in relation to neurologic outcome in very preterm infants. *Am J Obstet Gynecol.* 1993;169:169–175.

94. Degani S, Sharf M. Predictive values of Doppler criteria for intrauterine growth retardation in non-umbilical fetal vessels. *Isr J Obstet Gynecol.* 1991;2:138–142.

95. McCowan JME, Duggan PM. Abnormal internal carotid and umbilical artery Doppler in the small for gestational age fetus predicts an adverse outcome. *Early Hum Dev.* 1992;30:249–259.

96. Wladimiroff JW, Noordam MJ, Van Der Wijngaard JAGW, et al. Fetal internal carotid and umbilical ar-

tery blood flow velocity waveforms as a measure of fetal well-being in intrauterine growth retardation. *Pediatr Res.* 1988;24:609–612.

97. Nicolaides KH, Campbell S, Bradley KJ, et al. Maternal oxygen therapy for intrauterine growth retardation. *Lancet.* 1987;1:942–945.

98. Arduini P, Rizzo G, Mancuso S, et al. Short-term effects of maternal oxygen administration in blood flow velocity waveforms in healthy and growth-retarded fetuses. *Am J Obstet Gynecol.* 1988;159:1077–1080.

99. Arduini D, Rizzo G, Romanini C, et al. Fetal haemodynamic response to acute maternal hyperoxygenation as predictor of fetal distress in intra-uterine growth retardation. *Br Med J.* 1989;298:1561–1562.

100. de Rochambeau B, Poix P, Mellier G. Maternal hyperoxygenation: A fetal blood flow velocity prognosis test in small-for-gestational-age fetuses? *Ultrasound Obstet Gynecol.* 1992;2:279–282.

101. Caforio L, Caruso A, Testa AC, et al. Short term maternal oxygen administration in fetuses with absence or reversal of end diastolic velocity in umbilical artery: Pathophysiological and clinical considerations. *Acta Obstet Gynecol Scand.* 1998;77: 707–711.

102. Rizzo G, Arduini D, Romanini C. Cardiac and extracardiac flows in discordant twins. *Am J Obstet Gynecol.* 1994;170:1321–1327.

103. Gaziano E, Gaziano C, Brandt D, et al. Doppler velocimetry determined redistribution of fetal blood flow: Correlation with growth retardation in diamniotic monochorionic and dizygotic twins. *Am J Obstet Gynecol.* 1998;178:1359–1367.

104. Adams RD, Victor M, eds. *Principles of Neurology,* 3rd ed. New York: McGraw-Hill; 1985:463.

105. Hill A, Volpe JJ. Decrease in pulsatile flow in the anterior cerebral arteries is infantile hydrocephelus. *Pediatrics.* 1982;69:4–7.

106. Degani S, Lewinsky R, Shapiro I, et al. Decrease in pulsatile flow in the internal carotid artery in fetal hydrocephalus. *Br J Obstet Gynaecol.* 1988;95:138–141.

107. van den Wijngaard JAGW, Reuss A, Wladimiroff JW. The blood flow velocity waveform in the fetal internal carotid artery in the prescence of hydrocephaly. *Early Hum Dev.* 1988;18:95–99.

108. Kirkinen P, Muller R, Baumann H, et al. Cerebral blood flow velocity waveforms in hydrocephalic fetuses. *J Clin Ultrasound.* 1988;16:493–498.

109. Ben-Chetrit A, Anteby E, Lavy Y, et al. Increased middle cerebral artery blood flow inspedance is fetal subdural hematoma. *Ultrasound Obstet Gynecol.* 1991;1:357–358.

110. Guerriero S, Ajossa V, Mais A, et al. Color Doppler energy imaging in the diagnosis of fetal intracranial hemorrhage in the second trimester. *Ultrasound Obstet Gynecol.* 1997;10:205–208.

111. Sibony O, Fondacci C, Oury JF, et al. In utero fetal cerebral intraparenchymal hemorrhage associated with an abnormal cerebral Doppler. *Fetal Diagn Ther.* 1993;8:126–128.

112. Rizzo G, Arduini D, Colosimo C Jr, et al. Abnormal fetal cerebral blood flow velocity waveforms as a sign

of an aneurysm of the vein of Galen. *Fetal Ther.* 1987;2:75–79.

113. Johnson W, Berry JM, Einzig S, et al. Doppler findings in nonimmune hydrops fetalis and cerebral arteriovenous malformations. *Am Heart J.* 1988;115: 1138–1140.

114. Dan U, Shalev E, Greif M, et al. Prenatal diagnosis of fetal brain arteriovenous malformation: the use of color Doppler imaging. *J Clin Ultrasound.* 1992;20: 149–151.

115. Jeanty P, Kepple D, Roussis P, et al. In utero detection of cardiac failure from an aneurysm of the vein of Galen. *Am J Obstet Gynecol.* 1990;163:50–51.

116. Dörn M, Tercanly S, Holzgreve W. Prenatal sonographic diagnosis of a vein of Galen aneurysm: Relevance of associated malformations for timing and mode of delivery. *Ultrasound Obstet Gynecol.* 1995; 6:287–289.

117. Sepulveda W, Platt CC, Fisk NM. Prenatal diagnosis of arteriovenous malformation using color Doppler ultrasonography: Case report and review of the literature. *Ultrasound Obstet Gynecol.* 1995;6:282–286.

118. Mai R, Rempen A, Kristen P. Prenatal diagnosis of avein of Galen aneurysm assessed by pulsed and color Doppler sonography. *Ultrasound Obstet Gynecol.* 1996;7:228–230.

119. Goelz R, Mielke G, Gonser M, et al. Prenatal assessment of shunting blood flow in vein of Galen malformation. *Ultrasound Obstet Gynecol.* 1996;8:210–212.

120. Facchinetti F, Battaglia C, Benatti R, et al. Oral magnesium supplementation improves fetal circulation. *Magnesium Res.* 1992;5:179–181.

121. Mari G, Moise KJ Jr, Deter RL, et al. Doppler assessment of the pulsatility index of the middle cerebral artery during constriction of the fetal ductus arteriosus after indomethacin therapy. *Am J Obstet.* 1989;161:1528–1531.

122. Parilla BV, Tamura RK, Cohen LS, et al. Lack of effect of antenatal indomethacin on fetal cerebral blood flow. *Am J Obstet Gynecol.* 1997;176:1166–1169.

123. Degani S, Gonen R, Lewinsky RM, et al. Intracervical prostaglandin E$_2$ is associated with increased pulsatility in fetal cerebral vessels. *J Matern Fetal Invest.* 1994;4:171–173.

124. Mari G, Kirshon B. Doppler assessment of the fetal and uteroplacental circulation during nifedipine therapy for preterm labor. *Am J Obstet Gynecol.* 1989;161:1514–1518.

125. Cohen BJ, Stiger RH, Derks JB, et al. Absence of significant hemodynamic changes in the fetus following maternal betamethasone administration. *Ultrasound Obstet Gynecol.* 1996;8:252–255.

126. Arbeille P, Bose M, Vaillant MC, et al. Nicotine-induced changes in the cerebral circulation in ovine fetuses. *Am J Perinatol.* 1992;9:270–274.

127. Alahuhta S, Rasanen J, Jouppila P, et al. Ultraplacental and fetal haemodynamics during extradural anaesthesia for caesarean section. *Br J Anaesth.* 1991;66:319–323.

128. Brantberg A, Sonesson SE. Central arterial hemodynamics in small for gestational age fetuses before and during maternal hyperoxygenation: A Doppler velocimetric study with particular attention to the aortic isthmus. *Ultrasound Obstet Gynecol.* 1999;14: 237–243.

129. Potts P, Connors G, Gillis S, et al. The effects of carbon dioxide on Doppler flow velocity waveforms in the human fetus. *J Dev Physiol.* 1992;17:119–123.

130. Veille JC, Penry M. Effects of maternal administration of 3% carbon dioxide on umbilical and fetal renal and middle cerebral artery Doppler waveforms. *Am J Obstet Gynecol.* 1992;167:1668–1671.

131. Polvi HJ, Pirhonen JP, Erkkola RV. Nitrous oxide inhalation: Effects on maternal and fetal circulation at term. *Obstet Gynecol.* 1996;87:1045–1048.

132. Van Bel F, Sola A, Roman C, et al. Perinatal regulation of the cerebral circulation: Role of nitric oxide and prostaglandins. *Pediatr Res.* 1997;42:299–304.

133. Gramellini D, Folli MC, Raboni S, et al. Cerebral umbilical Doppler ratio as a predictor of adverse perinatal outcome. *Obstet Gynecol.* 1992;79:416–420.

134. Battaglia C, Larocca E, Lanzani A, et al. Doppler velocimetry in prolonged pregnancy. *Obstet Gynecol.* 1991;77:213–216.

135. Arduini D, Rizzo G, Romanini C. Changes of pulsatility index from fetal vessels preceding the onset of late decelerations in growth-retarded fetuses. *Obstet Gynecol.* 1992;79:605–610.

136. Weiner Z, Farmakides G, Schulman H, et al. Central and peripheral hemodynamic changes in fetuses with absent end-diastolic velocity in umbilical artery: Correlation with computerized fetal heart rate pattern. *Am J Obstet Gynecol.* 1994;170:509–515.

137. Cynober E, Cabrol D, Uzan M. Fetal cerebral blood flow velocity during labor. *Fetal Diagn Ther.* 1992;7: 93–101.

138. Chandran R, Serra-Serra V, Sellers SM, et al. Fetal cerebral Doppler in the recognition of fetal compromise. *Br J Obstet Gynaecol.* 1993;100:139–144.

139. Richardson BS, Carmichael L, Homan L, et al. Fetal cerebral circulatory and metabolic responses during heart rate decelerations aith umbilical cord compression. *Am J Obstet Gynecol.* 1996;175:929–936.

140. Gudmundsson S, Tulzer G, Huhta JC, et al. Venous Doppler in the fetus with absent end-diastolic flow in the umbilical artery. *Ultrasound Obstet Gynecol.* 1996;7:262–267.

141. Gembruch U, Baschat AA. Demonstration of fetal coronary blood flow by color coded and pulsed wave Doppler sonography: A possible indicator of severe compromise and impending demise in intrauterine growth retardation. *Ultrasound Obstet Gynecol.* 1996;7:10–16.

142. Baschat AA, Harman CR, Alger LS, et al. Fetal coronary and cerebral blood flow in acute fetomaternal hemorrhage. *Ultrasound Obstet Gynecol.* 1998;12: 128–131.

143. Zimmerman P, Alback T, Koskinen J, et al. Doppler flow velocimetry of the umbilical artery, uteroplacental arteries and fetal middle cerebral artery in prolonged pregnancy. *Ultrasound Obstet Gynecol.* 1995; 53:189–197.

144. Devine PA, Bracero LA, Lysikiewicz A, et al. Middle cerebral to umbilical artery Doppler ratio in post date pregnancies. *Obstst Gynecol.* 1994;84: 856– 860.

145. Carrol SG, Papaioannou S, Nicolaides KH. Doppler studies of the placental and fetal circulation in pregnancies with preterm prelabor amniorrhexis. *Ultrasound Obstst Gynecol.* 1995;5:184–188.

146. Sepulveda W, Shennan AH, Peek MJ. Reverse end-diastolic flow inn the middle cerebral artery: An agonal pattern in the human fetus. *Am J Obstet Gynecol.* 1996;174:1645–1647.

147. Respondek M, Woch A, Kaczmarek P, et al. Reversal of diastolic flow in the middle cerebral artery of the fetus during the second half of pregnancy. *Ultrasound Obstet Gynecol.* 1997;9:324–329.

148. Mari G, Wasserstrum N. Fetal flow velocity waveforms of the fetal circulation preceding fetal death in a case of lupus anticoagulant. *Am J Obstet Gynecol.* 1991;164:776–778.

149. Chandran R, Serra, W, Sellers SM, et al Fetal middle cerebral artery flow velocity waveforms—A terminal pattern, case report. *Br J Obstet Gyneacol.* 1991;98: 937–938.

150. Rizzo G, Capponi A, Pietropolli A, et al. Fetal cardiac and extracardiac flows preceding intrauterine death. *Ultrasound Obstet Gynecol.* 1994;4:139–142.

151. Nijhuis JG, Crevels CAI, van Dongen PWI. Fetal brain death; the definition of a fetal heart pattern and its clinical consequences. *Obstet Gynecol Surv.* 1990;46:229–232.

152. Hernandez MJ, Brennan RV, Boman GS, et al. Autoregulation of the cerebral blood flow in newborn dog. *Ann Neurol.* 1979;6:177–185.

153. Sonesson SE, Winberg P, Lundell BPW. Early postnatal changes in intracranial arterial blood flow velocities. *Pediatr Res.* 1987;22:461–464.

154. Gray PH, Griffin EA, Drumm JE, et al. Continuous wave Doppler ultrasound in evaluation of cerebral blood flow in neonates. *Arch Dis Child.* 1983;5: 677–681.

155. Archer LNJ, Levene MI, Evans DM. Doppler ultrasound examination of the anterior cerebral arteries of normal newborn infants: The effect of postnatal age. *Early Hum Dev.* 1985;10:255–260.

156. Perlman JM, Volpe JJ. Cerebral blood flow velocity in relation to intraventricular hemorrhage in the premature newborn infant. *J Pediatr.* 1982;100:956–958.

157. Pasternak JF, Gorey MT. The syndrome of acute near-total intrauterine aspphyxia in the term infant. *Pediatr Neurol.* 1998;18:391–398.

158. Archer LNJ, Levene MI, Evans DM. Cerebral artery Doppler ultrasonography for prediction of outcome after perinatal asphyxia. *Lancet.* 1986;2: 1116–1118.

159. Lou HC, Lassen NA, Friis-Hansen B. Impaired autoregulation of cerebral blood flow in the distressed newborn infant. *J Pediatr.* 1979;94:118–121.

160. Leaky FAN, Cates D, Mac Callum M, et al. Effect of CO_2 and 100% O_2 on cerebral blood flow in preterm infants. *J Appl Physiol.* 1980;48:468–472.

161. Costeloe K, Smyth DPL, Myrdoch N, et al. A comparison between electrical impedance and strain gauge plethysomography for the study of cerebral blood flow in the newborn. *Pediatr Res.* 1984;18:290–295.

162. Ley D, Marsal K. Doppler velocimetry in cerebral vessels of small for gestational age neonates. *Early Hum Dev.* 1992;31:171–180.

163. van Bel F, van de Bor M, Stijnen T, et al. Decreased cerebrovascular resistance in small for gestational age infants. *Eur J Obstet Gynecol Reprod Biol.* 1986; 23:137–144.

164. Scherjon SA, Costing H, Kok JH, et al. Effect of fetal braisparing on the early neonatal cerebral circulation. *Arch Dis Child.* 1994;7:F11–5.

165. Greisen GM, Hellstrom-Westas I, Low H, et al. Sleep–waking shifts and cerebral blood flow in stable preterm infants. *Pediatr Res.* 1985;19:1156–1159.

166. Martin CG, Snider AR, Katz SM, et al. Abnormal cerebral blood flow patterns in patients with a large patent ductus arteriosus. *J Pediatr.* 1982;101:587–593.

167. Archer INJ, Evans DH, Levene MI. The effect of indomethacin on cerebral blood flow velocity in premature infants. In: Sheldon CD, Evans DH, Salvage JR, eds. *Obstetric and Neonatal Blood Flow.* London: Biological Engineering Society; 1987:46–47.

168. Sung RY, Loong EP, Rok TF, et al. Topical prostaglandin E_2 gel for cervical ripening and closure of the ductus anterious in the newborn. *Arch Drs Child.* 1990;65:703–704.

169. Cowan F. Acute effects of indomethacin on neonatal cerebral blood flow velocities. *Early Hum. Dev.* 1986;13:343.

170. Perlman JM, McMenamin JB, Volpe JJ. Fluctuating cerebral blood flow velocity in respiratory distress syndrome. *N Engl J Med.* 1983;309:204–209.

171. Ando J, Takashima S, Takeshita K. Cerebral blood flow velocity in preterm neonates. *Brain Dev.* 1985;7:385–389.

172. Perlman JM, Volpe JJ. Suctioning in the preterm infant: Effects on cerebral blood flow velocity, intracranial pressure and arterial blood pressure. *Pediatrics.* 1993;72:329–334.

173. Hill A, Perlman JM, Volpe JJ. Relationship of pneumothorax to intraventricular hemorrhage in the premature newborn. *Pediatrics.* 1982;69:144–149.

174. Perlman JM, Volpe JJ. Seizures in the preterm infant effects on cerebral blood flow velocity, intracranial pressure and arterial blood pressure. *Pediatrics.* 1983;102:288–293.

175. Perlman JM Volpe JJ. Episodes of apnoea and trachycardia in the preterm newborn: Impact on cerebral circulation. *Pediatrics.* 1985;76:333–338.

176. Kurjak A, ed. *An Atlas of Transvaginal Color Doppler.* London: Casterton; 1994:77.

177. Orstrom K, Eliasson A, Horeide JH, et al. Fetal blood velocity waveforms in normal pregnancies. A longitudinal study. *Acta Obstet Gynecol Scand.* 1989;6: 8,171–178.

178. Degani S, Lewinsky RM, Shapiro I. Doppler studies in fetal cerebral blood flow. *Ultrasound Obstet Gynecol.* 1994;4:158–165.

CHAPTER EIGHTEEN

In Utero Surgical Interventions
of the Fetal Brain and Spine

Andrei Rebarber
Howard Weiner

This chapter reviews the recent advances in invasive therapies and techniques to treat, temporize, or cure various prenatally detected neurological malformations. Anomalies of the central nervous system are generally complex in nature, may be associated with other anomalies (i.e., syndromes), and are often not readily reversed through surgical means.

With the advent of high resolution ultrasound technology (2-dimensional and 3-dimensional) and transvaginal imaging investigators are able to better delineate fetal pathology prior to birth. With the expected advances in molecular biology and gene analysis, health care providers will soon be able to identify more precise etiologies for fetal malformations noted on ultrasound. A more accurate diagnosis will allow for an improved ability to predict whether certain therapeutic interventions would be deemed appropriate. The era of the fetus as a patient has dawned, and improvements in technology will allow treatment of congential anomalies prior to the beginning of life.

The ethical dilemmas involved in this decision making are complex and are dealt with in another chapter. Briefly, any intervention undertaken during pregnancy must take into account the risk/benefit ratio of two patients: the mother and the fetus. Additionally, whereas past invasive procedures have been limited to lethal conditions, recent advances in technology and operative techniques have raised the possibility that the entire spectrum of congenital anomalies might be amenable to antenatal repair. The risk to both mother and fetus associated with these invasive procedures must be weighed against the short-term and long-term benefit of the treatment, the latter of which may only be apparent in 10 or more years. The neonatal, pediatric, and adult brain is constantly remodeling itself. Therefore, the impact of fetal intervention on the brain's postnatal function is difficult to ascertain in a quantitative way and will continuously need to be reevaluated over time. These controversies will invariably subject this field to extensive criticism and scrutiny by both the scientific and lay community.

FETAL SURGERY FOR SPINA BIFIDA

Survivors of postnatal spina bifida surgery have significant physical and mental disabilities and must be prepared for a life time of associated problems such as chronic urinary tract infections associated with urinary incontinence, reduced intellect, shunt infections, scoliosis, sexual dysfunction, and psychosocial maladjustment. The purposes of postnatal surgery are to preserve intellectual, motor, and sensory function by restoring the spinal cord to its normal cerebrospinal fluid environment and to prevent central nervous system infection. Meningitis and ventriculitis produce intellectual and developmental delay. Attempts to avoid these complications are paramount. An additional purpose is to restore the normal contour of the back, which contributes to ease of care and future bracing.

The concept of fetal surgery for the repair of myelomeningocele is based on an increasing body of literature that supports a "two-hit" theory to account for some of neurologic deficits encountered after postnatal surgical correction. This suggests that in addition to the embryologic error of neuralation occurring at 22 to 32 days postovulation, secondary injury, either due to the *in utero* environment (i.e., chemical injury) or mechanical trauma during gestation to the exposed neural elements, allows for a more severe impairment.[1-3] Early fetal intervention would limit the impact of this secondary insult and possibly improve neurologic outcomes in these cases.

The potential benefit of *in utero* repair of myelomeningocele in humans is further substantiated by observations made in the various forms of neural tube defects. In situations where the spinal dysraphism is covered by a thicker element (e.g., lipomyelomeningocele or cervical dysraphism), neurological deficits are markedly decreased when compared with a myelomeningocele of the same severity exposed to the amniotic fluid. The most compelling argument is made when considering the hemimyelocele, where only half of the spinal dysraphism is covered by dura. The portion that contains covering appears to retain neurological function to a greater extent than the area that is more exposed. The deficit in these cases is limited to the limb ipsilateral to the exposed hemicord.[4]

Tulipan and Bruner first attempted to repair spina bifida *in utero* using a fetoscopic technique in 1994. Their presentation at the International Fetal Medicine and Surgery Society reported on four cases with disappointing results.[5] The first successful human procedure was performed in 1997 at Vanderbilt University by Tulipan and Bruner using an open technique. Details of this procedure were presented in 1997 at the International Fetal Medicine and Surgery Society.[6] Since this report, over 70 cases of intrauterine myelomeningocele repair have been described mainly at two centers in the United States. The following summarizes the work published from

these two centers and the possible future implications of this technique. A description of the actual technique of corrective spinal fetal surgery is beyond the scope of this chapter but can be found in the citations provided.

In 1999, Bruner and coworkers reported on 29 patients with isolated myelomenigocele who underwent prenatal surgical intervention between the gestational ages of 24 to 30 weeks. This group was compared to 23 control group patients matched for the diagnosis. Defects were repaired in the same standard fashion used for postnatal surgical therapy. In the first 22 cases, a shunt was placed to drain cerebrospinal fluid (CSF) out of the spinal area that was closed. The primary end points analyzed were: ventriculoperitoneal (VP) shunt placement, the presence of obstetrical complications (including hemorrhage, infection, preterm labor, chorioamniotic membrane disruption, intrauterine growth restriction, and oligohydramnios), gestational age at delivery, and birth weight. The secondary end points included: the age at shunt placement and degree of hindbrain herniation. The developmental outcomes of 26 study patients were followed up at a range of 2 to 18 months.[7]

In the prenatally treated group there was a statistically significant decreased requirement for ventriculoperitoneal shunt placement. In the cases where shunts were placed, the median age at shunt placement was also delayed. This was explained by the reduced incidence of hindbrain herniation in the prenatally corrected lesions. Regarding the obstetrical variables, however, there was an increased risk of oligohydramnios, preterm labor, preterm delivery, and as a result, lower birth weight in the study versus the control group patients at the time of delivery (Table 18–1).[7]

Despite promising results regarding hindbrain restoration and decreased VP shunt placement, the early assessment of these neonates revealed that "motor function has not exceeded expectations

TABLE 18–1.

Outcome Variables	Study Patients	Control Patients	*p* Value
Ventriculoperitoneal shunt placement	59%	91%	0.01
Age at shunt placement (median)	50 days	5 days	0.006
Hindbrain herniation	38%	95%	< 0.001
Oligohydramnios	48%	4%	0.001
Preterm labor	50%	9%	0.002
Preterm delivery	33.2 weeks	37.0 weeks	< 0.001
Birth weight (mean)	2171 g	3075 g	< 0.001
Talipes	28%	70%	0.005

Adapted from Bruner JP, Tulipan N, Paschall RL. JAMA. 1999; 282:1819.

based on the anatomical levels of the lesions."[8] Long term neurological outcome (i.e., lower extremity and bowel and bladder function) in these infants remains unknown.

Adzick and colleagues[9] and Sutton and coworkers[10] reported on a series of 10 patients who underwent fetal myelomeningocele repair between 22 to 25 weeks of gestation. Inclusion criteria for attempted surgical repair included: atrial diameter of less than 17 mm, ultrasound evidence of normal leg and foot motion without deformity, normal karyotype, and no other associated anomalies. The primary endpoints analyzed were: gestational age at delivery, birth weight, leg function in the neonatal period, need for shunt placement (head circumference and ventricular size at birth), and severity of the Arnold-Chiari malformation on each magnetic resonance imaging (MRI). Table 18–2 summarizes the data provided for the nine survivors of the surgery. One fetus died due to respiratory insufficiency secondary to prematurity with delivery occurring at 25 weeks of gestation. Figure 18–1 demonstrates the in-utero spina bifida repair of a fetus at 23 postmentrual weeks.

Interestingly, in this series of patients the authors noted that five out of the nine patients "had newborn lower extremity function better than expected by at least 2 spinal levels based on anatomic level as determined from the initial fetal MRI."[11] Bowel and bladder function could not be assessed due to the age of the infants at the time of publication.

In both studies, prenatal MRI was used as a crucial preoperative diagnostic method for defining the severity of the meningomyelocele defect. It is our contention that with transvaginal and transabdominal imaging using techniques described in the preceding chapters, that MRI may be an overly expensive, time-consuming adjunct that probably adds little more to characterizing the defects initially diagnosed by ultrasound. Critical to the use of ultrasound as a primary modality is intricate knowledge of the fetal anatomy and the transfontanelle scan-

ning techniques used to obtain the images, as discussed in previous chapters.

Fetal surgical intervention for myelomeningocele repair holds great promise. This surgery should still be regarded as an experimental procedure with unknown long-term effects. Although reversal of the hindbrain herniation is clearly apparent in both studies cited previously, how this translated into improved neurological performance and decreased long-term requirement for shunting is yet to be seen. The Chiari malformation consists of a complex

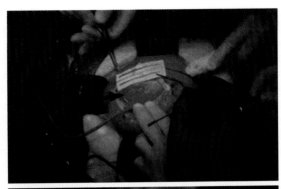
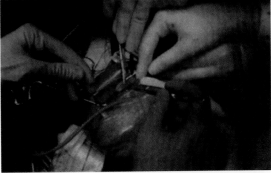
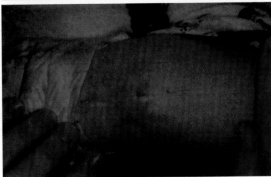

Figure 18–1. *In utero* spina bifida repair. **A.** Exposure of 23-postmenstrual week fetus through hysterectomy revealing spina bifida defect *(arrow).* **B.** Closure of skin flaps over the spinal cord; a cerebrospinal fluid shunt *(arrow)* with a one-way value had been inserted alongside the spinal cord. **C.** Healed back wound seen shortly after birth; the shunt tube has been removed.

TABLE 18–2. SURVIVAL DATA OF NINE PATIENTS UNDERGOING SURGERY

Outcome Variables	Study Patients
Ventriculoperitoneal shunt placement	59%
Age at shunt placement (median)	50 days
Hindbrain herniation	38%
Oligohydramnios	48%
Preterm delivery	40%
Birth weight (mean)	2171 g
Talipes	28%

set of anatomical defects (small posterior fossa, a beaked tectum, a large massa intermedia, polygyria, and downward herniation of the cerrebellar vermis and brainstem).[12] This set of anomalies can only partially be restored by fetal surgical intervention at 20 postmenstrual weeks or greater because they are created early in the embryologic period. A full description explaining the embryologic origin of the complete Chiari malformation is beyond the scope of this chapter but may be found in two published studies by McLone and coworkers.[13,14]

Finally, it is interesting to note that despite *in utero* surgical repair of a myelomeningocele, a communicating type of hydrocephaly develops. This may be the result of the impaired absorptive capacity of the arachnoid villi.[15] The mechanism by which this damage occurs is unclear. However, if this communicating type of hydrocephaly is the result of an early error in central nervous system development of the arachnoid granulations, then early fetal surgery will have limited potential for restoring normal CSF flow in the brain. Furthermore, because of the open fetal sutures and the presence of the anterior and posterior fontanelles, *in utero* hydrocephaly does not necessarily equate with impaired neurological function. Therefore, even in the setting of severe hydrocephaly, postnatal shunting may lead to "normal" developmental outcome in the absence of other central nervous system malformations.

To consider this approach, a health care provider must weigh the known postnatal short-term neurological benefits of fetal intervention (decreased shunting, possible improved neurological motor function) with the neurological risks of prematurity (i.e., interventricular hemorrhage, periventricular leukomalacia, infections, retinopathy of prematurity), as well as the non-neurologic risks of prematurity (i.e., respiratory distress, necrotizing enterocolitis, death). In fact, Adzick and colleagues[10] reported a 10 percent fetal/neonatal mortality rate associated with fetal myelomeningocele repair; a higher rate than that associated with its natural history during fetal life. The postnatal operative mortality rate of traditional surgical intervention is approaching zero, and 95 percent or greater survival rates for the first 2 years of life have been reported.

FETAL INTERVENTIONS FOR HYDROCEPHALY

Fetal hydrocephaly is a symptom with multiple underlying known etiologies. These etiologies have widely variable outcomes. Therefore, prenatal management of this clinical entity must include a careful search for other associated central nervous system

abnormalities using ultrasound technology, invasive testing for chromosomal analysis, and use of novel molecular techniques leading to the identification of causal gene defects for several neurogenetic disorders.[16–18]

Fetal interventions to relieve hydrocephaly during the 1980s met with dismal results secondary to the technologic limitations of the time, as well as poor patient selection. Birnholz and Frigoletto[19] are credited with the first attempted invasive therapeutic procedure that involved serial percutaneous cephalocentesis under ultrasound guidance in 1981. Six serial cephalocenteses, with withdrawal of 40 to 180 mL of ventricular fluid, were performed between 25 and 32 weeks of gestation in this fetus. Postnatal ultrasound documented a midline cyst (probable arachnoid cyst) and agenesis of the corpus callosum. Neurologically, this infant did poorly and at 16 months of life was diagnosed with Becker's muscular dystrophy. Clewell and colleagues,[20] in 1982, performed the first percutaneous ventriculoamniotic shunt placement in a fetus suspected of having X-linked aqueductal stenosis based on the family history and the ultrasound findings noted. Using ultrasound guidance, a ventriculoamniotic shunt was placed via a 13-gauge percutaneous approach at 24 weeks of gestation. The shunt appeared to work until the 32nd week when dramatic increase in ventricular volume was noted. The fetus was delivered at 34 weeks of gestation and various other anomalies were noted: bilateral flexion contractures of the wrist, duplication of the distal phalanx of the thumb, an atrioseptal defect, and bilateral inguinal hernias. Limited description of the neonatal follow-up is provided in the article.[20] Finally, Manning and coworkers reported on the dismal international experience of shunt procedures performed for obstructive hydrocephaly.[21] The international registry included reports from 21 centers from seven countries on 41 cases of ventriculoamniotic shunt placements for hydrocephaly. The procedure-related death rate was 10.25 percent, with 83 percent survivors in the postnatal period. In this cohort of patients only 77 percent of the fetuses were diagnosed with aqueductal stenosis in the postnatal period, however, shunts were placed in fetuses which later were identified to suffer from: holoprosencephaly, Dandy–Walker malformations, and various other malformations that currently would probably be exclusion criteria for performing such an invasive procedure. The only patients reported to be normal at follow-up were those diagnosed with aqueductal stenosis, therefore, subanalysis of this group of patients is warranted. Of the 32 treated fetuses with aqueductal stenosis in the registry, 28 survived (87.5 percent), but only 12 of the survivors (37.5 percent) were normal at follow-up. Reports from that time note that in neonates suffering from aqueductal stenosis "shunting early in the neonatal period improves the rates of survival (> 75 percent) and intellectual development (> 80 percent) of survivors."[21] This data suggests that the fetal intervention using the varied techniques of the international community may have improved survival slightly, however, outcome was not necessarily improved. The limitations of this report includes its study design, the poorly characterized techniques for shunt placement, a reliance on self-reporting of complications and/or only successful cases, the lack of clear assessment used in the postnatal period to evaluate neurological and developmental status, and the limited length of the postnatal follow-up.

Multiple case reports have been published over the past several decades describing cephalocentesis at term to allow for vaginal delivery to limit maternal morbidity in the setting of severe hydrocephaly associated with macrocephaly. This approach requires caution because the underlying etiology for the hydrocephaly is often not clearly delineated. Therefore, counseling parents regarding the prognosis for the unborn infant should not be overly pessimistic. Factors that can affect prognosis may include, but are not limited to, the following: type of hydrocephaly, underlying conditions, associated anomalies, and mode of delivery (i.e., breech presentation). In a cohort of 42 patients diagnosed with fetal ventriculomegaly between 20 to 38 postmenstrual weeks, one half of the 38 percent perinatal mortality rate was directly associated with a cephalocentesis.[22] Additionally, during a cephalocentesis signs of fetal distress on external fetal cardiac monitoring (i.e., fetal bradycardia) may be noted. These gradually resolve in most cases after the procedure is completed.[23] It is not clear whether or not this cardiac manifestation of neurological manipulation causes further neurological injury. Chervenak and McCullough[24] analyzed the ethical dilemmas involved in this management strategy and concluded that cephalocentesis and attempted vaginal delivery is permissible in cases where the mother refuses cesarean delivery despite proper counseling and/or in the setting where the hydrocephaly may be characterized to be due to an etiology that is incompatible with life or with virtual absence of cognitive function.

Ammar and coworkers[25] recently described prolonged intrauterine ventricular drainage using a maternal transabdominal approach. In this case, at 35 postmenstrual weeks the fetus was first diagnosed with massive ventriculomegaly in a breech presentation. Under sterile conditions, a catheter was placed into the ventricular cavity through a spinal needle, which was then connected to an external sterile drainage bag kept at the level of the maternal abdomen. Decompression over 53 hours was performed, with removal of 200 mL of cerebrospinal fluid. The procedure was apparently done to facilitate vaginal delivery. Limited outcome data is provided, however, the authors note that "no signs of interventricular or intracerebral hemorrhage were seen." The neonatal Apgar scores were extremely depressed, cord pH evaluation was not provided.

Bruner and Tulipan[26] performed an in utero-maternal transabdominal shunt procedure in a fetus diagnosed with "isolated" hydrocephaly on routine 20 postmenstrual weeks scanning. The procedure was performed at 24 postmenstrual weeks and delivery of the infant occurred at 35 postmenstrual weeks. The shunt procedure was described as having: "placed a shunt, a small tube that's about 2 mm in diameter, into the fluid space in the brain. The opposite end of the shunt is hooked to a small valve (about 2 inches long) that controls the flow of fluid that escapes through the top of the shunt. The valve is connected to another long, thin tube that is tunneled through the baby's skin between the shoulder blades. The fluid drains into the amniotic fluid." The report did not mention the prenatal and postnatal etiology for the hydrocephaly or define the prenatal parameters when such an intervention should be considered. Postnatal follow-up in a peer review journal of this case will allow for more critical assessment of the procedure and its basis.

Patient selection is clearly important in planning this therapeutic intervention. Ultrasound and MRI may be used to determine the presence of associated anomalies. However, certain syndromal stigmata may not be clearly delineated by these imaging modalities (i.e., ear deformity, webbing of the hands, lobulated tongue, genital anomalies). Preoperative endoscopic evaluation of the fetus may be warranted in these situations to ensure normality prior to attempting in utero shunting procedure, if this is even considered.

Several concerns have arisen regarding in utero intervention for hydrocephaly. It has been shown that "head enlargement at birth, ventricular size, and the age at the time of postnatal shunt placement are not related to later functional development"[27]. Whether, prenatal invasive therapy for fetal ventriculomegaly can improve the postnatal outcome of these infants with isolated hyrocephaly is as of yet unclear.

Lastly, questions remain regarding the safety of such techniques to the mother and fetus, and whether the theoretical benefits would outweigh the added risks. In conclusion, the most appropriate candidates for fetal hydrocephaly surgery include those with hydrocephaly due to pure aqueductal stenosis, or unilateral hydrocephaly causing mass effect in whom imaging studies demonstrate the remainder of the central nervous system to be normal.

Fetal Intervention for Arachnoid Cyst

We reported the first case of a prenatal cephalocentesis for an enlarging arachnoid cyst of the quadrigeminal cistern at the recent American Institute of Ultrasound in Medicine convention in San Francisco in 1999. Initial evaluation in our ultrasound laboratory diagnosed an interhemisphere

archnoid cyst measuring 2.5 cm × 5.0 cm. (Figs. 18–2 and 18–3). Amniocentesis was performed a normal karyotype returned. By 28 weeks the arachnoid cyst had grown (5.9 × 3.2 cm) resulting in new onset bilateral vetriculomegaly. Preoperative MRI and 2-D/3-D ultrasound imaging allowed for reassurance of normal brain anatomy, including identification of the corpus callosum. There are various types of cystic processes than can occur in the midline of the brain (e.g., porencephaly, arachnoid cyst, holoprosencephaly, and diencephalic cyst).[28] The differential diagnosis of these cysts is important from both the prognostic and therapeutic standpoint. To

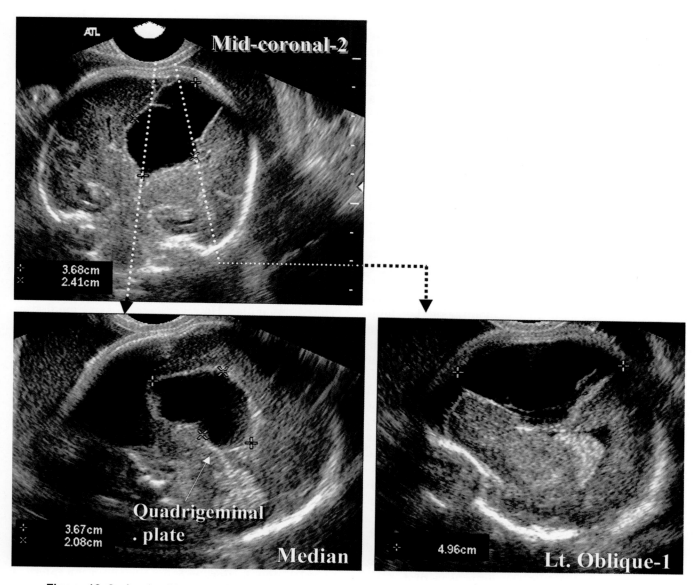

Figure 18–2. Arachnoid cyst at 23 postmenstrual weeks. **A.** Mid-coronal 2 plane depicts the interhemispoheric splaying noted secondary to the cyst location. **B.** Median plane reveals the origin of the cyst from the quadrigeminal plate. **C.** Left oblique view identifies the longest length of the arachnoid cyst.

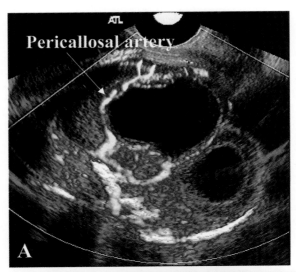

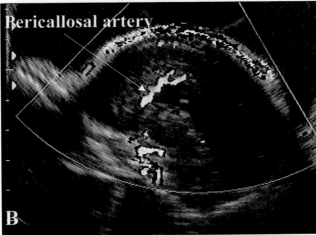

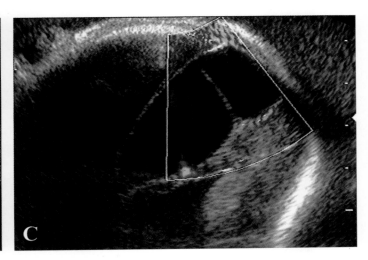

Figure 18–3. Arachnoid cyst at 28 postmenstrual weeks. **A.** A parasagittal plane depicting the displaced pericallosal artery along its entire length using power angiography Doppler mode. **B.** A median plane in which the anterior portion of the pericallosal artery is viewed with color Doppler. **C.** A coronal view evaluating the arachnoid cyst for vascularity with a septation.

clarify the embryology and pathogenesis, Mori proposed a classification to divide these cysts into four distinct entities. The patient's cyst was best classified as a B2 cyst, based on Mori's classification, a parasagittal cyst with an intact corpus callosum.[29] Although neurological outcome in most cases of arachnoid cysts are excellent, large arachnoid cysts, particularly those resulting in ventriculomegaly, have been associated with neurological impairment and the need for long-term shunting.

A transvaginal approach was performed using an automated needle-guided puncture device previously described.[30] The transvaginal approach via endovaginal probe guidance for cephalocentesis had previously been described but is limited to few cases.[31] This approach was chosen due to the fetal position and the assessment of the route that the needle would traverse to avoid cortical tissue and the vascular venous sinuses. This was identified using power Doppler imaging. Fetal intracystic (i.e., intracranial) pressure was noted to be 22 cm H_2O (normal = 5 cm H_2O) and approximately 120 mL of fluid was obtained. Initially the fluid was clear, however, it became blood tinged toward the end of the procedure. Intracystic hemorrhage was noted after the procedure (Fig. 18–4). The intracystic hemorrhage resolved over the next several weeks. Within 4 weeks, the arachnoid cyst reaccumulated. Evaluation of the fetal biparietal diameter shows in graphic form (Fig. 18–5) the persistently worsening macrocephaly, which was temporized by the procedure for 3 weeks, but reaccumuled fluid, increasing

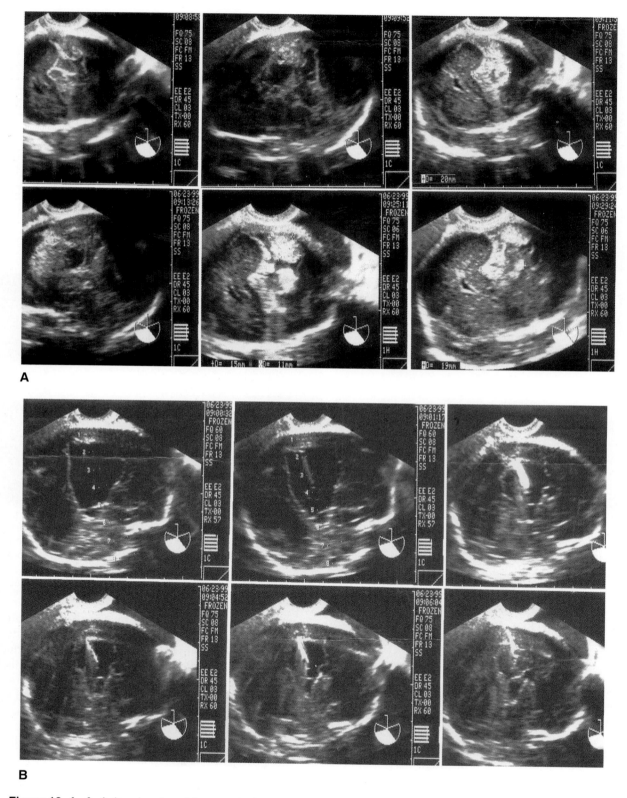

Figure 18–4. A. A timed series of transvaginal coronal sections of the fetal arachnoid cyst throughout the cephalocentesis from 9:00 AM until completion of the procedure at 9:08 AM. **B.** A timed series of transvaginal coronal sections after the cephalocentesis was performed with bleeding noted into the empty cystic cavity and clot formation without further expansion.

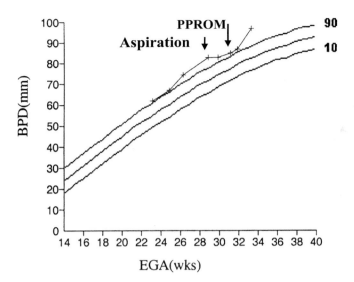

Figure 18–5. A graph depicting the biparietal diameter (BPD) along the *y* axis, and the increasing gestational age along the *x* axis. It reveals that the procedure temporized the enlarging BPD for approximately 3 weeks, however, reaccumulation of fluid was noted after the preterm premature rupture of membranes (PPROM) at 31 postmenstrual weeks.

head size once again, just prior to delivery. The mother's amniotic membranes ruptured at 31 post-menstrual weeks (3 weeks after the procedure had been performed), but there were no signs of infection. Expectant management allowed for vaginal delivery at 34 weeks of gestation. The neonate initially required cystoventriculoperitoneal shunting, however, the shunt was later removed due to infection. After the infection was treated, the child continued to experience progressive ventriculomegaly with cyst enlargement. An endoscopic fenestration of the cyst into the ventricles was performed successfully (Fig. 18–6). Follow-up head imaging studies revealed no hydrocephaly, a decreased cyst size, and normal developmental milestones at 1 year of age. The infant remains shunt free.

FUTURE DIRECTIONS FOR INVASIVE NEUROSURGICAL THERAPIES

Although there is growing enthusiasm for *in utero* treatment of meningomyelocele, significant controversy, based on a substantial body of animal and human data, still exists regarding the benefit of such early intervention. For other neurosurgical conditions, such as hydrocephaly, the controversy is even greater. Early attempts at fetal neurosurgery for hydrocephaly were met with uniformly disappointing results, and were therefore terminated. It has subsequently become apparent that the poor

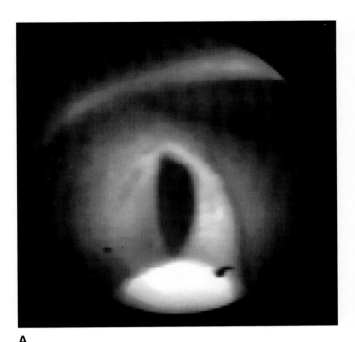

Figure 18–6. Intraoperative image of the endoscopic fenestration procedure of the arachnoid cyst in the postnatal period. **A.** Creation of the initial opening. **B.** The final image of fenestration.

neurodevelopmental outcome of these infants was undoubtedly related to the significantly high associated-malformation rate present in these patients in conjunction with the hydrocephaly. In addition, the shunt technology available for diverting cerebrospinal fluid into the amniotic fluid compartment was less than optimal. With these realizations, investigators have sought to define more optimal candidates for fetal neurosurgical interventions, such as those with aqueductal stenosis or isolated ventriculomegaly, and to use novel, less invasive approaches.

The most exciting prospects for fetal CNS interventions in the future include the introduction of specific genes of interest into the early developing human brain using molecular technology. At the New York University Skirball Institute of Biomolecular Medicine, researchers in developmental genetics are able to use ultrasound-guided injections of retroviral gene therapy vectors to obtain the widespread introduction of genes into the mouse CNS *in utero* as early as embryonic day 8.5.[32] For example, these investigators were able to inject a cell line engineered to express the secreted factor sonic hedgehog into early developing mouse brains.[33] As understanding of the molecular abnormalities underlying these various CNS malformations increases, so does the potential for novel genetic interventions.

Physician attitudes about treating children born with various impairments has evolved over the past 50 years. This is largely due to the technologic advances made to allow for medical and surgical treatments to improve quality as well as quantity of life for the infant. Pioneering work in this field will further these improvements starting from the beginning of life.

Medicine is a discipline with inherent prognostic uncertainty, where the risk and benefits of treatments are not always entirely predictable. Ethical decisions regarding controversial therapeutic interventions, therefore, must be made with this understanding in mind and full cooperation and consent of the patient and institutional review boards.

REFERENCES

1. Meuli M, Meuli-Simmen C, Yingling CD. *In utero* repair of experimental myelomeningocele saves neurological function at birth. *J Pediatr Surg.* 1996;31:397–402.
2. Drewek MJ, Bruner JP, Whetsell WO. Quantitative analysis of the toxicity of human amniotic fluid to cultured rat spinal cord. *Pediatr Neurosurg.* 1997;27(4):190–3.
3. Tulipan N, Bruner JP. Myelomeningocele repair *in utero*: A report of three cases. *Pediatr Neurosurg.* 1998;28:177–80.
4. Olutoye OO, Adzick NS. Fetal surgery for myelomeningocele. *Semin Perinatol.* 1999;23:462–473.
5. Adzick NS, Sutton LN, Crombleholme TM, et al. Fetal surgery for spinal bifida. *Lancet.* 1999;353:407.
6. Tulipan N, Bruner JP. Fetal surgery for spina bifida. *Lancet.* 1999;353:406.
7. Bruner JP, Tulipan N, Paschall RL. Fetal surgery for myelomeningocele and the incidence of shunt-dependent hydrocephalus. *JAMA.* 1999;282:1819–25.
8. Tulipan N, Bruner JP, Hernanz-Schulman M, et al. Effect of intrauterine myelomeningocele repair on central nervous system structure and function. *Pediatr Neurosurg.* 1999;31:183–8.
9. Adzick SN, Sutton LN, Crombleholme TM. Successful fetal surgery for spina bifida. *Lancet.* 1998;352:1675–6.
10. Sutton LN, Adzick SN, Bilaniuk LT. Improvement in hindbrain herniation demonstration by serial fetal magnetic resonance imaging following fetal surgery for myelomeningocele. *JAMA.* 1999;282:1826–31.
11. Tulipan N, Hernanz-Schulman M, Bruner JP. Reduced hindbrain herniation after intrauterine myelomeningocele repair: A report of four cases. *Pediatr Neurosurg.* 1998;29:274–8.
12. McLone DG, Knepper PA. The cause of Chiari II malformation: A unified theory. *Pediatr Neurosurg.* 1989;15:1–12.
13. McLone DG, Nakahara S, Knepper PA. Chiari II malformation: Pathogensis and dynamics. *Concepts Pediatr Neurosurg.* 1991;11:1–16.
14. Tulipan N, Hernanz-Schulman M, Lowe L, et al. Intrauterine myelomeningocele repair reverse preexisting hindbrain herniation. *Pediatr Neurosurg.* 1999;31:137–142.
15. Chervenak FA, Berkowitz RL, Tortora M. The management of fetal hydrocephalus. *Am J Obstet Gynecol.* 1985;151:933–6.
16. Gupta JK, Bryce FC, Lilford RJ. Management of apparently isolated fetal ventriculomegaly. *Obstet Gynecol Surv.* 1994;49:716–21.
17. Hollander NS, Vinkesteijn A, Schmitz-van Splunder P, et al. Prenatally diagnosed fetal ventriculomegaly; prognosis and outcome. *Prenat Diagn* 1998;18:557–62.
18. Birnholz JC, Frigoletto FD. Antenatal treatment of hydrocephalus. *N Engl J Med.* 1981;303:1021–3.
19. Clewell WH, Johnson ML, Meier PR, et al. A surgical approach to the treatment of fetal hydrocephalus. *N Engl J Med.* 1982;306:1320–3.
20. Manning FA, Harrison MR, Rodeck C. Catheter shunts for fetal hydronephrosis and hydrocephalus—Report of the International Fetal Surgery Registry. *N Engl J Med.* 1986;315:336–41.
21. den Hollander NS, Vinkestejin A, Schmitz-van Splunder P, Catsman-Berrevoets CE, Wladimiroff JW. Prenatally diagnosed fetal ventriculomegaly; prognosis and outcome. *Prena Diagn.* 1998;18:557–566.
22. Zimmer EZ, Jokobi P, Freidman M. Heart rate pattern of a hydrocephalic fetus during cephalocentesis. *Clin Exp Obste Gynecol.* 1986;13:12–15.
23. Chervenak FA, McCullough LB. Ethical analysis of the intrapartum management of pregnancy complicated by fetal hydrocephalus with macrocephaly. *Obstet Gynecol.* 1986;68:720–725.

24. Ammar A, Al-Jama F, Rahman S, Enizi AR, Mauzan Y, Sibai H. Prolonged intrauterine transabdominal ventricular external drainage. A method to decompress dilated fetal ventricles. *Minim Invasive Neurosurg.* 1996;39:1–3.

25. Humphrey N. Prenatal pioneer arrives. Vanderbilt University Medical Center Reporter June 25, 1999 (web page www.mc.vanderbilt.edu/reporter/index.html?ID=836 last modified March 30, 2000).

26. Reiner D, Sainte-Rose C, Pierre-Kahn A, Hirsch JF. Prenatal hydrocephalus: Outcome and prognosis. *Childs Nerv Syst.* 1988;4:213–222.

27. Jallo GI, Wisoff JH. Midline cysts in cerebrospinal fluid collections. Kaufman HH ed. Park Ridge, IL: The American Association of Neurological Surgeons Publications Committee, 1998:57–66.

28. Mori K. Giant interhemispheric cysts associated with agenesis of the corpus callosum. *J. Neurosurg.* 1992; 76:224–230.

29. Timor-Tritsch IE, Monteagudo A, Lerner JP. Ultrasound-guided transvaginal procedures. *Curr Opin Obstet Gynecol.* 1996;8:200–210.

30. Chayen B, Rifkin MD. Cephalocentesis. Guidance with an endovaginal probe and andovaginal needle placement. J Ultrasound Med. 1987;6:221–223.

31. Gaiano N, Kohtz JD, Turnbull DH, Fishell G. A method for rapid gain of function studies in the mouse embryonic nervous system. *Nat Neurosci.* 1999;2: 812–819.

32. Liu A, Joyner AL, Turnbull DH. Alteration of limb and brain patterning in early mouse embryos by ultrasound guided injection of Shh-expressing cells. *Mech Dev. 1998;75:107–115.*

Index

ISBN 0-8385-8859-X

90000

9 780838 588598

TIMOR/ULTRASONOGRAPHY
PRE & NEONATAL BRAIN